Fitness for Work

Fitness for Work
The Medical Aspects

4th EDITION

Keith T. Palmer
MRC Clinical Scientist
Honorary Reader and Consultant Occupational Physician
University of Southampton

Robin A. F. Cox
Consultant Occupational Physician

and

Ian Brown
Consultant Physician
Occupational Medicine and Toxicology
Southampton University Hospitals NHS Trust

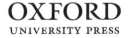

OXFORD
UNIVERSITY PRESS

OXFORD

UNIVERSITY PRESS

Great Clarendon Street, Oxford OX2 6DP

Oxford University Press is a department of the University of Oxford.
It furthers the University's objective of excellence in research, scholarship,
and education by publishing worldwide in

Oxford New York

Auckland Cape Town Dar es Salaam Hong Kong Karachi
Kuala Lumpur Madrid Melbourne Mexico City Nairobi
New Delhi Shanghai Taipei Toronto

With offices in

Argentina Austria Brazil Chile Czech Republic France Greece
Guatemala Hungary Italy Japan Poland Portugal Singapore
South Korea Switzerland Thailand Turkey Ukraine Vietnam

Oxford is a registered trade mark of Oxford University Press
in the UK and in certain other countries

Published in the United States
by Oxford University Press Inc., New York

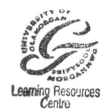

© Faculty of Occupational Medicine (except Chapter 2 [G. S. Howard] and
Chapter 3 [G. S. Howard and R. A. F. Cox]) 2007

The moral rights of the authors have been asserted

Database right Oxford University Press (maker)

First published 2007

Reprinted 2007

A catalogue record for this title is available from the British Library

Library of Congress Cataloging in Publication Data

Typeset by Cepha Imaging Pvt. Ltd., Bangalore
Printed in Great Britain
on acid-free paper by Biddles Ltd., King's Lynn

978–0–19–921565–2 (Pbk: alk. paper)   978–0–19–856822–3 (Hbk: alk. paper)

10 9 8 7 6 5 4 3 2

Foreword

By Dr Bill Gunnyeon

Much has changed in the world in general and in the world of work in particular since the 3rd edition of *Fitness for Work* was published. It is timely, therefore, that the content should be revised to ensure that it continues to provide appropriate and authoritative guidance to all who are involved in addressing the health issues associated with employment.

So how have things changed? Changing population demographics with an ageing population and historically low rates of unemployment are creating a diminishing labour market. At the same time the number of economically inactive people, many of them dependent on various forms of benefit, is high and many people over the age of 50 are opting to retire early rather than work even to normal retirement age. Easier movement across borders brings the challenges of a migrant workforce.

Industry has changed too. Manufacturing industry has been declining, replaced by service-based industries that bring potential new risks for the health of workers. More people now work from home than ever before. And job security is no longer guaranteed. Changes in medicine and health with the advent of new technologies and new forms of investigation and treatment have led to significantly improved outcomes for those with health problems, increasing the challenges when assessing fitness for work. Those improvements also mean that we will potentially spend a greater proportion of our adult lives in retirement.

At the same time work is increasingly recognized as important for people. We know that being out of work has negative health effects and can lead to social exclusion, health inequalities, and relative poverty for individuals and their families. Being in work brings positive benefits in building self-confidence, maintaining self-esteem, ensuring social contact, and allowing individuals to optimize opportunities for themselves and their families. And this in turn has benefits for communities and for society as a whole.

Against this background it is clear that we need to support people with health conditions and disabilities to help them remain in or wherever possible to return to work. For the future success of our economy employers will need to be able to ensure an available workforce with the right skills. We will need more people able to work; people at work for more of the time; people more effective when at work; people able to work until a later age; and people with health conditions or disabilities able to optimize work opportunities.

Thus the health and well-being of people of working age will become ever more important to us. If we are to be successful in meeting the challenges we face, our approach to assessing fitness for work will need to be more focused on supporting people to enter and return to work and helping people with health conditions or disabilities to remain in work, than perhaps it has been in the past. Flexible working, workplace adaptations, use of technology, better management of chronic disease, and recognition of the implications of ageing on work capability will all be essential.

Success will of course require all healthcare professionals involved in dealing with people of working age to approach this in a co-ordinated and mutually supportive way, recognizing the importance of work for individuals and of the relationship between work and health. Clinical specialists, Primary Care teams, occupational physicians, occupational health nurses, and a host of other healthcare professionals all have a role to play. Ultimate success, however, will only come if all those healthcare professionals work in partnership with employers, with individuals themselves and with their representatives. This edition of *Fitness for Work* recognizes all these challenges and will provide much valued advice and support for those who are seeking to rise to them.

Dr Bill Gunnyeon
Chief Medical Adviser
Department for Work and Pensions

Foreword

By Dr David Snashall

This is a unique publication. There is no book comparable to *Fitness for Work* in the world medical literature. The first edition in 1987 was born of an idea from the medical division of the Health and Safety Executive and published as a joint report of the Royal College of Physicians and its Faculty of Occupational Medicine, only ten years old at the time. From a joint report the book has progressed into a standard textbook where subsequent editions have been published exclusively by the Faculty.

Fitness for work was and is an important socio-economic issue especially when there are health considerations. The book was designed to help doctors, both occupational health specialists and others, other health professionals, employers, and trade unions understand the relationship between health and employability and to bring some common sense and some evidence (where it existed) to the decision-making process. There was some very fruitful working between experienced occupational physicians and specialists on this project. Most developed lasting respect for one another's expertise.

The book was read worldwide and deemed to be of value even in those countries where the processes involved in deciding who is fit and who is not fit for particular kinds of jobs is not the same as in the UK.

The second and third editions followed the format of the first, always retaining an editor from the previous edition to ensure continuity. This is still the case with the fourth edition.

Since 1987 however there have been massive changes in the nature of work, the way people are employed, attitudes to people with disabilities, and a growing realization that work is, in general, health promoting.

The most relevant milestone in this progression was undoubtedly the enactment of the employment provisions of the Disability Discrimination Act in 1997 whereby those deemed to be disabled in their everyday life (reckoned now to be one in five of the UK population) acquired some protection against discrimination by their employers. The resulting case law and a recent extension of the Act has changed previous perceptions of how people living with disabilities can be employed and that change is reflected in the present edition. Fitness standards are still prescribed, sometimes by statute, in certain hazardous industries where safety is of overriding concern, but in all other walks of employment the pendulum has swung towards anyone being considered fit for any job unless there is some substantial reason why they should not be.

Fitness for work can no longer be about exclusion of the unfit from jobs which could in fact be adapted to their disability. Occupational physicians' main contribution to the process is now to advise on how such employees can be safely employed and ergonomically supported.

Assessing fitness for work is a process conducted in a delicate, socio-political area and requires the use of evidence and judgement at a high level. That said, the chapter headings have hardly changed since the last (or even the first) edition; the approach however is constantly evolving to reflect changing medical fashions (stress, obesity, the biopsychosocial model of incapacity), medicines' success in prolonging the life of younger disabled people (for instance with congenital heart disease, cystic fibrosis), into their working years and a more civilized attitude to those with disabilities who want to work.

In closing this foreword, I must thank the contributors and in particular the Editor in Chief, Dr Keith Palmer, and Co-editors, Dr Robin Cox and Dr Ian Brown. This publication is an enormous undertaking and the editors are to be congratulated for producing a book of such comprehensive coverage and impeccable quality. The Faculty of Occupational Medicine and the book's innumerable readers are indebted to them.

Dr David Snashall
President
Faculty of Occupational Medicine

Preface to the fourth edition

Fitness for Work has grown out of a Report of the Royal College of Physicians to become an established and essential source of guidance to all those involved in the practice of occupational medicine, including occupational physicians, hospital doctors, general practitioners, and occupational health nurses. It has also become an important point of reference for non-medical professionals coming from many walks of life—personnel managers, safety officers, trades union officials, lawyers, and career advisers to name but a few.

A number of factors account for the book's enduring popularity, pre-eminent among which is the requirement for sound advice on fitness decisions in workers with health complaints. The need for such advice continues to grow with time, and is underpinned by changes in demography, changes in work practice, and changes in social and political policy.

Today's population is ageing and tomorrow's workforce will have more of the common, chronic age-related health problems that arise in older people. Equally, society needs such older workers to be kept gainfully employed. To achieve this ambition employers will have to become more flexible, to deploy with thought and understanding, and to accommodate health problems more often. There is no slack to discard valuable skills and experience. However, correct placement in jobs that match the older worker's capabilities may well require specific medical advice and assessment.

The agenda of the UK Government is shifting in step. A strong perception exists now that the State is spending too much money on supporting people who are off sick and too little on helping them to cope and remain at work, or to resume work quickly after illness. To redress the balance a number of initiatives have been launched (as described in Chapter 4). The new alignment of the Health and Safety Executive (HSE), within the Department of Work and Pensions has encouraged a more holistic approach to health problems in employment. While the important effort of controlling risks at work continues unchecked, greater attention is being paid to rehabilitation and surmounting barriers to vocational placement.

To an extent the current legislative framework also reflects the imperative. For example, the Disability Discrimination Act makes it unlawful for employers to discriminate against workers on grounds of medical disability, and requires that all reasonable steps are taken to accommodate health problems and preserve employment opportunities. Proper medical input is required to meet that obligation.

Thus, the demand side of the 'occupational health advice equation' favours more and better advice on health problems in employment. What can be said of the supply side? In fact, it is limited. Although occupational health provision continues to grow nationally, it still falls far short of matching the requirement. Many employers, especially those from small businesses, do not enjoy access to specialist advice. Moreover, most doctors cannot give it with confidence. There is little professional training on occupational medicine within the crowded curricula of medical schools, so doctors outwith specialist and Faculty-led postgraduate training programmes have to fend for themselves. Although general principles may support them in many situations, there is much to know about the practice of medicine in the workplace—not least the nature and demands of their patients' work and the ethical and legal framework in which communications with managers can securely be conducted. In short, GPs and hospital doctors can benefit from the availability of reference information. Occupational health nurses, personnel officers, and other managers are placed similarly.

The common but simplistic framework of thinking about health in employment—a black and white dichotomy in which those lacking perfect fitness for all duties should remain at home—has surely had its day. Illness, or the perception of it, is so common that most of us cannot claim to be perfectly fit for the majority of the time, but most people manage to attend work even with some health limitation. Doing so is beneficial for the individual and the employer, and necessary for society; work can be therapeutic, it is associated with lower morbidity and mortality, and it is economically and socially important; skills shortages require managers and health professionals to appreciate what is possible with good occupational health advice and to read around the subject.

These factors underpin the success of *Fitness for Work* and support the need for an updated formulation. In fact, given the growing importance of the topic the publisher has encouraged a text that is some 25% longer than its predecessor, a clear barometer of success.

Readers will find in this new edition some ingredients that are familiar and some that are new. In keeping with the book's tradition, most of the chapters are co-authored by a specialist occupational physician and a topic specialist—a happy alliance that draws on the skills of each party to deliver a product exceeding the sum of its parts. As in earlier editions, we have aimed to cover every significant medical problem likely to be found in the workforce and essential general issues such as the legal and ethical aspects of ill health at work. Every chapter has been updated, but changes in these last two areas are noteworthy, reflecting recent legal judgments on the one hand and revised guidance from the General Medical Council and the Faculty of Occupational Medicine on the other. A number of other significant changes have been made. A new chapter has been added on the principles and practice of health screening; two former appendices of particular importance to occupational health staff and employers (ill-health retirement and professional driving) have been promoted into full chapters; new appendices have been added on return to work after critical illness and health surveillance for vibration-exposed workers; and a chapter on women at work has been given a broader focus. Finally, authors throughout have been encouraged where possible to cite evidence-based advice and guidelines. Success in this area has been mixed, reflecting limitations in the current state of research knowledge; but management of low-back pain, occupational asthma, and surveillance for hand–arm vibration syndrome provide three instances in which new evidence is directing practice. More generally, *Fitness for Work* continues to provide a wealth of useful consensus guidance, codes of practice, and locally evolved standards with practical value to health and safety practitioners.

To an extent, occupational medicine, like medicine as a whole, is an art that tailors advice to individual patients under specific and unique circumstances. As with any clinical judgement, the medical advice that is given remains the responsibility of the doctor concerned, and the general guidance contained in this book must always be interpreted in that light. None the less, we believe this book will underwrite the considered opinions of clinicians and other professionals involved in the practice of occupational medicine.

K.T. Palmer
R.A.F. Cox
I. Brown

November 2006

Preface to the third edition

Fitness for work is now an established textbook for those doctors in training or practising as occupational physicians and an essential source of reference for non-medical professionals such as lawyers, personnel officers, and general managers who need information on the medical aspects of fitness for work. It is also mandatory reading for all occupational health nurses who may often work in isolation.

The words of the preface to the first edition of this book remain relevant:

Most firms, particularly small ones, still have no occupational health service or medical advice of their own. Medical guidance on fitness for work usually comes from the patient's family or hospital doctor. Unfortunately, inappropriate advice may be given, either because not enough is known by doctors about the jobs their patients do, or because employers are unaware of the way in which advances in medical treatment have improved prognosis.

The up-to-date specialist opinion and background information given here on a number of medical conditions should improve both the relevance and consistency of advice. It should also reduce discrimination, often on irrelevant health grounds, against those who are at work or seeking work. As with any clinical judgement, the medical advice that is given on a patient remains the responsibility of the doctor concerned, and the general guidance contained in this book must always be interpreted in the light, not only of the effect of the illness or disability on the individual patient, but also of the special requirements of the job.

Although access to occupational health services is still not as complete as it should be, the benefits of occupational health services are more generally recognized today by employers, employees, unions, and government. Indeed, through recent initiatives of the Health and Safety Executive (see *Developing an occupational health strategy for Great Britain*, Health and Safety Executive discussion document, 1998), the government has accorded very high priority to occupational health. As the demand for these services expands, more doctors and nurses trained in the specialty are required and there is a need to keep standard texts, such as *Fitness for work*, up-dated; it is equally important to take account of recent advances in medical practice. Of the 27 chapters on clinical topics, 26 have been written jointly by an occupational physician and by a clinician practising in the appropriate specialty. This new, revised edition includes a number of contributions from new authors.

The second main motivating force for revision has been the Disability Discrimination Act 1995, which came in to force in the UK in December 1996 and upon which sufficient experience and case law have now accrued to enable specific advice to be proffered. Each chapter refers to the Act where relevant, and a whole chapter is devoted entirely to this topic. It is hoped that the advice contained in the book will assist tribunals when considering cases brought before them under the Act.

The editors feel that the subject of ethics in occupational medicine is not only of great importance but is also often misunderstood by employers and even by occupational physicians. The previous edition of *Fitness for work* included the Faculty's *Ethics for occupational physicians* but, in this edition, a whole chapter has been devoted to ethical issues in occupational medicine written by the current Chairman of the Ethics Committee of the Faculty of Occupational Medicine. This is one of five new chapters. Another is a chapter on work and the older employee written in response to the increasing trend towards working in a self-employed capacity after the normal age of retirement. Older workers have special problems, particularly in adapting to change, which are addressed in this chapter. The other new chapters have been created by re-arranging the chapters on musculoskeletal disorders, the biggest single group of medical conditions affecting the working population, into separate chapters on spinal and general orthopaedic disorders, trauma, and rheumatology. Although this creates some overlap, the new format has allowed us to deal with the wide range of individual conditions in greater detail.

We have also included in the Introduction a contribution about no-fault compensation and the New Zealand experience of this practice in the hope that this wider publicity will give impetus to its implementation elsewhere, and so reduce the demands for prolonged and expensive litigation. Compensation and rehabilitation can both be expedited by the use of vocational assessment and so a new section on that subject is included in Chapter 4.

The Appendix on European Directives which appeared in the second edition has been excluded from the third edition because all the directives, where relevant, are referred to in the general text.

Although the contents of this book will be of particular use to doctors, managers, nurses, and personnel staff in the United Kingdom, we feel that most of the topics are covered in such a general way that they will help others elsewhere in the world who need to make informed decisions about the medical aspects of fitness for work; both of the previous editions have been shown to be of value in Europe and many other countries. It is particularly with this wider readership in mind that we are delighted that Professor Bengt Knave, Professor of Occupational Medicine at the National Institute of Working Life in Stockholm and the President Elect of the International Commission on Occupational Health (ICOH) has written the Foreword to this edition.

R. A. F. Cox
F. C. Edwards
K. Palmer

June 2000

Preface to the second edition

The first edition of this book was published as a Report of the Royal College of Physicians in 1988. It clearly fulfilled a very real need and we have been greatly encouraged by the favourable comments and reviews which it received. With changes both in clinical medicine and in employment practice the contents of the Report required updating. In so doing, the book has become a reference textbook and is no longer a report of a large steering group. The general format has been retained with each chapter written by an occupational physician and a practising clinician in the respective specialty, but some of the chapters in the first edition have been divided for functional convenience. For example, a separate chapter on trauma has replaced part of the previous chapter on orthopaedics, while disorders of the spine now have a chapter to themselves. In addition, there are new appendices on fitness for work overseas, European Community legislation, ill-health retirement and ethics. All the addresses referred to in each chapter will be found in the appendix of useful addresses (Appendix 9).

The editors feel that the subject of ethics in occupational medicine is not only of great importance but is also often misunderstood by employers and even by occupational physicians. The Faculty of Occupational Medicine's Ethics for occupational physicians, has recently been published and we believed that this should be included in its entirety apart from some minor editing to save space (see Appendix 6). Copies of the booklet are available from the Faculty of Occupational Medicine.

A further concession to the need to keep the size of the book within the publisher's limits was to prune the number of references. The references which the editors have included, therefore, are selected for their interest and relevance and we have abandoned any attempt to make the list at the end of each chapter comprehensive. We apologize to any authors who may be offended by this decision and to any readers who may feel that the style of the book has been diminished but the limitation of references has enabled us to expand the breadth of the book.

Although it will be of particular value to doctors, nurses, managers, and personnel staff in the United Kingdom, we feel that most of the topics are covered in such a general way that it will also be a great help wherever in the world there is a need to make informed dicisions about the medical aspects of fitness for work. It is particularly with this wider readership in mind that we are delighted that Professor Jean-François Caillard, Professor of Occupational Medicine, Director of Occupational Medicine in the University of Rouen, Chairman of the French Federation of Occupational Medicine, and the current President of the International Commission on Occupational Health (ICOH), has written the Foreword to this edition. We also feel that the book will have an even greater relevance and application in the United Kingdom in the light of the new DSS proposals on the medical assessment for Incapacity Benefit.

In fact, this book will be invaluable to anyone practising occupational medicine.

Although occupational medicine is one of the most rapidly expanding medical disciplines, and more doctors enter training for the specialty every year, the advice of occupational physicians is still not available widely enough, in the United Kingdom, to workers in industry and commerce, and to the self-employed. We hope that this book will, therefore, be of particular value to those people, whether general practitioners, nurses, personnel managers, trade unionists, or others such as the staff of the employment and careers services who need guidance on the medical aspects of employment and may not be able to obtain it from a specialist occupational physician.

R.A.F. Cox
F.C. Edwards
R.I. McCallum

February 1995

Preface to the first edition

The stimulus for this report came originally from the Health and Safety Executive's Medical Division, who approached the Royal College of Physicians of London and its Faculty of Occupational Medicine. A steering group, under the Chairmanship of the late Dr Peter Taylor, was set up by the College and the Faculty to plan and produce the report, with the requirements of hospital specialists, general practitioners, and occupational physicians particularly in mind.

Apart from specific activities for which detailed guidelines exist, such as heay goods vehicle drivers, airline pilots, and professional divers, the vast majority of jobs have no clear criteria of fitness and precise guidelines cannot be laid down. Thus the need for informed advice on medical aspects of fitness for work covering a wide range of medical conditions is evident. Some chronic diseases, while not excluding work altogether, can clearly limit the scope of employment, but the restrictions that may be imposed on such patients are often unnecessary and without any rational basis. While it must be accepted that there may be diverse views on employability in many medical conditions, such problems should always be the subject of informed discussion between the employer, occupational medical adviser, the patient's own doctor, and the patient. This report provides a basis for such discussions.

Occupational medicine is often thought of as being concerned only with the effects of work on health, i.e. the prevention of occupational disease and of the effects of exposure to various environmental hazards, but equally it is about the effects of health on work, the fitness for work, and the rehabilitation of the individual. Occupational medicine is essentially a clinical speciality and throughout this book authors emphasize the need for close collaboration between occupational physicians and their clinical colleagues. Each chapter has been written jointly by a clinician practising in the specialty and an occupational physician, and it is hoped that one outcome will be that clinicians and occupational physicians will be brought closer together, enabling them to see each other's point of view.

Most firms, particularly small ones, still have no occupational health service or medical advice of their own. Medical guidance on fitness for work usually comes from the patient's family or hospital doctor. Unfortunately, inappropriate advice may be given, either because not enough is known by doctors about the jobs their patients do, or because employers are unaware of the way in which advances in medical treatment have improved prognosis.

The up-to-date specialist opinion and background information given here on a number of medical conditions should improve both the relevance and consistency of advice. It should also reduce discrimination, often on irrelevant health grounds, against those who are at work or seeking work. As with any clinical judgement, the medical advice that is given on a patient remains the responsibility of the doctor concerned, and the general guidance contained in this book must always be interpreted in the light, not only of the effect of the illness or disability on the individual patient, but also of the special requirements of the job.

We hope that the report will be of use not only to doctors in occupational medicine, but also to those in general practice or hospital medicine, and of interest to occupational health nurses, managers, and personnel staff. It will provide an essential core of information and advice on the effects of health on work for doctors in training for the examination for Associateship of the Faculty of Occupational Medicine (AFOM).

It was decided to retain some overlapping sections in different chapters, for example those on haemophilia, cervical spondylosis, and ankylosing spondylitis, because these refiected the different approaches and expertise of the authors. In spite of the speed with which the picture of Acquired Immune Deficiency Syndrome (AIDS) is changing as further knowledge of the disease develops, the steering group felt strongly that it should be included in the book because of its importance in relation to public concern about employability and safety at work.

F.C.E.
R.I.McC.

April 1988

Acknowledgements

A book of this size, complexity, and significance would not be possible without tremendous effort on the part of many people and the support of many bodies. We would particularly like to acknowledge the Department for Work and Pensions which has sponsored this edition, and also to thank our many colleagues within the Faculty of Occupational Medicine of the Royal College of Physicians of London, for providing both direct and indirect support throughout the book's gestation. We thank these bodies and individuals, as we do the main contributors—in all 58 writers for this edition, who tread in the footsteps of previous authors making significant contributions to earlier editions of the work. These specialists have given freely of their time and shared their expertise and knowledge for the benefit of the health of working people and have helped to create this much enlarged fourth edition of what has become the Faculty's flagship publication. They have also borne patiently the enquiries of editors and publishers and can take credit for their individual chapters as we the editors take pride in the final book. As may be imagined, the co-ordination of such an endeavour is essential but a dauntingly large task; last but not least the editors thank Anna McNeil for taking on this job so ably and so well.

Keith T. Palmer
Robin A. F. Cox
Ian Brown

Contents

Contributors

Dr C. Astbury
MB, ChB, MRCGP, MFOM
Director of Occupational Health and Safety
Services
Isle of Man Department of Health and Social
Security

Professor T-C. Aw
FRCP, PhD, FFOM
Professor of Occupational Medicine
Kent Institute of Medicine & Health Services
University of Kent

Professor M. Aylward
CB, MD, FFPM, FFOM, FRCP
Director
UnumProvident Centre for Psychosocial and
Disability Research
Cardiff University

Professor H. A. Bird
MD, FRCP
Professor of Pharmacological Rheumatology
University of Leeds,
Consultant Rheumatologist,
The Leeds Teaching Hospitals NHS Trust

Dr D. Bracher
MRCGP, MFOM
Medical Inspector (HSE Diving Medical
Advisor)
Health and Safety Executive

Professor E. A. Brown
MA (Oxon), DM, FRCP
Consultant Nephrologist
Imperial College London
Hammersmith Hospital
London

Dr I. Brown
OBE, FRCP, FFOM
Consultant Physician
Occupational Medicine and Toxicology
Southampton University Hospitals NHS Trust

Dr O. H. Carlton
FRCP, FFOM
Head of Occupational Health
Transport for London

Dr J. T. Carter
PhD, FFOM, FRCP
Chief Medical Advisor
Department for Transport

Professor C. C. H. Cook
MD, MA, MRCPsych
Professorial Research Fellow
Durham University

Dr S. E. L. Coomber
MFOM
Consultant Occupational Physician
Director of Suffolk Occupational Health
The Ipswich Hospital NHS Trust

Dr R. A. F. Cox
FRCP, FFOM, DDAM
Consultant Occupational Physician

Dr M. P. Deahl
TD, Mphil, FRCPsych
Consultant Psychiatrist
Shropshire County PCT;
Visiting Professor
City University, London;
Commanding Officer
256 (City of London)
Field Hospital (V)

Dr J. M. Dixon
FRCA
Consultant in Anaesthesia and Intensive
Care Medicine
Norfolk and Norwich University Hospital
NHS Trust

Dr K. M. Doig
MSc, MBBS, MFOM
Manager Centre of Excellence
Chevron UK Ltd

Dr A. R. Erlam
MSc, FFOM
Senior Medical Inspector
Health and Safety Executive

Dr U. T. Ferriday
FFOM, MSc
Head of Occupational Health
British Sky Broadcasting Ltd

Dr I. S. Foulds
MB, ChB, FRCP, FFOM
Consultant Dermatologist and Senior
Lecturer in Occupational Dermatology
Institute of Occupational and Environmental
Medicine
University of Birmingham

Professor B. G. Gazzard
MA, MD, FRCP
Research Director for HIV
Chelsea and Westminster Hospital
London

Dr G. V. Gill
MSc, MD, FRCP
Reader in Medicine and Consultant Physician
University of Liverpool and University
Hospital Aintree

Dr H. N. Goodall
MBBS, MFOM
Senior Consultant Occupational Physician
The Preventative Healthcare Company Ltd

Professor C. G. Greenough
MD, MChir, FRCS
Consultant Spinal Surgeon
Director, Regional Spinal Cord Injuries Centre
Professor of Spinal Studies
The James Cook University Hospital
University of Durham

Professor Sir John Grimley Evans
MD, FRCP, FFPH
Professor Emeritus of Clinical Geratology
University of Oxford

Dr R. J. Hardie
TD, MD, FRCP
Consultant Neurologist
Frenchay Hospital
Bristol

Dr C. C. Harling
MA, FFOM, FRCP
Chairman, Ethics Committee
Faculty of Occupational Medicine

Mr P. A. Harris
FRCS, MRCOG
Consultant Obstetrician & Gynaecologist
West Suffolk Hospital NHS Trust

Dr J. Hobson
MB, ChB, MRCP, FFOM
Director of Occupational Health
MPCG Ltd
Stoke on Trent

Ms G. S. Howard
LLB, Dip Comp Law (Cantab), FFOM (Hon)
Employment Lawyer
Howard & Howard Solicitors

Mr K. B. Hughes
MBBS, FRCS
Honorary Consultant ENT Surgeon and
Associate Medical Director
Doncaster and Bassetlaw NHS Foundation
Hospital Trust

Dr S. B. Janvrin
MS, FRCS, FFOM
Former Chief Medical Officer
Civil Aviation Authority

Dr R. V. Johnston
FRCP (G), FFOM, MBA
Head Aviation Health Unit
UK Civil Aviation Authority

Dr R. S. Kaczmarski
MD, FRCP, FRCPath
Consultant Haematologist
Honorary Senior Lecturer
Hillingdon Hospital NHS Trust

Professor D. S. Q. Koh
MBBS, PhD, FFOM, FFPH
Professor and Head
Department of Community
Occupational and Family Medicine
Yong Loo Lin School of Medicine
National University of Singapore

Dr P. Litchfield
MSc, FRCP, FFOM
Chief Medical Officer
BT Group plc

Dr B. P. Ludlow
MBBS, FFOM, MMedSc
Chief Medical Officer
British Nuclear Group (Reactor Sites)

Dr H. G. Major
BSc, MBBS
Senior Medical Advisor
Driver and Vehicle Licensing Agency

Professor G. T. McInnes
MD, FRCP, FBPharmacolSoc
Professor of Clinical Pharmacology and
Consultant Physician
University of Glasgow

Dr N. K. I. McIver
OBE, FFOM
Occupational Health Physician
North Sea Medical Centre

Mr I. M. Nugent
MBBS, FRCS, FRCS(Orth)
Consultant Trauma and Orthopaedic
Surgeon
Royal Berkshire Hospital
Reading

Dr K. T. Palmer
DM, FRCP, FFOM
MRC Clinical Scientist
Honorary Reader & Consultant Occupational
Physician
University of Southampton

Dr S. B. Pearson
DPhil, DM, FRCP
Consultant Physician
Leeds Teaching Hospitals NHS Trust

Dr M. C. Petch
OBE, MD, FRCP
Consultant Cardiologist
Papworth Hospital
Cambridge

Mr J. Pitts
LLM, DAvMED, MRCP, FRCS, FRCOphth
Consultant Advisor in Ophthalmology to the
Civil Aviation Authority
Vision in Aviation (ViA) Ltd

Dr C. J. M. Poole
MD, FRCP, FFOM
Consultant Occupational Physician
Dudley NHS PCT

Dr M. C. Prevett
FRCP
Consultant Neurologist
Wessex Neurological Centre
Southampton University Hospitals NHS Trust

Dr A. E. Price
MB, ChB Hons, MFOM
Consultant Occupational Physician
Hinchingbrooke NHS Trust

Dr I. G. Rennie
FFOM, RCP
Medical Adviser
Kodak Ltd

Dr S. J. Ryder
OBE, FRCS(Ed), MFOM
Director of Occupational Health Services
NHS Highland

Dr A. M. Samuel
MSc, FRCP, FFOM
Chief Medical Officer, EDF Energy

Dr P. E. Sawney
MBBS, BSc, MRCGP, DGM (RCP),
DOcccMed, DDAM
Principal Medical Adviser
Department for Work and Pensions

Dr J. C. Smedley
DM, FRCP, FFOM
Director of Occupational Health,
Southampton University Hospitals NHS Trust

Dr J. L. Southgate
BM, BSc, MRCP
Consultant in Acute Medicine and
Gastroenterology
Norfolk and Norwich University Hospital
Trust

Professor E. L. Teasdale
FRCP, FFOM, FRCGP
Chief Medical Officer
Global Director of Health and Wellbeing
Consultant Occupational Physician
AstraZeneca and Lancaster University

Dr E. R. Waclawski
MD, FRCP (G), FFOM
Director of Occupational Health and
Consultant Occupational Physician
NHS Greater Glasgow and Clyde

Mr J. Mc K. Wellwood
MA, MChir (Cantab), FRCS (Eng)
Consultant Surgeon
Harley Street, London

Dr R. Willcox
FFOM, DTMeH
Consultant Occupational Physician
One Click Health, London

Dr S. Williams
MRCP, FFOM, MD
Consultant in Occupational Medicine
Royal Free Hampstead NHS Trust

Dr E. S. M. Ziegler
MFOM, MRCGP
Specialist Registrar in Occupational Medicine
Southampton University Hospitals NHS Trust

Chapter 1

A general framework for assessing fitness for work

K. T. Palmer and R. A. F. Cox

This book on fitness for work gathers together specialist advice·on the medical aspects of employment and the majority of medical conditions likely to be encountered in the working population. Though personnel managers and others will find it of great help it is primarily written for doctors so that family practitioners, hospital consultants, and occupational physicians, as well as other doctors and occupational health nurses, can best advise managers and others who may need to know how a patient's illness might affect their work. Although decisions on return to work or on placement must depend on many factors, it is hoped that this book, which combines best current clinical with occupational health practice, will be used by doctors and others as a source of reference and will remind them about the occupational implications of illness.

It must be emphasized that, apart from relieving suffering and prolonging life, the objective of much medical treatment in working-aged adults, whether it be a course of antibiotics or a renal transplant, is to return the patient to work. Much of the benefit of modern medical technology and the skills of physicians and surgeons will have been wasted if patients who have been successfully treated are denied work, through ignorance or prejudice, by employers or doctors acting on their behalf. A main aim of this book is to remove the excuse for denying work to those who have overcome injury and disease and deserve to work.

The book is arranged in chapters according to specialty or topic, the majority of chapters having been written jointly by a clinician and an occupational physician. For each specialty the chapter outlines the conditions covered; notes relevant statistics; discusses clinical aspects, including treatment that may affect work capacity; notes rehabilitation requirements or special needs at the workplace; discusses problems that may arise at work and any necessary work restrictions; notes any current advisory or statutory medical standards; and makes recommendations on the employment aspects of the conditions covered. A chapter on the possible effects of medication on work performance and additional chapters on ethics, the ageing worker, ill-health retirement, health screening, and fitness to drive are also included. Appendices describe the medical standards for civil aviation, merchant shipping, offshore work and diving, fitness for work overseas, and work with vibratory tools. A contribution on return to work following critical illness and a list of useful addresses and contacts conclude the book.

The first five chapters are applicable to any condition. This introductory chapter deals mainly with the principles underlying medical assessment of fitness for work, contacts between medical practitioners and the workplace, and confidentiality of medical information. Chapter 2 covers legal aspects, Chapter 3 focuses on the Disability Discrimination Act, Chapter 4 outlines the current provision for support, rehabilitation, and restoring fitness for work, and important ethical principles of occupational health practice are elaborated in Chapter 5 (which is written by the Chair of the Faculty of Occupational Medicine's Ethics Committee).

Health problems and employment

Workers with disabilities are commonly found to be highly motivated, often with excellent work and attendance records. When medical fitness for work is assessed, what matters is often not the medical condition itself, but the associated loss of function, and any resulting disability or handicap. It should be borne in mind that a disability seen in the consulting room may be irrelevant to the performance of a particular job. **The patient's condition should be interpreted in functional terms and in the context of the job requirements.**

Impairment, disability, and handicap

Handicap may result directly from an impairment (for instance, severe facial disfigurement), or more usually, from the resulting disability. To be consistent in the use of these terms, the simplified scheme of the *International classification of impairments, disabilities, and handicaps*[1,2] should be used as follows:

+ A disease, disorder, or injury produces an **impairment** (change in normal structure or function).
+ A **disability** is a resulting reduction or loss of an ability to perform an activity—for example climbing stairs, or manipulating a keyboard.
+ A **handicap** is a social disadvantage resulting from an impairment or disability, which limits or prevents the fulfilment of a normal role.

As examples:

+ A relatively minor impairment, the loss of a finger, would be both a disability and a serious occupational handicap to a pianist, although not to a builder's labourer.
+ A relatively common impairment, defective colour vision, limits the ability to discriminate between certain hues. This may occasionally be a handicap at work, although there are in fact very few occupations for which defective colour vision is a significant handicap.

Prevalence of disability and its impact on employment

Figures on the prevalence of disability and/or handicap in different populations vary according to the definitions and methods used and the groups sampled. An extra tier of uncertainty in assessing the numbers of disabled people in the workforce, or seeking work, arises from reluctance of people to admit their disability. Differences between surveys may also be due to the inclusion of non-physical handicaps and to different methods of reporting. Common to all is the rise in prevalence of disability with increasing age and, to a lesser extent, with manual as opposed to non-manual workers, social class, and/or occupational groups.

There is no doubt that, however measured, disabling illness is common and a major obstacle to gainful employment. One national population survey,[3] undertaken in Great Britain in 2001 by the Office of National Statistics as part of the Labour Force Survey, estimated that nearly one in five people of working age in private households had a long-term disability (3.7 million men and 3.4 million women). Some 3.4 million disabled people were in employment, although at a rate significantly lower than that of those without disabilities (48% vs. 81%). Roughly half of the disabled population was economically inactive (44% of men and 52% of women) as compared with only 15% of the non-disabled population. The overall proportion of people reporting long-term illness or disability that restricted daily activities was 18%, but the

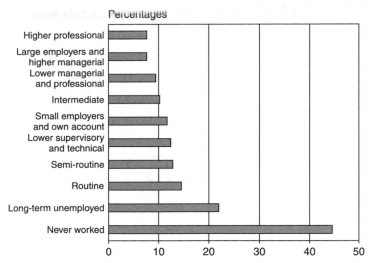

Fig. 1.1 Age-standardized rates of long-term illness or disability restricting daily activities: by socio-economic status, 2001, England & Wales (Office of National Statistics, reproduced with permission under the terms of the click-use licence).

age-standardized rate was three times higher in the long-term unemployed than in managerial and professional occupations (Figure 1.1).

Many other statistics paint a similar picture, of common illnesses that commonly erode work capacity:

◆ Sickness absence is estimated to have cost the UK economy almost £12 billion in 2004.

◆ Some 9% of adults in Britain suffer mixed anxiety and depression, 230 out of a thousand visit a GP every year with mental health problems and a tenth of these were referred to specialist psychiatric services in 2004.[4,5]

◆ The HSE estimates that in 2004/5 2 million working-aged adults in Britain were suffering from an illness which they believed was caused or made worse by work, contributing 28 million working days lost due to work-related ill-health and 7 million lost days arising from workplace injury.[6]

◆ One in four men and one in five women will suffer a critical illness before they are aged 65 years.[7]

◆ In England and Wales some 13 000 replacements of hip or knee joints are carried out each year on adults aged 15–59 years, representing nearly one in five of hip replacements and one in eight of knee joint replacements across all age bands.[8]

◆ The large European Community Respiratory Health Survey,[9] involving interviews with over 17 000 subjects, estimated that some 10% of adults aged 20–44 years wheeze at work, while 4% have work-related respiratory disability.

◆ A prospective population-based cohort study of 30 000 individuals in Manitoba, Canada, estimated that diabetics with complications were twice as likely as other workers to quit the labour force over follow-up;[10] people with diabetes are also more likely to experience problems in obtaining employment.[11]

◆ In a community-based survey in the north east of England[12] the unemployment rate for economically active patients with epilepsy was 46%, as compared with 19% in age and sex matched controls.

The experience in other countries is similar. Thus, according to the 2003 American Community Survey,[13] an estimated 11.5% of Americans aged 15–64 years (some 21 million people) had a disability, the majority of whom were unemployed.

Is this experience justified and reasonable? We would argue not, in many instances. Self-evidently, serious illness can prevent a person working in the short or long term; but many people with major illness *do* work with proper treatment and workplace support. Thus the relation with unemployment is not as constant and inevitable as these gloomy statistics suggest. Rather, the job prospects of people with common illnesses or disabilities can often be improved with proper thought, both about the work that *is* still possible and the reasonable changes that could be made to allow for their circumstances.

The Disability Discrimination Act 1995 (DDA)

These ideas are captured and distilled in primary legislation. The DDA has a major significance both for the disabled and for occupational physicians. In broad terms, and with certain important details of interpretation, the Act makes it unlawful for employers to discriminate against workers, irrespective of age, including job applicants, on grounds of medical disability; rather, it requires that all reasonable steps are taken to accommodate their health problems. This is a form of positive discrimination in favour of preserving employment opportunities. It is also the legal embodiment of good occupational health values and practice; long before the Act, occupational health professionals strove for the same outcome. However, employers are influenced very strongly by legal mandate and so the Act is an instrument for good, as judged from the viewpoint of the disabled.

Occupational physicians need a good working knowledge of the legislation. Such is the Act's importance that a whole chapter (Chapter 3) is devoted to its application and the recent development of case law, while references to the effects of the DDA in clinical situations are made throughout the rest of the book. Here only a few essential points are made.

In the Act, disability is not defined in terms of working ability or capacity but in terms of 'an adverse effect on the ability to carry out normal day to day activities'. Work itself does not, therefore, have to be considered in deciding whether an individual is disabled or not but of course it does have to be considered when a disabled person is in a work situation. It is in this circumstance that the opinion of the occupational physician will be required. The physician may be asked:

+ whether an individual's disability falls within the definition of the Act
+ if it does, what adjustments may be needed to accommodate the disabled individual in the workplace.

Adjustments may be to the physical and psychological nature of the work or to the methods by which the work is accomplished. It is for management, not the occupational physician, to decide in each individual case whether such adjustments are *reasonable*, although occupational health services may be well placed to *identify* potential adjustments. Before offering such opinions the occupational physician must make an accurate determination of the individual's disability, not in medical but in functional terms; this requires a detailed understanding of the work and the workplace in question—another abiding principle of good occupational health practice.

The ageing worker

One circumstance in which reasonable accommodation may be required is the employment of older workers. With increasing longevity and a growing shortfall in pension resources it will be necessary, in future, for people to work well past the current retirement age. This is likely to be beneficial to individuals both in terms of wealth and health, though some will need adjustments and modifications to their work or working time to accommodate some of the restrictions and impairments associated with ageing. Age, *per se*, should not be a bar to gainful employment, though the advice contained in this book or the advice of an occupational health professional, may be needed to integrate the older worker into employment effectively.

Some major issues surrounding practice in this area are aired in Chapter 26. Here we stress the importance of the topic and its close relation to occupational medicine. As the 'demographic time bomb' looms large, the slack to discard valuable skills and experience will diminish. Avoidance of ageist blanket judgements about work fitness, and greater flexibility and thought in job deployment will become commercially important; these are already basic values in occupational health practice, while the underpinning medical advice will come from health professionals with experience in the occupational setting.

Occupational health services

All employees should have access to occupational health advice, whether this is provided from within a company or by external consultants. Such advice may be provided by occupational health trained nurses or by specialist occupational physicians but, for some problems advice from one of the latter practitioners will be essential—e.g. in providing evidence for industrial tribunals or in other medico-legal cases. The exact nature and size of the occupational health service to which any company needs access depends on the size of the company and the hazards of the activities in which it is engaged. Some companies find it advantageous to share occupational health services.

The local Employment Medical Advisory Service (EMAS) of the Health and Safety Executive (HSE) is able to advise on the availability and sources of local occupational health services and occupational health practitioners. EMAS may give advice to individual employees, although the main role their medical inspectors (doctors) and occupational health inspectors (nurses) now fulfil is to support the general inspectors of the HSE.

In the main occupational health services advise on fitness for work, vocational placement, return to work after illness, ill-health retirement, work-related illness, and the control of

---

Box 1.1 Alternative models of service delivery

Although the demand for skilled occupational health advice continues to increase we are still far from reaching the ideal of access to occupational health for all the working population. If that objective is to be realized there will need to be far more resources in the form of trained and qualified occupational health nurses and physicians, a situation that seems highly improbable in the near future at least.

The alternative is to utilize the resources we have more effectively and efficiently by making use of modern technology. An initiative that is showing great promise is the use of nurse-led call centres supported by occupational health advisers and occupational physicians. This ensures that scarce resources are used only when necessary but that support and occupational health advice can be delivered to a much wider population, enabling significant reductions in lost time and earlier rehabilitation. The system is now well established and showing every sign of rapid expansion into a broad range of industries without compromising the present high standards of occupational health care.

occupational hazards. Some of these functions are statutory (e.g. certain categories of health surveillance) or advisable in terms of meeting legal responsibilities (e.g. guidance on food safety, application of the DDA). Some employers regard the main function being to control sickness absence. Although occupational health professionals, whether nurses or physicians, can help both managers and individuals to reduce sickness absence, its control is a management responsibility; occupational health practitioners should be careful to avoid the policing of employees who are absent for reasons attributed to sickness (see Chapter 5, Ethics).

Contacts between the patient's medical advisers and the workplace

The patient's own medical advisers have an important part to play. The importance of their contact with the workplace cannot be overemphasized. We suggest that consultants, as well as family practitioners, should ask the patient if there is an occupational health service at the workplace and, if so, obtain written consent to contact the occupational physician, or the occupational health nurse in the absence of a physician.

Where there is no occupational health service, early contact between the patient's doctor and management (usually the personnel manager) may also be valuable. It helps the employer to know when the patient is likely to return to work, and whether some work adjustment will be helpful, while family practitioners and consultants will be helped by having a better understanding of their patient's job.

Confidentiality

Usually, any recommendations and advice on placement or return to work are based on the functional effects of the medical condition and its prognosis. Generally there is no requirement for an employer to know the diagnosis or to receive clinical details. A simple statement that the patient is medically 'fit' or 'unfit' for a particular job often suffices, but occasionally further information may need to be disclosed, particularly, if limitations on work are being imposed. The certificated reason for any sickness absence is usually known by personnel departments, who maintain their own confidential records.

The patient's consent must be obtained, preferably in writing, before disclosure of confidential health information to third parties, including other doctors, occupational health nurses, employers, or other people such as staff of the careers or employment services. The purpose of this should be made clear to the patient; it may be to help with suitable work, and/or to maintain health and safety (their own and that of others). A patient who is found to be medically unfit for certain employment should be given a full explanation of why the disclosure of unfitness is necessary. Further advice may be found in the Faculty of Occupational Medicine's *Guidance on ethics for occupational physicians*[14] (see also Chapter 5).

Medical reports

When a medical report is requested on an individual, the person should be informed of the purpose for which the report is being sought. If a medical report is being sought from an employee's general practitioner or specialist, then the employer is required, under the Access to Medical Reports Act 1988, to inform the employee of their rights under that Act (which include the right to see the report before it is sent to the employer and the right to refuse to allow the report to be sent to the employer). If the report is sought from an occupational physician it will also come under the Access to Medical Reports Act if the occupational physician has ever had clinical care of the patient. Even if the occupational physician has not cared for the patient clinically, it is good ethical practice to follow the legal requirements of the Access to Medical Reports Act.

Employees are also now entitled to see their medical records, including their occupational health records, which would include any medical reports.

Any doctor being asked for a medical report should insist that the originator of the request writes a referral letter containing full details of the individual, a description of their job, an outline of the problem, and the matters on which the doctor's opinion is sought.

At the outset the doctor should obtain the patient's consent, preferably in writing, to examine him and furnish the report. Even if the patient has given consent the report should not contain clinical information, unless it is absolutely essential, and the contents should be confined to addressing the questions posed in the letter of referral and advising on interpreting the person's medical condition in terms of functional capability and their ability to meet the requirements of their employment. Gratuitous comment should be avoided, but the employer is entitled to be sufficiently informed to make a clear decision about the individual's work ability, both currently and in the future, any adjustments, modifications, restrictions, or prohibitions that may be required. The doctor should express a clear opinion and should offer a copy of the report to the employee. The employee can then request the doctor to correct any factual errors that they consider may have been included, but they are not entitled to require the doctor to modify the opinion expressed, even if they strongly disagree with it. A patient's return to work or his continuation in work may depend on the receipt of a medical report from his GP, consultant, or occupational physician. It is, therefore, in the patient's interest, and especially his financial interest, that such reports are furnished as expeditiously as possible without unreasonable delay.

When writing any medical report the occupational physician should always remember that the document will be discoverable if litigation subsequently ensues. It should be clear from the report, either from its content, the letter heading, or the affiliation under the signature, why the doctor is qualified to address the subject in question. For example, a doctor who does not possess recognized qualifications in occupational medicine should not purport to be an occupational physician and a doctor who is not on the GMC's Specialist Register should not call himself a 'consultant' occupational physician.[15]

Assessing fitness for work: general considerations

The primary purpose of a medical assessment of fitness for work is to make sure that an individual is fit to perform the task involved effectively and without risk to their own or others' health and safety.

Why an assessment may be needed

1. The patient's condition may limit, reduce, or prevent them from performing the job effectively (e.g. musculoskeletal conditions that limit mobility or carrying).

2. The patient's condition may be made worse by the job (e.g. excessive physical exertion in cardiorespiratory illness; exposure to certain allergens in asthma).

3. The patient's condition may make certain jobs and work environments unsafe to them personally (e.g. liability to sudden unconsciousness in a hazardous situation; risk of damage to the remaining eye or ear in a patient with monocular vision, or monaural hearing).

4. The patient's condition may make it unsafe both for themselves *and for others*, whether fellow workers and/or the community, in some occupational roles (e.g. road or railway driving in someone who is liable to sudden unconsciousness or to behave abnormally).

5. The patient's condition may pose a risk to the community (e.g. for consumers of the product, if a food handler transmits infection).

There is usually a clear distinction between the first-party risks of 2 and 3 and the third-party risks of 5. In 4, first- and third-party risks may both be present.

Thus, when assessing a patient's fitness for work, the doctor must consider the following factors:

- The level of skill, physical and mental capacity, sensory acuity, etc. needed for effective performance of the work.
- Any possible adverse effects of the work itself or of the work environment on the patient's health.
- The possible health and safety implications of the patient's medical condition when undertaking the work in question, for themselves, fellow workers, and/or the community.

For some jobs it should also be remembered that there may be an emergency component in addition to the routine job structure, and higher standards of fitness may thus be needed, on occasion, for the former.

When an assessment of medical fitness is needed

An assessment of medical fitness may be needed for those who are:

1. Being considered for a new job (e.g. at a recruitment or transfer/pre-placement assessment).
2. Already in employment (e.g. after significant illness).
3. Unemployed and seeking work in training, but without a specific job in mind.

For 1 and 2, the assessment will be related to a particular job, or to a defined range of alternative work in a given workplace. The assessment is needed to help both employer and employee, and should be specifically directed at the job in question. After a pre-placement or pre-employment medical examination, employers are entitled to know if there may be consequences from a medical condition that may curtail or restrict a potential employee's working life in the future. But, for 3, where there may be no specific job in view, the assessment must inevitably be more open-ended: health assessments may be required, for instance, by the employment or careers services in their attempt to find suitable work for unemployed disabled people. It is thus all the more important to avoid unnecessary medical restrictions or labels (such as 'epileptic'), as these tend to follow individuals in their search for work and may limit their future choice unduly.

Recruitment medicals

Employers often use health questionnaires as part of their recruitment process. Such questionnaires should be marked 'medically confidential' and should be read and interpreted only by an occupational physician or nurse. A questionnaire that has to be returned to a non-medical person—because an employer does not have an occupational health service, for example—is not protected by medical confidentiality and should not be so described.

Some individuals may be reluctant to disclose a medical condition to a future employer (sometimes with their own doctor's support) for fear that this may lose them the job. Although understandable, it must be pointed out that, should work capability be impaired or an accident arise due to the concealed condition, dismissal on medical grounds may follow. An industrial tribunal would be likely to support the dismissal if the employee had failed to disclose the relevant condition. It is not in the patient's interest to conceal any medical condition that could adversely affect their work, but it would be entirely reasonable for the applicant to request that the details be disclosed only to an occupational physician or nurse.

For some jobs (e.g. driving) there are statutory medical standards and for others employing organizations lay down their own advisory medical standards (e.g. food handling or work in the offshore oil and gas industry). For the majority of jobs, however, no agreed advisory medical standards exist, and for many jobs there need be no special health requirements. Job application forms should be accompanied by a clear indication of any health standards or physical qualifications that are required and of any medical conditions that would be a bar to certain types of job, but no questions about health or disabilities should be included on job application forms themselves. If health information is necessary, applicants should be asked to complete a separate health declaration form or questionnaire, which should be inspected and interpreted only by health professionals and only after the candidate has been selected, subject to satisfactory health.

The reason for a pre-placement health assessment, however that is performed, should always be assumed to be only for fitness for the proposed job and only medical questions relevant to that employment should be asked. If an employer wishes to know, for example, if the candidate can be expected to give 'long, healthy service', then such a request must be made clear at the outset as the nature of the assessment will be completely different, even if it is possible.

Recruitment and the company pension scheme

Many doctors and personnel managers in industry still believe that their company pension fund requires high standards of medical fitness for new entrants. Direct enquiry to the pension fund administrators themselves usually demonstrates that this is not the case. Fortunately, most pension funds follow the general principle recommended by the Occupational Pensions Board: 'Fit for employment—fit for the pension fund'.[16] It was the Board's view that 'The concern of an employer, when assessing a prospective employee, should be with ability to perform the job efficiently. There is no reason why pension scheme considerations should influence the employer's decision whether to employ him.' In general, a disease or disability should not be a reason *per se* for exclusion from pension schemes, nor should it be used as an excuse to deny employment, unless it adversely affects job performance or health and safety. For an approach to the calculation of disability pensions and current thinking on life underwriting the reader is referred to Brackenridge and Elder.[17] Where company schemes still operate against people with disabilities, attempts should be made to amend them. However, with recent changes in legislation pensions can now be personal, flexible, and mobile; anyone with a medical

Box 1.2 The status of medical standards

Medical standards may be advisory or statutory. They may also be local and tailored to specific job circumstances. Standards are often laid down where work entails entering a new environment that may present some hazard to the individual, such as the increased or decreased atmospheric pressures encountered in compressed-air work, diving and flying, or work in the high temperatures of nuclear reactors. Standards are also laid down for work where there is a potential risk of a medical condition causing an accident, as in transport, or transmitting infection, as in food handling. For onerous or arduous work such as in mines rescue or in fire-fighting, very high standards of physical fitness are needed. Specific medical standards will need to be met in such types of work: where relevant, such advisory and/or statutory standards are noted in each speciality chapter.

disability may be well advised to negotiate a personal policy that they can retain permanently irrespective of their employer.

Fitness assessment during employment

The stages at which a health appraisal may become necessary for someone in employment are as follows:

+ **Job change**. Although still working for the same employer, transfer or promotion may bring with it new demands and fitness requirements. The employee should be told of any special health requirements or qualifications for the new post and the health appraisal should relate to these. Job change may include more seniority or responsibility, for instance, or include overseas posting with a considerable increase in travel. All of these factors may have to be taken into account.

+ **Periodic review** of individual health may be undertaken in some circumstances and will relate to specific requirements (e.g. regular assessment of visual acuity in some jobs, statutory health surveillance for those working with respiratory sensitizers).

+ **Return to work after illness or injury** usually merits a health assessment and is discussed further below. Employees returning to work after **prolonged absence** often have special needs that should be taken into account where possible.

+ The question of **retirement on grounds of ill-health** may need to be considered (see also Chapter 27).

In any of these situations there is a legal requirement to consider 'reasonable adjustment' if the individual has a disability within the definition of the DDA, and it is good occupational health practice to do so in any case.

Special groups

Young people

Medical advice on occupation or training given to a young person who has not yet started a career often has a different slant from that given to an adult developing the same medical condition late in an established career. The later stages of a particular vocation may involve jobs incompatible with the young person's medical condition, or its foreseeable development and timely advice may avoid future disappointment. Conversely, a mature adult's work experience may enable them to overcome obstacles posed by a disease or disability in ways that a young worker could not.

It is particularly important that young people entering employment are given appropriate and consistent medical advice when it is needed. For instance, although a school-leaver with epilepsy might be eligible for an ordinary driving licence at the time of recruitment, it would be most inadvisable for them to take up a position where vocational driving was likely to become an essential requirement for career progression. A young person with atopic eczema may not wish to invest in training for hairdressing if advised that hairdressing typically aggravates hand eczema.

Severely disabled people

Where a medical condition has so reduced an individual's employment abilities or potential that they are incapable either of continuing in their existing work or of working in any open competitive employment, even with all appropriate adjustments, then sheltered work of some kind may be the only alternative to premature medical retirement, on the one hand, or to continued unemployment on the other.

The assessment of medical fitness for work

A general framework

As previously emphasized, the clinician's assessment should always be reported in terms of functional capacity; the actual diagnosis need not be given. Even so, an opinion on the medical fitness of an individual is being conveyed to others and the patient's written consent is needed for the information to be passed on, in confidence.

Each of the specialty chapters that follow outlines the main points to be considered when faced with specific health conditions. In this section we summarize a general framework, but emphasize that not all of the points raised will be relevant to any one individual, while some are relevant to more than one type of condition, or to more than one system or speciality. The key outcome measure is the **patient's residual abilities relative to the likely requirements at the workplace**, and so a proper assessment weighs functional status against job demands.

Functional assessment

To estimate the individual's level of function, assessments of all systems should be made with special attention both to those that are disordered and relevant to the work. As well as physical systems, sensory and perceptual abilities should be noted, as well as psychological reactions, such as responsiveness, alertness, and other features of the general mental state. The effects of different treatment regimes on work suitability should also be considered; the possible effects of some medication on alertness, or the optimal position of an arthrodesis, are only two of many examples.

Any general evaluation of physical and mental health forms the background to more specific inquiry. Assessment should also consider the results of relevant tests. The following factors may be material:

- **General:** stamina; ability to cope with full working day, or shiftwork; liability to fatigue etc.
- **Mobility:** ability to get to work, and exit safety; to walk, climb, bend, stoop, crouch, etc.
- **Locomotor:** general/specific joint function and range; reach of arms; gait; back/spinal function, etc.
- **Posture:** ability to stand or sit for certain times; any postural constraints; work in confined spaces, etc.
- **Muscular:** specific palsies or weakness; tremor; ability to lift, push or pull, with weight/time abilities if known; strength tests, etc.
- **Manual skills:** any defects in dexterity, ability to grip, or grasp, etc.
- **Co-ordination:** including hand-eye co-ordination if relevant.
- **Balance:** ability to work at heights; vertigo.
- **Cardiorespiratory limitations**, including exercise tolerance, and how this was tested; respiratory function and reserve; submaximal exercise tests, aerobic work capacity, if relevant.
- **Liability to unconsciousness,** including nature of episodes, timing, any precipitating factors, etc.
- **Sensory aspects:** may be relevant for the actual work, or in order to get about a hazardous environment safety.
  - **Vision:** ability for fine/close work, distant vision, visual standards corrected or uncorrected, any aids in use or needed. Visual fields. Colour vision defects may occasionally be relevant. Is the eyesight good enough to cope with a difficult working environment with possible hazards?

- **Hearing:** level in each ear; can warning signals or instructions be heard?
- For both **vision and hearing** it is very important that if only one eye or one ear is functioning, this should be noted so that thought can be given to protecting the remaining organ against possible damage.

- **Communication/speech:** two-way communication; hearing or speech defects; reason for limitation.
- **Cerebral function** will be relevant after head injury, cerebrovascular accident, some neurological conditions, and in those with some intellectual deficit: the presence of any confusion; disorientation; impairment of memory, intellect, verbal, or numerical aptitudes, etc.
- **Mental state:** psychiatric assessment may mention anxiety, relevant phobias, mood, withdrawal, relationships with other people, etc.
- **Motivation:** may well be the most important determinant of work capacity. With it, impairments may be surmounted; without it, difficulties may not be overcome. It can be particularly difficult to assess by a doctor who has not previously known the patient.
- **Treatment of the condition:** special effects of treatment may be relevant, e.g. drowsiness, inattention, as side-effects of some medication; implications of different types of treatment in one condition (e.g. insulin as opposed to oral treatment for diabetes).
- **Further treatment:** if further treatment is planned, e.g. further orthopaedic or surgical procedures, these may need to be mentioned.
- **Prognosis:** if the clinical prognosis is likely to affect work placement, e.g. likely improvements in muscle strength, or decline in exercise tolerance, these should be indicated.
- **Special needs:** these may be dietary; need for a clean area for self-treatment, e.g. injection; or relate to time, e.g. frequent rest pauses, no paced or shiftwork, etc.
- **Aids or appliances** in use or needed. Implanted artificial aids may be relevant in the working environment (pacemakers and artificial joints). Aids to mobility may have implications for work (e.g. wheelchair). Prostheses/orthoses should be mentioned. Artificial aids or appliances that could help at the workplace should be indicated.
- **Specific third-party risks** that could be conferred on other workers or members of the community, e.g. via the product such as infection in food handlers, etc.

Requirements of the job

The requirements of work may relate not only to the individual's present job but also to their future career. Always considering the possibility of 'reasonable adjustment', some of the following aspects may be relevant:

- **Work demands:** physical (e.g. mobility needs; strength for certain activities; lifting/carrying; climbing/balancing; stooping/bending; postural constraints; reach requirements; dexterity/manipulative ability, etc.); intellectual/perceptual demands; types of skill involved in tasks.
- **Work environment:** physical aspects, risk factors (e.g. fumes/dust; chemical or biological hazards; working at heights).
- **Organizational/social aspects,** e.g. working in small groups; intermittent or regular pressure of work; need for tact in public relations, etc.
- **Temporal aspects,** e.g. need for early start; type of shiftwork; day or night work; arrangements for rest pauses or breaks, etc.

- **Ergonomic aspects**; workplace (e.g. need to climb stairs; distance from toilet facilities; access for wheelchairs, etc.); workstation (e.g. height of workbench; adequate lighting; type of equipment or controls used, etc.). Adaptations of equipment that could help at the workplace should be indicated.

- **Travel**, e.g. need to work in areas remote from healthcare or where there are risks not found in the UK (see Appendix 5).

Too often, medical statements simply state 'fit for light work only'. The dogmatic separation of work into 'light', 'medium', and 'heavy' often results in individuals being unduly limited in their choice of work. A refinement of this broad grading is adopted by the US Department of Labor in its *Dictionary of occupational titles*.[18] Jobs are graded according to physical demands, environmental conditions, certain levels of skill and knowledge, and specific vocational preparation (training time) required, but current occupational health practice requires more specific adjustment of the job to the individual. The physical demands listed in Table 1.1 (adapted from the *Dictionary of Occupational Titles*) serve as a means of expressing both the physical requirements of the job and the physical capacities that a worker must have to meet those required by many jobs. The worker must possess a physical capacity that at least matches the physical demands made by the job. For example, if the energy or metabolic requirements of a particular task are known the individual's work capacity may be estimated and, if expressed in the same units, a comparison between the energy demands of the work and the physiological work capacity of the individual may be made. This has been used in assessing work capacity of patients with heart disease.[19] (See also Chapter 18, pp 413–4.) Energy requirements of various tasks can be estimated and expressed in metabolic equivalents, or Mets. (The Met is an arbitrary unit recommended by the American Heart Association: 1 Met is the approximate energy expended while sitting at rest, and is defined as the rate of energy expenditure requiring an oxygen consumption of 3.5 ml per kilogram of body weight per minute.) The metabolic demands of many working activities have been published and the equivalents for the five grades of physical demands in terms of muscular strength adopted by the US Department of Labor are listed for information. Work physiology assessments in occupational medicine provide a quantitative way of matching patients to their work[20] and are commonly used in Scandinavia and the US.

Factors influencing work performance

A functional assessment may need to consider factors that influence work performance. The ability to perform physical work, and even intellectual occupations involve some physical work, depends ultimately on the ability of muscle cells to transform chemically bound energy from food into mechanical energy. This in turn depends on the intake, storage, and mobilization of nutrient (fuel), and the uptake of oxygen and its delivery by the cardiovascular system to the muscles where it is oxidized to release energy. This chain of activities and processes is influenced at every juncture by other factors, both endogenous and external or environmental.

Factors which may influence work performance, directly or indirectly, include:

- training or adaptation
- the general state of health of the individual
- gender (e.g. the maximal strength of women's leg muscles is only 65–75% of that of men)
- body size
- age (the maximal muscle strength of a 65-year-old man is, on average, 75–80% of that when he was 20 and at his peak)

Table 1.1 The typical physical demands of work

---

1. Strength

Expressed in terms of sedentary, light, medium, heavy, and very heavy

Measured by involvement of the worker with one or more of the following activities:
  (a) worker position(s):
      (i) standing: remaining on one's feet in an upright position at a workstation without moving about
      (ii) walking: moving about on foot
      (iii) sitting: remaining in the normal seated position
  (b) Worker movement of objects (including extremities used):
      (i) lifting: raising or lowering an object from one level to another
      (ii) carrying: transporting an object, usually in the hands or arms or on the shoulder
      (iii) pushing: exerting force upon an object so that it moves away (includes slapping, striking, kicking, and treadle actions)
      (iv) pulling: exerting force upon an object so that it moves nearer (includes jerking)

The 5 degrees of Physical Demands are (estimated equivalents in Mets):

S **Sedentary work (<2 Mets):** lifting 10 lbs (4.5 kg) maximum and occasionally lifting and/or carrying such articles as dockets, ledgers, and small tools. Although a sedentary job is defined as one that involves sitting, a certain amount of walking and standing is often needed as well. Jobs are sedentary if walking and standing are required only occasionally and other sedentary criteria are met

L **Light work (2–3 Mets):** lifting 20 lbs (9 kg) maximum with frequent lifting and/or carrying of objects weighing up to 10 lbs (4.5 kg). Even though the weight lifted may be only negligible, a job is in this category when it requires walking or standing to a significant degree, or sitting most of the time with some pushing and pulling of arm and/or leg controls

M **Medium work (4–5 Mets):** lifting 50 lbs (23 kg) maximum with frequent lifting and/or carrying of objects weighing up to 25 lbs (11.5 kg)

H **Heavy work (6–8 Mets):** lifting 100 lbs (45 kg) maximum with frequent lifting and/or carrying of objects weighing up to 50 lbs (23 kg)

V **Very heavy work (8 Mets)** lifting objects in excess of 100 lb (45 kg) with frequent lifting and/or carrying of objects weighing 50 lbs (23 kg) or more

2. Climbing and/or balancing
  (a) **Climbing:** ascending/descending ladders, stairs, scaffolding, ramps, poles, ropes, etc., using the feet and legs and/or hands and arms
  (b) **Balancing:** maintaining body equilibrium to prevent falling when walking, standing, crouching, or running on narrow, slippery, or erratically moving surfaces; or maintaining body equilibrium when performing gymnastic feats

3. Stooping, kneeling, crouching, and/or crawling
  (a) **Stooping:** bending the body downward and forward by bending the spine at the waist
  (b) **Kneeling:** bending the legs at the knees to come to rest on the knee or knees
  (c) **Crouching:** bending the body downward and forward by bending the legs and the spine
  (d) **Crawling:** moving about on the hands and knees or hands and feet

4. Reaching, handling, fingering, and/or feeling
  (a) **Reaching:** extending the hands and arms in any direction
  (b) **Handling:** seizing, holding, grasping, turning, or otherwise working with the hand or hands (fingering not involved)
  (c) **Fingering:** picking, pinching, or otherwise working with the fingers primarily (rather than with the whole hand or arm as in handling)
  (d) **Feeling:** perceiving such attributes of objects/materials as size, shape, temperature, texture, by means of receptors in the skin, particularly those of the fingertips

Table 1.1 The typical physical demands of work—cont'd

5. Talking and/or hearing
   (a) **Talking**: expressing or exchanging ideas by means of the spoken word
   (b) **Hearing**: perceiving the nature of sounds by the ear

6. Seeing
Obtaining impressions through the eyes of the shape, size, distance, motion, colour or other characteristics of objects. the major visual functions are defined as follows:
   (a) **acuity:**
   far—clarity of vision at 20 feet (6 m) or more
   near—clarity of vision at 20 inches (50 cm) or less
   (b) **depth perception**: three-dimensional vision: the ability to judge distance and space relationships so as to see objects where and as they actually are
   (c) **field of vision**: the area that can be seen up and down or to the right or left while the eyes are fixed on a given point
   (d) **accommodation**: adjustment of the lens of the eye to bring an object into sharp focus; especially important for doing near-point work at varying distances
   (e) **colour vision**: the ability to identify and distinguish colours

Adapted from US Department of Labor.[18]

- nutritional state—particularly important when working in cold environments
- individual differences
- attitude and motivation
- sleep deprivation and fatigue
- stress
- nature of the work, workload, work schedules, work environment (heat, cold, humidity, air velocity, altitude, hyperbaric pressure, noise, vibration, air pollution).

These factors are well summarized in *The Physiology of Work* by Rodahl.[21]

Objective tests

The result of any objective tests of function relevant to the working situation should be noted. For instance, the physical work capacity of an individual may be estimated ergometrically using standard exercise tests, step tests, or different task simulations. Cardiorespiratory function may be relevant. Muscular strength and lifting ability can be assessed objectively by using either dynamic or static strength tests.

Matching the individual with the job

A functional assessment of the individual's capacities will be of most use when as much is known about the job as about the individual assessed. Sophisticated equipment is now available to make a functional capacity assessment that will match an individual to a task. Less formally, the requirements of the task can be categorized, so that a match can be made with the individual's capacity. There are wide variations in the practice of occupational medicine in different countries. In both France and Germany job matching is used formally in some work settings, but systematic job analysis and matching is currently rarely done at the workplace in the UK. However, an activity matching ability system (AMAS), which was developed in the UK, has been used by Remploy in a sheltered work setting. A comparable instrument is the work ability index (WAI), developed in Finland. In British industry, however, a pragmatic solution emerges when personnel staff and managers, company doctors, and supervisors discuss the placement needs of their disabled employees and, as both worker abilities and task requirements are well known to them, a theoretical match is often superfluous. Outside the workplace itself, more formal assessments may be made in medical rehabilitation or occupational therapy departments (see Chapter 4).

A comprehensive review of current approaches to the analysis of both the physical demands of jobs and the physical abilities of individuals, job matching and functional capacity assessment was published by Fraser in 1992.[22] Accommodation at the workplace is also discussed, and appendices include details of physiological and biomechanical techniques for work capacity measurement, as well as some schemata and scales in current use.

It is essential that the occupational physician or nurse who is assessing medical suitability for employment has an intimate understanding of the job in question.

Presentation of the assessment

If a written report is needed it should be legible, clearly laid out, signed, and dated. The report should mention any functional limitations and outline activities that may, or may not, be undertaken. Any health or safety implications should be noted and the assessment should aim at a positive statement about the patient's abilities. Any adaptations, ergonomic alterations or 'reasonable adjustments' to the work that would be helpful or required by the DDA should be indicated. Recommendations on restriction or limitation of employment, particularly for health and/or safety reasons, should be unambiguous and precise, and should be made only if definitely indicated.

Many standard functional profiles of individual abilities have been used in North America, Scandinavia, and the UK (mainly in the armed services). These profiles, which resemble each other, are known by acronyms of the initial letters of the parts of the body assessed, e.g. PULHEEMS, GULHEMP, PULSES. In the case of the GULHEMP profile each division is graded from 1 to 7. Other profiles have combined the evaluation of physical abilities with indications of the frequency with which certain activities may be undertaken. Although such profiles are relatively objective and systematic, and allow for consistent recordings on the same individual over a period of time, they take time to complete and much of the information may not be needed. Many doctors in industry who have tried to introduce a PULHEEMS type of system have found that it does not always help when dealing with the practical, and often complex, problems affecting individual employees.

Other simpler classifications are often used in clinical settings, e.g. the New York Heart Association's Impairment of Cardiac Functions. Graded in terms of symptoms, such classifications are of less use in assessing occupational fitness than in recording clinical progress or deterioration. Other scales (e.g. the Barthel Index) used to grade degree of damage or recovery after stroke, for instance, are used to assess outcome after different rehabilitation procedures, and often form part of occupational therapy assessments.

Recommendations following assessment

Recommendations following assessment depend on the circumstance of referral and the findings.

If the patient is employed, it should be possible to make a medical judgement on whether they are:

1. capable of performing the work with out any ill effects;
2. capable of performing the work but with reduced efficiency or effectiveness;

3. capable of performing the work, although this may adversely affect their medical condition;

4. capable of performing the work but not without unacceptable risks to the health and safety of themselves, other workers, or the community; and

5. physically or mentally incapable of performing the work in question.

For the employed patient, where the judgement is 2–5, the options of 'reasonable adjustment' may include work accommodation, alternative work on a temporary or permanent basis, sheltered work; or, in the last resort, retirement on medical grounds.

If the patient is unemployed but is being given a pre-employment assessment for recruitment to a particular job, options 1–5 will still be appropriate.

However, **if a patient is not being considered for a specific job** then the recommendation following the assessment cannot relate to specific job requirements and it is particularly important that **no unnecessary medical restrictions are imposed.**

The return to work

Even if the patient is assessed as medically fit for a return to their previous job without modification, medical advice may still be needed on the timing of return to work. A clear indication by the consultant or family practitioner to the patients, or to the employer or occupational physician, on when work may be resumed should be given wherever possible. Work should be resumed as soon as the individual is physically and mentally fit enough, having regard to their own and others' health and safety. Return to work at the right time can assist recovery, whereas undue delay can aggravate the sense of uselessness and isolation that so often accompanies incapacity due to illness, disability, or injury.

The contact between the patient's doctor and their employer or occupational physician, stressed earlier in this chapter, will ensure that preparations for the patient's return to work can be put in hand. Recommendations on when work may be resumed and on the patient's functional and work capacities should be clear and specific.

Patients who have been treated for cancer may have particular difficulties in integrating on their return to work, but, with modern treatment, many cancer patients return to full and productive employment. The advice of an occupational physician will be especially valuable in helping workers with cancer to return to their jobs as well as helping their employers and work colleagues to make any necessary adjustments. Close friends and relatives may also need advice when working at the same time as caring for a cancer patient. Many, but not all, patients who have been treated for cancer will be disabled, by definition, under the DDA. Doctors, employers, patients, and their carers can obtain information and advice on all aspects of cancer and including working with cancer, from CancerBACUP, whose address and telephone numbers are included in Appendix 8. They have recently introduced a support service for occupational health departments supporting workers with cancer.

Work accommodation

The patient's condition, which may or may not come within the DDA, may be such that their previous work needs to be modified. Both the physical and organizational aspects of the job must be considered. Simple features such as bench height, type of chair or stool, or lighting may need adjustment, or more sophisticated aids or adaptations may be required. The workplace environment may need to be adapted, for example by building a ramp or widening a doorway to improve access for wheelchairs. Financial assistance may be available from the Employment Service. Further details are included in Chapter 4.

Information on equipment may be available from several voluntary organizations such as the Royal Association for Disability and Rehabilitation (RADAR), the Disabled Living Foundation (DLF) and the Disability Information Trust (DIT) (see list of addresses in Appendix 8). The DIT has published a comprehensive volume, *Employment and the Workplace*.[23]

Certain organizational features of the work may need adjustment—for instance adjustment of objectives, more flexible working hours, more frequent rest pauses, job sharing, alterations to shiftwork or arrangements to avoid rush-hour travel. A short period of unpaced work may be necessary before resuming paced work. Sometimes the way in which the patient relates to fellow workers may need attention.

Alternative work

In many occupations, work accommodation or job restructuring is not possible and some type of suitable alternative work, possibly only temporary, may have to be recommended. This is usually judged on an individual basis by the occupational physician who can keep the employee under regular review. Where there are no occupational health services, the Employment Service's Disability Employment Advisers (DEAs) can visit the workplace to advise on work accommodation or alternative work (see Chapter 4, p 82). EMAS may be able to provide some advice to individual employees.

Premature medical retirement

Medical retirement is a last resort, if further treatment is impossible or ineffective, if suitable alternative or sheltered work cannot be provided, or if the employee will not accept such initiatives. If the 'threshold of employability for a particular job' cannot be reached, either through recovery of fitness, or adjustment of work, retirement on medical grounds may have to be considered. **A management decision on premature retirement on grounds of ill-health should never be made without a supporting medical opinion that has taken the requirements of the job fully into account**. Medical retirement is discussed more fully in Chapter 27. Other aspects of premature medical retirement in relation to the law are discussed in Chapter 2.

Recent developments and trends

Governmental initiatives

When judged in terms of vocational rehabilitation we live in exciting times. Rarely before (in peace time) has there been such an emphasis on preserving and maximizing fitness for work. The Government has the target of full employment firmly in its headlights. Described in Chapter 4 are several recent flagship policy documents, including *Our Healthier Nation*, *A Framework for Vocational Rehabilitation*, *Securing Health Together*, *Pathways to Work*, and the National Service Frameworks. Details are given also of recent initiatives and programmes, such as the 'Pathways to Work' and 'Job Retention and Rehabilitation' pilots and other services ('New Deal', the National Employment and Health Innovations Network, and 'New Deal for Disabled People') that complement long-standing arrangements (the Access to Work programme, Residential training, Jobcentre Plus, the Job Introduction Scheme, etc.).

Another exciting recent innovation has been the development of NHS Plus, a network of over 100 NHS occupational health departments offering quality assured occupational health support to local non-NHS employers.

Finally, the new alignment of the Health and Safety Executive, within the Department of Work and Pensions has encouraged a more holistic approach to health problems in employment.

The important effort of controlling risks at work continues unchecked, but greater attention is being paid to rehabilitation and the common health problems that serve as barriers to job retention and job placement.

These initiatives are to be welcomed. At present between 2% and 16% of the annual UK salary bill is spent on sickness absence. The costs of making reasonable adjustments to retain an employee who develops a health condition or disability are likely to be far lower than the costs of recruiting and training anew. Moreover, work brings with it health benefits to the individual—it can be therapeutic, it is associated with lower morbidity and mortality, and it carries important social benefits and a sense of well-being and integration with society. Thus, in both financial and in human terms (as well as in terms of legal responsibilities), these efforts are important.

Maintaining fitness for work

From the viewpoint of the occupational physician, fitness for work does not end with medical assessment. An employee must remain fit, which means attention to those factors that will prevent the deterioration of health. These may include policies or advice on smoking, exercise, diet, and alcohol consumption. A recent educational leaflet from the Faculty of Occupational Medicine and the Faculty of Public Health highlighted the importance of life-style factors in creating a healthy workplace and the costs to industry:

- an estimated 34 million days a year are lost in England and Wales through sickness absence resulting from smoking-related illness
- physical inactivity through its major health consequences (e.g. obesity, coronary heart disease and cancer) is estimated to cost the wider English economy over £8 billion per year
- alcohol misuse among employees in England costs up to an estimated £6.4 billion pounds a year in lost productivity (increased absenteeism, unemployment, and premature death).

The subjects of health promotion and general prevention of ill health are not discussed in this book, while health screening is touched on only in its occupational context. However, these activities are important ones in terms of the well-being of working aged people. The prevention of vascular disease—cardiac, cerebral, and peripheral—is particularly important as these diseases take a high toll in the working population and because simple initiatives can be effective. Doctors also have a duty to discourage smoking at work and smoking should be banned absolutely, on health grounds, in places where non-smoking employees would be subject to the tobacco fumes of others. (At the time of going to press this looks likely to be enshrined in legislation from 2007.) Finally, occupational physicians should encourage employers to provide facilities for employees to take regular exercise and be prepared to advise on sensible eating and the food that is available in eating places at work. The long-term prevention of ill-health, by whatever means, is as important to the prudent employer as ensuring that a new employee is fit for work.

Conclusions

Medical fitness is relevant where illnesses or injuries reduce performance, or affect health and safety in the workplace; it may also be specifically relevant to certain onerous or hazardous tasks for which medical standards exist. Medical fitness should always be judged in relation to the work, and not simply the pension scheme. It has little relevance in a wide range of employment situations: very many medical conditions, and virtually all minor health problems, have minimal implications for work and should not debar from employment. Medical fitness for employment is not an end in itself. It must be maintained.

References

1 *International classification of impairments, disabilities and handicaps.* Geneva: World Health Organization, 1980.

2 Wood PHN. The language of disablement: a glossary relating to disease and its consequences. *Int Rehabil Med* 1980; **2**: 86–92.

3 Smith A, Twomey B. Labour market experience of people with disabilities. Analysis from the LFS of the characteristics and labour market participation of people with long-term disabilities and health problems. *Labour Market Trends* 2002; **110**(8): 415–27.

4 Mind. Information Fact sheets. How common is mental distress? http://www.mind.org.uk/Information/Factsheets/Statistics/Statistics+1.htm#How%20many%20people%20in%20Britain%20experience%20mental%20health%20problems

5 Goldberg D, Huxley P. *Common mental disorders a bio-social model.* London: Routledge, 1992.

6 Health and Safety Commission. Health and Safety Statistics 2004/5. http://www.hse.gov.uk/statistics/overall/hssh0405.pdf

7 Health insurance: the online guide to critical illness insurance. Vital statistics. http://www.healthinsuranceguide.co.uk/statistics_mainbody.asp

8 Department of Health. Hospital Episode Statistics 2001–2. http://www.doh.gov.uk/hes/free_data/index.html.

9 Blanc PD, Burney P, Janson C, Torén K. The prevalence and predictors of respiratory-related work limitation and occupational disability in an international study. *Chest* 2003; **124**: 1153–9.

10 Kraut A, Walld R, Tate R, Mustard C. Impact of diabetes on employment and income in Manitoba, Canada, *Diabetes Care* 2001; **24**: 64–8.

11 Robinson N, Yateman NA, Protopapa LE, Bush L. Employment problems and diabetes. *Diabet Med* 1990; **7**: 16–22.

12 Elwes RD, Marshall J, Beattie A, Newman PK. Epilepsy and employment. A community based survey in an area of high unemployment. *J Neurol Neurosurg Psychiatry* 1991; **54**: 200–3.

13 US Census Bureau. American Community Survey 2003. http://factfinder.census.gov/servlet/MetadataBrowserServlet?type=dataset&id=ACS_2003_EST_G00_&_lang=en

14 *Guidance on ethics for occupational physicians*, 6th edn. London: Faculty of Occupational Medicine, Royal College of Physicians, 2006.

15 Palmer KT, Harling K, Harrison J, Macdonald EB, Snashall D. Good medical practice: guidance for occupational physicians. *Occup Med* 2002; **52**: 341–52.

16 Occupational Pensions Board *Occupational pension scheme cover for disabled people.* Cmnd 6849. London: HMSO, 1977.

17 Brackenridge RDC, Elder WJ. *Medical selection of life risks*, 4th edn. London: Macmillan, 1998.

18 US Department of Labor. *Selected characteristics of occupations defined in the Dictionary of Occupational Titles.* Washington: US Government Printing Office, 1981.

19 Long C (ed.). *Prevention and rehabilitation in ischemic heart disease.* Baltimore: Williams and Wilkins, 1980.

20 Erb BD. Applying work physiology to occupational medicine. *Occup Health Safety* 1981; **50**: 20–4.

21 Rodahl K. *The physiology of work.* London: Taylor & Francis, 1989.

22 Fraser TM. *Fitness for work: the role of physical demands analysis and physical capacity assessment.* London: Taylor & Francis, 1992.

23 *Employment and the Workplace.* Oxford: Disability Information Trust, 1994.

Chapter 2

Legal aspects of fitness for work

G. S. Howard

This chapter outlines some of the ways in which the law may affect the employment of people with health problems. There are three major legal sources relevant to employment in the UK—the common law, statute law, and European Directives.

Common law

The English legal system is based on the common law. This system developed from the decisions of judges whose rulings over the centuries have created precedents for other courts to follow and these decisions were based on the 'custom and practice of the Realm'.

The system of binding precedent means that any decision of the House of Lords (the highest court in the United Kingdom) will bind all the lower courts, unless the lower courts are able to distinguish the facts of the current case and argue that the previous binding decision cannot apply, because of differences in the facts of the two cases.

However, since the UK joined the European Union (EU), the decisions of the European Court of Justice (ECJ) now supersede any decisions of the domestic courts and require the national courts to follow its decisions.[1] The Human Rights Act 1998 became law in England and Wales in 2000 (in Scotland it became law in 1998) in order to incorporate the provisions of the European Convention on Human Rights into UK law. The two most important Articles applicable to employment law are Article 8(1)—the right to respect for privacy, family life, and correspondence and Article 6 the right to a fair trial.

The common law covers both the criminal and civil law. The law of negligence has grown out of the common law and forms part of the civil law of torts (civil wrongs). For centuries, the common law courts have held employers liable for negligence if the employer had not taken reasonable care for the health and safety of their workers. However, statute law since 1971 has developed to the point where there is a comprehensive regulatory framework of employment protection guaranteeing rights and freedoms of employees and imposing statutory duties on employers. This has been referred to by legal commentators as 'a floor of statutory rights'.

Common law duties of employers

At common law, employers have an obligation to take **reasonable care** of all their employees and to guard against reasonably foreseeable risks of injury. These duties are judged in the light of the 'state of the art' of knowledge of the employer—what they either knew or ought to have known.

Standard of care of occupational physicians

The **standard of care** expected of a professional, e.g. an occupational health specialist, is set out in a case that established the so-called '*Bolam*' test.[2] This held that a doctor could not be held to be negligent where he had exercised the standard of care 'of the ordinary skilled man exercising and professing to have that special skill'. A 'doctor was not negligent if he acted in accordance with a practice accepted as proper by a responsible body of medical opinion'.

However in *Bolitho*[3] the House of Lords held that *Bolam* would be followed only where that body of medical opinion had reached 'a defensible conclusion', i.e. where such conclusion could be rationalized and justified. If the groundswell of medical opinion was outdated and clearly erroneous, the judges would not accept the opinion even if it came from a respectable medical body.

The House of Lords held that:

> if, in a rare case, it had been demonstrated that the professional opinion was incapable of withstanding logical analysis, the judge was entitled to hold that it could not provide the benchmark by reference to which the doctor's conduct fell to be assessed. In most cases the fact that distinguished experts in the field were of a particular opinion would be demonstration of the reasonableness of that opinion.

In the case of an accredited specialist in occupational medicine the standard of care expected would be higher than for a GP who works part-time in occupational medicine.

Duty to inform and warn of risks to health and safety

Employers are obliged to inform their workers, including prospective employees, of inherent risks of the job so that they can accept or decline employment having made an informed choice.[4] Any warning does not of course relieve the employer of the duty to take all reasonable care to guard against reasonably foreseeable risks of injury. What it does is to provide employees with information they would otherwise have lacked. Sometimes, and possibly most effectively, this information is imparted through the company's medical advisers.

The principle of *volenti non fit injuria*, i.e. that the individual knew about the risk, understood the exact nature of that risk, and accepted that risk may conceivably be used by an employer in defence of a negligence claim. However, it has rarely proved to be a successful defence because the risk has to be accepted freely and without duress. If the only choice was between dismissal or accepting a particular risk at the workplace, the courts would not be slow to disallow the defence of *volenti*.

In one of the several cases brought against Bernard Matthews for work-related upper limb disorders (WRULDs), it was successfully argued by Mrs Mountenay and others[5] that she had not been given sufficient warning of the inherent risk of WRULDs associated with eviscerating chickens on a paced production line.

In the first case on 'stress' to reach the House of Lords (*Barber* v. *Somerset County Council*,[6] the leading case of *Stokes* v. *Guest Keen and Nettlefold* was cited as still being good law. In the latter, the company had been found liable for the scrotal cancers that eventually killed several of its workers. It had employed a doctor who lectured in industrial medicine. This doctor had failed to warn the men of the dangers of cancer associated with the oils that contaminated their overalls, as he had not wanted 'to alarm the men'. He could, and should, have circulated a leaflet to the men warning of the dangers of scrotal warts, and should have instituted periodic medical examinations. The employer was held to be vicariously liable for this act of negligence on the doctor's part. In *Barber's* case it was acknowledged by the House of Lords that:

> because of the nature of mental disorder it is harder to foresee than physical injury, but may be easier to foresee in a known individual than in the population at large …An employer is usually entitled to assume that the employee can withstand the normal pressures of the job unless he knows of some particular problem or vulnerability.

In summary, the employer's duties include obligations to:

- take positive and practical steps to ensure the safety of their employees in the light of the knowledge that they have, or ought to have;
- follow current recognized practice, unless in the light of common sense or new knowledge this is clearly unsound;
- keep reasonably abreast of developing knowledge and not be too slow in applying it;
- take greater than average precautions where the employer has greater than average knowledge of the risk;
- weigh up the risk (in terms of likelihood of the injury and the possible consequences) against the effectiveness and the cost and inconvenience of the precautions to be taken to meet the risk.

Balancing the risk

In essence a cost/benefit analysis must be done. In deciding what is 'reasonably practicable' to do in terms of eliminating risk and in determining what is reasonably foreseeable in terms of injury, the courts have determined a test that balances the quantum of risk against the time, trouble, and expense that the employer must go to avert that risk. The greater the risk of health or safety, the greater the time, trouble, and expense the law expects the employer to devote to mitigating that risk. In a leading case involving the National Coal Board,[7] the Court of Appeal held that the employer's obligation to discharge its duty of care would only be satisfied when the time, trouble, and expense required to avert the risk was grossly disproportionate to the risk involved. In other words, if the risk and gravity of harm is small or negligible, then the employer's duty to avert such risks would be considerably smaller,

Ignorance is no defence in law. Furthermore if one member of the employer's staff knows about a risk or a health or safety problem, then (whether this is shared with the employer or not) the employer is deemed to know about it. This is called **constructive knowledge** (see Chapter 3 on the Disability Discrimination Act 1995 for further discussion on this point).

The state of the art

The courts will look at the state of knowledge at the time of the alleged act of negligence in judging whether the employer ought to have acted or not.

Employers are not expected to be prophets, nor are they expected to remain ignorant of the growing knowledge of pertinent health and safety matters. Nor are they permitted to ignore advice and information given to them by their occupational health experts merely because other employers do not know about or concern themselves with these issues.

In cases concerning noise-induced hearing loss, the courts have investigated the state of knowledge among employers in the 1950s, even though the Ministry of Labour pamphlet *Noise and the worker* was not published until 1963. In *Baxter v. Harland and Wolff plc*,[8] the employer was held liable for noise-induced deafness as far back as 1953 because the employer failed to 'seek out knowledge of facts which are not in themselves obvious'.

Harland and Wolff had not sought or heeded medical, scientific, and legal advice between 1953 and 1963, despite there being evidence of several incidents of noise-induce deafness problems in the naval shipyards in Devon before the Second World War and medical reports and papers on this in the early 1950s. Evidence was produced that an advertisement in the *Lancet* on 28 April 1951 had featured a protective earplug.

The employer was held to be negligent because of its 'lack of interest and apathy... The defendants, knowing that noise was causing deafness among their workmen, should have applied their minds to removing the risk... (and) ...sought advice'.

Greater duty of care: 'eggshell skull' principle

The employer owes a higher duty of care to any particularly vulnerable employee with a known, pre-existing medical condition. Those with an 'eggshell skull physique' are more vulnerable to serious injury than others of robust physical health. Those with a fragile personality may suffer far greater psychological damage than those with a robust personality. This is defined as the 'eggshell skull' principle, a classic example of which can be seen in the case of *Paris* v. *Stepney Council*.[9] Here the Council employed a labourer with only one eye. They failed to ensure that he was wearing eye goggles and as a result he suffered an injury to his other eye at work and was blinded. The courts held that his employers owed him a much higher duty of care as he was an individual with extra risk of serious injury.

It is therefore important for employers to take informed advice from qualified occupational health professionals on fitness and placement decisions and the need for special arrangements or precautions. Failure to consider whether pre-employment medical checks are required and, if they are indicated, to arrange for them to be done by properly qualified and trained occupational health staff, may lead to a successful claim for negligence against the employer.

Duty owed in mental illness

In several cases the courts have extended the principle of the employer's common law duty to psychiatric injury. In a case that went to the House of Lords[10] the negligent party was held liable for the onset of chronic fatigue syndrome precipitated by a car accident.

Although not the first case to establish an employer's duty of care to look after the mental well-being of employees, *Walker* v. *Northumberland County Council*[11] was the first successful claim for damages for not safeguarding the mental health of the employee once he had suffered his first nervous breakdown. The High Court held that it was reasonably foreseeable that in returning to his former post without adequate help and resources, Mr Walker would again become mentally ill—especially in the light of the medical experts' opinions that the nature and the volume of his work was the major contributory factor for his first nervous breakdown. In *Barber's* case in the Court of Appeal[12] Lady Justice Hale laid down 15 useful propositions about an employer's duty of care in safeguarding its employees' mental health:

- There are no unique considerations applying to cases of psychiatric (or physical) illness or injury arising from the stress of doing the work the employee is required to do. The ordinary principles of employer's liability apply.
- The threshold question is whether this kind of harm to this particular employee was **reasonably foreseeable**. This has two components:
  - an injury to health (as distinct from occupational stress), which
  - is attributable to stress at work (as distinct from other factors)
- **Foreseeability** depends upon what the employer knows (or ought reasonably to know) about the individual employee. Because of the nature of mental disorder, it is harder to foresee than physical injury, but may be easier to foresee in a known individual than in the population at large. An employer is usually entitled to assume that the employee can withstand the normal pressures of the job unless he knows of some particular problem or vulnerability (staff who feel under stress at work should tell their employer and provide a chance to do something about it).

- The test is the same whatever the employment: there are no occupations that should be regarded as intrinsically dangerous to mental health.
- Factors likely to be relevant in answering the threshold question include:
  - *The nature and extent of the work done by the employee*
    - Is the workload much more than is normal for the particular job?
    - Is the work particularly intellectually or emotionally demanding for this employee?
    - Are the demands being made of this employee unreasonable when compared with the demands made of others in the same or comparable jobs?
    - Are there signs that others doing this job are suffering harmful levels of stress?
    - Is there an abnormal level of sickness or absenteeism in the same job or the same department?
  - *Signs from the employee of impending harm to health*
    - Has he a particular problem or vulnerability?
    - Has he already suffered from illness attributable to stress at work?
    - Have there recently been frequent or prolonged absences that are uncharacteristic of him?
    - Is there reason to think that these are attributable to stress at work, for example because of complaints or warnings from him or others?
- The employer is generally entitled to take what he is told by his employee at face value, unless he has good reason to think to the contrary. He does not generally have to make searching enquiries of the employee or seek permission to make further enquiries of his medical advisers.
- To trigger a duty to take steps, the indications of impending harm to health arising from stress at work must be plain enough for any reasonable employer to realize that he should do something about it.
- The employer is only in breach of his duty of care if he fails to take the steps that are reasonable in the circumstances, bearing in mind the magnitude of the risk of harm occurring, the gravity of the harm that may occur, the costs and practicability of preventing it, and the justifications for running the risk.
- The size and scope of the employer's operation, its resources, and the demands it faces are relevant in deciding what is reasonable; these include the interests of other employees and the need to treat them fairly, for example, in any redistribution of duties.
- An employer can only reasonably be expected to take steps that are likely to do some good; the court is likely to need expert evidence on this.
- An employer who offers a confidential advice service, with referral to appropriate counselling or treatment services, is unlikely to be found in breach of duty.
- If the only reasonable and effective step would have been to dismiss or demote the employee, the employer will not be in breach of duty in allowing a willing employee to continue in the job.
- In all cases, therefore, it is necessary to identify the steps that the employer both could and should have taken before finding him in breach of his duty of care.
- The claimant must show that that breach of duty has caused or materially contributed to the harm suffered. It is not enough to show that occupational stress has caused the harm.
- Where the harm suffered has more than one cause, the employer should only pay for that proportion of the harm suffered that is attributable to his wrongdoing, unless the harm is truly indivisible.

◆ The assessment of damages will take account of any pre-existing disorder or vulnerability and of the chance that the claimant would have succumbed to a stress-related disorder in any event.

In a more recent case—*Hartman* v. *South Essex Mental Health and Community Care NHS Trust* (and five other conjoined appeals)[13] the Court of Appeal took extensive guidance laid down by that Court in the *Barber* case but it noted that the House of Lords had held that it was guidance only and that each case must be determined on its own facts.

The overall test remains the conduct of the reasonable and prudent employer taking positive thought for his workers' safety in light of what he ought to know.

In *Hartman's* case, liability for her stress-related illness was not made out even though the occupational physician was aware of her heightened susceptibility to stress, as this information remained confidential. The critical issue in this case was whether the Trust should have appreciated that Mrs Hartman was at risk of succumbing to psychiatric illness. The Court of Appeal held that the case was not reasonably foreseeable.

Employees' duties

In common law, employees have implied duties, including the duty to work with reasonable care and competence and to serve their employer loyally and faithfully. They are also under a duty to be reasonably competent, to co-operate with their employer, and to obey reasonable lawful instructions. So for example, an unreasonable refusal to submit to a medical examination by a doctor of the employer's choice and to consent to the disclosure of a medical report could constitute a breach of the duty to co-operate or to obey a reasonable instruction.[14]

Statute law

Health and Safety at Work Act 1974

The Health and Safety at Work Act 1974 (HSAWA) is superimposed on earlier Acts and the duties imposed by some of these (e.g. the Mines and Quarries Act 1954, the Factories Act 1961, and the Offices, Shops and Railway Premises Act 1963) must still be met, although most of their enforcement provisions have been replaced in the new legislation.

The Health and Safety Commission (HSC) was set up by the Act and is responsible for policy; the Health and Safety Executive (HSE), together with local authority environmental health officers, are responsible for enforcing the Act's requirements.

HSAWA imposes criminal liability, and the company, individual managers, and employees can be prosecuted for breaches of their statutory duties. Lesser criminal cases brought under the HSAWA can be heard in the Magistrates Courts, which have the power to impose fines or commit a person to prison for up to 6 months. With the passage of the Offshore Safety Act 1992 the fines were increased to a maximum of £5000 for breaches of Sections 2–6 of the HSAWA and £20 000 for breaches of improvement or prohibition notices. If the HSE considers the breaches to be sufficiently serious, then the matter can be tried in the Crown Court, which has the power to impose an unlimited fine or a term of imprisonment.

There is provision in Section 47 of HSAWA to extend the jurisdiction of the Act to permit employees injured at work to sue for their injuries in the civil courts under the Act, but this Section has not been implemented to date. Employees who are injured at work as a result of a breach of any other statutory duties can sue in the civil courts, as the other statutory enactments impose both civil and criminal liability.

The Act covers everyone at work, including independent contractors and their employees, the self-employed, and visitors, but excludes domestic servants in private households.

Employers' statutory duties

HSAWA imposes general duties on employers under Section 2 to ensure, so far as is reasonably practicable, the health, safety and welfare at work of their employees. This specifically includes ensuring that:

+ there is a safe system of work;
+ there is a safe place of work;
+ staff are given information, instruction, and training on matters of health and safety, and are adequately supervised;
+ there is a safe system for the handling, storage, and transport of substances and materials;
+ there is a safe working environment.

Although there is no specific mention of a duty to conduct pre-employment medical examinations, part of a safe system of work could be interpreted as ensuring that the staff who have been recruited are fit to perform their duties where there is any question of medical fitness impinging on the work requirements. Adequate medical data on new members of staff is essential. However, due care must be taken to observe the employer's duties under the Disability Discrimination Act 1995 (DDA) (see Chapter 3).

Employees' statutory duties

Employees have duties under Sections 7 and 8 of the Act to 'take reasonable care' of their own health and safety, and the safety of others; to co-operate on any matter of health and safety; and to do nothing which could endanger their health and safety or that of others.

This duty could be taken to include the disclosure of a relevant medical condition when questioned. For example, an employee who failed to disclose that they had epilepsy, when working in a job where this could pose a hazard, might be in breach of their duty under Section 7 of the Act. Failing to disclose material health information on request may also constitute grounds for lawful dismissal (see 'Unfair Dismissal' below).

The institutions

The HSC was set up under the HSAWA as a tripartite body—Government, Confederation of British Industry (CBI), and Trades Union Congress (TUC)—and is responsible for national health and safety policy. The HSE is responsible for enforcing health and safety legislation, including the HSAWA. There are several divisions, the largest of which is Her Majesty's Factory Inspectorate (HMFI). The Employment Medical Advisory Service (EMAS) is the field force of the medical division of HSE, and will be described in Chapter 4.

Enforcement of the Act in offices, shops, railway premises, and warehouses is carried out by environmental health officers, who are employed by the local authorities. Their powers are the same as those of factory inspectors.

Employment protection legislation

Employees have been given statutory protection from being unfairly dismissed; the relevant provisions can be found in the Employment Rights Act 1996. Several aspects of these measures are important for those who develop illnesses or injuries while at work.[15]

Employees have been given protection from unfair dismissal provided that they satisfy certain qualifying conditions, such as 2 years' continuous service, being under the normal retirement age, ordinarily employed in Great Britain, etc.

Claims for unfair dismissal are heard by employment tribunals. The employment tribunals are chaired by a legally qualified solicitor or barrister of at least 15 years' standing and a panel of two lay members (one appointed by employers' organizations such as the CBI and one appointed by the TUC or other trades union bodies). The lay members advise the chairman as to good industrial practice. The chairman directs the lay members as to points of law.

Appeals on points of law or a perverse decision lie with the Employment Appeal tribunal (EAT), then with the Court of Appeal and the House of Lords on points of law only and where leave has been given. Cases are only granted leave by petition to appeal to the House of Lords on matters of public importance.

In cases involving questions of European Community law, cases may be referred directly from employment tribunals to the European Court of Justice (ECJ). Many of these referrals concern questions arising from the UK's anti-discrimination legislation, which, it is alleged, fails properly to implement the EU Directives.[16]

Grounds for dismissal

Section 98 of the Employment Rights Act 1996 sets our five potentially fair grounds for dismissal. They are conduct, capability, redundancy, illegality, and 'some other substantial reason'. The Employment Act 2002 and the Employment Act 2002 (Dispute Resolution) Regulations 2004 have radically changed the procedures that the employer must follow before dismissing an employee. The employer must use a standard dismissal procedure (in cases of capability the modified procedure would almost certainly never be applicable). When the employer considers the dismissal stage, there is a three-stage procedure:

1. the employer must write to the employee, giving the basis for which the employer considers that dismissal is appropriate together with all the evidence upon which the employer is considering dismissal;

2. there must be a meeting at which the employee and a union representative or work colleague can be present; and

3. following any decision to dismiss, the employee must be told about and given the right of an appeal on one of three grounds—unfair or prejudiced or biased hearing; new evidence that was not available at the original hearing; too harsh a decision.

'Capability': ill health cases

In order for an employer to justify the fairness of a dismissal on the grounds of ill health 'in all the circumstances of the case,[17] they must advance factual evidence of the 'ill health' preventing the individual from performing the jobs that they are employed to do, in order to justify the dismissal. In other words, the employer must obtain an up-to-date medical report from the clinician in charge of the employee's treatment. Tribunals also have to be satisfied that the employer acted reasonably in all the circumstances of the case, treating that reason as sufficient for dismissal, taking into account the size and administrative resources of the undertaking. In other words, large employers with Human Resources experts and extensive resources are expected to adopt all the good practices of a model employer, in contrast to a small employer who may be forgiven a failure to follow as thorough a dismissal procedure.

The tribunals have given guidance as to what constitutes reasonable conduct on the part of the employer in this regard (see below).

The mere fact that the individual is not prevented from performing all the duties that they are required to perform under their contract, does not affect a decision to dismiss for ill health, as long as the individual is unfit to perform some of the duties. This was stated in the case of *Shook v. London Borough of Ealing.*[18] Miss Shook was employed as a trainee residential care assistant, who strained her back and was off work for some 9 months. She was declared unfit to carry out her duties as a residential social worker because of the bending and lifting that was involved in her job and this was confirmed by both her general practitioner (GP) and the Council's medical officer. She was eventually dismissed after having been offered alternative posts, which she had rejected. She argued that her employers did not have any fair reason to dismiss her because she was not disabled from all her contractual duties as her contract actually contained a very wide flexibility and mobility clause and she worked in numerous posts within the Social Services Department of the Council.

The Court of Appeal ruled that the dismissal was fair and rejected this argument:

> ... The Tribunal were entitled to reject the submission that an employee is not incapacitated from performing ... the work which they are employed to do unless he is incapacitated from performing every task which the employers are entitled by law to call on him to discharge ...
> ... However widely that contract was construed, her disabilities related to her performance of her duties thereunder, even though her performance of all of them may not have been affected.

In other words, a dismissal on grounds of ill health can still be fair even where an employee is not incapacitated from undertaking all their duties, if they cannot undertake an important and primary duty (such as in this case lifting residents).

Lying about previous health conditions

Lying, as opposed to failing to volunteer information about material health problems, has been accepted as being a potentially fair reason for dismissal under the Employment Rights Act 1996,[19] being regarded as 'some other substantial reason for dismissal'.

The tribunals have distinguished between lying on a pre-employment medical questionnaire and failing to volunteer the information.[20] There is a subtle but important distinction. In some cases it has been held that there is no duty on employees to offer voluntarily medical information about themselves.

In Walton's case, the EAT held that:

> Although there was no need for the purposes of this appeal to decide whether the appellant should have disclosed his addiction when applying for employment, it could not be said that there is any duty on the employee in the ordinary case, though there may be exceptions, to volunteer information about himself otherwise than in response to a direct question.

It follows that prospective employees need to be asked direct questions in any pre-employment questionnaire, which should be designed on the advice of an occupational physician.

Failure to give an honest answer to a question of material importance can lead to a fair dismissal even if discovered after 1 year's service (the interval after which employees have a right to sue for unfair dismissal).

In *O'Brien v. The Prudential Assurance Co Ltd*[21] the EAT held that:

> In the present case, where the reason for dismissal was not merely the appellant's medical history (schizophrenia), but that medical history coupled with the fact that the appellant had deliberately misled the respondents about it in order to obtain employment, that could be put as a composite reason under the head of 'some other substantial reason of a kind such as would justify the dismissal'.

(NB: Since the introduction of the Disability Discrimination Act 1995, such a dismissal would almost certainly be an act of unlawful discrimination.)

Medical evidence and medical reports

In assessing fitness for work most employers rely initially on self-certificates for the first 7 days of absence and medical statements (MED 3) from the employee's GP, thereafter.

The Inland Revenue Guide to Employers when paying Statutory Sick Pay[22] suggests that employers may ask for any reasonable medical evidence of incapacity for work and this would include evidence from chiropractors, osteopaths, acupuncturists, etc.

If a MED 3 is provided, the Guide suggests that a MED 3 is

> strong evidence of incapacity and should usually be accepted as conclusive unless there is evidence to the contrary. Where there is evidence to the contrary, the Employment Tribunals have held that the employer is entitled to 'look behind' the medical 'certificate'[23] as the employer did in the case of Hutchinson v. Enfield Rolling Mills Ltd. Here Mr Hutchinson was signed off for a week with sciatica but was seen marching on a trade union demonstration in Brighton. His employers took the view that his presence in Brighton 'was not consistent with a person who was reputedly suffering from sciatica. In other words, if you were fit enough to travel to Brighton to take part in a demonstration, you were fit enough to report for work'.

The EAT agreed with the employer.

However, contrast Hutchinson's case with that of *Scottish Courage Ltd* v. *Guthrie*[24] (unreported) where a warning shot was fired across the bows of employers when they decided whether or not to pay sick pay in the face of an unchallenged MED 3. Mr Guthrie's GP had given him a MED 3 but the employer's medical advisers said that he was fit to return to work. Neither medical adviser had suggested that Mr Guthrie's sickness was other than genuine. The employer's sickness absence policy provided that: 'Employees who are absent from work as a result of genuine illness and who fulfill all the requirements of the scheme rules will be eligible for [sick pay]' and 'Payment for sickness absence is conditional upon all appropriate procedures being followed and on management being satisfied that the sickness absence is genuine'. Mr Guthrie had followed the relevant procedures and in the past the company had always paid sick pay where employees produced medical certificates from their GPs. The Company also agreed that Mr Guthrie did not have a bad sickness record. Mr Guthrie claimed that an unlawful deduction had been made from his wages. The EAT said that the tribunal was entitled to test whether the employer reached its decision in good faith. The decision to withhold sick pay was perverse, in that no reasonable employer could have reached it on the evidence gathered. Mr Guthrie was certified sick by his GP and, although the company's doctors differed as to when he could return to work, they had agreed that his illness was genuine. This case emphasizes the need for careful drafting of sick pay policies.

The advice from the Inland Revenue may appear to be at odds with the candid comment from one Oxfordshire GP who said: 'I fail to see any point in GPs signing sickness certificates. My professional relationship with my patient means that I am by no means unbiased. I invariably sign whatever the patient requests or I believe they would like.'[25] For an excellent definition of 'malingerer' see *Jeffries* v. *The Home Office*[26] in which the High Court held that: 'A malingerer is one who deliberately and consciously adopts the sick role, if necessary deceiving his medical advisers to persuade them that his complaints are true.'

Status of medical statements

If employers choose to rely upon medical statements (MED 3s), then they are entitled to do so, although they are provided for 'SSP purposes only' and they advise the patient to refrain from work (they do not direct any advice to the employer).

The NHS[27] from 2003 has attempted to try other methods of obtaining medical evidence for absence from work. One proposal was to allow Occupational Health Physicians to see the employee and to issue MED 3 statements. The Department for Work and Pensions[28] has published very useful advice to GPs regarding their patients' fitness for work: 'In summary, you should always bear in mind that a patient may not be well served in the longer term by medical advice to refrain from work, if more appropriate clinical management would allow them to stay in work or return to work'.

Not all duties are suspended when an employee is off sick

The definition of 'incapacity' for SSP purposes is inability to carry out *any* duties that it is reasonable to expect the employee to do under their contract. The definition requires consideration of the full range of the duties that it would be reasonable to expect the worker to carry out. So where for example an employee still has his ankle in plaster some 6 weeks after an operation, at a time when his consultant advises that he can place weight on that ankle and can walk with crutches or sticks, that employee could carry out sedentary tasks perhaps with adjustments to his working hours so that he can travel out of the rush hour. Clearly, if the GP continues to sign the employee off sick in such circumstances, careful and persuasive discussions need to take place between the occupational health physician and GP in order to try to resolve any concerns that the GP may have about his patient returning to work with his ankle still in plaster. In *Marshall* v. *Alexander Sloan Ltd*[29] the Employment Appeal Tribunal held that:

> The argument that all the appellant's obligations under the contract were suspended because she was off work ill so that her employers had no contractual authority to issue the order could not be accepted. Though a term has to be implied into a contract limiting the employee's obligation to perform all the terms of his contract when he is sick, such a term should be no wider than is necessary to give the contract business effect. Business commonsense requires only that when an employee is off sick, he is relieved of the obligation to perform such services as the sickness from which he is suffering prevents him from carrying out, not that all the employee's obligations are suspended.

In the present case, the Industrial Tribunal had found as a fact that the appellant could have complied with her employers' order and removed the stock from the car herself or got someone else to do so for her. Her sickness was not of a kind that prevented her from carrying out her obligation not to leave merchandise in the car. Therefore, she could be lawfully ordered to remove it.

Need for an up-to-date medical report

Employment tribunals have made it clear that employers should not rely on medical certificates alone. In *Crampton* v. *Decorum Motors Ltd* (unreported), the managing director received a MED 3 diagnosing Mr Crampton with 'angina pectoris'. Believing that this was a serious heart condition, the MD dismissed Mr Crampton on the basis of the MED 3 alone. This was held to be an unfair dismissal because a reasonable employer would have made further enquiries as to the seriousness of the condition, before taking such a drastic decision. In ill health cases (either long-term or acute) a full medical report should be sought by the employer from the occupational health physician or nurse who should have obtained an up to date medical report from the treating physician or surgeon. The employer is required to inform the doctor and the employee of the purpose for which the medical report is sought.[30] Typically, the employer will state that the report is required in order to plan for the work in the department, administer the sick pay scheme(s), and consider reasonable adjustments and alternative duties. A report could also be required for consideration for ill health retirement or permanent health insurance.

Doctors should always ensure that every employee who attends for an assessment clearly understands its purpose and the intended use of the report. In case of doubt, the occupational physician should explain the situation to the patient prior to any examination. If necessary, the doctor should write to the originator of the request seeking clarification.

When employers without any occupational health staff seek advice from an independent occupational physician, they should advise the doctor as to the purpose of their enquiry, the basic job functions of the individual, and length of the absence to date. The employer should obtain prior, written informed consent to do this from the employee. In most cases the report will be limited to non-clinical details and a functional assessment. If a medical report is being sought from the employee's GP or own specialist, then the employer is required under the Access to Medical Reports Act 1988 to inform the employee of their rights under that Act (which include the right to see the report before it is sent to the employer and the right to refuse to allow the report to be sent to the employer). In cases where a non-medically qualified person receives a medical report, they may not be able to understand it. Good practice dictates that they return it to the specialist seeking 'clarification and amplification'—*WM Computer Services* v. *Passmore* (unreported).

Data Protection Act 1998

Under Section 2 of the Data Protection Act 1998 (DPA), 'health data' is designated as 'sensitive data' for which 'explicit consent' is required before an employer can process such data. 'Processing' means obtaining, in-putting, storing, using, disclosing, amending, deleting, erasing, etc. Part 4 of the Code of Practice published by the Information Commissioner[31] provides essential information on how employers must treat health data and the rights of data subjects to give or withhold their explicit consent for such data to be processed. If explicit consent is obtained, employers (as opposed to occupational physicians or other treating doctors) may ask the specialist or GP a range of questions. If it is the case that the occupational physician seeks the medical report, then the employer is entitled to the answers to the following questions that disclose no clinical or confidential information. Answers should be limited to the list taken from the British Medical Association's model letter (Box 2.1).

Under Section 7 of the Act data subjects (i.e. job applicants, employees, and ex-employees and other third parties) have a right of access to such personal data whether in electronic or paper form subject to the restrictions and limitations placed on their rights in the Court of Appeal's judgment in *Durant* v. *Financial Services Authority (FSA)*.[32]

In brief, Mr Durant had been involved in litigation with Barclays Bank plc, which he lost. He then sought disclosure of documents (under Section 7 of the DPA providing for data subject access requests) held by the FSA and related to the complaint against him. The FSA refused to

---

Box 2.1 British Medical Association's model letter

1. When is the likely date of return to work?
2. Will there be any residual disability on return to work?
3. If so, will it be permanent or temporary?
4. Will the employee be able to render regular and efficient service?
5. If the answer is 'Yes' to question 2, what duties would you recommend that your patient does not do and for how long?
6. Will your patient require continued treatment or medication on return to work?

provide some of the documents on the grounds that they did not constitute personal data and/or were not part of a relevant filing system. Mr Durant brought a court action to seek disclosure of those documents. Following a decision at first instance that did not address fully the issues at hand, leave to appeal was granted. The appeal examined four issues:

+ the meaning of 'personal data';
+ the meaning of 'relevant filing system';
+ withholding personal data from a data subject on the grounds that third party personal data is present; and
+ the nature and extent of a court's discretion in deciding on subject access rights disputes.

The court concluded that **'personal data'** does not necessarily mean any and every document (and information contained in that document) that has the data subject's name on it. This is considered too wide an interpretation of the words 'related to' used in the definition of personal data in the Act. It was decided that the over-riding test is whether the information (not the document) in question affects a person's privacy, whether in his personal or family life, business or professional capacity. Whether or not information can be classed as 'personal data' will depend on where the information falls in the continuum of relevance or proximity to the data subject as distinct from matters in which he may have been involved to a greater or lesser degree. There are two 'notions' (as identified by the court) to help in this task:

+ is the information in itself significantly biographical?, and
+ does it have the data subject as its focus, as opposed to just being a 'bystander'?

In respect of the meaning of a **'relevant filing system'** the court has supported the view that has been widely held for some time now: information contained in manual papers should be contained in a structure that allows specific information (for example, health or performance history) about an individual to be readily accessible and identifiable from the outset of the search with 'reasonable certainty and speed'. A paper file on a named individual in which papers simply appear in date order, rather than by subject, is not a relevant filing system. The court stated that: 'It is plain … that Parliament intended to apply the Act to manual records only if they are of sufficient sophistication to provide the same or similar ready accessibility as a computerised filing system.'

When looking at withholding personal data from a data subject on the grounds that third party personal data is present the court concluded that it is acceptable to blank out references to third parties where they have not given consent for their identity to be disclosed. But if the reference to the third party is a part of the personal data there is a tension between the duty of confidentiality to the third party and the duty to comply with the rights of the Data Subject. In those situations the court must use its discretion based on the individual circumstances of the case.

The Information Commissioner has stated that he welcomes and supports the judgment of the court. His office has issued guidance to address the issues raised by this case, which is available on the Information Commissioner's website.[33]

Access to Medical Reports Act 1988

Under the Access to Medical Reports Act 1988 ('AMRA'),[34] employees are entitled to see any medical report that relates to them, if it has been prepared by a medical practitioner who is or has been responsible for their clinical care. It is clear that once an occupational physician (or a member of their staff) has treated an employee the Act will apply to all subsequent medical reports,[35] but it is less clear whether this may apply to other clinical reports such as a statement concerning fitness to work or placement assessments.

The Court has the power to order an individual to give their consent to the disclosure of clinical records and reports including any correspondence between the occupational physician, the consultant, and the management of the company.[36] However, the Courts and Employment Tribunals do not have the power to order disclosure of medical records without first obtaining the consent of the claimant, as this would breach both AMRA and the Data Protection Act 1998.[37]

Conflicting medical advice

In some cases employers receive conflicting medical opinions—the employee's own specialist or GP stating the individual is unfit to return to work and the occupational health practitioner confirming that the individual is fit to return to work. In such a dilemma, the tribunals have in the main accepted that a reasonable employer would reply upon the view of its occupational physician[38] unless:

- the occupational physician has not personally examined the individual but has merely written a report on the basis of the medical notes
- the occupational physician's report is 'woolly' and indeterminate
- the continued employment of the individual would pose a serious threat to the health or safety of the individual or to others
- the individual has been treated or is being treated by a specialist and the occupational physician has not received a report from that specialist
- the occupational physician recommends a 'third' opinion
- the employee asks the employer to allow him to present another specialist opinion.

The tribunals have accepted that an unreasonable refusal by an individual to return to work following the advice of the occupational physician constitutes misconduct on the part of the employee. The reason for dismissal is 'conduct'—refusing to obey a lawful and reasonable instruction. The Employment Tribunals have not been tolerant of employers who take decisions about the continued employment of the employee in haste, before the medical report is received.[39]

Consultation with the employee

The tribunals have ruled that in ill-health dismissal, the employer should normally contact the employee, either by telephone or personally, ideally by visiting them at home by appointment. The purpose of this contact is to consult the employee about the incapacity, to discuss any possible return date, the continuation or otherwise of company benefits and State benefits, the employment of a temporary or permanent replacement, and the future employment or termination of employment. Consultation in this case takes the place of warnings that employees are entitled to receive in poor performance or misconduct cases. This was stated in a number of leading cases.[40] Only in exceptional cases would an employer succeed in establishing that he had acted reasonably if he had failed to consult the employee in advance of making any decision.[41]

Seeking suitable alternative employment

The tribunals expect an employer to consider all alternatives other than dismissal, and this includes looking for suitable alternative employment within the organization or with any associated employers. The duty also includes considering whether any modification to the original job would be possible. (See Chapter 3 on the Disability Discrimination Act 1995 where, if the illness or injury, would be deemed to be a disability under the Act, there is a statutory duty to make reasonable adjustments to the workplace.) Failure by the employer to seek alternative employment will normally render any dismissal for ill health unfair. This proposition has received judicial approval in the House of Lords in *Archibald* v. *Fife Council*, albeit in a case involving the Disability Discrimination Act 1995 (see Chapter 3 for further details).

Permanent health insurance benefits

Practitioners who advise employers offering long-term disability (LTD) or permanent health insurance (PHI) schemes as part of their contractual benefits ought to be aware that a failure to consider offering such benefits in an appropriate case could well be challenged in the common law courts as a breach of the contract of employment, i.e. breach of the implied obligations of good faith.

The House of Lords ruled in the case of *Scally* v. *Southern Health and Social Services Board*[42] that there was a positive duty on employers rather than their medical advisors to inform their staff of those benefits for which the employee must make an application. In *Scally's case*, the employer was held to have been under an implied duty to explain to Dr Scally the details of the option offered to make additional voluntary contributions to the pension. The same principle could apply to the claiming of sick pay or PHI or LTD, maternity rights, etc. However, this implied duty on the employer does not extend to explaining to a sick employee the financial implications of resigning and taking long-term disability insurance scheme.[43] In the context of PHI and LTD schemes the duty may extend only to informing any employee in the relevant circumstances that they may be eligible for participation in such schemes. Consideration of eligibility for an LTD scheme or PHI scheme may also be viewed by the tribunals as an important factor in any unfair dismissal case as the tribunals could decide that there was an alternative to dismissal that was not properly considered by the employer—thus rendering the dismissal unfair. Company medical advisors should make themselves aware whether such benefits are offered so that they can advise effectively and appropriately. If such a scheme exists, the doctor (whether GP or occupational physician) ought to enquire of the employer whether the employee has been considered for such a scheme.

Early retirement on medical grounds

In some cases where the employee is permanently incapacitated from any further full-time, permanent employment with the employer, the individual may be dismissed and given an early retirement pension. The courts have also indicated that the employer must act in good faith in deciding such cases.[44]

It is essential for medical practitioners to read the exact wording of any pension scheme in this regard, particularly if a medical examination is to be performed in order to assess eligibility. It would be wise for medical practitioners to require a copy of the sick pay scheme, PHI scheme, and pension fund rules as they apply to early retirement pensions.

Management's role in sickness decisions

The tribunals have emphasized that the option to dismiss an employee off sick and unable to work is a management decision and not a medical one.[45] Doctors should therefore not allow themselves to be pressured into making such decisions for management. The doctor's role is to provide and interpret the medical information in order for management to be fully informed in order to make proper decisions about the employee's position.

Pre-employment medical assessments

Pre-placement medical questionnaires should ask suitable and relevant questions and gather only information which is pertinent.

Duty of care in writing pre-employment reports

A recent case in the Court of Appeal[46] has clarified to whom the occupational physician owes a duty of care when writing a report on the fitness for work of the job applicant. In *Kapfunde's* case, the Court made it clear that the person commissioning the report (i.e. the potential employer) was the only person to whom the occupational physician owed a duty of care when writing the report on the potential employee's fitness for work.

This was because there is no special relationship between a job applicant and the examining occupational physician. The disappointed job applicant will never see the pre-employment medical report nor would they rely on it for any purpose. Therefore the only person who could properly sue, if the report was negligent, is the employer as it would be they who had commissioned it and they who would rely on it.

Although the Kapfunde ruling has now clarified the occupational physician's duty vis à vis writing their pre-employment medical report, the doctor still owes to the patient the normal, standard of care and expertise in clinical matters. This includes ensuring that the actual examination and any tests carried out are conducted to the highest professional standards and that any abnormalities detected are notified to the patient and/or his GP with the subject's informed consent.

Duty to be honest

In a case brought before the ECJ, *X* v. *Commission of the European Communities*[47] it was ruled that prospective job candidates have the right to be informed of the exact nature of the tests to be carried out and to refuse to participate if they so wish.

In this case Mr X complained to the Court that he had been screened for HIV antibodies without his consent. The ECJ held that the manner in which the appellant had been medically examined and declared physically unfit constituted an infringement of his right to respect for his private life as guaranteed by Article 8 of the European Convention on Human Rights. The right to respect for private life requires that a person's refusal to undergo a test be respected in its entirety, but, equally, the employer cannot be obliged to take the risk of recruitment.

Confidentiality

Ethical questions including the duty of confidentiality are covered in detail in Chapter 5. Apart from the Article 8(1) right to respect for private life, doctors and nurses are under very strict ethical codes of conduct[48] and can be struck off the medical register for serious breaches.

Employers are not entitled to require their staff to undergo medical examinations without obtaining, **on each occasion,** the informed written consent of the individual. This means ensuring that the employee understands the nature of the examination and tests and the reasons for them. Medical staff should ensure that written consent forms are completed. Employers must also, **on each occasion**, obtain the employee's written, informed consent to disclosure of the results or a more detailed medical report to a named individual in the company.

In the absence of written consent no medical examination or disclosure should take place.

Expert evidence

Inevitably many occupational physicians will be asked at some time to give expert evidence in Employment Tribunals in ill-health dismissals or disability discrimination cases or in the High Court in personal injury claims. Expert witnesses give evidence of opinion as opposed to evidence of fact. Expert witnesses are governed by detailed rules and a Practice Direction in the Civil Procedure Rules (CPR).[49]

Pregnancy, discrimination, and the law

Any form of discrimination on the grounds of a woman's pregnancy is unlawful, constituting direct discrimination.[50] All aspects of pregnancy, pregnancy-related illness, and maternity are covered, including the notification of intention to take maternity leave, the taking of maternity leave, and intention to return to work following maternity leave. Under the Sex Discrimination Act 1975 and Management of Health and Safety at Work Regulations 1999[51] there is no ceiling on compensation for such discriminatory acts.

Furthermore, pregnant women and breast-feeding mothers are given statutory protection at work as employers are under a duty to carry out risk assessments and to have adequate control measures where possible. Failing adequate control measures, the woman has a right to be transferred to another, safer job or if this is not possible, she has a right to be suspended on normal pay.[52,53]

European law

Directives which are adopted by the Council of Ministers are binding on Member States and any emanations of the State, including former state bodies, such as nationalized industries, public utilities, and state schools are bound by the Directives.

Their employees may sue for breach of an article of the Directive directly in the UK tribunals. Employers in the private sector are not directly bound by a Directive, but Member States are required to adopt the Directive into their national legislation within a defined time-scale.

The Council of Ministers is represented by the appropriate minister from each Member State. Each Member State has a block vote, the number of votes depending on the size of its population. There are currently 25 Member States. Except on matters of health and safety and product safety, voting must be unanimous for a Directive to be adopted. The most important Treaty is the Treaty of Maastricht replacing the Treaty of Rome.

The Council of Ministers can also make recommendations.[54] Recommendations are generally adopted by the institutions of the Community when they do not have the power to adopt binding acts or when they think that it is not appropriate to issue more constraining rules under the Treaty. Although not legally binding, EU resolutions and recommendations have legal effect in particular when they clarify the interpretations of national provisions or supplement binding Community measures.

An important Recommendation in the field of employment is the European Commission Recommendation and Code of Practice on the protection of the dignity of women and men at work (92/131). This contains recommendations to employers, trade unions, and employees on avoiding and dealing with sexual harassment.

Working time directive

The Working Time Directive, which was adopted under the Qualified Majority Voting system (QMV) system, requires member states to legislate for a maximum of 48 working hours in any 7-day period, with rest breaks and restrictions on the number of hours of work that can be performed at night. It was adopted on 23 November 1993, with the UK abstaining. Draft regulations embraced by the Working Time Directive were published in April 1998 and became law in the UK in October 1998.

The Working Time Regulations 1998 (SI 1998/1833) provided workers with an entitlement to:

- a rest break where the working day exceeds 6 hours
- at least one whole hour off in each 24 hours
- at least 24 hours off in every week.

Other provisions include at least 4 weeks paid annual leave; restrictions on night work (including an average limit of 8 hours in 24); organization of work patterns to take account of health and safety requirements, and the adaptation of work to the worker; an average working limit of 48 hours over each 7-day period, calculated over a reference period of 17 weeks (Regulation 4(3) of the Working Time Regulations 1998).

A further Statutory Instrument, amending the first Working Time Regulations became law on 17 December 1999—The Working Time Regulations 1999. These Regulations simplified the meaning of the unmeasured hours and those workers who work unmeasured hours are now exempt from the 48-hour week; it also amended the requirement for employers to keep records of the hours worked by workers who had opted out of the 48-hour maximum working week.

The Directive is littered with 'derogations' that exempt certain types of work. There are some general exceptions that exclude workers in air, sea, rail and road, inland waterways and lake transport, sea fishing and other work at sea, as well as doctors in training. The major provisions for which there are no derogations are the 4 weeks of paid annual leave and the 48-hour working week.

Other exceptions may arise through national legislation or collective agreements for those whose working time is self-determined or flexible (e.g. senior managers or workers with autonomous decision-taking powers, family workers, and workers officiating at religious ceremonies). In addition, workers may agree voluntarily to work longer hours than those laid down in the Directive. In other cases, the workers must be permitted compensatory rest breaks if they work for more than 48 hours in a week (e.g. those whose job involves a great deal of travelling; security and surveillance workers; those whose jobs involve a foreseeable surge in activity such as tourism and agriculture; and emergency rescue workers). In *Landeshauptstadt Kiel* v. *Jaege*[55] the ECJ ruled that being on call even if not actually working constituted working time under the Directive. The ECJ held that:

> A period of duty spent by a hospital doctor on call, where the doctor's presence in the hospital is required, must be regarded as constituting in its entirety working time for the purposes of the Working Time Directive, even though the person concerned is permitted to rest at their place of work during periods when their services are not required.

> An employee available at the place determined by the employer cannot be regarded as being at rest during the periods of his on-call duty when he is not actually carrying on any professional activity.

Other health and safety directives

In January 1992, the UK introduced the 'Six Pack'[56] implementing EU Directives on a range of health and safety matters. These regulations made it mandatory for employers to carry out risk assessments in situations where there were 'significant and substantial' risks to health or safety and to appoint 'competent' people to assist them in this task. Employers are required to maintain and update these risk assessments and to document them. Other regulations require regular health surveillance such as under the COSHH Regulations.[57]

The Six Pack and in particular the Health and Safety (Display Screen Equipment) Regulations 1992 (the 'DSE' Regulations) and Code of Practice and Guidance Notes sought to regulate the use of Display Screen Equipment (more commonly known as Visual Display Units (VDUs)). The regulations lay down clear ergonomic rules relating to the work station, such as having adjustable chairs and suitable lighting. (These rules are set out in the schedule to the Regulations, covering screens, keyboards, desks, chairs, the work environment, and software.)

In addition, the Code of Practice and Guidance Notes recommend rest breaks for habitual VDU users of at least 5–10 minutes every hour before muscles become fatigued, rather than longer rest breaks after a longer working time. Employers in the UK have often based their health and safety policy in respect of VDU workers on these recommendations.

The Regulations also require employers to provide free eye sight tests and free spectacles if required for VDU use.

Employers are also required to undertake regular risk assessments of the workstation and the work in order to highlight any particular or individual problems before they become more serious.

The Control of Substances Hazardous to Health Regulations 2002 (COSHH) require employers (in brief) to take eight steps to control hazardous substances used in the workplace. These eight steps that employers using hazardous substances[61] take are:

1. to carry out a risk assessment, assessing risks to health arising from hazardous substances used or created by the workplace activities

2. to decide what precautions need to be taken

3. to prevent or adequately control exposure

4. to ensure that control measures are used and maintained

5. to monitor the exposure of employees to hazardous substances if necessary

6. to carry out health surveillance where the assessment has shown it is necessary or where the Regulations require it (an aspect of assessing fitness to work)

7. to prepare plans and procedures to deal with accidents, incidents, and emergencies involving hazardous substances, if necessary

8. to ensure that employees are properly informed, trained, and supervised.

Notes and references

1 In Scotland the legal system is quite different—its civil and criminal justice system being based on Dutch Roman law. However, in relation to employment law, everything in this chapter applies to the law of Scotland, save for differences in procedure in the Employment Tribunal.

2 *Bolam* v. *Friern Hospital Management Committee* [1957] 1 WLR 582.

3 *Bolitho* v. *City and Hackney Health Authority* [1997] 4 All ER 771.

4 *Stokes* v. *GKN* [1968] 1 WLR 1776.

5 [1994] 5 Med. LR 293.

6 [2004] IRLR 475.

7 *Edwards* v. *NCB* [1949] 1 ALL ER 743.

8 *Baxter* v. *Harland and Wolff plc* [1990] IRLR 516.

9 [1951] 1 All ER 42.

10 *Page* v. *Smith* [1995] 2 WLR 644.

11 [1995] IRLR 35.

12 Known then as *Sutherland* v. *Hatton (the first of the four conjoined appeals)* [2002] IRLR 263 at para 43.

13 B2/2002/1594; B3/2003/2144; B3/2004/0695; B3/2001/2474; B3/2002/2770.

14 The cases on breach of the implied duty to co-operate with the employer focus on the motive for the refusal—see *Langston* v. *AUEW* [1973] IRLR 82 and *BT* v. *Ticehurst* [1992] IRLR 219.

15 Section 98(2)(a) defines 'capability' in Section 98(3)(a), in relation to an employee, meaning his capability assessed by reference to skill, aptitude, health or any other physical or mental quality.

16 In *P* v. *S and Cornwall County Council* [1996] IRLR 347, the ECJ ruled that the word 'sex' in the Sex Discrimination Act 1975 led directly to the implementation of the Sex Discrimination (Gender Reassignment) Regulations 1999 SI 1999 1102.

17 Section 98(4) of the Employment Rights Act 1996.

18 [1986] IRLR 46.

19 Section 98 (1)(b) of the Employment Rights Act 1996.

20 *Walton* v. *TAC Construction Materials Ltd* [1981] IRLR 357.

21 [1979] IRLR 140.

22 Inland Revenue Guide to Employers (E14), on p. 18.

23 [1981] IRLR 318.

24 UKEAT/0788/03/MAA.

25 Grateful thanks go to Dr Clyde Webb for sending me one of his letters to the Society of Occupational Medicine. Dr Webb is participating in a pilot project organized by DWP to assess alternative models of sickness absence certification.

26 26 March 1999 (unreported).

27 The GP contracts from 2003 included the following clause: 'para 6.48(v) of the new GP contract— Furthering attempts to reduce certification work within general practice. National initiatives such as those established through the Cabinet Office will be implemented. Major local pilots in large companies and the NHS will be sought to evaluate the effectiveness of in-house occupational health services as an alternative to using general practice for certification. Should the pilots be successful the aim would be to allow the system to be refined so certification responsibility can be moved to occupational physicians and occupational health nurses, making significant progress towards national coverage by April 2006.'.

28 The DWP has published its Guide for GPs IB204 which can be found on the website www.dwp.gov.uk/medical/guides_ detailed.asp#IB204.

29 [1981] IRLR 264.

30 *Whitbread & Co plc* v. *Mills* [1988] IRLR 507.

31 The Code of Practice is in four parts. Part 4 consists of three publications—the Code, Supplementary Guidance and a Guide for Small Businesses.

32 Court of Appeal, LTL 8/12/2003.

33 www.informationcommissioner.gov.uk.

34 An excellent summary of the Act ('AMRA') can be found on the BMA website: http://www.bma.org.uk/ap.nsf/Content/accessmedreps.

35 See definition of 'clinical care' in section 2 of the Access to Medical Reports Act 1998 where 'care' is defined as including examination, investigation or diagnosis for the purposes of, or in connection with, any form of medical treatment;.

36 *Nawaz* v. *Ford Motor Company Ltd* [1987] IRLR 163.

37 *Hanlon* v. *Kirklees Borough Council* (see Chapter 3 for more detail).

38 *Jones* v. *The Post Office* [2001] IRLR 381 and *British Gas Plc* v. *Breeze* EAT 503/87 *Evers* v. *Doncaster Monks Bridge* (unreported).

39 *Rao* v. *CAA* [1994] IRLR 248.

40 *East Lindsay District Council* v. *Daubney* [1977] IRLR 181; *Spencer* v. *Paragon Wallpapers Ltd* [1976] IRLR 373.

41 *Eclipse Blinds Ltd* v. *Wright* [1992] IRLR 133; *AK Links Ltd* v. *Rose* [1991] IRLR 353.

42 [1991] IRLR 522.

43 *Crossley* v. *Faithful and Gould Holdings Ltd* [2004] IRLR 377 (Court of Appeal).

44 *Mihlenstedt* v. *Barclays Bank International Ltd and Barclays Bank plc* [1989] IRLR 522.

45 *The Board of Governors, The National Heart and Chest Hospitals* v. *Nambiar* [1981] IRLR 196.

46 *Kapfunde* v. *Abbey National and anor* [1998] IRLR 583.

47 [1995] IRLR 320.

48 Imposed by the regulatory bodies such as the General Medical Council (GMC) and Nursing and Midwives Council (MNC).

49 Part 1 and the Practice Direction.

50 *Webb* v. *EMO Cargo UK Ltd* [1993] IRLR 27.

51 SI 3242.

52 Regulation 16(1)(b). See also the case of *Hardman* v. *Mallon t/a Orchard Lodge Nursing Home* [2002] IRLR 516.

53 Regulation 16 (2) and (3).

54 See *Grimaldi* v. *Fonds Des Maladies Professionnelles* [1990] IRLR 400.

55 [2003] IRLR 804.

56 The Management of Health and Safety at Work Regulations 1992 replaced by the 1999 Regulations; Health and Safety (Display Screen Equipment) Regulations; Personal Protective Equipment at Work Regulations 1992; Provision and Use of Work Equipment Regulations 1992; Manual Handling Operations Regulations 1992; Workplace (Health, Safety and Welfare) Regulations 1992.

57 The Control of Substances Hazardous to Health Regulations 1999 SI No. 437, Regulation 11.

Chapter 3

The Disability Discrimination Act 1995

G. S. Howard and R. A. F. Cox

The Disability Discrimination Act 1995 (DDA) has now been in force for 10 years. Despite its shortcomings and ambiguities it has catalysed our social and corporate consciences to reject the outdated and discriminatory models of disability and it has introduced a realization that the disabled have a right to participate in society with opportunities equal to those of the able-bodied. More than any other factor, the Act has helped to change the public perception of those with impairments, whether physical, mental, or learning, from one of exclusion and intolerance to one of participation and integration. Prejudice and lack of understanding still linger, more intractably in some quarters than others, but the disabled are now welcomed into society in a way that would not have been contemplated 10 years ago. The occupational physician, however, is still required to determine disability within the law and to advise on the modifications and adjustments that the law demands from the employers of disabled persons.

The law

There are over 6.8 million disabled people of working age in Britain and the employment rate for disabled people is 51% compared with 81% for the non-disabled (Labour Force Survey Autumn 2004 www.statistics.gov.uk). The enactment of the DDA was a milestone for the disabled who for many years had lobbied for legislation to root out and destroy stereotyped ideas about disabled people and to stop unlawful discrimination in areas such as employment, the provision of goods and services, and education and transport. Nevertheless, those lobbying for the disabled were still not entirely satisfied with the new Act, which removed the quota scheme from employers as well as any requirement to register as a disabled person.

The Disability Discrimination Act 1995 has now been amended by the Disability Discrimination Act 1995 (Amendment) Regulations 2003,[1] which came into force on 1 October 2004[2] and which removed the small employers' (of fewer than 15 employees) exclusion and brought within the scope of the Act most of the currently excluded occupations (such as police officers, prison officers, and firefighters). The Act was also extended to cover qualification bodies such as the General Medical Council. The implication of this is not that competence standards for disabled medical students will be compromised but the methods of assessing or demonstrating those competencies must be subject to reasonable adjustment for disabled students.[3]

Furthermore, the justification defence for not making reasonable adjustments (Section 4B(1)) has been abolished and an additional definition of 'discrimination' has been added. Also for the first time a statutory definition of 'harassment' (Section 3B) has been given in the 2003 Regulations.

From 1 October 2004, service providers have also been required to take reasonable steps to remove, alter or avoid physical features of their premises (like steps or narrow doorways) that make it impossible or unreasonably difficult for disabled people to access their services.

The Act and its Regulations

The Act is drafted so as to leave many of the provisions to be 'interpreted' by Regulations, Guidance Notes, and Codes of Practice. The employment provisions of the DDA came into force on 2 December 1997 and the Codes of Practice and Guidance Notes were published originally in November 1996 but a new Code of Practice 'Employment and Occupation' was introduced in 2004.[4] Two sets of Regulations—the Meaning of Disability Regulations 1996 and the Disability Discrimination (Employment) Regulations 1996—also came into force in 1996 and as noted above, important amendments to the Act came into force on 1 October 2004 by way of The Disability Discrimination Act 1995 (Amendment) Regulations 2003. The Guidance notes remain the same.[5]

Summary of the Act

In order to qualify for protection under the DDA, a person must have, or have had in the past, a 'physical' or 'mental impairment' causing a substantial[6] and long-term adverse effect on their ability to carry out 'normal day to day activities'.[7] An impairment will only affect normal day to day activities if it affects one or more of the following:

- Mobility
- Manual dexterity
- Physical co-ordination
- Continence
- The ability to lift, carry, or otherwise move everyday objects
- Hearing, speech, or corrected eyesight
- Memory or ability to concentrate, learn or understand
- Perception of risk of physical danger

    'Long-term' is defined in Schedule 2(1) (2) of the Act as:

- 'lasting, or likely to last, for 12 months or more or
- for the rest of the affected person's lifetime
- or likely to recur if in remission'.

The Guidance to the Act gives helpful illustrations of what could be regarded as a normal day to day activity—but the Guidance merely provides examples and is not exhaustive.

In *Vicary* v. *British Telecommunications plc*[8] the Employment Tribunal erred in law in deciding that

> activities such as DIY tasks, filing nails, tonging hair, ironing, shaking quilts, grooming animals, polishing furniture, knitting and sewing and cutting with scissors were not normal day-to-day activities. It misunderstood the nature of the guidance given 'as set out in the Guidance to the Act'. Guidance makes it plain that the lists of examples are illustrative, not exhaustive. Making beds, doing housework, sewing and cutting with scissors, minor DIY tasks, filing nails, curling hair and ironing are normal day-to-day activities since they are all activities that most people do on a frequent or fairly regular basis.

Definition of 'discrimination'

There are now three definitions of 'discrimination' under the Act, as revised by the 2004 Regulations.[9] An employer discriminates against a disabled person if:

1. for a reason that relates to that person's disability he treats him less favourably than he treats or would treat others to whom that reason would not apply and that treatment cannot be justified

2. the employer discriminates against the disabled person by failing to make reasonable adjustments to the workplace

3. the disabled person is treated less favourably than the employer treats or would treat a person not having that particular disability whose relevant circumstances, including his abilities, are the same as, or not materially different from, those of the disabled person. This provides a third form of discrimination, direct discrimination.

New definition of 'harassment'[10]

For the first time in the antidiscrimination legislation, 'harassment' has been defined as conduct that is unwanted, which has the purpose or effect of either violating the disabled person's dignity, or creating an intimidating, hostile, degrading, humiliating, or offensive environment for him.

Whether such conduct could reasonably be viewed as harassment will be considered both subjectively and objectively in light of the disabled person's perception as well as whether it could reasonably be considered as having that effect. An illustration of harassment on grounds of disability can be found in the case of *Jenkins* v. *Legoland Windsor Park Ltd*[11] where the Employment Appeal Tribunal (EAT) held that the employer, which customarily gave employees plastic models of themselves as a 3-year merit award, had discriminated against a disabled employee by giving him a model that featured his disability. The employer made it clear that the model was a model of him, whereas the models given to other employees were identifiable by including some feature related to the work that each employee performed.

In this case Mr Jenkins had a withered left arm as a result of a motor-cycle accident and had his arm in a sling. The model he was presented was a man in a blue uniform with his right arm in a sling and with morose features on his face. Mr Jenkins was incensed as he had fought very hard over the years to come to terms with his disability. The psychiatrist who saw Mr Jenkins stated: 'This man is suffering from a depressive episode triggered by an insensitive experience at his place of work'.

Defences under the Act

An employer will only be able to justify discriminatory treatment where the reason for the discrimination 'relates to' that person's disability. Where the discrimination takes the form of direct discrimination (new Section 3A(5)) in comparison with an able-bodied person, there can be no justification (new Section 3A(4)). However, there will be no justification defence to a complaint of discrimination where the complaint relates to the new definition of discrimination, namely discrimination under Section 3A(5) where there is direct discrimination in comparison with an able-bodied person.

An employer may be able to defend a complaint of discrimination, even if the disabled person is treated less favourably for reasons relating to disability, if the employer can show that no reasonable adjustments could be made (Section 5(2)).

The former defence that it was 'justifiable' not to make any reasonable adjustments even if they could be made was repealed by the 2003 Regulations (Section 3A (6)). Now it will not be possible for an employer to argue that it was justifiable not to make reasonable adjustments if there are any that could be made.

Where any 'provision, criterion or practice' (previously 'an arrangement') made by an employer, or any physical feature of an employer's premises put a disabled person at a substantial disadvantage in comparison with an able-bodied person, then the employer is under an obligation to make reasonable adjustments to prevent that disadvantage arising (Section 4(A)(1)).

Provision is also made in the Act to enable employers who lease their property to obtain the landlord's permission to make alterations, in order to comply with their duty to make reasonable adjustments.

Discrimination against a disabled worker by other employees acting in the course of their employment will render employers vicariously liable unless they can show that they took all reasonable practicable steps to prevent the discrimination occurring.

The Act can only be enforced if an individual takes a complaint to an industrial tribunal.

Unlike other antidiscriminatory legislation, the DDA was not originally supported by a statutory enforcement agency such as the Equal Opportunities Commission (EOC) or the Commission for Racial Equality (CRE). However, the Disability Rights Commission (DRC) was set up in April 2000 and the Government has announced that in 2008 there will be a unified antidiscrimination regulatory body called the Combined Equality and Human Rights Commission (CEHR).

Meaning of disability

The Act defines a 'disability' as having a 'substantial and long-term adverse effect on that person's ability to carry out normal day to day activities'. **The definition does not include a person's ability to work unless the disability also affects '*normal day to day activities*'.** The loss of a little finger in a professional violinist would seriously impair their work, but it would not be a disability within the meaning of the Act because it would not substantially impair their ability to carry out 'normal day to day activities'.

In an early case concerning disability discrimination (*Goodwin* v. *The Patent Office*),[12] the EAT gave guidance on how tribunals should interpret a normal day-to-day activity and how, in general, tribunals should approach disability discrimination cases and what questions they should address. In this case the EAT ruled that, although Mr Goodwin was able to cope with ordinary, everyday activities at home, he was still disabled within the meaning of the Act because he was unable to hold a normal conversation and he had hallucinations and paranoid delusions, which impaired his ability to concentrate, learn and understand (Schedule 1. paragraph 4(g)) and this could have impaired his perception of the risk of physical danger (Schedule 1. paragraph 4(h)).

The EAT held that the words of Section 1 required a tribunal to look at the evidence by reference to four specific terms:

1. 'impairment'
2. 'adverse effect',
3. 'substantially' and
4. 'long-term' effect.

Tribunals might find it helpful to address each, while being aware of the risk of taking their eye off the whole picture.

In *Ekpe* v. *Commissioner of Police of the Metropolis*[13] the EAT stressed that: 'A tribunal inquiring as to whether an impairment affects the ability of the person concerned to carry out normal day-to-day activities should focus upon whether or not any of the abilities, or capacities, listed in paragraph 4(1)(a)–(h) of Schedule 1 to the Act have been affected. If they have, then it must be almost inevitable that there will be some adverse effect upon normal day-to-day activities. In most normal cases it is likely that the answer to the question 'has a paragraph 4(1) ability been affected?' will also answer the question whether there has been an impact on normal day-to-day activities. What is 'normal' for the purposes of the Act may be best understood by defining it as anything that is not abnormal or unusual (or, as in the Guidance issued by the Secretary of State, 'particular' to the individual applicant), just as what is 'substantial' may be best understood by defining it as anything that is more than insubstantial. What is normal cannot sensibly depend on whether the majority of people do it. The antithesis for the purposes of the Act is between that which is 'normal' and that which is 'abnormal' or 'unusual' as a regular activity, judged by an objective population standard.

In the present case, the tribunal erred in discounting the fact that the applicant could not put rollers in her hair and that she could not always use her right hand to apply makeup on grounds that neither was a 'normal day-to-day activity' because they are activities carried out almost exclusively by women. That reasoning, which would exclude anything done by women rather than men, or vice versa, as not being normal, was plainly wrong.

Anything done by most women, or most men, is a normal day-to-day activity. The errors that led the tribunal to this perverse conclusion were: to treat the borderline between that which is normal as a day-to-day activity and that which is not, as being determined by whether more or less than 50% of the population would do it, rather than by asking whether the activity can be considered as abnormal or unusual; and to regard the word 'particular' contained in the reference in the Guidance to a 'particular group of people' as meaning 'identifiable' rather than 'defined by some singular characteristic', and then apparently asking whether the group constituted the majority of the population'.

Tribunals are exhorted to refer explicitly to any relevant provision of the guidance or code that has been taken into account in arriving at a decision.

Terminal illness and 'recurring' illness

The definition of disability also includes those with terminal illnesses who are not expected to recover within the next 12 months and those with serious physical or mental disabilities who may become asymptomatic for part of the time but whose symptoms are likely to recur. Such periods of remission will form part of the requisite 12-month period (Schedule 1 paragraph 2(2) of 1995 Act). It is up to the Claimant to prove that the illness is likely to recur. In *Swift* v. *Chief Constable of Wiltshire Constabulary*[14] the Employment Appeal Tribunal held that the Tribunal must be satisfied that the illness is likely to recur and will again have a substantial adverse effect on the employee's ability to carry out normal day- to-day activities. 'Likely to recur' means whether, on the balance of probabilities the substantial adverse effect is likely to recur, not whether the illness alone is likely to recur.

Severe disfigurement

The definition also includes people with 'severe disfigurements' such as facial scars or burns (Schedule 1 paragraph 3). The Code of Practice suggests that in deciding whether a severe disfigurement ought to be regarded as a disability, account should be taken of its location (e.g. whether it is on the back or on the face).

Exceptions

The Act excludes deliberately acquired disfigurements from the scope of 'severe disfigurements'. The Meaning of Disability Regulations 1996 excludes people with tattoos that have not been removed and piercings of the body for decorative or non-medical purposes, including any objects that may be attached through such piercings. Other exclusions include those with addiction problems with illicit substances and alcohol, those who have a tendency to set fires, a tendency to steal, a tendency to physical or sexual abuse of other persons, exhibitionism, and voyeurism. It also excludes those with seasonal allergic rhinitis. In *Murray* v. *Newham Citizens' Advice Bureau Ltd*,[15] the EAT held that it was a breach of the Disability Discrimination Act 1995 to refuse to employ a volunteer at a Citizen's Advice Bureau because at a pre-selection meeting, he had disclosed that he had been in prison for stabbing a neighbour with a knife in 1993, at which time he was diagnosed as a paranoid schizophrenic. Thereafter, he received treatment and appropriate medication. The EAT held that the exclusion in the Regulations referred to freestanding conditions, and not to those conditions that are the direct consequence of a physical or mental impairment within the meaning of S1(1).

Where the consequence of a recognized illness is a tendency to violence, a potential employer may only treat the disabled person less favourably than other persons if the discrimination can be justified under S5(1)(b).

In the above case, the Claimant's tendency to violence was a consequence of paranoid schizophrenia and thus a manifestation of his disability. The employment tribunal should have held that if the applicant was treated less favourably by reason of a tendency to violence, that amounted to discrimination on grounds of his disability that the respondents were required to justify under S5(1)(b).

However, in *Butterfield's* case the EAT held that the distinction made in *Murray's* case was not helpful. Mr Butterfield had committed crimes of indecent exposure—exhibitionism in the exclusion provisions of the Regulations. Yet he was also chronically depressed. The EAT held that he may have both a legitimate impairment and an excluded condition and 'but for' his mental illness he may never have committed the crime.

In any event the Tribunal had to consider 'causation'—What was the reason for the less favourable treatment? A *prima facie* case of discrimination may be made out if the impairment was an effective cause of the discrimination.

Perceived disability

One Minister's view was that the Act would apply 'only once symptoms have appeared'. This is not, however, made explicit in the Act. There appears to be confusion between the symptoms and clinical signs of a condition that has not yet produced any impairment (and may never do so), and asymptomatic carriers of conditions such as HIV or Huntington's chorea who will inevitably become impaired in due course. However, the Government has stated that people who are perceived to have a disability but who have no symptoms will not be protected by the Act. Under this interpretation a person with mild cerebral palsy or a diagnostically confirmed but latent neurological condition or someone genetically destined to develop Huntington's chorea or a person infected with HIV would not be protected until the condition caused an impairment of normal day to day activities. The situation was clarified in some respects by the Disability Discrimination Act 2005. The Act is mainly concerned with matters relating to issues outside the employment relationship, but it includes an extension to the definition of disability to cover automatically people with three progressive conditions—HIV, cancer, and multiple sclerosis from the point of diagnosis without the need to establish whether they have any adverse effect on their ability to carry out day-to-day activities.

A consultation document was published by the Department for Work and Pensions (DWP) on 16 December 2004 on whether, among other things, the Bill should exclude certain cancers from the scope of the extended definition. The document proposed excluding some common cancers that are not considered to require substantial treatment and it identified a list of the cancers to be excluded (e.g. basal cell carcinomas and Bowen's disease).

The Act came into effect in December 2005. Under its provisions any persons affected by any of these conditions will be protected under that Statute (notably DDA 1995 Schedule 1(8)) as from the point of diagnosis, even if they do not count as disabled under the normal DDA provisions because they can still carry out normal day to day activities.

On the other hand, a condition such as Type I diabetes, also being a progressive disease, will continue to be covered under Schedule 1, paragraph 8 because its adverse effects on day-to-day activities will be substantial. Type II diabetes would be regarded as a disability under this paragraph if it is considered that it will have a substantial adverse effect, either at the time of diagnosis or in the future. Under Schedule 1, paragraph 6 both Type I and Type II diabetes will still be regarded as disabilities because they are controlled by insulin or oral hypoglycaemic agents. People with other progressive conditions that are likely to have a substantial adverse effect on day-to-day activities, with or without treatment, will continue to be protected by the DDA under Schedule I.

Additional duty on employer

The Act (Section 5(2) as amended) states that an employer also discriminates against a disabled person if he fails to comply with a Section 6 duty (the duty to make reasonable adjustment) imposed on him in relation to the disabled person. In *Collins* v. *The Royal National Theatre Board*[16] the Court of Appeal (overturning its previous decision in *Jones* v. *The Post Office*[17]) virtually ruled out the possibility of the defence of justification where the employer had failed to make any reasonable adjustment when it was reasonably practicable to do so.

Employer's ignorance of the disability—a common sense approach

New Section 4A(3) only imposes a duty on an employer to make reasonable adjustments if the employer knows or could reasonably be expected to know that the person is disabled and would be substantially disadvantaged unless a reasonable adjustment is made. This includes both actual and 'constructive' knowledge (where one person in the organization knows about the disability or has information to realize that there might be a disability and that the disabled person would be placed at a substantial disadvantage). In most cases, this will be a matter of fact to be determined by the employment tribunal. In other words, did the employer have enough information about the fact of and the details of the disability, and should they have realized from that knowledge that a duty to make reasonable adjustments existed? Often this will depend on the size of the employing organization and the expertise of the staff that it employs. Small employers are less likely to be expected to have a high standard of constructive knowledge, particularly where there is no occupational health service or where the MED 3 does not contain a helpful or an accurate diagnosis.

The knowledge that occupational health staff may have about an employee's disability is often the key to this question. The 2004 Code of Practice at paragraph 5.15 provides an example of how a physician should approach the sensitive matter of disclosure of an employee's disability to the employer (Box 3.1).

A tribunal will not require disabled people to give long and detailed explanations as to the effects of their disability merely to cause the employer to make adjustments that it probably should have made in the first place. On the other hand, it is equally undesirable that an employer should be required to ask a number of questions as to whether a person with a disability feels disadvantaged merely to protect themselves from liability. Common sense is what the Employment Tribunals expect. In *A. M. MacCarthy* v. *Russell Jones & Walker (2004)*,[18] the EAT held that in this case (the Respondents are a highly regarded firm of solicitors, specializing in personal injury work) the employer could be expected to make reasonable adjustments under the Disability Discrimination Act 1995 (S6) if its human resources officer was deemed to be an 'agent or employee' under the Code of Practice (1996) (paragraph 4.62. is the same

Box 3.1 **Disclosure of a disability to an employer**

An occupational health adviser is engaged by a large employer to provide it with information about its employees' health. The occupational health adviser becomes aware of an employee's disability, which the employee's line manager does not know about. The employer's working arrangements put the employee at a substantial disadvantage because of the effects of her disability and she claims that a reasonable adjustment should have been made. It will not be a defence for the employer to claim that it did not know of her disability. **This is because the information gained by the occupational health adviser on the employer's behalf is imputed to the employer.** The occupational health adviser's knowledge means that the employer's duty under the Act applies. If the employee did not give consent for the occupational health adviser to pass on personal information to the line manager, it might be necessary for the line manager to implement the reasonable adjustment without knowing precisely why he/she has to do so.

paragraph as 5.15 above). In this case, Mrs MacCarthy complained that the HR officer had refused to wait for her psychologist's report that was to form part of her evidence for her grievance and had refused to allow her psychologist to attend her grievance to give evidence on her behalf. This, said the EAT, could be considered a failure to make reasonable adjustments under S6 of the Act. She had even requested that, at the very least, her employers should consider this report before deciding on her grievance.

When the report was considered by the Respondent's head of human resources on September 25, Mrs MacCarthy was immediately contacted and told that they had agreed to her psychologist attending the meeting. Mrs MacCarthy declined the offer, resigned and complained of constructive dismissal and discrimination under the Disability Discrimination Act 1995.

The EAT held that the Respondents had not received Mrs MacCarthy's resignation letter until 23 September. That raised the question of whether the Respondents had sufficient knowledge of Mrs MacCarthy's disability within those 3 days to raise a Section 6 duty to make reasonable adjustments. In order to decide that, the tribunal ought to have looked at whether the HR Officer was an 'agent or employee' under the *Code of Practice for the elimination of discrimination in the field of employment against disabled persons or persons who have had a disability (1996) paragraph 4.62*. This would have defined whether receipt of the report was sufficient to determine that the Respondent had the necessary knowledge of its contents to raise a Section 6 duty to make reasonable adjustments.

The matter was remitted to the same tribunal so that it could consider whether the HR officer could be regarded as an 'agent or employee' and to decide whether there was a breach of Section 6 between 20 and 23 September.

In *HJ Heinz Co Ltd* v. *Kenrick*[19] the EAT took the view that the employers, through their medical adviser, had sufficient knowledge of the manifestations of the applicant's disability at the time they dismissed him for it to be held that they had treated him less favourably for a reason that related to his disability within the meaning of Section 5(1)(a) of the DDA. This was notwithstanding that his condition was not identified by name as chronic fatigue syndrome or medically confirmed until shortly after his dismissal.

> Section 5(1) (a), in any event, does not require the employer to have knowledge of the disability as such ... The correct test is the objective one of whether the relationship between the disability and

the treatment, (in this case dismissal) exists, not whether the employer knew of it. This requires employers to pause to consider whether the reason for some dismissal that they have in mind might relate to disability and, if it might, to reflect on the Act and the Code of Practice before implementing. Unless the test is objective, there will be difficulties with credible and honest yet ignorant or obtuse employers who fail to recognise or acknowledge the obvious.

(Here dismissal, though perhaps the commonest consequence, is used as an example. Disability might also be related, knowingly or unknowingly, to failure to reward or to promote for example.)

Examples of more subtle discrimination

An example of more subtle, 'institutionalized' discrimination would be a blanket requirement to hold a current, full UK driving licence, whether or not a driving licence was essential for a particular job. This would clearly discriminate against people with certain physical or mental disabilities.

Employers must ensure that only essential requirements are imposed as critical at recruitment. Standard contracts with ill-considered clauses on mobility and requirements for a driving licence render them vulnerable to charges of discrimination.

Practical example

Consider an example of how the Act might apply in practice. A competent secretary who has been disabled from rheumatoid arthritis for 15 years applies for a job. She cannot type at a normal speed but she can type with the help of an arm rest and with repeated and constant breaks from the keyboard, although her typing speed is lower than that of an average secretary. Will it be unlawful to refuse to employ this candidate because of her arthritis? It appears so, if she would have been suitable save for her disability. Would it be unlawful to refuse to employ her because she could not type at the normal speed? Again, Yes—unless the employer could justify, as an absolute necessity, that this particular job required normal typing speed and that no reasonable modifications could be made to the job, such as sharing some of the duties. This secretary would fall into the definition of someone who was physically disabled, and if she were rejected because she could not type at normal speed, then this would fall within the definition of discrimination under Section 5(1) of the Act, namely a reason relating to her disability.

It would not matter for the purposes of the Act if a secretary were recruited who suffered from another disability, say depressive illness, which did not affect her typing speed but did affect her moods and her attendance record. Neither would it matter that all able-bodied recruits who could not type at the normal speed were also rejected for the job. The reason for refusing to employ this particular woman would have related to her disability.

Causal link

The Courts have made it clear that if the disability is causally linked with the impairment, then any discrimination relating to that impairment may be unlawful. In *Kirton* v. *Terosyl Ltd*[20] the Court of Appeal ruled that the impairment of urinary incontinence, as a result of surgery for prostate cancer, was brought about 'as a result of' the cancer, within the meaning of the statutory definition of disability, notwithstanding the intervening act of the surgical treatment of the cancer. According to Lord Justice Pill, the words 'as a result of that condition' should not be 'so narrowly construed as to exclude an impairment which results from a standard and common form of operative procedure for the cancer.' Lord Justice Scott Baker added that 'impairment' in this context 'also includes the ordinary consequences of an operation to relieve the disease.'

Discrimination occurring after the employment has terminated

Discrimination can occur before, during or after employment. In six conjoined appeals, *Rhys Harper* v. *Relaxion Group plc, etc.*,[21] the House of Lords ruled that the Disability Discrimination Act 1995 makes it unlawful to discriminate against former employees, as well as current employees, if there is a substantive connection between the discriminatory conduct and the employment relationship, whenever the discriminatory conduct arises. In some cases, the issue relates to the giving or refusing to give a reference. The House of Lords saw no distinction between the giving or refusing to give a reference the day before the employment ends and the day after.

> If it is the employer's practice to give references to former employees, then the employer must not discriminate. If the employer's practice is to cease giving references after a given interval, then the refusal of a reference to a particular individual after that interval has passed will not, without more, (*sic*) be discriminatory. Failure to provide a non-contractual benefit will not constitute discrimination unless the non-contractual benefit is one which normally is provided, or would be provided, to others in comparable circumstances.

Duty to make reasonable adjustments

One of the central duties on employers under the Act 'is to make reasonable adjustment to the workplace', if a provision, criterion, or practice applied by or on behalf of an employer, or any physical feature of premises occupied by the employer, places the disabled person concerned at a substantial disadvantage in comparison with persons who are not disabled '

The Act lists in Section 6(3) examples of the kinds of adjustments that employers might be expected to make, including:

* adjustments to their premises
* allocating some of the duties to able-bodied employees
* transferring the disabled person to another vacancy
* altering the employee's working hours
* assigning the employee to a different workplace
* allowing the employee time off during work for rehabilitation, treatment, or assessment
* giving the employee training, or acquiring or modifying equipment (e.g. a simple device on a telephone for someone who has impaired hearing would suffice if that was all that was needed).

In the example of the typist with rheumatoid arthritis, the claimant could show that she would be at a 'substantial disadvantage' compared with workers who are not disabled. To avoid discrimination it would be necessary to make reasonable adjustments to the workplace, such as allocating some of the typing duties to others so that the typing duties were reduced and, perhaps, making this employee responsible for more non-typing duties such as making travel arrangements, keeping the diary, preparing expense claims etc.; or even offering an adapted keyboard if this would overcome the problem. Moving the individual to another vacancy where there is less typing is another adjustment that would avoid potential discrimination.

In other cases more sophisticated adjustments may be necessary, such as providing a voice-operated software program, modifying manuals and instructions, providing readers or interpreters, providing extra supervision, and so on. The duty to make reasonable adjustments does not include the provision of a personal carer to take a disabled employee to the toilet[22] as the duty relates to work-related adjustments, not to the provision of additional staff.

An example of this arose in the case of *Paul* v. *National Probation Service*[23] where the claimant had chronic depression for which he was under the care of a consultant psychiatrist. An offer of employment to him was withdrawn after an occupational health adviser wrote to his GP and, on the basis of that report, decided that the employment might be too stressful. The EAT made clear that in many cases, having a disability does not adversely affect an individual's general health. They held that

> In many cases, having a disability does not adversely affect an individual's general health and an occupational health assessment will not lead to a refusal of employment unless the disability affects the applicant's ability to do the work and no reasonable adjustments can be made. The existence of a disability does not of itself therefore substantially disadvantage a disabled person who is subject to this general requirement and, in the present case, the applicant was not placed at a substantial disadvantage in comparison with persons who are not disabled merely because of the need for occupational health clearance.

Instead, what the tribunal should have considered (but did not) was whether there were reasonable steps that the employers could have taken to comply with their duty to prevent disadvantage to the applicant. These included obtaining specialist advice from the applicant's consultant on his fitness for the post, and taking steps in relation to adjusting the job they had offered.

In this case the EAT found that the occupational health adviser failed to advise on the correct steps to take when making 'arrangements' that may substantially disadvantage a disabled person. She had only sought the GP's advice on the applicant's psychiatric condition. The GP had not been treating his patient for this condition so his report said nothing about his fitness for the post or his ability to cope with stress. The occupational health adviser should, therefore, have consulted the psychiatrist for his views on the fitness of his patient for the supervisor post, his ability to cope and what reasonable adjustments, if any, should be made. The Employment Tribunal in this case found that the employer had not discriminated because they had not failed to make 'arrangements' that placed Mr Paul at a substantial disadvantage as compared with people who are not disabled. The EAT reversed the Tribunal's decision. They found that the Tribunal had 'misidentified' the 'arrangement' that placed the applicant at a substantial disadvantage. The Employment Tribunal had found that the arrangement was the employers' requirement that all posts would be offered subject to occupational health clearance.

The EAT held that the 'arrangement' was in fact the assessment by the occupational health adviser as to the challenging and stressful nature of the post for which he applied and his unfitness for it. This was part of the arrangements for determining to whom employment should be offered and placed the applicant at a substantial disadvantage in comparison with persons who are not disabled.

The EAT held that Mr Paul had been discriminated against because the prospective employer had not made reasonable adjustments—i.e. had not obtained specialist advice from the applicant's consultant on his fitness for the post in question, had not spoken further to the applicant and if appropriate had not referred the matter back to the occupational health adviser to take steps to adjust the job they had offered.

Transfer to slightly higher graded, higher paid job without having to compete

The House of Lords has given a very helpful and progressive decision in *Archibald* v. *Fife Council*[24] in which they held that a reasonable adjustment could be the offer of an alternative job (at a slightly higher graded, higher paid rate) without having to compete. In this case a road sweeper became seriously disabled (affecting her mobility) following an unsuccessful operation on her ankle, thus disabling her from her road-sweeping duties. She could have taken on a clerical job but was not successful in any of her 100 or so interviews. The House of Lords held that:

> The Disability Discrimination Act is different from the Sex Discrimination and Race Relations Acts in that employers are required to take steps to help disabled people which they are not required to take for others. The DDA does not regard the differences between disabled people and others as irrelevant. It does not expect each to be treated in the same way. The duty to make adjustments may require the employer to treat a disabled person more favourably to remove the disadvantage which is attributable to the disability. This necessarily entails a measure of positive discrimination.

The duty to make an adjustment is triggered where an employee becomes so disabled that she can no longer meet the requirements of her job description. The term 'arrangements' made by an employer in Section 6(1) is undefined and applies to the job description for a post and the liability of anyone who becomes incapable of fulfilling the job description to be dismissed, as much as it applies to an employer's arrangements for deciding who gets what job or how much each is paid.

The employer's 'arrangements' in the present case placed the applicant 'at a substantial disadvantage in comparison with persons who are not disabled' within the meaning of Section 6(1) because the job description required her to be physically fit, which she was no longer able to meet, and that exposed her to another 'arrangement' or condition, which was that if she was physically unable to do the job she was employed to do she was liable to be dismissed. The comparison under Section 6(1) with persons who are not disabled is not confined to non-disabled people doing the same job. Therefore, the steps that the employer might have to take in order to prevent the arrangements placing a disabled employee at a substantial disadvantage in comparison with non-disabled persons include transferring her to another job, a possibility expressly contemplated by Section 6(3)(c).

The duty to take such steps as it is reasonable in all the circumstances for the employer to have to take, could include transferring, without competitive interview, a disabled employee from a post she can no longer do to a post that she can do. The employer's duty may require moving the disabled person to a post at a slightly higher grade. A transfer can be upwards as well as sideways or downwards. Section 6(3)(c) is just an example of an adjustment. What steps are reasonable depends on the circumstances of the particular case.

In the present case, therefore, transferring the applicant to a sedentary position that she was qualified to fill was among the steps that it might have been reasonable in all the circumstances for the employers to have to take once she could no longer walk and sweep. The employment tribunal wrongly thought that transferring the applicant without requiring her to undertake a competitive interview would be preferential treatment and not a reasonable step for the employers to have to take in light of Section 6(7), which provides that 'nothing in this Part is to be taken to require an employer to treat a disabled person more favourably than he treats or would treat others.' Section 6(7) is prefaced by the words, 'subject to the provisions of this section', so that, to the extent that the duty to make reasonable adjustments requires it, the employer is not only permitted but obliged to treat a disabled person more favourably than others.'

Continuing sick pay

In another progressive decision, *Nottinghamshire County Council* v. *Meikl*[25] the Court of Appeal held that a 'reasonable adjustment' could include the consideration of extending full sick pay past the normal entitlement for full pay. The implications of this case for employers are considerable. What this means is that an employer's obligation can extend to not reducing a disabled employee's sick pay where her entitlement to full pay under a sick-pay scheme would otherwise be exhausted, if the tribunal decides that that would have been a reasonable adjustment for the employer to make. That is particularly likely to be the case where, as in *Meikle*, the employer has failed to make other reasonable adjustments, which would have reduced the disabled employee's absence.

In this case Mrs Meikle had lost the sight of one eye and some sight in the other. She made various requests to the school for adjustments, including moving her classroom locations, increasing the amount of preparation time she was given, and enlarging written materials and notices. Few of these steps were taken. Eventually she resigned, claiming constructive dismissal and disability discrimination.

This case also held that a 'detriment' under the Act also included 'constructive dismissal' entitling the employee to resign, where the detriment complained of amounted to a repudiatory breach of contract—in this case, the persistent failure of the employer to carry out reasonable adjustments amounted to a fundamental breach of the obligation of trust and confidence.

Listening to occupational physicians

Employers should take note of advice given to them by an Occupational Physician. In *Beart* v. *HM Prison Service*[26] the Court of Appeal held that the employment tribunal was entitled to find that there was a duty on the employers to make an adjustment by relocating the applicant to a different prison after she became ill with depression because of difficulties she encountered at work.

The Court of Appeal pointed out that the test of reasonableness under Section 6 of the DDA is directed to the steps to be taken to prevent the employment from having a detrimental effect on the disabled employee. Here there was medical evidence that there was a relationship between the difficulties the applicant encountered at work and the onset of her illness. An occupational health consultant had recommended that she should be relocated and the tribunal's finding that the step of relocation would have been a reasonable one was directed to the extent to which taking the step would prevent the effect in question. In *Surrey Police* v. *Marshall*[27] the EAT went so far as to say that by ignoring 'so senior a man as Dr Lipsedge', the employment tribunal had made such a serious error of law, that the employment tribunal should re-hear the case and consider his expert evidence.

Knowledge of disability

In a landmark claim for personal injuries (for stress-related illness) the Court of Appeal (CA) in *Harman* v. *South Essex mental Health and Community Care Trust* [2005] IRLR 293 has decided that an employer will not be 'deemed' to have constructive knowledge when the occupational physician knows about the disability.

This conflicts somewhat with the Disability Rights Commission's (DRC) Employment Code of Practice, which states that: 'It will not be a defence for the employer to claim that it did not know of her disability. This is because the information gained by the occupational health adviser on the employer's behalf is imputed to the employer. The occupational health adviser's knowledge means that the employer's duty under the Act applies. If the employee did not give consent for the occupational health adviser to pass on personal information to the line manager, it might be necessary for the line manager to implement the reasonable adjustment without knowing precisely why it has to do so.

In this case, Mrs Hartman's previous medical history was held by the Occupational Health Department. This included details of her having previously suffered a nervous breakdown and the fact that she had still been on medication—which might have allowed the employer to foresee her eventual relapse. The Court of Appeal held that this knowledge could not be deemed to have been available to the employer because it had been supplied to the OH department, in reply to a questionnaire, on a 'personal and confidential' basis.

The significance of this decision may be limited in the context of the duty on employers to make reasonable adjustments (one form of discrimination under Section 5(2) under the Disability Discrimination Act 1995). An employer has no duty to make an adjustment 'if the employer does not know, and could not reasonably be expected to know' about the disability (S6(6) of the Act).

But the DRC's Code of Practice 2004 warns that: 'If an employer's agent or employee (such as an occupational health adviser, a personnel officer or line manager or recruitment agent) knows, in that capacity, of an employee's disability, the employer will not usually be able to claim that it does not know of the disability, and that it therefore has no obligation to make a reasonable adjustment.'

One of the most interesting dicta in the *Hartman* case is that it is not correct in law to attribute to an employer knowledge of confidential information disclosed by an employee to the employer's occupational physician, whether the physician is a direct employee or self-employed or contracted through an external agency.

In *Hartman's* case the Court of Appeal held that her employers could not be deemed to have the knowledge that she was vulnerable to further psychiatric illness because of her previous history, because she had disclosed this on a pre-employment medical questionnaire and the questionnaire said that it was '*for use by the occupational health service only*' and in addition that it was '*personal and confidential*'.

The BMA's publication *Medical Ethics Today*, 2nd edition (chapter 16, p. 587) says,

> the fact that a doctor is a salaried employee gives no other employee of that company any right of access to medical records or to the details of examination findings. With the employee's consent the employer may be advised of any relevant information relating to a specific matter on a strictly need to know basis, the significance of which the employee clearly understands. If an employer explicitly or implicitly invites an employee to consult the occupational physician, the latter must still regard such consultation as strictly confidential.

But the DRC's Code draws a distinction between the knowledge of an in-house occupational physician and that of an independent occupational physician providing a service external of the company.

Paragraph 4.16 states that 'Information will not be imputed to the employer if it is gained by a person providing services to employees independently of the employer. This is the case even if the employer has arranged for those services to be provided.'

This is now clearly wrong in light of *Hartman*, where the Court of Appeal drew no distinction between directly employed occupational physicians or those employed on a contract for services and held that in either case the employer cannot be imputed with knowledge through their occupational physicians.

Employees and prospective employees should therefore be advised to tell their employer or prospective employer that they have a disability under the Disability Discrimination Act 1995 that requires the employer to make some reasonable adjustments.

This may mean that the employee will have to tell their employer or prospective employer much more about their disability in order for the employer's duty to make reasonable adjustments to be fulfilled. Then the employer will have actual knowledge and will be able to obtain sensible advice on what reasonable adjustments can be made. In effect, in future, individuals with a disability may have to waive their right to confidentiality at least in part.

On the other hand the occupational physician is clearly under a professional, if not a legal, obligation to inform an employer, with the employee's consent, if he or she is aware that an employee, or prospective employee, has a disability within the DDA and may require adjustment to his or her workplace or working practice.

What is 'reasonably practicable'?

An adjustment might be 'practicable', i.e. physically possible, but not 'reasonable'. The tribunals will weigh which measures are actually reasonable, and whether they would help to overcome the difficulty faced by the disabled person. The cost and disruption to the employer, and the availability of resources and financial assistance, will be taken into account.

Employers are not allowed to plead ignorance about external sources of finance and support: they have an obligation to find out about access to agencies and resources for the disabled.

There is no longer any 'justification' defence if the employment tribunal finds that the adjustment was reasonably practicable.

Definition of mental impairment

A 'mental impairment' was defined in the original Act as a mental illness only where that illness was a 'clinically well-recognised illness'. The 2005 amendment removed from the DDA's definition of disability the requirement that mental illnesses must be 'clinically well recognised'. How this will affect the definition of mental illness remains to be established.

Currently, the courts and tribunals regard a mental illness as falling within the Disability Discrimination Act 1995 if it appears within the *World Health Organization, International Classification of Diseases (ICD 10)* or within the *Diagnostic and Statistical Manual of Mental disorders (DSM IV)*. When the 1995 Act was in preparation, examples of mental impairment that were given included schizophrenia, manic depression, severe and extended depressive psychoses and a 'range of other conditions well-recognised by clinicians, psychiatrists and psychologists'. The Minister indicated that moods or mild eccentricities would not be covered by the Act. The necessity of having a proper clinical diagnosis for a mental illness has been endorsed by the Courts in cases such as *Morgan* v. *University of Staffordshire*[28] where the EAT held that words such as 'anxiety', 'stress', and 'depression' used in GP notes will not suffice in order to prove a mental impairment under the Act. They held that:

> ... copies of medical notes which referred to 'anxiety', 'stress' and 'depression'. The occasional use of such terms, even by medical men, will not amount to proof of a mental impairment within the Act, still less as to its proof at some particular time.'
>
> The possible routes to establishing the existence of mental impairment within the DDA are as follows:
>
> (i) proof of a mental illness specifically mentioned as such in the World Health Organization's International Classification of Diseases (WHO ICD).
>
> (ii) proof of a mental illness specifically mentioned as such in another professional publication such as the Journal of Psychiatry; British Medical Journal, The Lancet and the like;
>
> (iii) proof by other means of a medical illness recognized by a respected body of medical opinion;
>
> (iv) proof by substantial and specific medical evidence of a mental impairment that neither results from nor consists of a mental illness.
>
> If a claimant relies upon falling within the WHO ICD, many parts of its classification require specific symptoms to be manifest over a minimum specified period or with a minimum specified frequency. Thus, 'clinical depression' without more is insufficient. The term has no such simple category.
>
> In the present case, therefore, for the applicant to have pointed to occasional references in the medical notes and to the indices in the WHO ICD, without any informed medical evidence beyond those notes, was to invite failure.

Phobias such as agoraphobia and claustrophobia are covered under the Act along with syndromes such as autism and Asperger's syndrome and conditions such as schizophrenia and bipolar affective disorder as well as learning difficulties such as dyslexia.[29] Although addiction to drugs is not covered by the Act any addiction which was originally the result of the administration of medically prescribed drugs or other medical treatment will be covered and, as we have seen, these conditions excluded in the Regulations may not have to be free-standing and not symptoms of an existing psychiatric condition (see note 15 above).

Conditions that may fall within the Act's scope

At any given time there are a number of physical and mental complaints whose clinical basis is not strictly proven or defined. Often such cases arise when emerging conditions engender controversy and a genuine dispute within the medical profession. Sometimes these are regarded as falling within the definition of mental illness.

The tribunals have accepted that chronic fatigue syndrome (sometimes erroneously called ME) is a mental impairment, though a cautious employer may deem it wise to give a wide meaning to the word 'impairment' and treat conditions such as 'obesity' and 'stammering'[30] as impairments falling within the Act.

Other difficult cases

Another example would be the case of someone suffering from schizophrenia or bipolar affective disorder, who could do a job perfectly well as long as they take their medication but cause considerable difficulties at work when they fail to do so. Such an employee is definitely disabled within the meaning of the Act, but what adjustments would be reasonable for an employer to make in order to accommodate their occasional lapses in receiving their regular medication? Perhaps it would be reasonable to make it a term of continued employment that they self-refer every month to the occupational physician or nurse to be given their injection or tablets?

What the Act does not cover

To reiterate a point made earlier, the disability must have an adverse and long-term effect on one of the listed day to day activities (set out in Schedule 1 paragraph 4 of the Act).

The Guidance Notes give advice on how an employer should judge whether an impairment has a 'substantial' effect on the carrying out of 'normal day to day activities' and give several practical examples of substantial effects. One of the normal day-to-day activities is 'memory or ability to learn, concentrate or understand' Thus, if a person with dyslexia is either unable to write a cheque without assistance or has considerable difficulty in following a short, written sequence such as a simple recipe or a brief list of domestic tasks, then this could constitute a substantial effect. Merely being unable to remember the name of a familiar person once in a while or not being able to concentrate on a task requiring application over several hours, in themselves, would not be seen as having a substantial effect.

However, the Guidance Notes do state that if two or more conditions which, taken individually, would not be regarded as having a substantial effect were present, then their summated consequences might constitute 'a substantial effect'. Further information is provided in the appendix to this chapter.

Effects of medical treatment

Disabled people are still protected against discrimination even if they have successfully controlled or corrected their disability by medication or the use of a prosthesis or other aid. People wearing hearing aids are covered by the Act. Epilepsy corrected by medication or diabetes controlled by insulin are other examples, and the Act would cover people disabled by osteoarthritis of the lip, even when they no longer have any impairment following the successful insertion of a prosthesis.

Exclusion for corrected sight

People whose sight impairments are correctable by spectacles or contact lenses are not protected by the Act. According to the Government 'people who wear spectacles or contact lenses would not generally think of themselves as disabled'. The word 'correctable' implies that those who choose not to wear spectacles or contact lenses and those whose sight is consequently impaired will not enjoy the protection of the Act.

What should employers ask?

Should an employer 'quiz' job candidates or employees returning from sick leave to determine if they have a substantial, long-term disability? If such enquiries are relevant to the job it is entirely appropriate for them to be raised, but the Government's advice is not entirely clear.

Paragraphs 7.16–7.24 of the Code of Practice[31] recommend good practice in obtaining information about disabilities prior to interview and during the interview and selection process in order to avoid placing the disabled person at a substantial disadvantage.

Dangers of not asking

The employer may subsequently be deemed not to have taken reasonable steps to ascertain whether an employee had a disability within the meaning of the Act.

Dangers of asking

The potential danger of employers asking such questions would be to give to the dissatisfied job applicant or dismissed employee *prima facie* evidence against the employer that the disability, or a reason relating to it, may have been the reason for the non-engagement or the dismissal.

If the job candidate or employee does declare the disability voluntarily, then some employers may seek to marginalize them either into lower graded, less well-paid jobs or may find some other reason not to employ them.

It is also possible that some employers may attempt to look for a 'medical' excuse for refusing to recruit or for dismissing, particularly where there has been a history of 'nervous breakdown' or stress-related illness.

'Wording' on application forms

It might be wise to include a statement on application forms, so that the tribunals may see that the employer has made clear the reason for asking about disabilities. It could read in the following terms:

This organization is committed to its policy of equal opportunities and in particular its duties under the DDA. This organization seeks to offer employment opportunities irrespective of physical or mental disabilities wherever possible, as long as they do not compromise your health and safety or the health and safety of other workers, contractors, or members of the public.

These questions are asked in order to assist any person with a physical or mental disability in order to accommodate their needs.

The answers to any questions on disability will not be used in any way adversely to affect or discriminate against any job candidate in any employment decisions that will be made about you, either now or in the future.

The information contained on this form will be kept strictly confidential within the personnel/occupational health department and will not be used or disclosed to any other people without the written consent of the person to whom the information relates.

Using the appropriate experts

Because the need to establish a medical condition rests with the applicant in disability cases, the evidential burden is very similar to personal injury claims. This means that both parties will wish in many cases to have the evidence of expert witnesses.

Unfortunately, the tribunals still have no power to order a claimant to submit to a medical examination and to stay the proceedings if the applicant refuses. This matter will need to be addressed in the future in order to give those powers to tribunal chairmen. Taking dyslexia as an example, tribunals would need to address the following matters with the help of expert witnesses:

- Has the applicant established that they have dyslexia?

- If yes, does the condition have a substantial effect on the carrying out of one or more of the normal day to day activities in Schedule 1, paragraph 4?

The fact that dyslexia is a recognized impairment would be confirmed by reference to the ICD or DSM definitions and its presence in the individual should be tested with the WAIS R III test, 1997, administered by a qualified and expert educational psychologist.

Whether the dyslexia has a 'substantial' effect on the ability to learn or concentrate or memorize would depend on the results of the WAIS R or any other tests administered. **The tribunals have emphasized the need for employers to take expert occupational health advice in disability cases**.

In *Holmes* v. *Whittington & Porter*,[32] the Tribunal held that: 'The General Practitioner should not have signed himself "Company Medical Adviser" as he was neither a specialist in occupational medicine nor a specialist with regard to epilepsy.'

The employer admitted to the tribunal that it did not address its mind as to whether their medical advice was the best medical advice, or whether the doctor had any qualifications in occupational medicine or any specialty with regard to epilepsy. It did not address its mind as to whether they should have gone further than their doctor's report and taken further advice from a medical professional who was a specialist in occupational medicine and someone who was a specialist in epilepsy to see whether they had the same view as the company's doctor. They had not determined whether an occupational physician and/or a specialist in epilepsy could have made any suggestions about Mr Holmes, about his treatment and about how he should be treated at work or any adjustments that might be made to his working conditions. The employers had come to the decision that no reasonable adjustments could be made for Mr Holmes but that decision was made without knowing the full picture because it did not have sufficient information on which to make those sorts of decisions in the absence of the best medical advice from specialists.

It is not true to say that it is an enormous imposition on the employer, it just means the requirements of this Act are different from what has been required of employers before and that they just have to take more steps so that employees who are disabled persons are protected.

Orders for consent to disclosure of relevant medical records

The Courts and Employment Tribunals are limited to ordering that the claimant gives his/her consent to disclosure of relevant medical records. Failure to give consent can lead to the claim being struck out despite any argument that the claimant may put forward about such an Order being a breach of his/her right to respect for privacy under Article 8(1) of the Human Rights Act 1998. In *Hanlon v. Kirklees Borough Council*[33] Mr Hanlon's case for disability discrimination was struck out by the EAT after he failed to give his consent to disclosure of his relevant medical records. He argued that by striking out his claim, this had breached his right to respect for privacy guaranteed under Article 8(1) of the Human Rights Act 1998. The EAT held that:

> In any event it is not an absolute right of privacy but it is subject to a protection and rights of others and it seems to me that the balancing exercise which was clearly performed by both Chairmen clearly balances up the right for privacy as regards medical records with the proper conduct of the litigation in this case and I am satisfied that no human rights Articles were unfairly breached.

Disability policies and strategies

A dismissal can be fair in cases of disability, if the reason for dismissal is material and substantial and reasonable accommodation is not possible. Avenues that should be explored include seeking suitable alternative employment, modifying the duties, hours, or place of work, etc. Written advice from an occupational physician will be vital. Such documents may be viewed by the dismissed employee under complaint procedures so it is important to ensure that reports are factual and accurate.

Advice from the occupational physician

At recruitment

Although some disabilities are clearly apparent to anyone, such as a person who is blind, on crutches or in a wheelchair, there are many that may be known only to the disabled people themselves.

The status of some conditions under the DDA will often not be apparent without medical advice. Those with disabilities will need the protection of medical confidentiality when it comes to interpreting the disability in functional terms and in advising on the 'reasonable adjustments' that may be needed to accommodate them.

The overall responsibility for compliance with the employment provisions of the Act rests firmly with the employer, but employers will need professional help in many cases in interpreting the definitions and in determining what adjustments are needed. Employers will normally call on occupational physicians to provide expert advice.

At the recruitment stage the occupational physician should advise an employer on the nature of any disability as it might affect the particular job applied for and advise on any reasonable adjustments, including consideration of other vacancies if necessary. (See *Paul v. National Probation Service*, above.).

When disabilities are revealed in the recruitment process whether by completion of a medical questionnaire, or in an examination, the occupational physician will need to evaluate them and to advise the employer whether the disability will affect the person's work capability or work attendance and, if so, what adjustments are required.

The Act requires an employer to accommodate a higher level of sickness absence in a disabled individual. If a disabled candidate is otherwise suitable in terms of competence, experience and qualifications, and is no threat to the health and safety of themselves or others (the Act does not oblige an employer to take on a person whose disability may be a hazard to themselves or others in a particular work situation) then an employer would be in contravention of the Act if they rejected the person solely on the basis of a predicted greater sickness absence.

A possible exception might arise in jobs whose nature required full availability for work at all relevant times (e.g. emergency rescue team members).

In order to give appropriate advice on necessary adjustments, the occupational physician should have an intimate knowledge of the job and its requirements for which the applicant is being recruited and a broad knowledge of the company. The occupational physician is also uniquely placed to determine whether the applicant's disability is compatible with considerations of health and safety.

It is entirely justified to deny employment where a disability may compromise the health and safety of the applicant or third parties and where no reasonable adjustments can be made.

In summary, the occupational physician will need to address three questions:

* Does the individual have a disability within the definition of the Act, i.e. a physical or mental impairment that has a substantial and long-term adverse effect on normal day to day activities?
* Is the person fit for the particular employment, i.e. can they fulfil the job requirement without risk to their own health or safety or that of others?
* Are any adjustments needed in the workplace to accommodate the individual's disability and of so what are they?

During employment

There will be occasions when, in order to avoid inadvertent discrimination, management will need to know whether a current employee has a disability within the meaning of the Act. The occupational physician's expertise will be called on in those circumstances and they may need to examine the employee or obtain medical information from other sources such as the employee's general practitioner (GP). **In conveying an opinion to managers, the doctor must observe the normal rules regarding confidentiality and informed consent.**

Is it the duty of an occupational physician to advise whether a medical condition falls within the DDA?

If, as sometimes happens, an occupational physician is asked by an employer to advise whether a particular employee's illness or injury is likely to fall under the Disability Discrimination Act 1995 or not, this is a perfectly legitimate question. However in law, it is not the duty of any occupational physician to tell an *Employment Tribunal* whether or not an impairment has or has not a substantial and adverse effect upon a normal day-to-day activity. This is the primary duty of the Employment Tribunal to determine. In practice the answer may be very different. In the *Abadeh* and *Vicary*[34] cases, two different employment tribunals referred to the role of an occupational health physician when giving evidence at a hearing in a DDA case. In *Vicary's case* the Employment Appeal Tribunal referred to evidence from the employers' Regional Medical Officer, Dr Macaulay, and noted that she had attended a number of training courses on the DDA and then went on to say:

> 'We understand from Dr Macaulay that driving is not regarded by those doctors who specialise in the operation of the Disability Discrimination Act as a normal day-to-day activity, and that writing letters, reports and taking minutes are not so regarded.' The tribunal also noted Dr Macaulay's opinion, based on her observations, that Mrs Vicary's impairment was not 'substantial'.
>
> It is not for a doctor to express an opinion as to what is a normal day-to-day activity. Nor is it for the medical expert to tell the tribunal whether the impairments which had been found proved were or were not substantial. Those are matters for the employment tribunal to arrive at its own assessment.'
>
> In Abadeh's case the EAT said this: 'The employment tribunal erred in finding that the applicant's impairments did not have a substantial adverse effect on his ability to carry out normal day-to-day

activities, so that he was not a disabled person within the meaning of S.1 of the DDA. The tribunal were over-influenced by the employer's regional medical officer's opinion of whether or not the impairments were 'substantial' under the Act, and in effect adopted her assessment instead of making their own.

It is not the task of the medical expert to tell the tribunal whether an impairment was or was not substantial. That is a question that the tribunal itself has to answer. The medical report should deal with the doctor's diagnosis of the impairment, the doctor's observation of the applicant carrying out day-to-day activities and the ease with which he was able to perform those functions, together with any relevant opinion as to prognosis and the effect of medication.

However in practice, it is highly relevant and often appropriate for an occupational physician to advise an employer or prospective employer whether in the occupational physician's opinion, the individual:

1. has a disability of any kind;

2. is one that is likely to fall within the Disability Discrimination Act 1995—i.e. has lasted or is likely to last for 12 months or more and has a substantial effect upon normal day to day activities;

3. affects in any way the individual's ability to perform the job in question (or to continue to do their job);

4. what reasonable adjustments could be made in order for the individual to perform their job efficiently and effectively.

Confidentiality

At times the occupational physician may be in an ethical dilemma. For example, a disabled person may reasonably refuse to allow the occupational physician to reveal information about their disability to the employer. However, employers may be deemed to know what their agents know, and so knowledge of an individual's disability gained by an occupational physician working on behalf of the employer, could be imputed to the employer. In these circumstances the occupational physician should explain to the disabled person the reasons and the benefits of disclosing non-confidential information about the latter's functional ability to the employer. If consent is still refused, careful note of the fact should be recorded in the medical record and a copy given to the individual. If the disability would require adjustments to the workplace, the doctor should inform the employer of that fact alone without revealing the medical diagnosis or the nature of the disability.

A disability need only be disclosed to an employer if it may affect the person's functional performance, or jeopardize health and safety. If, in the occupational physician's opinion, a disability will not affect functional performance and no adjustment is necessary, disclosure to the employer is not needed. Employers may reasonably request to be made aware of any employee who may have a disability within the meaning of the Act so that they can avoid inadvertent discrimination. If that is an employer's policy it should be made plain to all employees or prospective employees so that they can give written, informed consent or withhold permission for disclosure of such information if they wish.

The occupational physician must do everything possible to promote the employment of disabled people and to protect them against discrimination, and should not hesitate to emphasize this. Their role should be that of a scrupulous arbiter, to ensure that the disabled are treated equitably and without discrimination. Their duty is not solely to protect the employer against charges of discrimination, though this will be the natural sequel of an established professional trust between the doctor, employer, and employee.

Justification

An action may only be brought under the Act if discrimination has occurred. It may be entirely justified to treat a disabled person less favourably if the person's disability limits their ability to fulfil the demands of the job effectively, either through physical or mental impairments that affect functional performance or for reasons of health and safety. The occupational physician's assessment will be crucial in these circumstances[35] and they may be required subsequently to justify their opinion in a tribunal. Tribunals that consider cases of alleged discrimination against the disabled are likely to depend heavily on the expert evidence of occupational physicians.

Early retirement on ill health grounds

An employee is most unlikely to bring an action if they have voluntarily chosen to retire on grounds of ill health and such medical retirement has been sanctioned by the doctor advising the pension trustees. If, however, early retirement is proposed on medical grounds by an employer or by a doctor acting on behalf of the employer, then this is regarded in law as a dismissal—see *Catherall* v. *Michelin Tyre plc.*[36]

In this case the issue was whether the employee had been dismissed in law or had resigned. The employee agreed to retire on medical grounds during a redundancy situation. The employment tribunal took the view that he chose early retirement, which was more bene-ficial to him financially than redundancy. The EAT remitted the case back to the tribunal to re-examine the cause of the termination. As Mr Justice Nelson explained: 'if the choice was between redundancy or retirement through ill health, the appellant was not being asked whether he wanted to terminate his employment but only how it was to be terminated. This effectively gave him no choice at all and could in itself be said to amount to a dismissal.' Even if there was not an express dismissal, a further issue arose as to whether the redundancy selection procedure was operated in such a way as to entitle the employee to claim that he had been constructively dismissed and bring a claim in respect of a discriminatory dismissal under the DDA

It is essential to ensure that 'reasonable adjustment' has been carefully and rigorously considered and rejected for justified reasons before recommending retirement on grounds of disability. Medical retirement may be discriminatory against a disabled individual (see above) unless the reasons for it are substantial and material. The occupational physician will need to establish this before sanctioning retirement to the pension trustees.

In dealing with cases that may be covered under the DDA, occupational physicians must ensure that they have fully investigated and understood the functional implications of an individ-ual's disability. They must also have a full understanding of the job in question so that their advice on adjustment is based on sound information and not speculation and if necessary after taking expert medical advice (see *Paul* v. *National Probation Service* note 23). Finally, they must follow the well-defined path of professional ethics at all times while protecting the interest of the disabled individual as their primary responsibility. Occupational physicians should always bear in mind that their actions, advice, and opinions may be the subject of cross-examination in an industrial tribunal at a later date.

Appendix: Definitions

The DDA states that 'an impairment is to be taken to affect the ability of the person concerned to carry out normal day to day activities only if it affects one of the following', which the new Guidance Note expands on the list recorded in the Act by providing definitions as follows:

- **Mobility** covers moving or changing position in a wide sense. Thus account will be taken of the extent to which a person can get around unaided or using an appropriate means of transport, can leave home with or without assistance, walk a short distance, climb stairs, travel in a car or on public transport, sit, stand, bend or reach or get around in an unfamiliar place. An impairment that has a substantial effect on mobility would include an inability to travel a short journey as a passenger in a vehicle; inability to walk other than at a slow pace or with unsteady or jerky movement, and difficulty in going up and down stairs.

- **Manual dexterity** covers ability to use hands and fingers with precision. Account will be taken of ability to pick up and manipulate small objects, write, type, or operate a range of equipment manually. Loss of function in the dominant hand would be expected to have a greater effect than the equivalent loss in the non-dominant hand.

  An impairment that has a substantial effect on manual dexterity would be loss of function in one or both hands such that the person cannot use the hand(s); inability to use a knife and fork at the same time; ability to press the buttons on a keyboard or keypad in an ordered way but only much more slowly than is normal for most people.

  Physical co-ordination covers balanced and effective interaction of body movement, including hand and eye co-ordination.

  An impairment that has a substantial effect on physical co-ordination would be ability to pour liquid into another vessel only with unusual slowness or concentration; inability to place food into one's own mouth with a fork or spoon without unusual concentration or assistance.

  This definition does not cover 'mere clumsiness'.

- **Continence** covers the ability to control urination and/or defecation. Account should be taken of the frequency and extent of loss of control and the age of the person. For example, infrequent loss of control of the bowels or loss of control of the bladder while asleep at least once a month would be regarded as having a substantial effect.

- **Ability to lift, carry or otherwise move everyday objects**. Account should be taken of a person's ability to repeat these functions or, for example, weight bear over a reasonable period of time. Everyday objects might include such items as books, a kettle of water, bags of shopping, briefcase, an overnight bag, a chair, or other piece of light furniture.

  An impairment that has a substantial effect on ability to lift and carry etc. would include ability to pick up an object of moderate weight with one hand but not with the other; inability to carry a loaded tray steadily.

- **Speech, hearing, or eyesight**
  - **Speech**: Account should be taken how far a person is able to speak clearly at normal pace and rhythm and to understand someone speaking normally in their native language. It is necessary to consider any effects on speech patterns or which impede the acquisition or processing of one's native language, for example by someone who has had a stroke.

    An impairment that has a substantial effect on speech if the person is unable to give clear instructions orally to colleagues or providers of a service or is unable to ask specific questions to clarify instructions would be regarded as substantial.

  - **Hearing**: If a person uses a hearing aid or similar device, what needs to be considered is the effect experienced if the person is not using the hearing aid or device in normal environmental conditions such as a level of background noise of such a range and of such a type that most people would be able to hear adequately.

An impairment that has a significant effect on hearing where there was an inability to hold a conversation in a noisy place such as on a factory floor or an inability to hear and understand another person speaking clearly over the telephone would be regarded as substantial.

- **Eyesight**: Schedule 1, paragraph 6(2) (a) clearly states that where the impairment of a person's sight is 'correctable' by spectacles or contact lenses they will not be deemed to have a physical impairment: **but** a sight impairment which has a substantial effect would be an inability to recognize by sight a person across a moderately-sized room; inability to distinguish colours (i.e. total colour blindness); inability to read ordinary newsprint.

- **Memory or ability to concentrate, learn, or understand**: account should be taken of the person's ability to remember, organize their thoughts, plan a course of action and then execute it, or take in new knowledge. This includes whether the person learns to do things more slowly than others. An impairment that has a substantial effect on the memory or ability to concentrate, learn or understand would be a persistent inability to remember the names of familiar people such as family or friends; inability to adapt to minor change in the work routine.

- **Perception of the risk of danger**: this includes both the underestimation and overestimation of physical danger by a disabled person, including danger to their well-being. Account should be taken of matters such as whether they are inclined to neglect basic functions such as eating, drinking, sleeping, keeping warm and personal hygiene; reckless behaviour that puts the person at risk; or excessive avoidance behaviour without a good cause.

An impairment that has a substantial effect on perception of the risk of danger would be where there was an inability to operate safely properly maintained machinery or an inability to nourish oneself. Fear of heights, or underestimating dangerous hobbies such as mountaineering would not be regarded as substantial impairments.

The Code of Practice explains that this list is meant to take into account the activities that are normal for most people on a daily or regular basis. It is not intended to include activities that are normal only for a particular person or a group of people. The Guidance gives examples that it describes as 'indicators' and not 'tests'. They do not mean that if a person can do an activity listed in the Guidance then they do not experience a substantial effect. The person may be inhibited in other activities that may indicate a substantial effect.

Notes and references

1   SI 2003 No. 1673.

2   A report published by the Department for Work and Pensions (DWP) 'Disability in the workplace: Employer' and Service Providers' responses to the Disability Discrimination Act 1995 in 2003 and preparation for changes in 2004' found a significant lack of awareness of the new Regulations.

3   Cohen D and Hebert K. Training in undergraduate and postgraduate medicine for people with disabilities; BMJ Careers. *BMJ* 2004; **329:** 123–5. (http://careerfocus.bmjjournals.com/search-dtl)

4   The Disability Discrimination Codes of Practice (Employment and Occupation, and Trade Organizations and Qualifications Bodies) Appointed Day Order 2004, SI 2004/2302.

5   Disability Discrimination Act 1995. Guidance on matters to be taken into account in determining questions relating to the definition of disability. London: The Stationary Office 1996.

6   New Section 4A. 'Substantial' means 'more than minor' according to the Parliamentary debates.

7   Paragraph 4 of Schedule 1 of the Act.

8   [1999] IRLR 680.

9   New section 3A of the amended 1995 Act.

10 New section 3B of the amended 1995 Act.

11 Unreported -Appeal No. EAT/1155/02 MA.

12 [1999] IRLR 4.

13 [2001] IRLR 605.

14 [2004] IRLR 540.

15 [2003] IRLR 340 *Edmund Nuttall Ltd* v. *Butterfield* [2005] IRLR 751.

16 [2004] IRLR 395.

17 [2001] IRLR 284.

18 Unreported UKEAT/0102/04/CK.

19 [2000] IRLR 144.

20 [2003] IRLR 353.

21 [2003] IRLR 484.

22 *Kenny* v. *Hampshire Constabulary* [1999] IRLR 76. In this case the EAT ruled that 6(2), which refers
    to 'any term, condition or arrangements on which employment, promotion, a transfer, training or any
    other benefit is offered or afforded', directs employers to make adjustments to the way the job is
    structured and organised so as to accommodate those who cannot fit into existing arrangements.
    Employers are not under a statutory duty to provide carers to attend to their employees' personal
    needs, such as assistance in going to the toilet. A line has to be drawn on the extent of the employer's
    responsibilities in providing adjustments to accommodate a disabled employee. Although an employer
    is required by Section 6(1) to consider making physical arrangements for a disabled person to use the
    toilet and physical adjustments to accommodate the presence of a personal carer, had Parliament
    intended to impose on employers the duty to cater for an employee's personal needs in the toilet it
    would have said so, and the Code of Practice would have laid out the criteria to be applied.

23 [2004] IRLR 190.

24 [2004] IRLR 651.

25 [2004] IRLR 703. At the time of writing, the Council has petitioned the House of Lords for leave to
    appeal.

26 [2003] IRLR 238.

27 [2002] IRLR 843.

28 [2002] IRLR 190.

29 Case on agoraphobia is *BT* v. *Pelling* 25th May 2004; Appeal No. EATS/0093/03; case on claustrophobia
    is *Freer Bouskell* v. *Brewster* UKEAT/0377/03/DM; case on Asperger's syndrome is *Hewitt* v. *Motorola Ltd*
    [2004] IRLR 545; case on schizophrenia is *EDS* v. *Travis* Appeal No.UKEAT/0476/03/ILB and bipolar
    disorder is *Surrey Police* v. *Marshall* (above). Dyslexia is cited in the Code of Practice as an example
    of a learning disorder falling within the term 'mental impairment' in Section 3.3 and other numerous
    sections in the Code.

30 The DRC believes that someone with a stammer which substantially disadvantages that person is a
    sensory impairment of speech and would fall within the definition of 'speech' which is a normal day
    to day activity that could be affected.

31 In paragraph 7.22 the Code recommends that 'employers should think ahead for interviews. Depending
    upon the circumstances, changes may need to be made to arrangements for interviews or to the way in
    which interviews are carried out.'

32 Unreported.

33 Appeal Nos. UKEAT/0119/04/ILB & UKEAT/0120/04/ILB.

34 [2001] IRLR 23 and [1999] IRLR 680.

35 See *Surrey Police* v. *Marshall* and the EAT's view of Dr Maurice Lipsedge's expert evidence.

36 [2003] IRLR 61.

Chapter 4

Support and rehabilitation (restoring fitness for work)

M. Aylward and P. E. Sawney

Introduction

How should vocational rehabilitation be best defined to describe its most essential elements that will inform and guide occupational health professionals and other key stakeholders to assist people with health-related problems and disabilities to gain optimal social functioning and return to the world of work? At a time when, despite improvements in most objective measures of health, levels of disability and health-related work absence continue to increase there is a pressing need to identify and successfully address psychological and societal factors that constitute obstacles to recovery and barriers to (return to) work rather than reducing sickness and disability to a personal pathology. Moreover, the great majority of people in receipt of state incapacity benefits, and indeed very many patients who consult their general practitioners (GPs), report non-specific and subjective health complaints that have a high prevalence in the general population. Working age people who are most likely to lose their job and be excluded from work thus do not fit the traditional model by having severe bodily or mental impairments. For these people sickness and incapacity for work are personal (psychological) and social problems rather than a medical one.

Rehabilitation cannot be a second stage after healthcare has failed. Biopsychosocial factors aggravate and perpetuate sickness and disability and act as obstacles to recovery and barriers to return to work. Vocational rehabilitation should address these impediments. The essential components of such an approach are described in this chapter, together with the underpinning reasoning and accumulating evidence of their effectiveness. Too often one or more of these elements are ignored and attempts at return to work fail. The role of the individual stakeholders and key players in the return-to-work processes are described with a particular emphasis on the interface between occupational health professionals and these key stakeholders. Examples of current rehabilitation service provision are given together with an Annex describing recent UK Government strategic developments and practical initiatives in vocational rehabilitation.

The relationship between work and health

Work forms a large part of most peoples lives. It brings a range of benefits to individuals, in addition to the financial benefits of a wage and pension. Work can provide people with a sense of dignity and purpose, brings opportunities to meet new people, develop new skills, and give something back to the community, all of which can help boost an individual's confidence and self-esteem. In short, work allows full participation in our society.

The way we work has changed over the years—these days more women work, there is more shift work and greater use of flexible hours. People may choose or need to work for longer. Jobs are no longer for life and during a working lifetime an individual is likely to do a variety of jobs and may work either full-time or part-time at different stages. In a broad sense, work need not be for financial gain: voluntary or charity work brings many of the non-financial benefits of employment.

Just because someone has an illness, injury, or disability does not necessarily mean that they cannot work. There are many examples of people who work despite severe illness or disability. Likewise, most people with disabilities, whether these arise from ongoing illness or not, who want to, can work. Too often health professionals and others have equated the presence of an illness, injury, or disability with being unable to work.

On the other hand being out of work leads to poorer health and a shorter life.

Poor working conditions may cause illness and poor health but it is now clear that unemployment is damaging to both mental and physical health at all ages: people who are out of work have more illnesses and are likely to die younger. These health effects are discussed in more detail later. This poorer health leads to a greater need for health services. Re-entry into work leads to an improvement in health. Worklessness and the problems it can bring is now recognized as an important public health issue in the UK as highlighted in a recent Government White Paper on ways of improving the health of the nation.[1]

Only 50% of people with disabilities are in work compared with about 75% of the able-bodied working age population; the figure for those with a mental health problem is only 21% in employment.

The present costs of worklessness and incapacity are considerable. Physical or mental incapacity for work, particularly where this is long term, can have far reaching implications for individual patients, employers, and the overall economy. Sickness absence is estimated to cost employers over £11 billion per year,[2] although this may be a gross underestimate. Approximately 10% of long-term sickness absence accounts for three-quarters of these costs. Extra costs benefits (Disability Living Allowance, Care Allowance) and state incapacity benefits now cost about £20 billion a year (of which £6.7 billion is spent on Incapacity Benefit itself) compared with about £3.5 billion for unemployment benefits. This represents a fifth of UK benefit expenditure or 5.6% of total government expenditure. 2.7 million people are in receipt of state incapacity benefits with 700 000 people moving on to these benefits each year. Moreover, a substantial number of people on incapacity benefits do not fulfil the National Insurance entitlement criteria and thus receive no cash benefit. Instead these people receive 'credits only', which permit access to a range of other social security benefits, including NI contributions. The costs to individuals may be long-term social exclusion, ill health, and poverty. In addition, the cost to business is reflected in the recent steep rise in Employers Liability Insurance premiums. And there is a substantial though unquantified cost to the NHS and social services of managing the attendant physical and mental health problems associated with worklessness.

The effects of unemployment and worklessness in terms of health are only now been fully recognized. Unemployment causes poor health and health inequalities, and this effect is still seen after adjustment for social class, poverty, age, and pre-existing morbidity. Some of the key adverse effects are listed in Box 4.1. A person signed off-work sick for 6 months has only a 50% chance of returning to work. By 1 year it is 25% and by 2 years about 10%. One study showed that by 6 months off-work certified sick the majority of people were suffering from depression, whatever the initial presenting problem. Most importantly regaining work may reverse the adverse health effects of unemployment.

While it is right to consider the health consequences of worklessness and unemployment we also need to remember that despite the UK's comprehensive health and safety legislation too many people are still injured or made ill as a result of their work. Unsafe working conditions may be a direct cause of illness and poor health; improvements in health and safety risk management could prevent much avoidable sickness and disability.

Box 4.1 Adverse effects on health associated with worklessness include:

♦ Reduced psychological well being with a greater incidence of self harm, depression and anxiety.

♦ Increased smoking at the onset of unemployment. The prevalence of smoking is considerably higher among those who are unemployed.

♦ Increased alcohol consumption with unemployment especially in young men.

♦ Weight gain.

♦ Reduced physical activity and exercise.

♦ The use of illicit drugs in the young who are without work.

♦ Increased sexual risk taking in young men.

These facts should all be of concern to health professionals, particularly those practising in the field of occupational and disability assessment medicine, and underline the need to ensure that work is safe and healthy.

Legal framework

By law employers have a duty to provide a safe system of work for all employees. In the UK, under the Health and Safety at Work Act 1974(1) all employers have a legal duty to ensure the health, safety, and welfare of their employees. The Management Regulations give guidance to employers on meeting this duty to provide safe working practices. They require an employer to make a suitable and sufficient assessment of the risks to the health and safety of their employees.

Box 4.2 Examples of illness or injury in the UK attributed to work (Health and Safety Commission,[3] Health and Safety Executive[4])

♦ 2 million people suffer an illness that they believe has been caused by, or made worse by their work

♦ 24% of GP consultations with working age people are work related

♦ about 4% of all cancers have an occupational cause

♦ 0.5 million people have been made deaf by their work

♦ 0.5 million people believe that their job caused them to suffer mental illness and mental ill health causes 13.5 million lost working days a year

♦ musculoskeletal conditions cause 12.3 million lost working days a year, though not all of these episodes can be attributed to work

♦ more than 150 000 people have lung problems they believe to be work related.

The Approved Code of Practice (ACOP) to the Regulations states that employers, in undertaking their risk assessment, should identify groups of workers who might be particularly at risk, for example, disabled people.

The Disability Discrimination Act (DDA) 1995 aims to eliminate discrimination against disabled people—a group that may include many of those who have long-term health conditions or impairments. Apart from a general principle of non-discrimination in employment the act imposes a duty on employers to make reasonable adjustments to working arrangements. In many cases the 'reasonably practicable adjustments' to reduce workplace risks required under health and safety legislation will be the same as 'reasonable adjustments' under the DDA. Employers need to aware that they must fully explore the potential of both duties in order to avoid unfair treatment of an employee, or potential employee, with a health condition or disability. In discharging those duties employers and managers will often seek expert advice from occupational health professionals.

What is meant by the term 'vocational rehabilitation'?

An employment goal must be at the heart of vocational rehabilitation (VR), which is aimed at overcoming obstacles to work, i.e. to remain in or return to work, or access employment for the first time. This could relate to full-time or part-time employment, self-employment or even voluntary work. Those with a key interest in rehabilitation, the stakeholders, include individual workers and their families, healthcare providers, employee representatives, employers, insurers, and government. All these stakeholders need to start from the basic premise that the individual is 'employable' until proven otherwise. In short any form of rehabilitation needs to consider the personal and social needs of the individual as well as any physical or mental functional needs. The necessary medical, social, and psychological interventions, to help the individual overcome obstacles to work then need to be identified by assessment. A discussion of 'obstacles' and how to address them follows in the next section.

The British Society of Rehabilitation Medicine (BSRM) report *Vocational Rehabilitation: the way forward* (2nd edition)[5] defined VR as 'a process whereby those disadvantaged by illness or disability can be enabled to access, maintain or return to employment, or other useful occupation'. The BSRM saw rehabilitation as:

- An active process by which people disabled by injury or disease regain their former abilities or, if full recovery is impossible, achieve their optimum physical, mental, social, and vocational capacity and are integrated into the most appropriate environment of their choice.

- The use of all means aimed at reducing the impact of disabling and handicapping conditions and at enabling disabled people to achieve optimal social integration.

- A process of active change by which a person who has become disabled acquires the knowledge and skills needed for optimal physical, psychological, and social function.

This may involve rehabilitation, (re)training and resettlement.

The Government's Framework for Vocational Rehabilitation[6] states that VR:

- Is a process to overcome the obstacles or barriers an individual faces when accessing, remaining, or returning to work following injury illness or impairment. This includes the procedures in place to support the individual and/or the employer or others (e.g. family carers) including help to access rehabilitation services and manage their delivery.

- Also includes a wide range of interventions to help individuals with a health condition and/or impairment overcome obstacles to work, e.g. assessment of needs, retraining and capacity building, return to work management by employers, reasonable adjustments and control measures, disability awareness, condition management, and medical treatment.

The Government's Framework for Vocational Rehabilitation[6] reviewed current evidence and summarized stakeholder views. The review of research on VR found that although there is good evidence related to restoring function, particularly for some health conditions such as back pain, evidence for what is effective VR in the UK is contradictory and inconclusive. Specifically:

◆ Much of the research on VR is small scale and difficult to apply more generally; there are few longitudinal studies that track the employment and relate this to any VR interventions received; there are few randomized control trials that measure impact on employment outcomes that are not influenced by unobserved individual, economic, and social characteristics.

◆ The factors that affect entry into employment and return to work for people with health conditions and/or impairments are still not fully understood.

◆ The influence that VR service and delivery processes have on gaining or retaining employment over and above other factors that affect employment outcomes are not clear.

◆ The evidence on what types of intervention help people return to work after a period of sickness absence is contradictory and inconclusive and cannot provide a definitive guide to effective practice for VR.

Who might be helped by vocational rehabilitation?

It is also worth considering the people for whom VR interventions could be an option to help them gain or retain employment. These include people of working age:

◆ Currently in employment who are experiencing difficulty retaining employment because of a health condition or impairment.

◆ Temporarily absent from work because of a health condition or impairment.

◆ With a health condition or impairment for whom absence becomes longer term and who may become unemployed as a result.

◆ Who have not worked for some time, or never worked, because of a health condition or impairment.

Moreover, in relation to ill health caused by work where compensation becomes a factor, minimizing the extent and adverse effects of injuries can be a better and fairer solution for all parties than simply trying to put a financial value on the harm done. There is a strong moral case for ensuring that when workers are injured, impaired, or made ill as a consequence of workplace activities, they receive appropriate support and not just financial compensation.

Why a biopsychosocial approach to rehabilitation?

The traditional concept of rehabilitation is a secondary intervention to *restore* patients as far as possible to their previous condition after disease or injury (within the limitations imposed by pathology and impairments), to develop to the maximum extent their (residual) physical, mental, and social functioning, and, where appropriate, to return them to (modified) work. This is a medical approach assuming persisting physical or mental impairment due to a serious medical condition, and that rehabilitation is a separate stage distinct from medical treatment and carried out after treatment which fails to achieve full recovery is concluded.

However, that approach does not fit most conditions that underpin incapacity for work in the UK. The population of working age people who are most likely to lose their job and be excluded from work do not fit the traditional model of severe bodily or mental impairment (leading to a long-term disability)—they are much more likely to have a health condition with essentially subjective features that impact on the ability to work.[7,8] Leading examples include mild to moderate mental health problems and painful conditions, such as low-back pain and upper limb disorders. The goal for such people is not just clinical recovery but restoration of functioning and participation, including work. Many people with severe medical conditions do work; conversely many workless people with a 'health condition' have little objective evidence of disease and/or impairment. In fact the more severe medical conditions account for a minority of disability and incapacity benefits recipients in the UK;[8] some 75% of benefit recipients of working age have less severe health conditions, for example mental health, musculoskeletal and cardiorespiratory conditions, referred to here as *common health problems*.

This is not to say that rehabilitation from severe medical conditions such as stroke, head injury and spinal trauma is not important. Such impairments usually require the input of specialist professionals with their own body of knowledge and expertise with a considerable medical element. The following discussion is of relevance to those people with more severe conditions as well as those with common health complaints.

It is necessary to reconsider the theoretical and conceptual basis of rehabilitation, using the biopsychosocial framework to relate components of disability, obstacles to recovery, and rehabilitation interventions to overcome these obstacles (Table 4.1). The biopsychosocial model is an individual-centred model that considers the person, his or her health problem, and social context. 'Biological' refers to the physical or mental health condition, 'psychological' recognizes that personal/psychological factors (e.g. beliefs, attitudes, perceptions, etc.) also influence functioning, and 'social' recognizes the importance of the social context, systems, culture and pressures and constraints on behaviour and functioning. The model suggests that there can be biological, psychological, and social obstacles to employment that can interact, and, in the case of rehabilitation prevent a return to employment.

This approach lends itself particularly well to common health complaints such as low-back pain and non-psychotic mental health disorders. This area has recently been extensively reviewed by Waddell and Burton whose conclusions are summarized below.[9] In examining the evidence for the effectiveness of biopsychosocial interventions for different types of health conditions, Waddell and Burton show how such multidimensional interventions are most effective in rehabilitation.

Obstacles to recovery and return to work

Recovery from common health problems is generally to be expected, and long-term incapacity is not inevitable. A high prevalence of subjective health complaints has been reported among Nordic adults:[10] 'tiredness' featured in half of the population sample questioned; at least 25% reported 'worry' and 'depression', and musculoskeletal complaints featured prominently, with 'neck pain' in 41% of women. More than 50% of those sampled reported two or more health

Table 4.1 Elements of a rehabilitation programme: addressing disability and obstacles to recovery

Components of disability	Obstacles to recovery	Elements of a rehabilitation intervention
Bio-	[Medical condition] Activity level versus job demands	[Healthcare] Increasing activity levels and restoring function
Psycho-	Individual psychological factors Perceptions of work	Shifting beliefs, attitudes + behavioural change
Social	Socio-demographic Work-related [Organizational, System]	Modified work involving the employer; all players on side. [Policy]

complaints in the preceding 30 days. Moreover, the prevalence of substantial complaints when rated for severity ranged from 4% for headache in men to 26% for tiredness in women. Substantial musculoskeletal complaints ranged from 9% to 17% across genders. Similar findings have been reported in Great Britain.[11] Most acute episodes settle quickly. The great majority affected by these common health problems remain at work or return to work; only about 1% go on to long-term incapacity.[12] Essentially these are ordinary people with manageable health problems if given the right opportunities, support and encouragement.[12] In other words there is often no biomedical reason for being permanently 'disabled'. Thus, in summary, the epidemiology of common health problems shows that: (1) prevalence rates are extremely high in the general population of working age; (2) most episodes resolve uneventfully, or at least most people do manage to cope despite some persistent or recurrent symptoms; (3) most people remain at work most of the time, and the large majority of those who do take sickness absence manage to return to work quite quickly, with or without formal healthcare; and (4) for only a few do the symptoms become intolerable and incapacitating. Thus, these health conditions on their own do not explain long-term incapacity.

So why do some people not recover as expected? To answer this question requires a shift of focus from aspects of the health condition, towards factors that may be acting as hindrances or impediments to normal recovery, restoration of function, and (return to) work. More explicitly, these factors may be conceived as 'obstacles to recovery' and 'barriers to (return to) work' that are potential targets for some form of rehabilitation intervention.[13,14]

The concept of 'obstacles' was developed clinically, and initially focused on clinical and psychological factors. Extending that concept to rehabilitation is a logical step, but obstacles to clinical recovery are not necessarily the same as obstacles to returning to work; the latter include a broader range of non-clinical, work-related, and social factors.

Biological (health condition), psychological, and social (especially work-related) obstacles to return to work all appear to be important, accepting that there is overlap and interaction between the different dimensions, and that their relative importance may vary in different individuals and settings, and over time.[15] Individual assessment of these obstacles may provide a problem-oriented approach to rehabilitation that can: (1) guide clinical evaluation; (2) identify obstacles to return to work; (3) develop targeted interventions to overcome these obstacles; (4) facilitate rehabilitation interventions.[12,16]

The emerging consensus from research is that rehabilitation for the more common health conditions usually requires a combination of therapeutic and social interventions that address the clinical problem *and* issues in the individual's physical and social environment. Most importantly rehabilitation needs to be seen as a *process*; it is a function of services and not necessarily a separate service.

Rehabilitation has often been described as multidisciplinary, but that places too much emphasis on the professional input and perspective. To understand and develop rehabilitation for the common health complaints, it is more helpful to focus on the elements of the intervention. Taking the biopsychosocial model and the WHO framework[17] as the starting point, it follows that biopsychosocial issues can constitute obstacles to recovery, either singly or in combination. Thus, to address health-related incapacity for work and overcome these obstacles, a rehabilitation intervention should address all three of these dimensions. Too often one or more of these dimensions is ignored and attempts at rehabilitation fail.

Biological interventions for increasing activity levels and restoring function

Modern clinical management of the majority of health complaints emphasizes the importance of restoring function as the best means of relieving symptoms. Most people recover rapidly and return to their normal activities and work, and for them it may be argued that routine healthcare effectively does rehabilitate. For those who do not recover rapidly, healthcare and continued symptomatic treatment alone is not enough. In longer-term incapacity, the biological dimension and healthcare are only part, and often the lesser part, of the problem.

For example almost all successful rehabilitation programmes for musculoskeletal and cardiorespiratory conditions include some form of active exercise or graded activity component. The key element is activity *per se*, with the immediate goal of overcoming limitations and restoring activity levels: the ultimate goal is to increase participation and restore social functioning. The same principles then seem equally applicable to mental health conditions, where increased physical activity has been shown to improve depression and general mental health.[18–20]

In principle, there should be steadily increasing increments of activity level, which are time-dependent rather than symptom-dependent. Properly implemented, a programme of increasing activity will increase a sense of well-being, confidence, and self-efficacy, which in turn will promote adherence. There is a clear paradox between medical advice to rest and rehabilitation activity. Contrary to traditional thinking, there is now strong evidence that inactivity leads to physical and mental deterioration,[21] while work is good for general physical and mental health and well-being. Shifting erroneous perceptions and beliefs about rest and activity can lead to new perspectives on the therapeutic value of (controlled) work.

Cognitive-behavioural and educational interventions

Attitudes, beliefs, and behaviour can aggravate and perpetuate symptoms and disability, so addressing these issues is an essential part of management. This principle seems to apply generally across all rehabilitation for physical and mental symptoms, stress, distress, and disability.

Most psychological and behavioural approaches now combine *cognitive-behavioural* principles.[22,23]

- Cognitive approaches focus on mental events—changing how patients think about and deal with their symptoms; behavioural approaches focus on changing patients' illness behaviour. Cognitive approaches try to teach patients to re-think their beliefs about their symptoms, and what they do about them, building confidence in their own abilities and skills.

- Behavioural approaches try to extinguish symptom-driven behaviour by withdrawal of reinforcements such as medication, sympathetic attention, rest, and release from duties, and to encourage healthy behaviour by positive reinforcement.

- Cognitive-behavioural approaches try to address all psychological and behavioural aspects of the illness experience, in order to: change beliefs, change behaviour, and improve functioning. There is accumulating evidence for the applicability of the cognitive-behavioural approach across all the common health complaints.[24–26]

Changing beliefs and behaviour may also share some educational principles around developing skills and confidence, including concepts of engagement, enablement, and empowerment.

Social and occupational interventions

For many of the common health complaints, work-related interventions may be as appropriate and effective as healthcare for helping workers to remain in, return to, or move into work. The minimum social component of a rehabilitation intervention appears to be agreement by all the stakeholders (patient, all health professionals, and the employer) that the primary goal is job retention or reintegration. The setting of the rehabilitation intervention may carry important, implicit messages: healthcare commonly removes workers from the workplace and may actually act as a barrier to work; locating rehabilitation interventions in the workplace may conceptually, and in practice, link them closer to their ultimate goal.

Physical and mental demands of work are a potential barrier, which may be reduced by ergonomic interventions, physical or psychosocial accommodations, or modified work. Modified work may take the form of (temporary) individual adaptations to reduce demand, or it may be a matter of changing the work organization, with the primary goal of facilitating return to work—i.e. a route to sustained, regular work. The provision of modified work is a workplace intervention by the employer, not a healthcare intervention: inappropriate advice about modified work by doctors and therapists may be counter-productive and actually create a barrier to return to work. A review of 29 empirical studies has strongly demonstrated the success of modified work as an intervention[27] that halved the number of work days lost and the number of injured workers who went on to chronic disability.

Addressing psychosocial and inter-personal issues around return to work may be as important as modifying physical demands. The importance of the employer and a structured return to work programme has been recognized. In such a programme: the employer contacts the absent worker soon after the onset of sickness absence; the supervisor informs the sick person's co-workers about the situation; adjustments to tasks performed by the sick worker upon return to work are considered (and co-workers are made fully aware); there are clear routines for the programme and everyone knows who is responsible; the supervisor or line manager create a positive emotional atmosphere.

The principle of structured return to work should be a part of any rehabilitation intervention for common health complaints. Communication is an absolute prerequisite for a co-ordinated intervention[28–30] and demands a common model and language, involving 'getting all the players on side'.

In terms of the biopsychosocial model of disability, as adopted by the International Classification of Function,[17] personal and environmental factors may have even greater influence on functioning than any underlying impairment when it comes to incapacity for work and sickness absence.[31] There is now considerable evidence that the development of chronicity and incapacity depend even more on psychosocial factors. Disability is restricted activity, which is ultimately a matter of behaviour. As Waddell and Burton[9] put it: 'Behaviour depends on personal attitudes and beliefs, coping strategies, emotions and psychological distress, but is also a matter of free will and personal responsibility'. Environmental factors exert powerful feedback and constraints on behaviour.

The role of the health services and healthcare professionals

Traditional healthcare may provide symptomatic relief and be sufficient for most patients, but trends of sickness absence and incapacity for work suggest it is not always sufficient in itself for successful re-entry into work. Based on the above analysis any proposed rehabilitation intervention/programme should:

- Have primarily vocational goals and outcome measures.
- Should be multidimensional in nature (which may, but does not necessarily, mean multidisciplinary), and address the biological, psychological, and social components of sickness, disability, and work incapacity, which feature obstacles to recovery and barriers to (return to) work.
- Be designed to additionally answer the following questions:
  —How does any healthcare element increase activity levels and restore function (as opposed to purely symptomatic management)?
  —What does the intervention do to shift beliefs and behaviour?
  —How does the intervention overcome obstacles and facilitate return to work?

There is a pressing need to shift attitudes to health and work rehabilitation needs to encompass the concept of prevention of long-term disability and work incapacity by parallel interventions from healthcare and workplace rehabilitation. In this context healthcare professionals should strongly challenge two incorrect assumptions:

◆ First, the assumption that work will be harmful—current evidence suggests that work is a minor contributory factor for most common conditions and that work is generally good for physical and mental health.[13]

◆ Secondly, there is an assumption that rest from work is part of treatment—on the contrary, modern approaches to clinical management stress the importance of continuing ordinary activities and early return to work as an essential ingredient of treatment.[32]

General medical practitioners (GPs) as non-occupational health specialists in fact play a key part in relation to fitness for work advice and back-to-work decisions by employers. Additional rehabilitation services—whether NHS or private—are needed to manage the conditions presented by their patients of working age. Sick certificates issued by doctors (usually GPs) undertaking the clinical care of patients record the medical advice to refrain from work. Most doctors who issue certificates and give such advice do not have adequate training or expertise in occupational health or disability evaluation and are therefore often unable to consider the real grounds for incapacity. For the majority of patients who return to work rapidly, this may provide a good enough approximation, but for those who receive repeated and long-term certification it is not. Surveys estimate[33] that over 70% of employers make decisions on fitness for work on the basis of a doctor's certificate. Patients and doctors are often unaware of and fail to consider the likely long-term implications: sick certificates initially issued almost casually for acute illness may then label people as sick and disabled, and actually promote long-term incapacity. Most patients and doctors do not realize that a proportion of those who remain off work will lose their jobs—and a medical certificate does not protect them.

We suggest that the health aspects of rehabilitation need to encompass:

◆ The concept of clinical management aimed at restoring maximal function (work capacity) from day 1 of illness or injury, i.e. it is an integral part of the business of every healthcare professional who treats patients.

◆ Restoring function and ability rather than just restoring health. Results of a recent Government Consultation exercise[6] indicate that a substantial majority of respondents agree that the core objective of rehabilitation is restoration of effective social integration and functioning which includes work.

◆ Integration of therapeutic and other interventions.

◆ Timely availability of help, responsive to users' needs.

◆ Rehabilitation as a function of services rather than a separate service (which has been the traditional NHS approach).

◆ Recognition that sickness and work incapacity are fundamentally social problems, in the resolution of which healthcare, though important, offers no solution on its own.

This thinking about rehabilitation is very different to the traditional model but many doctors, patients, and employers still seem to be stuck somewhere around the traditional model. The shift from a predominantly medical model of disability to a social model and the accompanying re-definition of the relative roles of health professionals and people with disabilities is reflected in the concept of 'enablement', which is now seen as central to rehabilitation. Enablement has been defined as: 'an individual-centred, individual-driven process for achieving individual goals'. This transfers the balance of power from health professionals to the person with disabilities.

The person with healthcare needs and/or disabilities moves from being a relatively passive recipient of healthcare and rehabilitation processes to achieve health service goals, to a more active role as an active user of health service and rehabilitation resources to achieve their own rehabilitation goals. Correspondingly, the role of health professionals becomes more one of supporting and facilitating that process.

Vocational assessment

VR is clearly dependent on labour market opportunities, including availability, quality, pay levels, and security of employment; as well as personal capabilities related to the physical and psychological demands of work. Vocational assessment refers to the process of recruitment and placement of people who face health or disability obstacles to work and is part of the general management of disability in the workplace. At an individual level it is the process of determining a person's vocational assets, limitations, behaviour, and physical and mental tolerances usually in a specific type of work environment. In order to do this an analysis of core requirements of the job usually needs to be undertaken so as to match the suitability of the person to the job. From the previous discussion it will be apparent that the ideal rehabilitation process is one where the medical and vocational elements are phased into one with assessment as a continuous part of these activities. Box 4.3 sets out some important elements of vocational assessment.

Box 4.3 Terms relevant to vocational assessment

- **Job description**: description of the tasks of the job as outlined by the employer; it should be as objectively and factually based as possible and must include any core medical or statutory criteria, which must be met along with health and safety standards.

- **Job analysis**: an objective ergonomically based evaluation of the job, both the essential and peripheral tasks, and the workplace usually provided in a standardized format.

- **Functional capacity assessment (FCA)**: refers to the evaluation of the employee or potential employee in terms of their capacity to perform the essential duties of the job. Standardized FCAs have been developed which use highly sophisticated apparatus to provide assessments with a high level of objectivity, validity, reliability, and predictive power. A FCA may, for example, assess an individual's capacity and performance in walking, standing or manual dexterity.

- **Psychological assessment**: assessment by an occupational psychologist can determine the impact of psychological factors on an individual's ability to perform a job and may comprise part of a FCA.

- **Work hardening**: simulates dynamic job functions and demands to ensure that the relevant capabilities are properly developed to meet job demands; this may be done by using work samples or 'on the job'.

- **Reasonable accommodation**: the DDA imposes a legal obligation to make reasonable adjustments to facilitate the employment of disabled people. Such adjustments may also make good business sense if they help the employer to avoid the costs of sickness absence and ill-health retirement. They may include: adjustments to premises; modifying equipment; providing support staff; altering working hours; reallocating duties; and providing additional training.

The interface between occupational health professionals and other stakeholders

A new approach to VR within the UK will require the engagement of Government and all stakeholders building upon current best practice, pilots, and research. The UK has the best overall workplace safety record in Europe but the record on occupational health does not compare so well. Illness or disability is treated as an 'on/off' switch all too often leading to prolonged absence, unemployment, or long-term inactivity. The current evidence suggests that much of this inactivity and absence could be avoided.

All stakeholders have to respond with a better service to those whose health conditions places them at risk of unemployment or inactivity. This will help individuals and their families, control costs, grow capacity in the labour market, and realize the benefits of the social inclusion and other material and psychological advantages that employment can bring. Although, far from comprehensive, there is an increasing body of evidence to support the proposition that managed and carefully structured intervention can help tackle the most common and important problems, including mental health, cardiovascular, and musculoskeletal conditions.

This is not just a health led, medically focused, agenda—all stakeholders must play a new part (see below)—but in any policy initiative with 'rehabilitation' in the title, there will always be a public expectation that the health services (both state and private) will play a major part.

The role elements in Box 4.4 are suggested as a minimum.

Box 4.4 **The role of stakeholders in vocational rehabilitation**

Vision

GPs, hospital doctors, occupational physicians, and employers, and wider society working together to facilitate optimal workplace rehabilitation for all ill or injured persons.

Aims and objectives

For the ill or injured person rehabilitation will aid and support physical and mental recovery and will aim to restore function. The objective will be a return to optimum participation in daily activities, including work. This outcome will best be achieved when all stakeholders work together to ensure that there will be, as required: fair recruitment, workplace adjustments, redeployment and adequate support. In turn this will be achieved when healthcare professionals, particularly GPs, hospital doctors, and occupational physicians, work together and with other stakeholders.

Returning to work

Healthcare professionals have an important role in helping their patients to return to work following an injury or illness. The doctor's role must go wider than diagnosis and evidence based clinical management of the patient's condition. Doctors should provide and communicate appropriate information to the patient and employer and should work closely with all stakeholders, including other health professionals, to facilitate the patient's safe and timely return to the most appropriate employment. This role requires doctors to recognize, and support, the employee–employer relationship and to have a good working knowledge of

Box 4.4 The role of stakeholders in vocational rehabilitation *(continued)*

the many support services and interventions that can assist the return to work, the elements of which:

- require that the employee's functional capabilities at least match the physical and psychological requirements of the job.
- may be hastened by a managed increase in activity before the patient is fit to resume work at full capacity.
- primarily involve a dialogue between the employer and employee, where necessary informed by expert medical advice.
- require advice and guidance from a range of health professionals such as: occupational physicians, GPs, hospital specialist doctors, occupational health nurses, physiotherapists, and psychologists. Illness, sickness, and disability are not a matter for healthcare alone; they are equally a matter of occupational health.

The role of the employer

- To make early contact and maintain frequent contact with the sick or injured employee. (This contact should preferably be by a manager or supervisor closely involved with the employee's work.)
- To seek to elucidate which aspects of work the patient is unable to perform and to discuss modifications to enable an early return to work.
- To take action to put these aspirations into effect in a planned and co-ordinated fashion.

The role of the patient's own doctor (GP or hospital specialist)

- To be aware of the limitations and restrictions imposed by the patient's condition both at home and at work.
- To incorporate a timely return to work into an evidence-based care plan for each patient.
- To identify and address obstacles to such plans.
- To recognize the possible consequences of inactivity for the patient.

The role of the occupational health specialist

- To combine an understanding of the medical issues with an understanding of the requirements of the specific work and the workplace.
- To provide experience in addressing barriers to return to work by advising the employee, the employer, the GP, and other health professionals on the full range of occupational health issues.

The key elements of a return to work plan which require action by healthcare practitioners are:

- **Communication**: e.g. the GP should encourage early communication between the patient and the employer who should keep in early and frequent contact with a sick employee.

Continued

Box 4.4 The role of stakeholders in vocational rehabilitation *(continued)*

- **Recognition of obstacles to recovery and barriers to a return to work**: e.g. early recognition of potential obstacles to recovery of function and barriers to participation in work allows active intervention including appropriate adjustments.

- **Knowledge of support services**: e.g. the availability of multidisciplinary support in facilitating the safe and timely return to work is important. Such support may include health interventions, such as physiotherapy, or other work-based interventions.

- **Active management (rather than a passive 'wait and see' approach)**: e.g. *(with employee consent)* the GP could provide the employer with key factual information on the employee's **fitness** status; also whether there are likely to be functional limitations or restrictions that are temporary or permanent, with an estimate of recovery time.

- **A positive outlook**: a working life should be a realistic expectation for most people, even those with considerable functional restrictions or limitations. It will very rarely be appropriate for a doctor to advise a patient of working age that they will be unable to ever work again.

- **A patient-centred approach**: patients should be encouraged to take an active role in, and to take appropriate responsibility for, their return to work, and to communicate directly and with their manager/employer wherever possible.

Examples of current rehabilitation service provision for people with health conditions or disabilities

Recent Government initiatives

At a strategic and policy level a great deal of attention is at last turning to the challenges of VR. Some recent and current Government initiatives are set out in the Annexe that concludes this chapter.

Department for Work and Pensions (DWP) Jobcentre Plus Services

In Great Britain the state funded Jobcentre Plus provides a range of well-established employment and training measures to help disabled people into employment. Working from the premise that some 70% of unemployed disabled people are helped through the mainstream activities and programmes of Jobcentre Plus, that leaves the remainder requiring help through specialist disability support run by Jobcentre Plus. These are detailed below.

Disability Employment Advisers (DEAs)

DEAs aim to provide coherent employment advice and assessment for employers and disabled people. Their services are accessed through the local jobcentre or Jobcentre Plus office.

The function of DEAs is to help disabled people select, obtain and keep jobs and help employers develop good recruitment policies. This includes offering support to employers to retain employees who become disabled, or for whom a worsening disability poses a threat to continued employment. They have access to the full range of Jobcentre Plus disability and mainstream programmes. (See below.)

Work Preparation

For those disabled people who are not yet ready for work, Work Preparation provides a tailor-made package of help designed to assist them to return to work. The purpose of the programme is to help jobseekers to:

+ understand the effects of their disability on work-related activities
+ build their confidence to pursue work opportunities effectively
+ make an effective occupational choice
+ improve interpersonal skills at work
+ re-learn basic skills.

About 9000 people a year are helped by Work Preparation.

Vocational Training

This is available for those disabled people who need it. Most will take their place alongside non-disabled people but where no suitable local provision is available, residential training may be offered at 14 colleges or providers.

Residential training providers (RTPs) have become specialist providers of training for disabled people. These are more likely to be able to cater for the often complex needs of disabled people than mainstream provision. The client group includes those with a physical and/or sensory disability; a deteriorating medical condition; mental disabilities; and behavioural and learning difficulties (and frequently a combination of the four).

The providers enable trainees to move towards social inclusion through an inclusive approach to meeting their individual training, support, and caring needs. This incorporates: psychological and counselling support; specialist medical facilities and expertise; therapeutic support; technical support; assessment and employment preparation advice and guidance; enhanced staff expertise; and specially designed buildings and facilities.

The providers consist of four large and three small residential training facilities catering for all disabilities, one specialist residential training adviser for people with hearing impairments, and six for adults with visual impairment.

Access to Work (AtW) programme

This is delivered by Jobcentre Plus, and aims to provide support to overcome the effects of disability at work so that disabled people can participate in mainstream employment. Disabled people apply through their local DEA or by going directly to an AtW Adviser at a regional AtW business centre.

The AtW programme provides support tailored to the needs of individual disabled people to enable them to overcome the effects of their disability in the workplace. Applicants must be in, or about to enter, *paid work*. Support can take the form of help with the cost of getting to work, help with the cost of aids and adaptations to equipment, computers or the workplace and with the cost of a support worker. The latter can take many forms, e.g. carer, driver, job coach, advocate, job-aide, counsellor, travel buddy, communicator/note-taker for deaf people, personal reader/helper for those with a visual impairment and job designer. Jobcentre Plus expects to help about 18 000 new applicants a year with this programme.

An AtW Adviser will work together with the applicant and the employer to arrive at the most effective solution to meet the needs of the disabled person in the workplace. The support agreed by Jobcentre Plus continues for a maximum of 3 years, when it is reviewed. If continuing help (e.g. support worker) is still needed, then further grants will be for less than 100% of the cost, as detailed in the following paragraphs.

Access to Work pays 100% of the approved costs for anyone entering paid employment from unemployment or who has been in paid employment for less than 6 weeks. Unemployed people do not have to be on Job Seekers Allowance. People who change jobs get 100% funding. AtW can also meet 100% of approved costs for help with fares to work and with communicator support for deaf people at a job interview whatever the employment status of the disabled applicant.

For all other employed people (including cases reviewed at the 3-year stage) a system of cost sharing applies under which AtW does not pay the first £300 in any 3-year period; it meets 80% of costs between £300 and £10 000; and it pays for all costs over £10 000. Self-employed people are not asked to contribute towards the cost of their support.

Job Introduction Scheme

This provides a weekly grant of £75 in 2005 towards the cost of employing people with disabilities for a trial period of employment. This is usually 6 weeks but may be extended to a total of 13 weeks. The scheme is for use at the discretion of Jobcentre Plus staff in situations where a disabled applicant is considered suitable, but the employer has genuine doubts about the individual's ability to cope with the proposed job or place of work. It is expected that 3000 people a year will be helped by this measure.

WORKSTEP

Jobcentre Plus also manages WORKSTEP, the Government's **supported employment programme.** The programme was introduced in April 2001 and provides support for about 26 000 people. The aim of WORKSTEP is to provide tailored support to find, secure, and retain jobs for people with disabilities who have more complex barriers to finding work and keeping work. WORKSTEP provides the support and opportunity for people to progress to open employment where this is the right option for the individual. The programme also retains its role in providing longer-term support for people who need it.

WORKSTEP provides a wide range of supported work opportunities that meet the differing needs of disabled people. Supported employees work in jobs or in supported factories and businesses.

The programme is delivered in partnership with over 240 local authority, private sector, and voluntary organizations, including Remploy Ltd and The Shaw Trust.

Jobcentre Plus has adopted the Business Excellence Model to continuously improve its services including work preparation/employment rehabilitation; for example there is an expectation of 50% positive outcomes (into jobs, training or education) from work preparation/employment rehabilitation contracts.

New Deal for Disabled People (NDDP)

This is the first programme specifically designed to support people on disability and health-related benefits into employment. Participation in NDDP is entirely voluntary.

NDDP pilots ran from September 1998 to June 2001 and helped over 8000 people into work. Based on this success, and building on the best practice from those pilots, NDDP was extended from July 2001 across England, Scotland, and Wales with the introduction of a network of Job Brokers from private, voluntary, and public sector organizations or combinations of these in partnership who:

- help customers understand and compete in the labour market;
- agree with each customer the most appropriate route into employment for them;
- support customers in finding and keeping paid employment;

- work closely with providers of training and other provision where a customer needs additional support;
- work with local employers to identify their needs and match them with the skills of their customers; and
- support customers during their first 6 months in employment.

The programme is aimed at unemployed and economically inactive people, including those with disabilities, in receipt of benefit for 6 months or more and their dependent partners. The programme is voluntary and offers:

- a guaranteed minimum take home income of £170 a week or £9000 a year for those taking up full-time employment;
- flexible support for part-time and full-time work and self-employment;
- a tax and national insurance free Employment Credit (paid to the individual) of £60 a week for up to 12 months (£40 for part-time work);
- personal advice;
- In-work Training Grant of up to £750;
- jobsearch help.

Pathways to Work pilots

Launched at the end of 2003 in pilot areas the 'Pathways to Work' approach offers enhanced support to those who are in receipt of a state incapacity benefit, including specialist personal advisers, a series of six work focused interviews and a £40 per week return to work credit and a 'Choices Package'. These voluntary components include a Condition Management Programme (CMP), delivered by the NHS, to help clients better manage their condition and to reduce the disability produced by chronic illness/injury. From 2006 the pilots are being extended to cover 30% of the country.

Private and voluntary sector

In addition the private and voluntary sector provide a huge range of rehabilitation services and support, often in close partnership with the state (NHS, Jobcentre Plus). Leading examples include Shaw Trust and Remploy.

Guidance to healthcare professionals

The DWP Chief Medical Adviser has issued a guide for medical practitioners and other health professionals (IB 204—*A Guide for Registered medical Practitioners*, DWP, 2004), which contains full details of the statutory certification process for fitness to work and also information on other benefits and services designed to help people get back to work. It is available on-line at www.dwp.gov.uk/medical.

Summary

- Prolonged absence from normal activities, including work, is often detrimental to a person's mental, physical, and social well-being, whereas a timely return to appropriate work benefits the patient and his or her family by enhancing recovery and reducing disability.
- An approach to rehabilitation based upon a biopsychosocial model is necessary to identify and address the obstacles to recovery and barriers to (return to) work. It should also meet the

needs of those with common health problems who do not recover in a timely fashion and identify the roles of key stakeholders.

♦ Rehabilitation is dependent on labour market opportunities, including availability, quality, pay levels, and security of employment; as well as personal capabilities related to the physical and psychological demands of work.

♦ A patient's return to function and work as soon as possible after an illness or injury should be encouraged and supported by employers, occupational and other health professionals, fellow employees, and rehabilitation service providers.

♦ A safe and timely return to work also preserves a skilled and stable workforce for employees and society, and reduces demands on health and social services, as well as on sickness absence schemes and disability payments.

Annexe: Vocational rehabilitation—some examples of recent UK Government strategic developments

At a strategic and policy level a great deal of attention is at last turning to the challenges of VR. Some recent and current government initiatives are set out here.

Securing Health Together (2000)

A 10-year, cross-government occupational health policy that aims to achieve: a 20% reduction in the incidence of work-related ill health; a 20% reduction in ill health to members of the public caused by work activity; a 30% reduction in the number of work days lost due to work-related ill health; and that everyone currently in employment but off work due to ill health or disability is, where necessary and appropriate, made aware of opportunities for rehabilitation back into work as early as possible. The initiative also recognizes that everyone currently not in employment due to ill health or disability is, where necessary and appropriate, made aware of and offered opportunities to prepare for and find work. There is an associated website with further information on the policy at www.ohstrategy.net.

Pathways to Work

There are 2.7 million people of working age that receive incapacity benefit because of a health condition. We know that about three-quarters of them say they would like to work. Launched at the end of 2003 in pilot areas, the 'Pathways to Work' approach offers enhanced support to those who are in receipt of incapacity benefit, including specialist personal advisers; provides a series of six work focused interviews and a £40 per week return to work credit and a 'Choices Package'. These voluntary components include a Condition Management Programme (CMP), delivered by the NHS, to help participating clients better manage their condition and to reduce the disability produced by chronic illness/injury.

National Service Framework for Mental Health

This National Service Framework addresses the mental health needs of working-aged adults up to 65. It is founded on knowledge-based practice and partnership working between those who use and those who provide services; between different clinicians and practitioners; across different parts of the NHS; and between the NHS and local government. It also reaches out to the community, to individual groups and organizations, including the voluntary, independent, and business sectors. 'Standard One' aims to combat discrimination against individuals and groups with mental health problems, and to promote their social inclusion. Mental health problems can result from the range of adverse factors associated with social exclusion and can itself also be a cause of social exclusion. For example, in relation to health and work:

◆ unemployed people are twice as likely to have depression as people in work;

◆ children in the poorest households are three times more likely to have mental health problems than children in well off households;

◆ half of all women and a quarter of all men will be affected by depression at some period during their lives.

NHS Plus

This is a network of over 100 NHS occupational health departments that meet a number of quality standards and provide occupational health (OH) support to non-NHS employers locally. In addition, the NHS Plus website (www.nhsplus.nhs.uk) is an open source of information on occupational health matters for the both employees and employers. NHS Plus sponsors research and runs an evidence-based guidance project.

Job Retention and Rehabilitation pilots (JRRP)

This ground breaking 5-year randomized controlled trial has been working to evaluate the effectiveness of a number of interventions aimed at job retention. The interventions are directed at health, the workplace, or a combination of the two. The aim is to establish what works best, for whom, and in what circumstances, and is directed towards those who have been off work for between 6 and 26 weeks.

National Employment and Health Innovations Network

Funded by the Departments of Health and DWP, this brings together those who are active in a wide range of work-related health projects related particularly to employment issues, allowing best practice to be shared and demonstrating the range of initiatives.

New Deal

The DWP provides a range of rehabilitation-focused services for people of working age, providing financial help and support. **New Deal** is a key part of the Government's strategy to get people back to work. It gives people on benefits, including those with health problems or disabilities the help and support they need to look for work, including training and job preparation (www.dwp.gov.uk).

References

1 *Choosing health: making healthier choices easier.* CM 6374. London: Department of Health, The Stationery Office, 2005.

2 Tyler A. The costs for industry. In: *What about the workers?* Conference Proceedings. London: Royal Society of Medicine Press, 2004.

3 Health and Safety Commission. *Management of health and safety at work.* Regulations, 1999. Approved Code of Practice. Sudbury: HSE Books, 2000.

4 Health and Safety Commission. *A strategy for workplace health and safety in Great Britain to 2010 and beyond.* MISC 643, CIO 02/04, 2004

5 Frank AO. *Vocational rehabilitation—the way forward,* 2nd edn. London: British Society of Rehabilitation Medicine, 2003.

6 *A framework for vocational rehabilitation.* London: Department for Work and Pensions, 2004.

7 Waddell G, Aylward M, Sawney P. *Back pain, incapacity for work and social security benefits: an international literature review and analysis.* London: The Royal Society of Medicine Press, 2002.

8 Aylward, M. Needless unemployment: a public health crisis? In *What about the Workers?* Conference Proceedings. London: The Royal Society of Medicine Press, 2004.

9 Waddell G, Burton AK. *Concepts of rehabilitation for the management of common health problems.* London: The Stationery Office, 2004.

10 Eriksen HR, Svendsröd R, Ursin G, Ursin H. Prevalence of subjective health complaints in the Nordic European countries in 1993. *Eur J Public Health* 1998; **8:** 294–8.

11 Wessely S. Mental health issues. In: *What about the workers?* Conference Proceedings. London: Royal Society of Medicine Press, 2004.

12 Waddell G, Aylward M. *Scientific and conceptual basis of incapacity benefits.* London: TSO, 2005.

13 Howard M. *An 'interactionist' perspective on barriers and bridges to work for disabled people.* London: IPPR, 2003. www.ippr.org/research/index.php?current=24&project=90

14 Burton AK. Back injury and work loss: biomechanical and psychosocial influences. *Spine* 1997; **22:** 2575–80.

15 Feuerstein M, Zastowny TR. Occupational rehabilitation: multidisciplinary management of work-related musculoskeletal pain and disability. In *Psychological approaches to pain management. A practitioners' handbook* (eds Gatchel RJ, Turk DC), pp. 458–85. London: The Guilford Press, 1999.

16 Main CJ, Burton AK. Economic and occupational influences on pain and disability. In *Pain management. An interdisciplinary approach* (eds Main CJ, Spanswick CC), pp. 63–87. Edinburgh: Churchill Livingstone, 2000.

17 World Health Organization. *International classification of functioning, disability and health.* Geneva: WHO, 2000. http://www3.who.int/icf/icftemplate.cfm

18 Schneider J. Work interventions in mental health care: some arguments and recent evidence. *J Mental Health* 1998; **7:** 81–94.

19 Boardman J. Mental health and employment. *Mental Health Rev* 2001; **6:** 6–12.

20 Crowther RE, Marshall M, Bond GR, Huxley P. Helping people with severe mental illness to obtain work: systematic review. *BMJ* 2001; **322:** 204–9.

21 Acheson D. *Inequalities in health report.* London: The Stationery Office, 1998.

22 Main CJ, Spanswick CC. *Pain management. An interdisciplinary approach.* Edinburgh: Churchill Livingstone, 2000.

23 Linton SJ. *New avenues for the prevention of chronic musculoskeletal pain and disability.* Amsterdam: Elsevier Science, 2002.

24 Vlaeyen JW, Linton SJ. Fear-avoidance and its consequences in chronic musculoskeletal pain: a state of the art. *Pain* 2000; **85:** 317–32.

25 Crombez G, Eccelston C, Baeyens F, van Houdenhove B, van den Broek A. Attention to chronic pain is dependent upon pain-related fear. *J Psychosom Res* 1999; **47:** 403–10.

26 Von Korff M. Fear and depression as remediable causes of disability in common medical conditions in primary care. In *Biopsychosocial medicine* (ed. White P). Oxford: Oxford University Press, 2005.

27 Krause N, Dasinger LK, Neuhauser F. Modified work and return to work: a review of the literature. *J Occup Rehabil* 1998; **8:** 113–39.

28 Sawney P, Challenor J. Poor communication between health professionals is a barrier to rehabilitation. *Occup Med* 2003; **53:** 246–8.

29 Beaumont DG. Rehabilitation and retention in the workplace—the interaction between general practitioners and occupational health professionals: a consensus statement. *Occup Med* 2003; **53:** 254–5.

30 Beaumont DG. The interaction between general practitioners and occupational health professionals in relation to rehabilitation for work: a Delphi study. *Occup Med* 2003; **53:** 249–53.

31 Wade DT, de Jong BA. Recent advances in rehabilitation. *BMJ* 2000; **320**: 1385–8.

32 Waddell G. *Models of disability: using low back pain as an example.* London: Royal Society of Medicine Press, 2002.

33 Kazimirski JC. CMA Policy Summary. The physician's role in helping patients return to work after an illness or injury. *Can Med Assoc J* 1997; **156**: 680A–680C.

Chapter 5

Ethics for occupational physicians

C. C. Harling

'Ethics is a generic term for various ways of understanding and examining the moral life. ...morality refers to norms about right and wrong human conduct that are so widely shared that they form a stable (although usually incomplete) social consensus.'[1] Thus a study of ethics and the application of ethical theory should provide action guides for human behaviour.

The application of ethics to healthcare work—usually termed biomedical ethics—is not an entirely abstract issue: neither is it unchanging dogma. While there is a strong logical and academic base to the study of biomedical ethics the practical application of such ethics ought to build upon a consensus from within society, expressed by democratically elected government. This leads to laws, professional rules of behaviour and collective agreements, which in turn can be analysed in an ethical manner, leading to a complete cycle of development. In liberal democracies, there is a prior presumption that compliance with the law will result in ethical behaviour. This is, however, not invariably the case.

Doctors may not have a sexual relationship with their patients. Such behaviour between two consenting adults is not forbidden by the law of the UK but will lead to punishment by the General Medical Council (GMC). In the practice of occupational medicine, the courts have decided that a doctor does not owe a legal duty of care to an applicant for a job when conducting a pre-employment examination and therefore cannot be sued. The doctor does, however, have a professional duty of care to all those who consult him or her: a poorly or incompetently conducted assessment could result in action by the GMC.

There are many competing ethical theories which may be applied to the study of biomedical ethics. This chapter is not the place to describe each theory in full and debate their strengths and weaknesses. Readers interested in a more general discussion and critical analysis of ethical theories as applied in the biomedical field are recommended to read Beauchamp and Childress (*Principles of biomedical ethics*, 5th edn).[1]

The basis of biomedical ethics in liberal democracies lies in common morality-based ethical values and uses four main principles or shared moral beliefs.

Respect for the autonomy of an individual has been at the centre of medical ethics for decades. This is more easily seen within the traditional treatment aspect of healthcare. Here it is accepted that a competent adult has the right, for example, to decline treatment even where that decision may cause them serious harm or even death. There is no doubt, in English law, that a follower of the Church of Jehovah's Witnesses may decline a blood transfusion even though death may result.

Two further ethical principles are closely related. The concept that a physician should do no harm (non-malficence) is linked in the contrary sense with the concept that healthcare professionals should do good for their patients (beneficence): these principles can be readily identified in the Hippocratic declaration and remain fundamental to the modern delivery of health care.

Finally, the concept of justice, or more properly of distributive justice, involves the ideas of fairness and the equitable distribution of both rights and responsibilities within a society. The emergence of the importance of this principle is a relatively modern development compared with the acceptance of the previous three. It allows us to balance the rights of the individual, which are to some extent pre-eminent in our society, with their corresponding responsibilities when analysing biomedical ethical issues.

These four principles are further illuminated or specified by ethical rules such as truthfulness, privacy, fidelity and confidentiality. For example, health professionals are expected to be honest in what they say and do. In many societies, higher standards of behaviour are expected of doctors than the general public. Although there may be a pragmatic justification for such rules, they are founded in ethical analysis. Thus these rules help us in applying the principles to practical activity and hence to derive moral action guides from our shared moral principles.

The need for a special consideration of ethical standards in the practice of occupational health arises because occupational physicians adopt different roles from other specialists or from general practitioners. In addition to their traditional contacts with patients, they give advice on the health aspects of products, processes, and practices of companies to managers and employees—including their representatives. In their relationships with people in the workplace, occupational physicians must demonstrate, by their behaviour and their conduct, that they clearly appreciate in which capacity they are acting at the time, and should ensure that others fully understand their position.

The traditional doctor–patient relationship may cause particular difficulty unless there is transparency and openness during the consultation. It is the responsibility of the occupational physician to ensure that those whom he sees on an individual basis fully appreciate the nature and boundaries of the relationship.

It would be inconvenient at the least to have to analyse each set of circumstances afresh each time they occur; there would be no consistency. Although each doctor remains personally responsible for their own actions, codes of conduct have been produced to guide doctors in their actions.

In the UK, the GMC sets out the 'standards that the public have a right to expect of their doctors' in several booklets.[2] These are of necessity general in their application and set out basic principles of behaviour. Others in the UK also publish guidance on ethics such as the British Medical Association and the medical Royal Colleges.

The Faculty of Occupational Medicine of the Royal College of Physicians of London first published its *Guidance on Ethics for Occupational Physicians* in 1980: it is currently reviewing the publication and the sixth edition[3] was published in 2006. Although the focus has been primarily on UK practice, the principles espoused will be more widely applicable.

Ethical practice does not constitute a fixed and universally applicable code of conduct. Even within a single country, regulations and attitudes constantly change and so the rules of 'acceptable practice' must be re-appraised regularly. This is of importance for occupational physicians with increasing globalization and movement of people around the world. Nevertheless, the basic principles noted above underpin the ethical practice of occupational physicians. The International Commission on Occupational Health (ICOH) has published a Code of Ethics[4] that applies to all occupational health professionals, and which forms a valuable basis for a national approach. The International Labour Office (ILO)[5] also gives guidance in which it recommends national associations to prepare and review their own codes of ethics.

General principles

Ethics, as a code of moral conduct, should take account of change, including changing attitudes and behaviour in society, changes in the law, and changes as a result of research and technical developments.

Changes in the law in particular may influence the behaviour of occupational physicians. The law as it applies to the practice of occupational health in the UK is reviewed elsewhere in this book and will not be repeated here. Compliance with the law or behaviour permitted under the law is not necessarily ethical. Examples such as the Abortion Act are well known; more recently medical involvement in 'intelligence gathering' and proposed 'assisted suicide' legislation produce widely differing views of the ethical position.

In recent years in the UK there have also been fundamental changes in the organization and management of occupational health practice. Many more independent practitioners offer services on a contract basis and fewer physicians are directly employed by companies. Because of these changes, and because of the different roles they are required to play in respect of their patients, their employer, the patient's employer, trade unions and the public, occupational physicians may find that they face conflicts of interest and loyalty. Ethical axioms though not universally agreed, provide a map to help in the resolution of such conflicts. There may be more than one 'correct' course of action—or there may appear to be none. Ethical behaviour thus depends on the exercise of judgement, but the views of experienced colleagues may prove invaluable in such circumstances.

In the last edition of this book, the view of a senior UK judge, Lord Woolf, speaking in 1997, was quoted:[6] 'The general approach of the courts is to apply the standards that the medical profession adopts …the courts do not impose their ethical standards on the medical professions. Wisely, they leave the medical profession to determine what is, and what is not, ethical behaviour.'

More recently, in the matter of which risks should be disclosed by a surgeon when obtaining informed consent for a procedure, the Courts have reduced the size of the risk that must be discussed below that generally practised by doctors. Although relating to surgical practice, the implications for 'informed consent' in all aspects of medical practice, including occupational medicine, are clear. For example, when discussing the consequences of allowing a report to be sent to the employer, the occupational physician will need to be explicit about possible adverse effects of that decision. The test will be what is likely to be important to the individual, not a generic, pre-prepared list.

As much of occupational health advice is provided by doctors who also work as general practitioners, doctors sometimes find themselves in a position where they give occupational medical advice to companies and, at the same time, provide primary medical care to some or all of the employees of that company. This may give rise to a conflict of interest. In these circumstances they must put the interests of the individual patient first. They should invite the company to seek alternative occupational health advice, rather than jeopardize the primary care doctor–patient relationship.

Occupational physicians may be called on to advise on the nature or extent of work-related health risks to individuals, to the workforce, to the environment or to the public. It is their responsibility to assist in the risk assessment process but not to decide on the acceptability of the risk. They are also likely to be part of a team that determines the means whereby such risks may be controlled but will commonly not lead in such activity. Some doctors may find a subsidiary role less comfortable than the primacy that is normally assumed in medical practice. Acting as one of a team is an essential part of the role of any occupational physician.

There is increasing pressure from society for greater transparency. Legislation on data protection, human rights and, more recently, freedom of information has been enacted in recent years, though the lack of case law does not always make the interpretation straightforward. The advice of senior colleagues and the use of national professional guidelines are valuable in such circumstances.

As a general principle, physicians should be as open as possible in the disclosure of records and reports to the subjects not only as required by legislation but based on the ethical position of respect for the autonomy of the individual. Only very rarely will the possible adverse impact on the patient's health prevent such openness. There are moves in medicine generally to copy all correspondence, including doctor to doctor letters, to the patient. Already this is normal practice in some occupational health departments. Employers should be advised that the subjects of reports will normally be told of the contents.

Where medical practitioners act as independent advisers (and, therefore, outwith the Access to Medical Reports Act 1988)[7] to third parties such as insurance companies or lawyers, it may not be appropriate for the subject of the report to receive a copy of it, unless this is required by a court or has been agreed in advance by the third party. If this is the case, the occupational physician must ensure that the subject of the examination/report is fully aware that they will not be able to have access to the report and has the opportunity to withdraw in advance.

The occupational physician in an organization must act as an impartial professional adviser, concerned primarily with safeguarding the health of employed people and others who may be affected by work activity. Demonstrable professional competence, independence, and integrity, as well as openness in matters of concern, are necessary to command the confidence and respect of management, employees, and their representatives. Without these the doctor cannot be effective.

Guidance on ethics inevitably strays into areas of practice, because advice on behaviour is seldom readily available in technical publications. Occupational health advice is commonly given not only by specialist occupational physicians, but by general practitioners and by doctors in other specialties. All must ensure that they have the necessary competence. Acting outside the limits of professional competence is likely to place the practitioner's registration at risk, as well as compromising the health and safety of the individual or organization to whom advice is given.

Occupational physicians commonly have responsibilities for staff working in another country, have themselves to work abroad, or are accountable to business or occupational health management based in another country. Legal and ethical standards vary from country to country. Occupational physicians must ensure that practices and standards imposed from abroad conform, at the minimum, to those in the country in which they are working. When they are working abroad themselves, the standards must be compatible with those of the host country, always ensuring that the highest standards prevail.

Medical records and confidentiality

General principles

The occupational physician or nurse is responsible for all clinical information, whether it is held manually or electronically, and must ensure the security of that information at all times. The principles of confidentiality within medical practice, on which guidance is issued by the GMC, apply equally in occupational health. Changes in the standards of storage of medical records in other clinical practice should be taken into account. In the UK's National Health Service (NHS) the principle that the patient 'owns' clinical information about themselves has led to a system of guardianship of information in hospitals. Forthcoming electronic records will, it is agreed, have an audit trail to see who has accessed clinical information and a requirement that those who access information will have to use the highest security and validation systems such as those developed for internet trading.

Medical records

Occupational physicians should take and maintain full, factual, contemporaneous, and dated notes. Not only is this good practice, but these notes may be required for disclosure or litigation.

Although unrestricted access to clinical data should be confined to the doctor and the nurse, other members of an occupational health department will need some access. All such staff must be made fully aware of their personal responsibility to keep all clinical information confidential, and where they do not belong to a professional group, which requires adherence to clinical standards of confidentiality, they should sign an undertaking that they will abide by the rules of confidentiality. Temporary staff must be included in this arrangement.

The informed consent of the subject is required before access to clinical information may be granted to others. 'An informed consent occurs if, and only if, a patient or subject with substantial understanding and in substantial absence of control by others, intentionally authorizes a professional to do something'.[1] For consent to disclose medical records to be valid, the subject must know:

- what information is to be disclosed
- to whom the information will be disclosed
- for what purpose the information will be transferred
- the consequences of consenting or refusing to such disclosure.

Further, consent is not a 'one-off' process: rather it is a dynamic process. Obtaining a signature on a consent form may be a means of demonstrating at a future date that the individual consented to disclosure at the time the document was signed. It is not an everlasting permission to disclose any medical information about the individual.

Clinical data and other information obtained by occupational physicians may only be disclosed without such consent if:

- the disclosure is clearly in the patient's interest, but it is not possible or it is undesirable to seek consent
- it is required by law
- the demands of the public interest outweigh the presumption of confidentiality.

Disclosure, other than with consent or where required by law, requires the balancing of competing ethical rights and needs very careful consideration. It may often be relevant to consult with others including, where appropriate, senior colleagues or a professional indemnity organization. In considering the public interest, the physician needs to assess the risk of serious harm, or death, to the patient or others, national security, and the prevention or detection of serious crime. A decision to disclose clinical information without consent may need to be justified at some time in the future.

It is the responsibility of the physician to ensure that the patient has personally given informed consent. A signature on a paper presented by a third party is no guarantee that it is even genuine or that consent has been obtained by due process and is fully informed.

Access to records

There is a presumption that everything learned by a doctor in the course of his or her professional activities will be held confidentially and not released to third parties, save with the consent of the individual. There are a number of specific exemptions (see above) but they are few and limited. This does not prevent occupational physicians coming under substantial pressure to release information inappropriately.

Within the European Union the protection and confidentiality of personal information is the subject of a Data Protection Directive. In the UK this has been implemented by a revised and extended Data Protection Act 1998.[8] This repeals all the provisions of the Access to Health Records Act 1990 as they relate to living people. These Acts are a manifestation of the increasing tendency towards greater transparency and more rights for individuals in relation to information held about them. The law has been extended from electronic data to all data held manually in filing systems allowing identification of personal data, and also extends the rights of subjects to access information held about them and to control its processing. Processing includes obtaining the data in the first place and covers its handling in many ways, including its transfer to another data controller: transfer of data to controllers outside the jurisdiction of the EU who do not have data protection laws at least as stringent as those in Europe is specifically precluded. This may have implications for multinational companies.

Occupational physicians must have an understanding of the law relating to records, their confidential maintenance, and the rights of individuals to access and control, and should ensure that their own behaviour conforms to the ethos underpinning this approach. Although professional associations can give more detailed guidance as case law and experience develop, there remains an onus on the individual to develop a broad understanding of the issues and to act appropriately.

Access to reports for employment or insurance purposes provided by medical practitioners who are responsible for the clinical care of a patient is the subject of the Access to Medical Reports Act 1988. When an occupational physician seeks such a report from a general practitioner or hospital specialist, this Act will apply, and the employee's rights under the Act must be explained and respected as a part of the process of obtaining informed consent.

Although there is doubt about the application of the 1988 Act to reports generated by occupational physicians—do they provide care ('care' includes examination, investigation, or diagnosis for the purposes of, or in connection with, any form of medical treatment) to the individual—changes in other legislation have made this argument largely academic. Sensitive personal information can only be released with consent and consent may be withdrawn at any time that such a decision can be effective; though a decision to withdraw consent previously given cannot be made after the report has been sent.

Occupational physicians who see an individual for a 'one-off' examination or report would not be considered to be providing care and the Act would not apply to such reports: the ethical need for consent would of course remain. Occupational physicians providing long-term occupational health services to a workforce may well be seen to provide care by, for example, giving immunizations, treatments, or other interventions. They may therefore come within the provisions of the Act. Other healthcare professionals are not subject to the Access to Medical Reports Act but are subject to the full force of the Data Protection Act and professional codes of conduct.

The ethical position is clear. Provision of a health report to a third party needs consent, which requires that the individual knows what is in the report, to whom it is being sent, for what purpose the report is required and the likely consequences, both beneficial and adverse, of the decision to allow or refuse consent to disclosure.

Occupational physicians may act as line managers within their own department. They must claim no special privilege of access to medical information about colleagues and staff over and above that available to other line managers. If a report is required an independent occupational medical assessment of a member of staff may well be appropriate to ensure the protection of the individual's privacy and confidentiality.

Disclosure in legal cases

There are many circumstances where medical records may be required for legal purposes. The procedures to be adopted by occupational physicians will vary from country to country, depending on local regulation, and it is commonly prudent for physicians to seek advice from their medical defence organization or professional association. As a general rule clinical information on individuals should not be released without written informed consent. There may well be pressure from lawyers on either side of a case to allow greater access to an individual's complete medical records and the physician should ensure that the person concerned understands exactly what is to be released and to whom. In general, however, the consent should relate to records relevant only to the case.

A court of law, an employment tribunal, or similar body may require the disclosure of all or part of a patient's medical records. In that case the physician should comply but must inform the individual.

Transfer, retention, and archiving of records

Occupational health records should be stored in such a way as to facilitate their transfer to another occupational health provider, their archiving, or their destruction. The detail will vary but consideration must be given to the possibility of the individual changing employer, dying, or transferring to a different part of the same company, as well as to any changes of occupational health provider. It is necessary also to take account of the circumstances in which a company ceases to exist or is taken over by another company. Storage and transfer arrangements must ensure security and confidentiality and must take account of the rights of individuals in respect of data protection and access and the requirement for consent to any change. The physician must ensure that the new holder of the records is an appropriate person for this role. Where there is a transfer of occupational health records from one provider to another, it is sufficient to advise the workforce generally by circular letter but the system must allow individuals to opt out of the transfer arrangements.

Some occupational health records may be required, by law, to be retained for a set period. These may be the records of the results of health assessments such as those for asbestos or lead workers, rather than the actual clinical records. It is the employer's responsibility to retain such records, rather than that of the physician, and they should be kept separate from the clinical records.

Fitness for work

Pre-employment health assessment

Pre-employment health questionnaires are often the only health screening undertaken at the time of employment. Several legal and ethical issues arise over the wording, interpretation, and handling of such questionnaires. If applicants have to post them back, obscurities cannot be clarified by direct questioning, so the design must take this into account. It is usual to include in the pre-employment system the facility to have telephone conversations with the applicant and an appropriate examination where doubt remains. Questionnaires should be sent for completion only when a conditional offer of employment has been made.

The content and format of the questions must be scrutinized carefully to ensure that they do not encourage any form of discrimination or contravention of the Disability Discrimination Act 1995 (DDA).[9] Applicants should not be expected to reveal clinical details to those who are not bound to observe medical confidentiality. Only if questionnaires are returned to qualified medical or nursing staff can there be any assurance that clinical details will be handled with appropriate confidentiality.

Questionnaires for the purpose of, and marked as, pre-employment health assessment should seek only information relevant to the decision of suitability for the post and not extraneous medical matters that might be of interest. The test that should be applied is 'does the answer to this question affect the decision about suitability for the proposed employment' or not: if not, the question should not be asked. Routine queries about height and weight rarely if ever affect decisions about employment and should not be asked. They run the risk of being seen as having been used as an unfair discriminant by those turned down, which may lead to unnecessary argument or even litigation.

The forms may include general information on disabilities, as this may be necessary if the employers are to fulfil their obligations under the DDA. These obligations include considera-tion of reasonable adjustments to the workplace to enable a disabled person to work. If there are specific medical conditions that would preclude employment, these should be defined in advance. This may include reference to drugs, whether prescribed or not. It is at the pre-employment stage that the employer should advise potential applicants if health screening will include drug tests, and whether a positive result would be a bar to employment. Potential applicants then have the option to proceed on an informed basis.

Sometimes it may be necessary to apply to an applicant's general practitioner or specialist medical adviser for specific information relevant to employment. This should only happen with the individual's informed consent. It can never be justified to ask for disclosure of the applicant's medical records in general. The request must specify the information, and the purpose for which it is required.

At a pre-employment health assessment, the primary responsibility of the occupational physician is to the employer. The UK Court of Appeal has ruled that the doctor owes no legal duty of care to the applicant. Although this ruling clarifies the legal situation, ethically the physician has a professional duty to act with due care and competence in undertaking a pre-employment health assessment. This includes taking appropriate action if a clinical abnormality is discovered, even if this has no relevance to employment.

The physician should ensure that the applicant understands the role of the doctor or nurse in acting for the employer. Medical examination by a physician is justified ethically only where risk assessment, which may include financial risk to the potential employer, shows it to be appro-priate though the laws relating to such examinations vary in different countries and must be adhered to. If the work requires a specified and justifiable standard of physical or mental health, or the health of the applicant may affect the health or safety of others, a medical examination is likely to be necessary. Rarely, there may be a need for a medical examination by a physician to ascertain fitness for a company pension scheme, or to advise the trustees of any limitations, although normal practice is 'fit for employment, fit for the pension scheme'.

Sickness absence

The management of 'sickness absence', now commonly described as managing attendance, is a clear management responsibility and not a function of an occupational health service. The occupational physician is responsible for providing impartial advice within the limits of medical knowledge, avoiding unsupportable medical speculation: they may also have a role in monitoring 'absence attributed to sickness' and its causes. The dual responsibility—professional to the individual and contractually to the employer—requires the highest standards of objectivity and evidence-based practice.

The physician's assessment will include not only the medical causes and prognosis of health-related absence but also any work adjustments that may be necessary; the question of whether or not a particular adjustment is reasonable is a matter for the employer.

Increasingly occupational health services are actively involved in the process of rehabilitation rather than just providing reports and advice for others to implement. This wider role requires additional skills and operating arrangements.

Retirement on health grounds

In order to advise on ill health retirement, the occupational physician must be fully conversant with the rules relating to pay during sickness absence, the rules and definitions of the company pension scheme, and the fitness requirements of the job. These rules vary widely between organizations and the physician must take care that he understands the rules under which the employee works. The physician's task includes the determination of disability and its likely duration, in relation to the requirements of the individual's work. This must be done by personal assessment of the employee and after having consulted the family doctor or attending specialist where appropriate. Having confirmed the nature of the condition and the degree of disability, and before making a recommendation, the physician should consult with the management on what reasonable adjustments can be made to the workplace to accommodate the employee, or whether alternative employment is available. This is required under the DDA. The physician should ensure that the advice given is impartial and objective, and related to the medical facts, rather than to any other employment considerations (see also Chapter 27).

It is often helpful for physicians to anticipate likely problems relating to ill-health and employment or retirement and to have discussed these in advance with personnel and pension staff. Difficulties arising over the employment of people with chronic conditions or serious communicable diseases (see below) can often be resolved in advance, ensuring the optimum placement of such staff and satisfactory arrangements for early retirement should this become necessary.

Health screening and special tests during employment. Health promotion

Occupational physicians may undertake a variety of health screening tests, often unconnected with the risks of work. Voluntary health promotion programmes must be clearly differentiated from those that are required by law, or, rarely, as a condition of employment. There should be clear procedures for the handling of results and for the employment consequences of any abnormalities discovered. If the anonymized and grouped results of such programmes are to be passed on to the employer, this must be agreed with the participants in advance.

Biological monitoring

Programmes for biological monitoring and biological effect monitoring must have a clear purpose and be well planned and implemented. The outcome should be improved control of hazards and reduction of risk. Participation should include informed consent even when monitoring is required by law.

Although the purpose of the programme may be to use the grouped results to assess and improve control measures, individual results falling outside agreed parameters will require specialist interpretation. Arrangements should be in place to refer, if considered necessary.

Planning such programmes must include the communication of results. The release of grouped results to all those with an interest in the control of the risks must be agreed in advance. Occasionally it may be necessary to release an individual's results to a third party to achieve the objective but this can only be with their informed consent.

Genetic screening

Although consideration of family history is a form of genetic assessment, the use of genetic screening tests has had little impact in the field of employment in the UK so far. It has been used to deny employment to those at risk of developing berylliosis and as a screening test for propensity to develop carpal tunnel syndrome. The only known application in the UK is in the armed forces, where candidates for flying are screened for the sickle cell trait, because of the risk hypoxia may pose.

There are many objections to third party use of genetic screening. Given the uncertain or probabilistic nature of the information, ethical principles suggest that such testing should be entirely at the discretion of the individual who should have complete control of the use of information so obtained. It is difficult to see how informed consent, particularly in terms of the consequences, could be truly obtained. The difficulty of interpreting such information in an employment context means that the probability of unfair discrimination is high.

In the UK, there is a moratorium on the use of genetic screening for insurance purposes (until 2006). In the field of employment, it is recognized that there is no systematic use of genetic screening for employment purposes—the one example usually quoted of testing for sickle cell trait in military aircrew is reported to be under review. The government decided that the use of genetic information to make a general assessment of an individual's health would not be acceptable and that the right of an individual not to know their genetic makeup should remain. It is proposed to use the concept of genetic discrimination to control activities in employment though a review of genetic screening in employment was promised for 2005 thus leaving open the possibility that such testing may be useful and justified in the future.

Serious communicable diseases

The UK GMC has published guidance on the ethical considerations of dealing, particularly, with those with HIV, hepatitis B or C, and tuberculosis. Guidance has also been published by the Department of Health. Occupational physicians in the healthcare industry should be conversant with such publications. Wherever occupational physicians work, they are themselves healthcare workers and must therefore follow national guidance. Where new information or research is published before an official guideline is changed, the new information must be considered. Even when they believe their own work will not jeopardize patients, they must not rely on their own assessment of the risk, but must seek and follow professional advice. Policies and procedures must be in place to ensure that their own staff comply with guidance.

Some countries require proof of freedom from infection with HIV before allowing visitors to work in that country. Where HIV testing is essential, expert counselling on the implications must be given to ensure fully informed consent, and post-test counselling must be available.

Immunization programmes

Where immunization programmes may be required at work, consent can only be regarded as informed if the risks are quantified and communicated. The policy should consider the implications of refusal to be immunized or to seroconvert and must cover the situation where a worker proves to be a carrier of infection. This will include issues arising from a failure on the worker's part to inform their manager or to comply with reasonable restrictions at work.

Testing for alcohol and drugs

Occupational physicians may be involved in screening and testing for alcohol and drugs. It is important to differentiate between tests for the clinical benefit of the individual and those undertaken primarily to protect the company and third parties. Physicians should avoid participation in policing procedures wherever possible, as this is likely to compromise their relationships with both workers and management. Tests for alcohol consumption undertaken as part of a company programme need not be performed by physicians or nurses. Breath analysis equipment, made to the appropriate specifications, can be used. Physicians should be involved in setting up such programmes and should advise on the appropriate action levels for blood alcohol and ensure that proper respect is given to the rights and dignity of individuals.

Where tests for drugs are instituted as part of company policy it is important that the purposes and procedures, the criteria for testing, the taking and handling of samples and the reporting and outcome of results are clearly specified in advance. The Faculty of Occupational Medicine has published detailed guidance. It is important, if medical and nursing staff are involved, that they are properly trained and that their roles are clearly understood by staff and managers. The physician can play a significant role in ensuring that properly informed consent is given to obtaining samples and that, at all stages, ethical practice is allied to carefully defined and controlled procedures.

Medical and nursing staff who are involved in taking and processing biological samples, and in the handling and reporting of results, act as agents for the employer. They must avoid using such occasions to give personal medical advice to individuals. This will reduce the risk of confusion between their role as agents for the employer and their traditional role as confidential medical advisers.

Business ethics

Business codes

Occupational physicians are expected to abide by the codes of business ethics followed by their employers and contractors. However, as registered medical practitioners they must comply with the rules of the GMC. They must ensure that there is no conflict between these obligations and resolve differences at the outset. They should strive to influence company policies in ways that take account of the health of employees and others affected by the organization's activities.

Contracted services

Increasingly, occupational health services are provided by staff who are not directly employed by the organization they serve. The commercial pressures inherent in this type of market can lead to particular ethical difficulties. It is important that occupational physicians abide by sound principles of business ethics in their dealings with client companies and each other, in order to safeguard their own reputations and that of the specialty as a whole. When occupational physicians act as managers, they must also recognize that the ethical standards by which they will be judged will be those standards that would apply to their dealings and relationships with patients.

Advertising

Occupational physicians in the UK, like other doctors, have to be registered with the GMC and abide by its rulings. Similar obligations may exist for medical practice abroad. In the UK, this limits advertising to the provision of factual information and services. Organizations employing occupational physicians are not restricted in this way, but doctors must dissociate themselves from marketing that does not meet the standards of the GMC, and ensure that advertising literature does not make claims that are not factual and verifiable.

Competence

Occupational physicians should only accept duties that are within their competence. When tendering for work, they must assess the level of specialist skills required and refer to a higher level of expertise if that is appropriate.

The term 'occupational physician' is often misused. Only doctors with postgraduate training in occupational medicine should describe themselves as occupational physicians, and the use of the terms 'consultant' or 'specialist' in occupational medicine within Europe should be reserved for doctors who are eligible for inclusion on the specialist register established under the European Specialist Medical Qualifications Order 1995.

Competitive tenders

Competition in the provision of occupational health services can be a healthy stimulus towards improving standards. Tendering exercises should be conducted honestly and fairly. Great care must be taken not to damage the reputation of competitors. It is improper either to offer inducements in order to secure business, or to make approaches to the staff of a competitor or existing service provider in order to obtain commercial advantage. Occupational health staff who are employed by an occupational health provider to work with a particular client should not use their position to gain personal advantage by, for example, offering the same service independently at a lower rate, or by disclosing commercially sensitive information to a competitor. Such action constitutes a breach of contract and could render the individual liable to a claim for damages.

Occupational physicians who act as technical advisers in tender evaluations must not have a commercial relationship with any of the competitors. They should declare any personal or professional interests and must provide objective advice on the merits of each proposal.

Transfer of services

Services may be transferred from one occupational health provider to another in a variety of circumstances. The abiding principle must be to safeguard the health, safety, and welfare of those to whom the service is being provided. The outgoing provider should make every reasonable effort to facilitate the handover. The cost of special equipment or programmes, which may be the property of the outgoing provider, should be agreed in advance if they are to be handed over. There are a number of legal considerations relating to the transfer of staff from one employer to another. Occupational health records should be transferred if practicable (see above).

Research

Research is essential for the development of occupational health practice. Most research is conducted by academics but the practice of occupational medicine offers particular opportunities.

The general ethical principles of research are that the subject must give informed consent to participation (which they may withdraw at any time), that no harm or detriment (to their care or employment) should come to the participant, and that the laws and ethical principles of data protection should be rigorously observed.

Occupational health research often involves the use of records or data that was collected for other purposes. Use of such data requires informed consent unless there is no alternative and under special arrangements. Such data collection and processing in the NHS may be authorized under so-called 'section 60' arrangements. In other cases, it will be necessary to take detailed advice as complex judgements will be required.

In keeping with data protection principles, data should be anonymized as early in the process as possible. Employee subjects are likely to be concerned about the possibility of data leakage and appropriate steps must be taken to secure both physical and electronic data.

All research can only be conducted with the approval of a research ethics committee (REC). Such committees are established within the NHS and other research organizations. Local RECs give approval for research within the organization: where research is conducted in a number of different organizations, multicentre RECs have been established with a central contact point to facilitate applications. Again, the rules are complex and competent advice is essential for those planning to conduct research.

Audit, or the review of information for the purposes of operational monitoring, does not require the same arrangement as research but it may be difficult to distinguish between the two activities on occasion. As the audit at least should be carried out by all occupational physicians, those attending occupational health departments should be told at first contact that data that they provide may be used for audit, and where appropriate, research. The wishes of those who do not wish to participate must be respected.

Communication of results poses particular difficulties and sensitivities in occupational medical practice. Forward planning and involvement of all stakeholders from an early stage is essential.

Relationships with others

General principles

Occupational physicians have an ethical obligation to put the interests of their patients first. Their obligations to others, including their employers, the workforce as a whole, and the general public, must also be recognized.

Particular attention should be paid to the role of the general practitioner, especially where this concerns treatment and referral, and consent to release clinical information. Occupational physicians in the healthcare sector must be especially careful that the general practitioner is not bypassed.

Other health professionals

Nurses play an important part in occupational health and physicians must ensure that they understand the ethical requirements for nursing. In many situations the nurse may be the occupational health manager and that role must be respected.

The occupational physician will work closely with other health and safety professionals such as occupational hygienists and safety officers, as well as with managers and engineers. Exchange of information is important but scrupulous care must be taken to safeguard confidential medical information.

Managers and workpeople

Managers may not always appreciate the physician's ethical duty to individuals and his independent position on clinical matters. The limits of accountability to managers need to be clarified before difficulties arise. Conflicts of interest between obligations to individuals and to managers or the company can usually be resolved by discussion, but conferring with senior professional colleagues may often assist.

It should be normal practice for occupational physicians to discuss health and safety issues with workpeople or their representatives. A good working relationship with trade unions, where they represent the employees and while respecting the confidentiality of individuals, will resolve many issues.

The public and the environment

The occupational physician has a duty to society, and occasionally must put the public interest before that of a patient. When safety or public health may be endangered, the physician may, legally and ethically, breach confidentiality. It will be the physician's conscience which will dictate action, but advice from senior colleagues should be sought if possible. Ultimately, physicians may be required to justify their course of action in a court of law.

References

1 Beauchamp TL, Childress JF. *Principles of biomedical ethics*, 5th edn. Oxford: Oxford University Press, 2001.

2 Ethical Guidance, General Medical Council, London. At www.gmc-uk.org/standards/default.htm

3 The Faculty of Occupational Medicine. *Guidance on ethics for occupational physicians*, 6th edn. London: Faculty of Occupational Medicine, 2006.

4 International Code of Ethics for Occupational Health Professionals. Singapore, 2002. www.icohweb.org/cose_docs.html

5 International Labour Organisation at http://www.ilo.org

6 Lord Woolf. Medics, lawyers and the courts. *J R Coll Physicians Lond* 1997; **3b1**(6): 686–93.

7 http://www.opsi.gov.uk/acts/acts1988/Ukpga_19880028_en_1.htm

8 http://www.opsi.gov.uk/acts/acts1998/19980029.htm

9 http://www.opsi.gov.uk/acts/acts1995/Ukpga_19950050_en_1.htm

Further reading

The BMA's handbook of ethics and law, 2nd edn. London: BMA, 2004.

Directive 95.46 of the European Parliament and the Council of 24 October 1995 on the protection of individuals with regard to the processing of personal data and on the free movement of such data. *Official J European Communities* L2811995; 38, 23 November: 31–55.

Kapfunde v. *Abbey National and Dr Daniel*. London: Industrial Relations Law Reports 583, 1998.

Human Genetics Commission at www.hgc.gov.uk; (look under 'genetic discrimination')

Serious communicable diseases. (see www.dh.gov.uk)

Guidelines on testing for drugs of abuse in the workplace. London: Faculty of Occupational Medicine, 1994. (revision due 2006)

Westerholm P, Nilstun T, Ousetueit J (eds) *Practical ethics in occupational health*. Oxford: Radcliffe Medical Press, 2004.

Chapter 6

Neurological disorders

R. Willcox and R. J. Hardie

Introduction

This chapter deals mainly with common acute and chronic neurological problems, particularly as they affect the special needs of affected employees and job applicants. The complications of occupational exposure to neurotoxins and putative neurotoxins will also be covered in so far as they relate to fitness of an exposed employee to continue working.

In addition to a few well-known and common conditions such as migraine and stroke that will be familiar to all occupational physicians, many uncommon but distinct neurological disorders may present infrequently. Fortunately for the occupational health specialist, fitness for work in these disorders is generally determined by the person's functional neurological abilities and not by the precise diagnosis. This will also need to be put into the context of the job in question, as the basic requirements for a manual labouring job may be completely different from something more intellectually demanding. Indeed, even an apparently precise diagnostic label such as multiple sclerosis (MS) or a brain tumour, can encompass a complete spectrum of neurological disability from one who is entirely asymptomatic to another who is totally incapacitated for work.

Furthermore, reports by treating clinicians and general practitioners and even specialist neurologists and neurosurgeons may describe the past history and symptoms in detail without analysing functional abilities at all. These colleagues may also fail to appreciate occupational aspects, particularly in relation to potential hazards in the workplace, and blithely assert that they see no reason why their patient should not return to work when they have no concept of the associated risks and limitations.

Many neurological patients have more than one problem and the number and range of disabling neurological disorders and symptoms is very large. There are over 100 disabling neurological symptoms, in marked contrast to other specialities, e.g. respiratory and cardiac disease, which each only cause six or seven disabling problems.[1]

It is not just the widely ranging clinical aspects of a person's neurological disorder that must be considered systematically, but also their variability and their susceptibility to environmental factors in the workplace; the effects of specific medication commonly used; the need for assistive technology of various types; and the incapacitation risks as well as various ethical and legal considerations.

Size of the problem

Neurological disorders are an important cause of disability in modern Western society (Table 6.1). Estimates from the Neurological Alliance, an umbrella organization of all the main neurological charities in the UK, suggest that about 10 million of the UK population have a neurological condition that has a significant impact on their lives.[2] This figure includes 2–3 million people with

Table 6.1 Incidence, prevalence, and consequences of the major disabling neurological disorders. Expressed as a rate per 1000, all ages, unless otherwise specified. Ordered by age at peak onset, where possible

Peak onset	Condition	Incidence	Prevalence	Disability
0–15	Cerebral palsy*	2	3	3
	Meningitis	0.07		
	Muscular dystrophy		0.09	
16–24	Head injury†	3		
	Epilepsy	0.7	5	
	Migraine		70	7
25–54	Multiple sclerosis	0.04	1	0.7
	Cerebral tumour	0.16	0.45	0.16
	Guillain–Barré	0.01		0.002
55–74	Stroke	2	15	6
	Parkinson's disease	0.15	1.2	
	Motor neurone disease	0.01	0.05	0.05
75+	Dementia‡	15	67	

Notes: *Per 1000 live births; †requiring hospital admission; ‡aged 65 years and over. Redrawn with permission from Langton Hewer and Tennant (2003).[1]© Psychology Press, 2003.

recognized pathology as well as single seizures, essential tremor, etc., and the remainder with migraine and other headache disorders. Most of them are able to manage their lives on a daily basis, but over 1 million of them, 2% of the entire population, are disabled and likely to be excluded from full-time employment. This figure includes most people with congenital conditions such as cerebral palsy, those who have recently had a brain injury or stroke, and some people living with motor neurone disease, MS, Parkinson's disease (PD), and various forms of dementia. It also includes some of those with epilepsy or migraine. Nearly two in five of all those people most severely disabled report a neurological cause. It is difficult to make valid comparisons with other major disease groupings, partly because many neurological diseases are age related. Mortality and morbidity also vary by condition. Diseases that are commonest below 65 years and have prolonged morbidity have far greater relevance to work ability than either rapidly fatal diseases or those whose main clinical impact occurs late in life. About one-quarter of those aged between 16 and 64 with a chronic disability have a neurological condition.[2]

Table 6.1 compares incidence, prevalence, and disability rates for some of the more important neurological diseases. They are usefully stratified by age groups that separate young children up to 15 years, and school leavers and younger people (16–24 years) from those with families, jobs and careers (25–54), and those reaching the end of their working life and entering active retirement (54–74 years). The rates cited are estimates and not confined to the working age group, but they provide some indication of the burden of the commoner problems.[1]

With the exception of malignant brain tumours and motor neurone disease, relatively long survival rates mean that the prevalence and disability rates are much greater than incidence. Compared with that of stroke, the overall health impact of most other neurological diseases is small. Although generally thought of as a disorder of the elderly, about a quarter of the 100 000 people suffering their first strokes each year in Britain are below age 65 years.

Occupational causes of neurological impairment

Occupational causes of neurological impairment are rare, and are considered further below. The occupational physician is more often involved with the job adaptation and rehabilitation of patients with neurological disabilities than with eliminating the small number of known occupational neurotoxins from the workplace, but should also be aware of possible work-related factors that may exacerbate a pre-existing neurological disorder. Potential occupational exposure to organic solvents or heavy metals, for example, needs to be particularly carefully considered in employees who already have mild neurobehavioural problems or a neuropathy.

Clinical assessment

By the time the occupational physician sees an employee, the diagnosis is likely to have been established. In these circumstances, it is more important at interview to assess the individual's ability either to continue to perform or to return to the job held before the illness began, or else to adapt to alternative employment.

In normal subjects, perception and recognition of sensory stimuli and executive mental functions are intact; normal posture, balance, and gait can be maintained; there is good delicate control of movement and normal control of vasomotor and sphincter functions. Normal subjects should also have an absence of any positive symptoms or signs such as involuntary movements, pain or other abnormal sensations, or hallucinations.

Disturbances of awareness include blackouts and seizures as well as alterations in the ability to stay awake. Neurobehavioural disorders following head injury, stroke, or encephalitis may range from mild and transient to severe and permanent. Someone may be left with communication disabilities from dysarthria or dysphasia, a visual field defect or more global cognitive problems of which they may not even be aware. Dysphasia and dyspraxia can preclude employment that requires regular communication with other workers or the general public. Disturbance of spatial relationships may prevent the patient from driving, and efficient integration of all cognitive functions is important for those with intellectually demanding jobs.

Disturbances of posture, balance, or gait are usually easy to establish. Subjects complain of dizziness, unsteadiness, or spatial disequilibrium and their co-ordination may be impaired. PD is a classic example of a movement disorder. Adjustment of antiparkinsonian drug treatment may minimize work problems, but jobs that involve rapid hand co-ordination may still be difficult. Similarly, muscle spasticity associated with upper motor neurone disorders may prevent fine manual work or even the ability to stand for long periods.

The consequences of neurological dysfunction are clearly different for manual and non-manual workers. Manual jobs require good muscle power and peripheral sensation but a degree of impairment in intellectual function might not be so serious. Lifting or moving objects—particularly if repeated frequently—can be a problem for those with disorders of muscles and peripheral nerves. If there is a radiculopathy, repetitive movements involving movement of the vertebral column may exacerbate the original cause of the disability. By contrast, an employee with complete paraplegia or a hemiparesis may still be able to undertake a desk job, although commuting to work may be a bigger problem than doing the job itself.

The impact of prognosis and rehabilitation on work

The impact of neurological problems on work may be considered in three stages. The first stage covers workers with no previous health or disability problems who develop a condition, whether or not it is work-related, that has the potential to affect job performance in the future if their condition deteriorates. The second stage represents the person who has a condition that is already affecting job performance. Thirdly, attendance at work may start to become affected. The impact on work will depend on the extent of any recovery, the availability of treatment to cure or alleviate the residual effects and whether the employer, after becoming aware of the condition, is willing and able to introduce workplace adjustments that offset any potential for aggravation by work activities.

Some slowly progressive neurological conditions may move predictably from the first stage through the second to the third, but in others the clinical course may be unpredictably episodic, transient, or static. Such prognostic considerations are important for the patient's job prospects. Although some diseases such as epilepsy (see Chapter 8) have their own unique statutory medico-legal implications, with which the physician must be familiar, most disorders must be dealt with on an *ad hominem* basis.

For example, the prognosis of MS is difficult to evaluate, especially at the outset. The disease may never cause more than a transient episode of blurred vision or it may progress rapidly and inexorably to tetraplegia. Similarly, cerebrovascular disorders may range from a catastrophic intracerebral bleed to transient ischaemic episodes with full resolution. Most stroke patients recover at least partially, so it is important wherever possible to keep their original job open, albeit in a modified form if necessary. Such modifications may be temporary or permanent and will require periodic re-evaluation. The occupational physician should be actively involved by directly intervening in matching the job to the disabled worker and by advising on appropriate rehabilitation interventions as well as reasonable adjustments.

After an acute episode the neurologically disabled employee should not expect, or be expected, to have made maximum or full recovery before work is resumed. The rehabilitation process will be enhanced if the patient can return to the job part-time initially. The process of going to work and performing a job is a worthwhile outcome in itself, and ongoing rehabilitation will allow problems to be identified at an early stage. Therapy at the place of work can be of benefit to both the employee and employer. Recruiting and training new employees to a task can be expensive and it may be far more cost-effective to rehabilitate a trained but disabled worker. Small changes in posture and ergonomics at work, external aids and simple adjustments to office layout, for example, can make a big difference to functional capacity. The type of rehabilitation needs to be carefully planned by the therapists and doctor working together, but the outcome is often rewarding. Similarly those in whom slowly progressive disability is anticipated deserve careful planning to review their needs at timely intervals appropriate to the underlying pathology. Continuing at work may be a source of great psychological strength to someone recently diagnosed with an incurable neurological disease, but both the patient and the employer must also be protected from unnecessary risk. In more severe cases environmental control systems and other assistive technology may enable a disabled person to use office equipment and continue at work.[3]

Regrettably, however, rehabilitation tends to be undervalued and underfunded, even for acute disorders such as strokes and traumatic brain injuries, and yet should ideally follow through ultimately into the workplace. When the NHS proves inadequate, occupational medical facilities may be able to fill the gap. Specialist vocational rehabilitation services are available in the private sector and hopefully the National Service Framework for long-term neurological conditions (2005) will facilitate expansion of comparable statutory services in the UK.[4]

Lay attitudes and influences on employability

The commitment of the occupational physician to 'do something' for the employee who has developed a neurological disorder can be undermined, curtailed, or even prevented by uninformed lay opinion in the guise of management decisions. Managers should refer all disabled employees to their occupational health provider. In a well-organized company the health provider will become aware of such people, because there will be a review procedure triggered by their sickness absence. The occupational physician should ensure that managers harbour no misconceptions based on inadequate lay knowledge.

Many people, for example, believe that MS inevitably leads to an incontinent wheelchair-bound existence. Likewise, they often greatly underestimate the improvement in functional ability that can follow a stroke, either from the natural recovery process itself or from an appropriate and effective rehabilitation programme. The term 'brain tumour' conjures up all manner of misconceptions that may not apply at all to indolent acoustic neuromas, for example. Managers may also be puzzled by the problems of nominal dysphasia, or the variable nature of the disability of myasthenia or PD in a single day. It is the occupational physician's role to explain, to make the relevant clinical assessment, and to advise on the necessary job modifications and fitness to drive where driving is an integral part of the job.[5]

Ethical considerations

Apart from general principles covered elsewhere in this volume, neurological disorders present some particular ethical challenges to the occupational physician, mainly surrounding genetics (Box 6.1), expectation of progression, and confidentiality. Genetic problems usually begin once carrier status becomes apparent, either from the family history in a dominantly inherited condition, or after presymptomatic gene testing in the laboratory.[6] Huntington's disease is perhaps the best-studied example, where the mutant gene is fully penetrant and all carriers eventually become affected. However, symptom onset may be delayed for decades and attendant anxiety may be extremely hard to distinguish from true neuropsychiatric problems.[7]

There are many similarities with HIV testing, where seroconversion does not necessarily denote the onset of clinically relevant disease. The diagnosis itself of a neurogenetic condition may be perfectly compatible with full-time working, but usually carries with it the inevitability of progression and, depending on the expected time course, possibly premature retirement. Indeed, this inevitability of progression is not unique to genetic disorders, for neurodegenerative diseases and malignant cerebral tumours also deteriorate inexorably.

As a general rule, the rate of symptom progression prior to diagnosis is a reasonable guide to the future in individual employees and should determine the frequency of any regular occupational screening programme. The physician must be careful not to pre-judge a person's employability based on the pathological diagnosis alone.

Box 6.1 Important ethical problems in gene carriers

- ◆ Popular misunderstanding of the consequences of having an abnormal gene
- ◆ Unpredictable age of symptom onset
- ◆ Variable gene penetrance alters prognosis
- ◆ Impact of knowledge of pathological genotype on a person's self-identity,
- ◆ Disclosure of genetic information to third parties
- ◆ Use of genetic information to deny access to employment and insurance
- ◆ Antidiscrimination legislation

Normally clinical ethics requires that the patient with sufficient mental capacity is the ultimate medical decision-maker. Neurological disorders affecting the brain, however, may impair that person's capacity and judgement to assess the seriousness of their condition, to plan, and to appreciate the connections between their own disability and their productivity as well as hazards at work. Patient autonomy is limited when there is a risk of serious injury to them or their work colleagues, which may override the normal demand for confidentiality. An example would be a vocational driver with impulsiveness, a recent diagnosis of a cerebral glioma, or Huntington's disease in someone who has already had one minor accident at work.

Summary

In summary, neurological disease can create a wide variety of disabilities. The objective clinical assessment of the symptoms and signs and the review of the patient's functional work capacity are much more important than the diagnostic label. In the past the label itself may have been an impediment to future gainful employment through misconceptions about the neurological disability as much as failure to provide energetic and intelligent rehabilitation. The Disability Discrimination Act 1995 now requires employers to make active, reasonable adjustments and in all these matters the occupational physician plays an important role.

When making recommendations about medical retirement, the occupational physician must collect and weigh all the facts of the case meticulously and critically, deliberately examine possible objections to their own view, and consider seeking advice from colleagues. Taking all of the facts into account, a decision must usually be made in the face of some uncertainty that demands an astute combination of clinical judgment, occupational insight, and common sense. Ultimately, the decision rests with the physician's wisdom and commitment to the common good of the employee and their employer.

How neurological illnesses may influence work

The disability that a patient suffers is dependent on the symptoms and signs that the disease produces and not the disease itself. Certain disorders, and particularly brain injuries caused by a variety of pathologies, can lead to loss of function anywhere in the nervous system. Occupational physicians must be familiar with the characteristics of particular employees and the nature of their disease as well as their specific work duties before they can determine their work capability.

The following headings can provide a checklist to ensure comprehensive consideration of the key potential clinical aspects of any given neurological disorder. The physician should identify those clinical features that may be present, and actively seek to exclude their presence or assess the extent of any impairment in order to evaluate the occupational implications.

Very often it is not possible with brain disease to decide how much of the employee's disability is physical and how much psychological, and it can even be a disadvantage to attempt to be precise in separating them.

Higher cerebral functions

Many neurological diseases affect mental functions, but their influence on work depends very much on the job. A labourer can continue to work with a moderate, or sometimes even a severe intellectual impairment, but an executive cannot. There are no guidelines that can be used generally.

Cognitive function and psychometrics

Possibly the most important consideration is the likelihood of a person with any kind of cerebral pathology suffering cognitive impairment that may mean they are unreliable at work. In one community-based occupational survey, frequent or very frequent cognitive failures (e.g. problems of memory, attention, or action) and minor injuries were reported by about 10% of the workers, and work accidents requiring treatment by almost 6%.[8] The extent to which these could be attributable to organic neurological disease is not known, as minor injuries are not recorded by official sources but could have implications in productivity and worker health.

Detailed and objective psychometric evaluation may be necessary in the presence of some neurological disorders affecting the brain, depending on the person's responsibilities. For those with unskilled jobs, it may be sufficient for a good line manager to be satisfied that an employee is capable of understanding and following basic instructions satisfactorily. On the other hand, a team leader, an executive, or professional person may require careful assessment: both to protect themselves from premature return to work and the risk of failure and loss of reputation and self-esteem; and also to protect their employers from incompetence. An important feature of some cerebral pathologies is lack of insight into one's own limitations, so it is imperative not to rely wholly on the patient.

The patient may already have undergone cognitive assessments, in which case the relevant reports should be obtained. It will be necessary to distinguish between results of screening tests, often administered by occupational therapists, for example using certain validated instruments such as the Rivermead Behavioural Memory Test and Chessington OT neurological assessment battery, and more definitive standardized neuropsychological tests by trained clinical psychologists.

The physician must consider the available data and when they were obtained in the light of the pathology and prognosis. For example, trends of improvement may be apparent after a single-event brain injury, or conversely of deterioration in someone with a cerebral tumour or degenerative condition. The relevance of the results must also be considered in the light of the demands of the specific job under consideration.

The term 'ecological validity' has been coined to refer to the relevance of performance under formal test conditions to the subject's behaviour in 'the real world', which may of course be better or worse than expected from the tests. For example, a subject may perform well on specific tests of verbal memory in quiet conditions in an outpatient setting, but be incapable of taking telephone messages reliably in a noisy and hectic office environment. Conversely, poor performance on tests thought to be sensitive to frontal lobe dysfunction may be irrelevant to someone's ability to return to undemanding work they have been doing for many years. It may often be better if at all practicable to allow an employee the opportunity for a work trial under careful but unobtrusive observation and supervision. This may allow insight to develop on both sides and, in cases of failure to cope, will lead to better acceptance of a negative decision, otherwise precautionary safeguards can be formalized or dispensed with.

Simple memory aids are universally used at home as well as in the workplace, from the basic written 'To Do' list or note stuck in a prominent position, to sophisticated paper-based organizers, electronic personal digital assistants, programmable mobile phones and computer software. The demands of many jobs require such great powers of cognitive processing that they would be beyond most average people without such aids. Paradoxically, their greatest limitation is the person losing the portable aids or just forgetting to use them, which is by no means confined to those with organic neurological disease! Nevertheless, behavioural approaches can be beneficial to the training of all employees, and certain cognitive rehabilitation techniques applied in particular to those with organic impairment.[9]

Memory loss can seldom be improved pharmacologically, but it can arise or be made worse by drugs, in which case a reduction in medication may be beneficial. For example, anticonvulsants and psychotropic medication may impair memory. It is not uncommon for a patient to be discharged from hospital, for example after a life-threatening stroke or infection, on large doses of multiple drugs that are not then critically reviewed thereafter as spontaneous improvement occurs.

Behaviour and impulse control

Even if rigorous neuropsychological testing reveals no abnormality, any cerebral pathology can give rise to disturbances of normal behaviour and impulse control that can have serious implications for employability. Sometimes these are obvious to lay colleagues and managers, particularly if they knew the employee before a traumatic brain injury or the onset of a neurological condition. Lack of attention to personal hygiene, appearance, and presentation at work may be a clue to the onset of frontal lobe dementia. Occasionally, and especially in MS, euphoria may limit an employee's motivation to overcome associated physical disability and to maintain their work potential.

Other changes can be more subtle or variable and unpredictable, with outbursts of offensive language, physical aggression or sexually inappropriate behaviour towards colleagues or customers giving rise to serious concern and perhaps disciplinary action. Such neurobehavioural changes can be associated with secondary problems such as marital breakdown or substance misuse that may be mistaken for the primary cause unless the connection is made by gathering information from a variety of sources with the necessary consent. They may be helped by specific behavioural approaches in neuropsychological rehabilitation.[9]

Disturbances of arousal and consciousness

Fixed deficits of alertness and attention are usually obvious at basic personnel interviews, but certain conditions can give rise to variable deficits, particularly where sleep is disturbed. Epilepsy is dealt with elsewhere in this volume. Here the key occupational considerations are the risk of lapses in attention or awareness occurring at work, and the possible adverse effects of medication (see p 117).

Sleep

We live in an increasingly sleep-fragmented society with up to 20% of the population working outside the regular 0800–1700 hour day.[10] Some major accidents have been related to sleep deprivation while the daily toll on the roads is such that lack of sleep is as much a contributor as alcohol—and the combination is particularly lethal.[11]

Sleep disturbance is not uncommon in neurological conditions affecting cerebral function or associated with chronic pain or immobility, effects that can be magnified by stimulants and antiparkinsonian drugs. Perhaps because the definition of 'normal sleep' remains elusive, as do the determinants of normal sleep, the use of drugs to treat insomnia is rising despite evidence of harm and little meaningful benefit, and the correlation of psychopathology with poor sleep satisfaction is strong.[12] Accurate diagnosis of the causes of poor sleeping is seldom achieved and simple effective measures are often not tried first.[13]

Obstructive sleep apnoea (4% men, 2% women) is of increasing importance because of neurocognitive and cardiovascular sequelae.[14] It is associated with work deficits[15] and early treatment can be justified on economic grounds.[16]

Shift work has been well reviewed as has fatigue and its implications.[10] Joint guidelines for shiftworker assessment are published by the Faculty of Occupational Medicine and the Society of Occupational Medicine (1999).[17]

Shift work is associated with changes in metabolism and older employees tend to fare less well but there is great variation among individuals. There are no neurological disorders that present an absolute contraindication to night and shift work, and thus require a permanent assignment or transfer to day work. However, relative contraindications would include seizure disorders and PD. Prevention of jet lag is increasingly well understood and simple measures to reduce fatigue are available for those who travel as part of their work.[18]

Paroxysmal pain disorders

Certain neurological conditions may be entirely benign and yet associated with intense paroxysms of pain. The simplest example is trigeminal neuralgia, characterized by lancinating facial pain, but the evidence for most treatment options is poor.[19] Postherpetic neuralgia and migraine are other common pain disorders. Here the key occupational considerations are the risk of incapacitation occurring at work, and the possible adverse effects of medication.

Speech, language, and communication

Speech disorders, whether dysphasia, dysphonia, or dysarthria, can be helped by speech therapy but it is rare for major improvement to occur without recovery of the underlying condition to enable the employee to return to work. Moreover, apart from those who earn their living by talking, such as teachers, broadcasters, or politicians, these problems affect social and home function far more than work, which may even be precluded altogether. It is often more effective to reduce the importance of speech in the job and to provide aids such as a word processor possibly with text-to-speech software. Speech amplifiers can be used if the voice is very weak, as can occur in laryngeal dystonia. Dysphasia can be associated with other language problems such as dyslexia, dysgraphia, and dyscalculia, and therefore the communication needs must be considered as a whole in such cases with a speech and language therapist.

Emotional state

Changes in mood state can occur with some neurological diseases. PD in particular is associated with a high incidence of depression. It is not uncommon to develop secondary depression if the condition is incurable, for example, and progressive disability naturally tends to be very frustrating. This can be helped by antidepressants, particularly those with stimulant rather than sedative properties, provided that unwanted effects on mental function can be avoided.

The main exception is MS, in which depression can certainly occur but its absence is often striking in contrast to the physical state of progressive disability. While euphoria may be accompanied by denial of problems as part of a psychological defence mechanism, it may also be a sign of incipient cognitive failure with frontal lobe dysfunction, with obvious implications for employers.

In addition to the physician's usual choice of pharmacological interventions, it is usually worth considering other therapeutic approaches ranging from simple counselling and cognitive behavioural therapy to formal neuropsychological rehabilitation.[9]

Symptoms related to cranial nerves

Problems relating to the nerves of the eye and ear are considered in Chapters 9 and 10 respectively. Impaired olfaction from a neurological cause occurs most commonly after head injuries, although local rhinological conditions, heavy smoking, and advancing age are more likely causes in the general working population. In occupations using noxious substances, an employee with impaired olfaction might be at greater risk of hazardous exposure. Few jobs specifically require a good sense of smell, but with anosmia there is usually a concomitant loss of taste apart from the four primary tastes of sweet, acid (sour), bitter, and salt, the sensory perceptions of which are located on the tongue. Cooks and professional tasters would therefore be handicapped by such a disability.

Lesions of the trigeminal nerve rarely influence work capacity, although the risk of corneal trauma should be considered when sensation is impaired. In contrast, the pain of trigeminal neuralgia, combined with the sedative effects of analgesia, can interfere greatly with concentration at work.

Bell's palsy is a fairly common cause of acute painless facial weakness. It usually improves with time, but is disfiguring and can be embarrassing if the work involves talking to and meeting the public. The only danger is to the eye, when the cornea is at risk from drying and abrasion due to problems with lid closure and the tear mechanism. Fortunately eye closure nearly always recovers, even if the lower facial paralysis does not. Bell's palsy and other facial palsies should rarely be a cause of a long-term inability to work. Synkinesis and facial spasm, common features of partial recovery, can be effectively managed with botulinum toxin injections. Plastic surgery techniques such as weighting of the upper lid may improve eye closure and cosmesis too.

Corneal protection is important in employees working with machinery or in dusty atmospheres after either trigeminal or facial nerve deficits. They should be educated to report new findings such as eye pain, discharge, or change in vision. Wearing goggles or large protective glasses with side guards helps exclude draughts and dust. Lubricating drops can be applied regularly by day and a simple eye ointment used at night. Those occupations necessitating the wearing of face masks or breathing apparatus may require special assessment.

The lower cranial nerves principally control swallowing and articulation (see Speech section above). Difficulty with breathing and paralysis of the respiratory muscles are also matters rarely requiring special consideration at work. However, the development of portable ventilators has enabled some people with high cervical cord injuries to return to work part-time with the appropriate safeguards.

Motor symptoms related to the trunk and limbs

Patients with problems related to their trunk and limbs often find it difficult to describe their symptoms. This makes it difficult to categorize the problem. Often the word 'weakness' is used to describe incoordination and sensory symptoms and phrases like 'my hand feels numb' are used to express weakness when there is no sensory change, and careful clinical assessment is necessary. In making an assessment for work the doctor can often be guided by a physiotherapist or occupational therapist.

Weakness can be due to many causes including lesions of the upper or lower motor neurones or neuromuscular junction, muscle disease (myopathy), or psychological mechanisms. These can usually be distinguished from one another clinically. The management of the different causes and their effects on work capability are different.

Upper motor neurone lesions, extrapyramidal disorders, and hypertonia

In acute upper motor neurone lesions, for example after a stroke, difficulties can often be helped by rehabilitation. Physiotherapy aims to retrain movement patterns, posture and trunk control as the central nervous system (CNS) adapts, and hence function can be improved. Pure muscle strengthening exercises are usually contraindicated. Hypertonia in long-standing upper motor neurone lesions leads to poor posture and clumsiness of movement that often affects fine hand movements or gait. Spasticity is often present, and causes problems with pain, involuntary spasms and contractures that may require specific treatment.[20]

In PD and other parkinsonian syndromes, increased tone and rigidity is associated with bradykinesia. It is the slowness of movements that is usually the greatest disability.[21] For example, a patient may walk easily for long distances in the open but with great difficulty in a crowded workshop requiring frequent changes of direction. Fine motor skills are considerably impaired and unfortunately are not easily helped by physiotherapy. Drug treatment is usually more rewarding.

Employers sometimes assume that a lighter or sedentary job might be easier to perform, but this is not always the case because weakness may not be the problem. Instead the patient needs a job that requires less skilful movements: for example, assembling small components would be more difficult than a heavier but less precise activity.

Ataxia and incoordination

The results of ataxia and incoordination can be similar to those of peripheral sensory loss, but the disability is likely to be worse because other sensory input, for example vision, cannot be used in compensation. Unless the cause of the ataxia can be corrected, no amount of retraining will help. In these circumstances the environment must be changed if the ataxia is a cause of danger to the employee or if it limits their work.[22]

Lower motor neurone lesions

With lower motor neurone diseases the situation is different. Unless there is very severe weakness and joint instability, decreased tone does not cause a problem and the main difficulty is loss of power. In contrast to upper motor neurone lesions, physiotherapy should aim to strengthen the appropriate muscles. If there is complete paralysis of a muscle, other muscles may be strengthened and trick movements learnt. The long-term prognosis depends on the pathology. In acute Guillain–Barré syndrome full recovery can occur. In progressive diseases where treatment cannot halt the decline, excessive physiotherapy can lead to exhaustion and worsen symptoms but orthoses may help localized sites of weakness.[3]

Disorders affecting the neuromuscular junction and muscle

Disorders affecting the neuromuscular junction and muscle are much less common than other neurological diseases. The former is characterized by fatiguability, exercise makes the weakness worse, and so muscle-strengthening exercises are inappropriate. The typical pattern of weakness has a proximal emphasis in all these conditions. The problem at work is usually confined to weakness and therefore with appropriate mobility aids for travelling to and moving about the workplace, employees doing sedentary work may have little or no difficulty apart from coping with stairs, low toilet seats and reaching files from high shelves.

Somatosensory impairments

The effects of somatosensory loss in the limbs can be more disabling than motor lesions, and a major handicap to employees. Humans rarely exert their maximum muscle power and have considerable motor reserves if they wish to use more force. However, all modalities of sensory input are often used to the full. It is difficult to compensate for even mild cutaneous sensory loss in the fingers caused by a neuropathy or cervical myelopathy for example, and no amount of therapy or retraining will restore completely normal function.

If joint position sense is impaired, therapists can provide education about the disability and compensatory strategies; for example, using vision more when walking with diminished proprioception in the legs. Employees are likely to encounter difficulty with skilled movements of the hands, but may be helped by better lighting, or simply using a different type of pen or a word processor.

Loss of spinothalamic, pain, and temperature sensation produces different problems. If light touch and position sense are preserved, the patient's skilled use of the hands and walking are unaffected but the normal protective response of withdrawing from dangerous stimuli may be impaired. Those with loss of pain sensation are at risk of thermal injury if they come into contact with particularly hot or cold materials at work and remain exposed for a long time without realizing. Similarly, ill-fitting footwear may not be appreciated, resulting in skin damage. These difficulties occur most frequently in diabetic patients or those with other chronic neuropathies.

In more severely disabled employees with paraplegia, loss of sensation in the buttocks and legs results in increased risk of pressure sores. Proper seating to prevent trauma, both in the wheelchair and at the workstation, is important. Occupational therapists specialize in prescribing posture aids, seating cushions, and appropriate chairs.

Loss of sphincter control

Poor sphincter control is a symptom of many neurological diseases. It will be a problem at home and at work, and the management in both places is identical. By controlling fluid intake and having easy access to toilets it is usually possible for an employee to remain continent and cope at work. However, they may have other disabilities that limit work effectiveness. During the acute stage of an illness that causes urinary retention or incontinence, a catheter may be necessary, but usually the patient learns how to stimulate bladder reflex activity by abdominal pressure or other means and thereby regains control of micturition. This is more likely to be successful with a spinal cord lesion above the conus, and less successful when there is a more peripheral root lesion. If control cannot be achieved, either the use of a catheter with a drainage bag, or intermittent self-catheterization, will minimize embarrassment and permit continuation at work.

Neuropathic bowel dysfunction may result in extremes of faecal incontinence or chronic constipation, sometimes alternating unpredictably between the two. Neither is desirable, but unfortunately these problems are often poorly managed and cause considerable distress despite being entirely avoidable with a careful bowel management regimen. Laxatives help to overcome constipation but may be avoided because they are assumed to make incontinence more likely. One method is to use bulk softeners and laxatives but to aim for a regular bowel action at a conveniently planned time. This may rarely require an enema or digital rectal stimulation, but usually it can be achieved with regular suppositories.

Fatigue

Fatigue is a vague and imprecise term, and a normal phenomenon and consequence of work.[23] Rather than weakness, which is the inability to activate muscle power, physical fatigue denotes the inability to sustain power output and so can theoretically be measured objectively. However, fatigue can also affect mental performance and be influenced by factors such as motivation, attention, and arousal. It is also a subjective symptom that can be pleasant but is usually regarded by patients as unpleasant tiredness, weariness, or even exhaustion.

Fatigue can be a symptom of virtually any medical or psychiatric condition, and is susceptible to innumerable other factors. It affects many with organic neurological disorders, simply because mental and physical performance may already be impaired physiologically. For example, people recovering from simple concussion, let alone severe traumatic brain injuries, commonly complain of mental fatigue that is made worse by any form of sustained concentration. Those with corticospinal motor impairment from myelopathy or after stroke suffer from inefficient co-contraction of agonist and antagonist muscles, spasticity and mass motor activation. PD, other involuntary movements and cerebellar ataxia are all associated with greater energy demands, and of course myasthenia is characterized by objective muscle fatigability. However, it is MS that is most commonly associated with complaints of disabling fatigue and leading to high unemployment rates, even in the absence of severe physical disability, probably reflecting generally inefficient neurotransmission in the presence of demyelination.[24]

Simple measures may assist a neurological patient who is struggling to cope at work because of excessive fatigue. They may benefit from extra assistance at home with personal care that may be unduly time-consuming, or with mobility aids and transport. Sometimes gentle persuasion to accept provision of a wheelchair or motorized scooter can help someone previously determined to remain ambulant at all costs. Cardiovascular fitness can sometimes be improved with an appropriate exercise programme, and relative immobility is not an exclusion criterion because paraplegics can work out using a hand bicycle for example. Flexible work practices should be considered, with reduced hours and increased rest periods. Relaxation techniques, sleep hygiene and psychological interventions may also be beneficial.

Drug management

Patients with neurological disease are sometimes given excessive drug treatment, which can limit their capacity for work. As a general rule, any drug acting on the CNS will interfere with arousal, awareness, and cognitive function to some degree, particularly when given in higher doses. Therefore, it is important to review any medication and liaise with medical colleagues responsible for the clinical management about stopping any non-essential treatment. Not infrequently, multiple drugs are initiated by specialists in an acute setting, but not revised and tapered once the patient is discharged. The general practitioner may be reluctant to interfere with treatment initiated in hospital, yet be content to issue repeat prescriptions inappropriately. The occupational health interview prior to a return to work may be the ideal opportunity to rationalize the medication.

Antiepileptic medication is a good example, particularly when started by general physicians or neurosurgeons in hospital rather than electively by a neurologist. Co-ordination and balance problems may only become apparent when someone returns to work, and be the first clue to incipient phenytoin toxicity started inappropriately as prophylaxis after a craniotomy.

Analgesia requires particular care, as patients do not always appreciate the potential adverse effects as much as the benefits. It is rare for pain alone to prevent an employee working, but it is common for unrelieved pain to reduce the employee's work effectiveness. Clearly the underlying cause of the pain must be treated, but skill is required in selecting the correct analgesia.[25] Certain types of neuropathic pain may respond to particular therapies, such as carbamazepine. Minor tranquillizers can be particularly helpful when taken at night to improve sleep, which itself may ameliorate pain. Tranquillizers should be used with caution during the daytime as drowsiness can make driving dangerous and reduce efficiency at work. They are best used for a limited duration, when the patient is going through a particularly stressful period, to prevent habituation.

Explicit advice must be given about dose frequency, because some patients tend to take too much, while others get inadequate pain relief. Any disabling pain preventing efficient working should be controlled with sufficient prophylactic medication wherever possible. If the pain is continuous or regular then the therapy needs to be taken regularly. An employee who refuses to take analgesia until breakthrough pain impedes their work has probably waited too long. On the other hand, medication overuse is thought to be a significant factor perpetuating chronic headache and possibly backache in some patients. Opiates are seldom if ever justified for non-malignant pain.

Antispasticity medication with baclofen or tizanidine can relieve painful and disabling muscle spasms. The dose may have been carefully titrated against functionally relevant criteria, but not infrequently is increased simply because spasticity is still detectable on examination without taking into account possible adverse effects. These include increasing muscle weakness, which is actually the mechanism of action, and sedation that may interfere with work capacity.[20]

Drug treatment is relatively straightforward in the early stages of PD, but special neurological expertise is required to manage longer-term complications of antiparkinsonian medication such as fluctuations in motor response and drug-induced dyskinesia.

Although rare in absolute terms, immunosuppressive therapy is being used more frequently for certain neurological disorders. There is increasing evidence of its efficacy in some acquired neuropathies as well as inflammatory myopathies and autoimmune conditions such as myasthenia and vasculitis. The occupational physician will need to be mindful of relevant potential side-effects such as anaemia, leucopenia, skin changes, steroid-induced diabetes, myopathy, and osteoporosis in those who return to work on treatment.

Driving

> In the interests of road safety, those who suffer from a medical condition likely to cause a sudden disabling event at the wheel or who are unable to safely control their vehicle from any other cause, should not drive.[5]

Decisions on fitness to drive can be extremely difficult for patients with neurological conditions.[26] This is particularly for vocational licences for which the regulations are stricter. The standards of medical fitness to drive and the role of the Driving and Vehicle Licensing Agency (DVLA)[5] are discussed in Chapter 28, and the particular problems arising in relation to epilepsy are also discussed in Chapter 8. With trauma or other pathology affecting the nervous system, the challenge is to determine whether the resulting neurological deficit itself or the future risk of seizures constitute unacceptable driving hazards.

The commonest conditions where licence holders should not drive include following any unprovoked seizure or unexplained blackout, and immediately after a craniotomy, severe traumatic brain injury or acute stroke. Those with either static or progressive or relapsing neurological disorders likely to affect vehicle control because of impairment of co-ordination and muscle power may continue to drive providing medical assessment confirms that driving performance is not impaired.

Doctors have a duty to advise their patients of their statutory obligation to notify the DVLA of any medical condition if there is the slightest possibility that driving might be impaired. Ideally the doctor should personally assess the ability of the patient to operate car controls and to respond quickly, accurately, and intelligently to driving conditions. In practice, referral to a specialist assessment centre for disabled drivers is advisable if there is any doubt, not least because a detailed professional report will be prepared after more relevant and objective assessment, together with any recommendations about appropriate driving adaptations. Sophisticated vehicle adaptation is now possible and varies from automatic transmission to joysticks and infrared controls for people with severe disabilities. Contact details of disabled drivers' assessment centres are available on the DVLA website.[5]

Employers have a responsibility to ensure that their vocational drivers are medically fit. It is important that their motor insurance covers any disabled drivers. Generally, if the employee's driving ability is acceptable to the DVLA, when they have all the information, the employee should not be prevented from driving. In rare neurological cases where the occupational physician judges there to be a significant risk to the public, the patient may refuse to inform the DVLA. This is usually because of pathological loss of insight, for example in dementia or after frontal lobe injury. If doctors are uncertain about the risks of driving in a particular case, they should contact the DVLA, who take specialist advice from a panel of honorary medical advisers that always includes several experienced neurologists. The physician should consult Chapter 28 for further information.

How workplace factors influence neurological function

In considering neurological fitness for work, the most important thing is to review disability in relation to the work demands, and to assess the patient's current status. Nevertheless, it is useful to review specific workplace exposures that can cause or exacerbate neurological disease and which can influence work function. Workplace exposures can be classified as physical, psychological, and chemical. The exposures will be dealt with in turn, distinguishing where necessary between factors that exacerbate pre-existing disease from those that are specific causes of neurological deficit.

Psychological factors

Psychiatric disorders are dealt with in Chapter 7, but it should be remembered that a number of adverse psychological effects from work could influence patients with neurological disorders. An internal state of stress is an almost universal experience at some times in the workplace, reflecting conflicting influences and demands on our time and motivation. It is widely held that stress can be good or bad, depending on the tonic state of psychophysiological arousal acting on the cerebral cortex. Below a certain level, under conditions of boredom or through pharmacological effects, attention, cognitive processing, and task performance are all inefficient. Conversely, performance also deteriorates and people start to make errors if arousal levels are too high because of a narrowing of attention to multiple inputs. There is an intermediate level of arousal that should result in optimal task performance, and it is likely that this parabolic relationship is altered adversely in the presence of neurological conditions affecting brain function.

Sleep and fatigue

Apart from stress and boredom, there are effects from shift work that could either mimic or exacerbate neurological disorders. The main adverse effect of shift work is fatigue. Many workers complain of it, and it can result in tiredness or even drowsiness at work with insomnia when attempting to sleep.[23] In practice these symptoms may be more noticeable, in the short term, than the gastrointestinal or cardiovascular effects found in large-scale longitudinal surveys of shift workers. The circadian rhythm disruption caused by rotating shift work, although measurable, is rarely translated into overt symptoms other than fatigue. For the patient with pre-existing neurological disease this may worsen work performance whatever the nature of the original deficit (motor, sensory, or cerebral function). Obviously a patient with myasthenia or narcolepsy would be particularly affected. The financial pressures to continue shift work may be considerable and it must be remembered that some shift patterns (particularly the 10- or 12-hour shift) do provide opportunities for a second job on the days off shifts.

Physical agents

As for psychological stress, exposure to moderate levels of various environmental stressors results in deteriorating work performance. Repeated exposure can bring about adaptations to reduce this adverse impact, i.e. training. It seems reasonable to assume that a fully trained employee who acquires a new neurological diagnosis is more likely to return to work in such a stressful environment than a new recruit is likely to succeed in being trained.

Noise

Noise may actually help to improve or maintain performance in conditions of low arousal. However, excessive noise can cause irritability, restrict attention to other stimuli and disrupt task performance. The sounds used for warnings in locomotive cabs and aircraft cockpits can lead to excessive physiological startle responses, even in healthy people, so the occupational physician should consider the likely interaction between the ambient noise levels in the workplace and the particular diagnosis with these factors in mind.

Although noise-induced hearing loss is the most obvious problem associated with excessive noise levels, other effects such as headaches, diminished ability to concentrate and communicate, and even perceived difficulties with balance can be important, particularly in a patient with imperfect neurological function.

The deafness caused by noise is due to damage to the organ of Corti in the inner ear, but patients with pre-existing deafness (whether conductive or perceptive, and unilateral or bilateral) should be protected from further damage. This is considered in greater detail in Chapter 10 on hearing.

The problems with communication in noisy environments are twofold. First, it is difficult to communicate at all with high ambient noise levels and while wearing hearing protection. Secondly, someone may already have a neurological dysfunction that limits communication. This could be an impairment of articulation, speech production or language. Such employees, in particular, should avoid noisy work situations that may worsen their ability to communicate safely and effectively.

Vibration

Vibration is widespread in industry and often accompanies noise. The health hazards generally occur at vibration frequencies between 1 and 1000 Hz. There is no doubt that operating in vibrating environments for any length of time affects visual and psychomotor performance, as anyone will testify after a long car journey. The vibration may be whole body, as occurs in van and truck drivers where the vibration is generally at the lower end of the range (1–10 Hz). Hand-transmitted vibration from 10 to 1000 Hz occurs when holding a vibrating tool, such as a chain saw or pneumatic drill, or holding the work-piece to a vibrating machine as in some metal finishing processes.

Little is known about the chronic effects of whole-body vibration (apart from specific influences on body organ resonance and perhaps an association with low back pain), but the effects of hand–arm vibration are well recognized and can be disabling (see Appendix 6).

Temperature and humidity

Extremes of temperature may cause subjective discomfort and a variety of effects but particular interest lies in the influence of temperature on patients with pre-existing neurological disease. At high ambient temperatures the symptoms of MS worsen temporarily as core temperature rises slightly because of slowing of nerve conduction through demyelinated plaques, but recover when the body is cooled. A similar adverse effect occurs with low ambient temperatures, which also slow peripheral nerve conduction and neuromuscular actions generally, posing a particular problem for those with neuropathic, myotonic, and other myopathic disorders. Such patients should, wherever possible, avoid working where extremes of ambient temperature are likely to occur.

Little has been written about any clinical consequences of disordered sweating in neurological patients, although idiopathic hyperhidrosis does feature in the index of the British National Formulary. Excessive facial sweating can occur with cluster headache, and after incomplete lesions of the spinal cord when it will also affect the upper trunk, but this is unlikely to present practical problems. Of greater significance may possibly be those with widespread impaired sweating and hence thermoregulation, because of damage to either the spinal cord, autonomic pathways, or peripheral nerves.

Light

Poor lighting at work is a particular problem for the visually impaired (Chapter 9). Both poorly lit and dazzlingly bright workplaces may cause headaches. It is thus important that the employee has optimum refractive correction. Photosensitive epilepsy is considered in Chapter 8. Flashing lights in working environments can also precipitate migraine.

Atmospheric pressure

In general, someone with established neurological disease should avoid exposure to hyperbaric and hypobaric pressure. Recreational diving, if carefully managed, need not be barred absolutely unless there is a significant risk of incapacitation. However, the possibility of exacerbating existing neurological deficits underwater must always be anticipated, with any attendant risk, for example difficulty in carrying out safety-critical checks or emergency drills. (See also Appendix 4.)

Chemical factors

Naturally occurring or synthetic chemical agents in the environment, including the workplace, may sometimes cause changes in neurological structure or function. For example, parkinsonism can certainly be a feature of poisoning by carbon disulphide, carbon monoxide, and manganese, while chronic mercury exposure causes cerebellar ataxia. Many potentially toxic agents can persist for many years in the body, especially those that are lipid soluble. More often non-occupational neurological disorders mimic neurotoxic syndromes such as encephalopathy, movement disorders, and peripheral neuropathy. Patients with a non-occupational neurological deficit may also have their symptoms exacerbated by workplace exposure, or attribute symptoms to such exposure and seek confirmation and reassurance that their concerns are valid.

Furthermore, there have been many health scares concerning putative neurotoxicity where numerous factors confound interpretation of hard facts and fuel considerable controversy. Validated biomarkers are seldom available, except for example measuring red blood cell acetyl cholinesterase inhibition after exposure to organophosphates. In view of the vague nature of many of the effects, objective data from neurophysiological or psychometric testing has proved useful to augment epidemiological studies, but prospective studies and valid controls are often lacking. It is rare for clinical conditions from neurotoxins to cause inability to work. Clearly, adequate protection and regular clinical assessment are important. The whole field of neurotoxicology is beyond the scope of this chapter, but four topical areas will be covered as examples of the relevant issues to be considered. The reader should consult specialist texts for further details.[27]

Toxic neuropathies The clear-cut peripheral neuropathies induced by inorganic lead compounds and the organic solvents n-hexane and methyl-n-butyl-ketone are relatively easy to evaluate. Other industrial agents also cause neuropathy, normally mixed sensory and motor in type, but inorganic lead is exceptional in causing a pure motor neuropathy. Regeneration usually follows slowly and uneventfully provided exposure is halted in affected employees. Clearly it would be inadvisable for any employee with a pre-existing neuropathy of any aetiology to be exposed knowingly to such an additional hazard, regardless of the standard safety precautions in the workplace.

Heavy metal toxicity and organic solvents The acute encephalopathy associated with exposure to aluminium first described in smelter workers was known as 'pot room palsy', and characterized by incoordination, poor memory, and impaired abstract reasoning. Permanent neuropsychological impairment has been reported following occupational exposure to high doses of heavy metals utilized in many industrial processes, either involving inhalation or after accidental ingestion.

There may also be concomitant symptoms referable to other organs. Dementia from occupational or environmental exposure is rarely considered, but it is important as symptom progression may be halted or possibly reversed if the diagnosis is identified early.

Even more controversial is whether low-level chronic exposures to heavy metals, either in the workplace or the environment could be responsible for cognitive dysfunction and dementia. The literature includes various papers assessing neuropsychological function in workers at risk. In some studies, researchers have assessed subclinical endpoints, as workers have non-specific symptoms or no symptoms. It remains uncertain whether continued occupational exposure may lead to frank clinical and possibly irreversible problems.

This is also true of organic solvents that are widely used in manufacturing industry, dry-cleaning, degreasing, and paint production and application. The acute effects of organic solvents range from mild fatigue to frank psychosis. The weight of evidence suggests that chronic exposure to hydrocarbon solvents at current limits does not appear to cause adverse neurobehavioural effects. Nevertheless, there is still controversy over the severity of effects that can arise from workplace exposure. Psychosis, dementia, and compensatable disability appear to be frequent in Scandinavian studies but less severe effects have been described in other Western countries.[28]

Organophosphate pesticides and sheep dips Well-established acute toxic effects of organophosphate pesticides and sheep dips arise from their capacity to inhibit acetylcholinesterase in the central and autonomic nervous systems and at the neuromuscular junction. They have only been seen after clearly excessive exposures that should not occur if the substances are used in the approved manner. A more controversial possibility is that organophosphates might cause long-term illness, even when there has been no obvious acute toxicity. In particular, a syndrome of chronic organophosphate-induced neuropsychiatric disorder (COPIND) has been proposed, including personality changes, impulsive suicidal thoughts, and frank cognitive impairment.

The Department of Health concluded in 1999 that subtle neuropsychological abnormalities probably could occur as a long-term complication of acute organophosphate poisoning, especially if the poisoning were severe.[29] However, long-term memory appeared not to be affected. Persistent peripheral neuropathy can sometimes follow acute poisoning by certain organophosphates that inhibit an enzyme known as neuropathy target esterase, but these have not been used in the UK for some years.[30]

In contrast, the balance of evidence did not support the occurrence of peripheral neuropathy or clinically significant neuropsychological impairment from low-level exposure to organophosphates in the absence of overt acute poisoning. Nor was such exposure thought to be a major factor in the excess mortality from suicide that had been demonstrated in British farmers.

Several outstanding gaps in knowledge were identified, including uncertainty as to whether low-level exposure to organophosphates might cause disabling neuropsychological illness in a small minority of exposed persons who for some reason, either genetic or environmental, are unusually sensitive to these chemicals. In support of this, farmers with chronic illness that they attributed to work with sheep dips have been found to differ from controls in the prevalence of a polymorphism of an enzyme involved in organophosphate metabolism.[30]

Identification and prevention of occupational neurotoxicity

A detailed occupational and environmental history is mandatory when considering exposure as a possible aetiology or a potential aggravating factor for a neurological condition. This should include specific aspects of the employee's tasks, the use of personal protective equipment and contact with specific chemicals, if applicable. Specific enquiries should be made and if possible documents, such as Control of Substances Hazardous to Health (COSHH) Regulations, occupational exposure limits and chemical hazard alert notices requested.

Questions about the use of specific natural remedies, recreational drug use, and routine household products as well the source of residential water supply are also important. Obtaining exposure data and estimating the likely dose and duration is part of a risk assessment. A comparison of this dose and duration with available literature from individual, group, or animal data published by regulatory agencies is an important next step. Working with a professional toxicologist or industrial scientist is recommended when managing such a patient.

Preventive procedures may be applied to the chemical process, the workplace or to the individual worker. Effective engineering controls and devices have included ventilation systems, ergonomic changes, safer tools, and the isolation of areas for dangerous exposures. Preventive practices directed at the workers are less effective as they do not reduce the absolute potential for exposure. Education and advice about work hazards and the provision of personal protective equipment may not always reduce accidents and exposures as these garments may not fit properly, or be uncomfortable to wear, and poor compliance may limit protection. Pre-placement medical examinations can identify those with risk factors for relevant medical conditions, e.g. diabetics with neuropathy, and reduce their exposure by reassigning work. Screening and surveillance is also important and should aim to identify or document early adverse health effects.

Assistive technology

With environmental control systems, it is often possible to set up a workstation that will allow the disabled employee to use a word processor or a telephone, and even initiate simple mechanical tasks. An environmental control system is a computer with links to peripheral equipment, such as doors, telephones, and light switches. The patient can control the equipment from a keyboard, hand-held remote infrared controller, or more sophisticated switching devices that, although slower, can be operated by small movements of the limbs, head, lips, or tongue. Regional environmental control co-ordinators based at major rehabilitation units can advise. The systems are available for home use under the NHS but at work they may allow a disabled person to continue useful work. Their provision would be best made after advice from the co-ordinator and with the help of an occupational therapist. With adequate access even the weakest person can use an electric wheelchair, of which there is a wide range. Specialist help should be sought in choosing the most appropriate one.[3]

Table 6.2 summarizes some of the general occupational considerations relevant to vocational fitness assessments, together with some of the specific disorders considered in the next section.

Specific neurological disorders

Earlier in this chapter the relation between symptoms and signs of neurological disease and work were considered. Although the symptoms and signs often give a better assessment of generic work capability, the underlying diagnosis is important in assessing the prognosis and guiding decisions about whether a person should be employed, what adjustment(s) should be made, or recommending medical retirement.

Headache disorders

Daily in the UK more than 90 000 are absent from school or work on account of headache.[31] Eighty per cent of the population have tension type headache, 2–3% of adults have chronic tension type headache (on more than 15 days per month), 10–15% have migraine, and 4% have chronic daily headache, with 1 in 50 having medication overuse headache.[32] Organic disease is

Table 6.2 Occupational considerations in neurological conditions

Clinical aspects of neurological function
Cognitive function and psychometrics
Disturbances of arousal and consciousness
Paroxysmal pain disorders-migraine, trigeminal neuralgia
Language and communication
Behaviour and impulse control
Emotional state
Special senses
Olfaction
   Neurological aspects of vision
   Visual acuity
   Colour perception
   Visual fields, e.g. hemianopia, central scotoma
Taste
Hearing and vestibular function
Swallowing and nutrition
Mobility and gait
Upper and lower motor neurone functions—spasticity, weakness
Cerebellar function—limb co-ordination and balance
Extrapyramidal functions—tremor, bradykinesia, involuntary movements
Neuromuscular
Somatosensory—touch, pain, temperature
Neurogenic sphincter disturbance

Medication for neurological conditions and side-effects thereof
Anti-epileptic
Antispasticity
Antiparkinsonian
Analgesia, including antimigraine
Immunosuppresive therapy

Special considerations in the workplace
Incapacitation risk, including driving
Intrinsic variability
   Short-term fluctuations
   Unpredictable relapses
Progression: risk and rate of future deterioration
Exacerbating environmental factors
   Noise
   Vibration
   Extremes of temperature
   Illumination and photosensitivity
   Atmospheric pressure
   Sleep deprivation
   Psychological stress
Assistive technology
   mobility aids
   environmental control systems
   communication aids, etc.

Ethical and legal considerations
Pre-symptomatic testing-HIV, genotyping
Stigma, stereotyping, and discrimination
Neurological disorders of particular relevance
Multiple sclerosis

Table 6.2 Occupational considerations in neurological conditions—cont'd

Stroke, subarachnoid haemorrhage and vascular brain injury
Traumatic and other non-vascular (hypoxic) brain injury
CNS infections
    Meningitis—viral, bacterial, etc.
    Encephalitis
Extrapyramidal disorders
    Parkinson's disease
    Dystonia
    Huntington's disease
Dementia incl. SDAT, CJD
Neurosurgical
    Brain and spinal tumours
    Craniotomy
Hydrocephalus and shunts
Headache and other paroxysmal pain disorders
    Migraine
    Tension-type headache
    Cluster headache
    Trigeminal neuralgia
Cerebral palsy
Myelopathies and spina bifida
Anterior horn cell diseases
    Poliomyelitis
    Motor neurone disease
Peripheral neuropathy
Neuromuscular junction disorders—myasthenia gravis
Muscular disorders
    Polymyositis
    Metabolic myopathies
    Progressive muscular dystrophies
Neurotoxic exposure, e.g. organophosphorus compound poisoning
Chronic fatigue syndrome
Sleep disorders
    Obstructive sleep apnoea
    Narcolepsy

a very uncommon cause unless the headache is of recent origin, or has changed its character, or if there are abnormal physical signs. In the older worker temporal arteritis should also be considered.

Migraine may occur with or without aura, typically a visual disturbance although other transient focal neurological deficits may occur simultaneously or sequentially, such as dysphasia or sensory disturbance. It then progresses to a unilateral or generalized headache with nausea and/or vomiting. It is not uncommon for the aura to occur without the headache. The manifestations of the migraine can change with time, and it is most unlikely that the migraine is symptomatic of any underlying localized pathology.

Headache in general and migraine in particular leads to sickness absence but workplace underperformance is at least as significant financially as absence. In one study, 40% of migraineurs caused the majority of both absence and underperformance.[33] Conversely, a high proportion of workers attribute headaches to their work.[32]

In spite of advances in medication and management guidelines[34] migraine and other forms of headache are underdiagnosed and undertreated. A variety of questionnaire instruments have emerged to manage headache and migraine better both from an individual clinical perspective and the corporate workplace viewpoint to reduce disability. There is evidence that migraine intensity but not frequency is related to disability.[35]

It is increasingly recognized that co-morbidity has occupational significance and clinical history taking should pay particular attention to coexisting depression, anxiety, stress, and psychometric features. Thus depression and stress are often features of morning headaches that prevent people getting to work.[36] An individual's perceived capacity to exercise self-control is a factor in the impact of stress in the aetiology of headaches and can be improved with the deployment of cognitive behavioural therapy.[37]

The principle of stratified care ('right first time' care) in contrast to stepped care (initially trying simpler medication and then gradually moving to more powerful medications at subsequent consultations) has enormous occupational consequences. Stepped care tends to lead to less satisfied, more frustrated employees and unnecessary time away from the workplace attending consultations.[38] The use of an assessment instrument improves diagnostic accuracy, treatment effectiveness, and patient satisfaction.[34] Also, chronic headaches are often the result of medication overuse, including triptans (5HT-1a agonists), which needs to be born in mind in sickness absence reviews. Acupuncture can reduce days off sick from headache.

Modern headache management is regularly reviewed and updated by the British Association for the Study of Headaches.[31] Precipitant factors such as workplace chemicals (including perfume or deodorant), oscillating temperature, humidity or light, irregular meal patterns and irregular sleep patterns (particularly sleeping in late) should be elicited in an occupational history. There are now a wide variety of modes of medication delivery including nasal sprays, injectable and sublingual formulations and suppositories, and regular prophylaxis with pizotifen, beta-blockers, and amitriptyline such that effective treatment is available for the majority to reduce sickness absence and boost workplace performance. As important as the medication, managers should be well educated about the condition because anecdotal evidence suggests that unsympathetic management prolongs time off and induces fear of returning to work.

In general, migraine is unlikely to fall under the DDA. However there is wide variation in its effects and for those who need regular preventative medication it may fall within the definition. Workplace adjustment may require changing lighting or temperature and providing a quiet, dark room if possible when a sufferer needs to rest. Migraineurs are likely to be precluded from some safety-critical jobs such as airline pilots, air traffic controllers and aerial climbers.

Disorders of awareness and sleep

Disturbances of awareness include blackouts and seizures as well as alterations in the ability to stay awake. A practical approach to restricting driving after episodes of loss of consciousness is set out in the guidance from the DVLA, depending on the results of cardiovascular as well as neurological examination.[5] These guidelines can reasonably be applied in other occupational settings where incapacitation risks must be minimized.

Daytime somnolence is a perfectly normal physiological phenomenon, particularly soon after a heavy lunch. However, obstructive sleep apnoea is increasingly being recognized as a cause of excessive daytime somnolence, and is most common in middle-aged men. Obstructive sleep apnoea is important because of its neurocognitive and cardiovascular sequelae and potential to interfere with work.[39] Sleep disruption is frequent with carbon dioxide retention causing headaches on waking, with poor concentration and consequent impairment of work. It can also cause drowsiness when driving. Establishing the existence of obstructive sleep apnoea can be difficult and depends on clinical suspicion. Patients frequently contend that night time sleep is normal—the problem, in their view, is in the daytime—unless their partner complains of loud snoring, which is not an invariable feature anyway. Sufferers are particularly intolerant of rotating shiftwork, and should lose weight and avoid alcohol. In severe cases continuous positive airways pressure at night is often very effective. Screening tools are available and early treatment can be justified on economic grounds. In an occupational context a two-stage approach has been recommended in a workforce of commercial drivers, using symptoms plus body mass index for screening everyone for the presence of severe sleep apnoea, followed by overnight oximetry that can be done at home for those at high risk.[40]

The classical narcolepsy syndrome is very rare, comprising cataplexy, hypnogogic hallucinations, and sleep paralysis as well as irresistible sleep attacks. Cataplexy is the sudden decrease or loss of voluntary muscle tone following emotion and may itself present just as much of a hazard at work. Effective treatment involves optimizing nocturnal sleep duration, and allowing planned daytime naps as well as appropriate medication.

Return to work following stroke and transient ischaemic attacks

The effects of an acute stroke are determined by the combination of the volume of brain tissue that is damaged and its location. This combination will determine the rate of recovery and the occupational prognosis. Clinically however, it is more relevant for the occupational physician to use the Oxford clinical classification of stroke, or something similar (see Box 6.2), without needing direct access to imaging results.[41] It follows that the prognosis of a total anterior circulation infarct is worst, and that of lacunar and posterior circulation infarcts best because they are the smallest, with partial anterior circulation infarcts intermediate.

Box 6.2 Anatomical diagnosis of stroke

Lacunar syndromes (LACS)

- pure motor stroke
- pure sensory stroke
- ataxic hemiparesis, including dysarthria/clumsy hand syndrome
- sensorimotor stroke.

Lacunar syndromes typically involve a complete hemi-body distribution, or at least the whole of the face and arm (brachiofacial), or the whole of the arm and leg (bachiocrural). More restricted deficits are likely to be of cortical origin.

Total anterior (carotid) circulation syndrome (TACS)

Combination of all three below at time of maximum deficit:

- hemiplegia or severe hemiparesis contralateral to the cerebral lesion
- homonymous heminanopia contralateral to the cerebral lesion
- new deficit of higher cerebral function, e.g. visuospatial disorder, dysphasia.

Continued

> ### Box 6.2 Anatomical diagnosis of stroke *(continued)*
>
> ## Partial anterior circulation syndromes (PACS)
>
> - combination of two of three features above of TACS, or
> - new deficit of higher cerebral function only, or
> - pure motor/sensory deficit less extensive than for LACS, e.g. one limb only.
>
> ## Posterior (vertebrobasilar) circulation syndromes (POCS)
>
> At time of maximum deficit, any of:
>
> - ipsilateral cranial nerve III–XII with contralateral motor and/or sensory deficit
> - bilateral motor and/or sensory deficit
> - disorder of conjugate eye movement
> - cerebellar dysfunction
> - isolated hemianopia or cortical blindness.

Cerebrovascular disease results in two pathologies, either ischaemia or haemorrhage, with infarction, gliosis, and atrophy as the end result of both. Typically haemorrhage is intracerebral, but it can be subarachnoid from either aneurysms or vascular malformations. The method of stroke management depends as much on the clinical state as on the underlying pathology.

By definition, TIAs cause focal neurological disturbance for less than 24 hours and thus in themselves are unlikely to have more limited occupational implications. However, it is not uncommon for incomplete neurological assessment or clinically silent cerebral infarction to occur in this context. For these reasons, the occupational assessment should adopt the same systematic approach for any employee who has suffered any form of cerebrovascular event. This assessment needs to take into account the following factors.

Risk factors

The employee's treating physicians should have conducted a thorough search for modifiable risk factors. The occupational physician will need to consider the significance of these in the workplace, and may be able to reinforce the importance of their control. Underlying cardiac disease or poorly controlled hypertension must be identified with any adverse consequences, for example, vigorous exertion or safety-critical time pressures.

Risk of recurrence/incapacitation

It would be wrong to prevent a person returning to work just because the employer is concerned that a further episode might occur. Each employee needs to have the prognosis assessed individually and reasonable adjustment made in work practices. The absolute risk of a first stroke following a single TIA, or of a second stroke following a first one, is statistically quite low. Nevertheless, the risk of recurrent TIAs is highest within the first 6 weeks of an initial event, and a second stroke twice as likely to occur compared with those who have never had a first stroke. Such analysis may have implications for those who work in geographical isolation or entirely alone. There is a small but significant risk of sudden incapacitation from a recurrence, hence the DVLA regulations requiring certain periods off driving depending upon the clinical features and the nature of the licence (see Chapter 28).[5]

Medication

As with all employees, any potentially adverse effects of prescribed medication should be identified. Poorly controlled hypertension is occasionally only identified for the first time following a cerebrovascular event, requiring treatment with several different antihypertensive agents and a cholesterol-lowering drug, multiplying the risks of interactions. Postural hypotension and cognitive slowing are particularly important. Antithrombotic medication itself may be relatively harmless, but the occupational physician should be aware of those who are on formal anticoagulation and consider their risk of exposure to potential hazards. For example, members of the uniformed services might be restricted to administration and training rather than frontline duties.

Functional deficits

The time to maximum recovery varies widely, but can be a year or more. However, after about 4 months it is usually possible to give a reliable prognosis as by then the functions that are recovering can clearly be discerned and any function that has not started to recover is unlikely to do so completely. However, a final prognosis should not be given until the employee has received optimum rehabilitation, which requires considerable skill.

Physical deficits such as a residual hemiparesis are usually apparent to everyone, including the employee, their managers and work colleagues. Standard assessments will determine any reasonable adjustments to the workplace that may be required, with appropriate advice from a physiotherapist or occupational therapist as necessary. Of greater importance, however, is the potential for other focal neurological deficits to co-exist that may not be so obvious but have important consequences for employability.

Subtle deficits of cognitive function may occur, particularly following non-dominant hemisphere strokes affecting frontal lobe executive functions and non-verbal abilities. Those who have had a dominant hemisphere lesion may not only have residual dysphasia with word-finding difficulties apparent in normal conversation, but the coexistence of dysgraphia, dyslexia, and dyscalculia must be sought. Finally, visual field deficits, whether absolute or for simultaneous stimuli presented in opposite visual fields, may require careful assessment, together with other tests for visual agnosia or other perceptual difficulties in certain occupations.

Cerebral tumours

Unlike tumours elsewhere in the body, intrinsic cerebral and spinal cord tumours do not metastasize outside the CNS. Their histological grade can still vary from benign to rapidly malignant, but ultimately the anatomical site determines prognosis. Even the most benign tumour can be incurable if it is deeply inaccessible within the brain. Fortunately most benign tumours can be treated successfully by surgery, some of the malignant ones can be halted by radiotherapy, and a few are amenable to chemotherapy.

After treatment, an assessment of the employee's function and information about the prognosis usually facilitates decisions about work. If function is good, return to work should be automatic but if it is not then the decision to return will rest on two opposing trends:

◆ the natural improvement that will occur with rehabilitation and recovery after treatment such as subtotal excision, not dissimilar to recovery from a stroke.

◆ the natural history of the tumour, which, if malignant or liable to recur, makes the long-term prognosis worse.

Occupational physicians may need to consider the risk of symptomatic seizures arising in the future, particularly after craniotomy or with any tumours affecting the cerebral cortex (e.g. glioma, meningioma).

Parkinson's disease

PD is, after stroke, the second most common cause of acquired physical disability from a neurological condition in later life. Its incidence increases progressively with age, and affects about 1% of the population above retirement age. Nevertheless a significant minority of cases occur at younger ages, occasionally even under 40 years. The cardinal clinical features of parkinsonism are well known, namely the classical triad of slowness of movement or bradykinesia, rest tremor, and cogwheel rigidity, together with impairment of postural righting reflexes.

Before reaching a diagnosis of primary parkinsonism, i.e. idiopathic PD characterized by Lewy body neuropathology, the physician must attempt to rule out secondary causes of so-called symptomatic parkinsonism (Box 6.3).[21]

Environmental neurotoxicity hypotheses

Although the aetiology of idiopathic PD is unknown, one popular hypothesis concerns one or more hitherto unidentified environmental toxins, probably affecting only those exposed subjects with a particular genetic susceptibility.[21] Epidemiological studies have suggested that drinking well water, exposure to industrial chemicals or living near industrial chemical plants, or exposure to pesticides or herbicides increases the risk of PD.[42] Of interest, MPTP, a selective dopaminergic cell toxin associated with parkinsonism, was industrially developed as a potential herbicide with a structure resembling paraquat but was never produced commercially. The herbicide rotenone is a potent inhibitor of mitochondrial activity of particular research interest in animal models of parkinsonism.

The occupational physician is best placed and should always consider any potential neurotoxic exposure in the employee's workplace.[43] For example, manganese poisoning was first described in 1837 from France in men grinding manganese dioxide, and continues to be the subject of reports from several parts of the world. Long-term exposure to manganese dust mainly affects the CNS, parkinsonism is the typical presentation, and clinical progression continues even 10 years after cessation of exposure.[44] A current controversy with substantial medicolegal implications is whether welding increases the risk of PD. Racette *et al*.[45] reported a prevalence of parkinsonism 10 times higher within a sample of active male welders studied in Alabama compared with the general male working population. These authors speculated that exposure to manganese-containing flux either increases the prevalence at all ages or may shift the distribution of PD to a younger age in those exposed.

Box 6.3 Causes of symptomatic parkinsonism

- Any acute cerebral pathology, e.g. encephalitis, traumatic brain injury, anoxia, or ischaemia

- Parkinsonism-plus syndromes associated with non-Lewy body neurodegenerative disease

- Chronic exposure to prescribed medication that blocks dopamine receptors in the brain, e.g. major tranquillizers, and other phenothiazines such as prochlorperazine and metoclopramide given as antiemetics or for vertigo

- Environmental toxins.

Occupational considerations

The main occupational considerations in someone with PD are:

- their functional capacity in relation to the degree of motor impairment;
- concomitant cognitive and emotional factors;
- optimizing symptomatic control with medication while minimizing adverse effects;
- periodic review in anticipation of disease progression.

In the early stages of PD, motor impairments may be completely corrected with dopamine replacement therapy, although problems with micrographia and a slow shuffling gait may gradually become more apparent. In those occupations dealing directly with members of the public, prominent tremor can be embarrassing for both parties, although patients can sometimes be remarkably resourceful in disguising their disabilities using a variety of trick manoeuvres. When speech is impaired through dysphonia, the use of a voice amplifier, for example on the telephone, may need to be considered.

Cognitive impairment is rarely a feature of PD unless it has been present for a decade or more, but depression is remarkably common and may have a similar neurochemical basis of catecholamine deficiency to the motor impairments. Effective drug treatment is available and can be extremely rewarding in improving both productivity and quality of life.

As the underlying disease progresses slowly after the first few years, the requirement for medication may increase. A significant proportion of patients, particularly younger ones, also develop fluctuations in motor performance during the course of a day that often coincides with the cycles of drug absorption and metabolism, resulting in its extreme form in the 'on–off phenomenon'. This can result in spectacular oscillations between someone who is totally immobile and frozen to the spot one minute, and moving freely and almost normal the next. Sometimes this latter phase is associated with drug-induced dyskinesia with troublesome involuntary movements that can be embarrassing and disconcerting to colleagues. Careful titration of the timing of oral medication may be insufficient to control these motor fluctuations. Specialist neurological advice may be sought concerning other available strategies, such as the use of longer-acting dopamine receptor agonist drugs; modified-release levodopa formulations; the use of subcutaneous apomorphine either by intermittent injection or by infusion; and even deep brain stimulation.

Most antiparkinsonian drugs, particularly with the larger doses required in the later years of the condition, have the potential to cause psychiatric side-effects including impaired attention, confusion, visual hallucinations, and frank delusional states. These can arise idiosyncratically with certain powerful dopamine receptor agonists, and may resolve completely following withdrawal of the drug.

Although disability in PD does steadily progress, normally it does so only slowly over the course of a decade or more. This may be sufficient for the employee to reach retirement age. The occupational physician should be proactive in arranging to review the employee and his changing circumstances at appropriate intervals. The Parkinson's Disease Society of the United Kingdom (see Appendix 8) takes a particular interest in providing advice and support for sufferers who are still in active employment, and its network of regional officers and branches can also provide information and training for employers.

Essential tremor

Essential tremor is another idiopathic condition, often familial and dominantly inherited, that is 10 times more common than PD, but not associated with bradykinesia or rigidity. It almost always affects both upper limbs symmetrically, and less commonly the head, lower limbs, tongue, and voice. Older textbooks referred to it as a benign condition, but it is a lifelong disorder that gradually worsens. It can certainly cause significant interference with handwriting, employment, and activities of daily living, and also with social function because of embarrassment.

Many patients with essential tremor require nothing more than an accurate diagnosis and reassurance that a more sinister disease is not present. The impact of social embarrassment, depression, and anxiety must not be overlooked. The avoidance of stimulants such as caffeine and the judicious consumption of ethanol at social events are helpful to some patients and there appears to be little increased risk of alcoholism. Approximately half benefit from either primidone or beta-adrenergic blockers such as propranolol. Response to one does not predict response to the other, but complete suppression of tremor is rare.[22]

Dystonia

There are various forms of dystonia but, rather like essential tremor, they are probably under-diagnosed, usually idiopathic but with a significant genetic component, and poorly understood. Primary generalized dystonia normally starts in childhood and gives rise to severe motor dysfunction ('dystonia musculorum deformans') that is seldom compatible with work. Secondary causes are extremely rare except as a side-effect of drugs such as major tranquillizers.

However, focal forms of adult-onset dystonia are probably more common than PD in those of working age, and are classified according to their anatomical involvement. They usually cause some form of irregular involuntary muscle spasms resembling tics such as dystonic writer's cramp, torticollis, dysphonia, or blepharospasm. They are usually persistent and remission is uncommon but they do vary in severity and can be controlled to some extent by voluntary strategies such as trick movements. Formerly they were classified erroneously as psychogenic conditions for this reason, but there is now good evidence that they are associated with basal ganglia dysfunction. They respond poorly to anticholinergic medication such as benzhexol, but the introduction of botulinum toxin treatment has revolutionized their management.

Return to work after traumatic head and brain injuries

Occupational medical advice is typically sought after head injuries in one of two different situations. The first, seemingly straightforward, request comes from employees who consider that they are ready to return to work but have been instructed to obtain medical clearance before doing so. The other concerns an employee who has already returned to work following such an injury and who, either in their own opinion or that of their colleagues, is experiencing difficulties. Although superficially these appear to require different approaches, the same careful systematic analysis must be applied following any significant head injury because of the extremely wide variety of factors that require consideration.[46]

The first step is to estimate the severity of the injury to the brain, which is the best indicator of prognosis (Table 6.3). Most people use the term 'head injury' loosely to refer to any traumatic event, but the authors recommend use of term 'traumatic brain injury' to underline this distinction. A variety of data can be used to estimate the severity, of which the Glasgow Coma Score (GCS) on admission, and the durations of coma and of post-traumatic amnesia (PTA) are most useful prognostically, providing they are not prolonged by anaesthesia, sedative medication including opiates, or systemic factors. PTA of 2 weeks or more predicts inevitable measurable residual cognitive problems, of variable impact as far as employment is concerned; a month of PTA predicts at best a reduced work capacity; and a PTA of 3 months makes voluntary or subsidized work a likely best outcome while at worst residential placement may even be needed.[46]

Table 6.3 Severity grading of traumatic brain injuries

Severity	Initial GCS	Duration of coma (GCS<9)	Duration of PTA	Duration in hospital	Duration of recovery	Return to work
Complete recovery usual						
Very mild	14–15	<5 min	<5 min	0	<1 month	<1 month
Mild	13–15	<15 min	5–60 min	<2 days	1 month	<2 months
Moderate	9–12	15 min–6 h	1–24 h	7 days	1–3 months	1–4 months
Some permanent impairment expected						
Severe	<9	6–48 h	1–7 days	>7 days	3–9 months	6–12 months
Very severe	<9	>48 h	>7 days	>7 days	9–12 months	>12 months
Extremely severe	<9	>48 h	>28 days	>14 days	24+ months	Never

PTA, post-traumatic amnesia; GCS, Glasgow Coma Scale.

However, there are many patients whose injuries are not obviously very severe yet who have difficulty in returning successfully to their previous work. There are two possible explanations for this: either the severity of the underlying brain injury has been underestimated; or there are associated non-organic factors that contribute to a vicious cycle of ongoing subjective cognitive difficulties, low mood and self-esteem, and physical inactivity. While it is possible to adopt the entirely pragmatic approach that the explanation doesn't really matter, it can have important therapeutic and medico-legal implications.

Eventual outcome is the result (see Table 6.4) of complex interaction between injury severity, intrinsic recovery, and individual personal and environmental factors from the *International Classification of Functioning, Disability and Health* (ICFDH).[47] The latter include increasing age over 50 years, coping styles, social background, family support and relationships, pre-existing problems, past experiences, current attitudes and future expectations and genetic make-up, particularly the possession of at least one apolipoprotein E4 allele, which is associated with a poorer long term outcome.[46]

Table 6.4 Influences on outcome after traumatic brain injury

Pre-injury	Primary*	Secondary	Recovery
Genotype	Diffuse	Mass effects	• Recovery of neuronal excitability
Age	Axonal	Ischaemia	
Sex	Vascular	Seizures	• Network and neuronal reorganization and regrowth
Psychosocial status	Focal	Infection	
Comorbidities	Contusions	Systemic factors	
Nutrition	Haematomas (EDH; IDH)	BP, O$_2$, °C, etc	• Behavioural adaptations and substitutions
Alcohol			
Drugs	↓	↓	
	Biochemical mediators of necrosis and apoptosis		• Systemic and contextual limitations

*Apart from primary injuries after traumatic brain injury, the table illustrates factors influencing outcome after many sorts of brain injury. BP, blood pressure; EDH, extradural haematoma; IDH, intradural haematoma (subdural and intracerebral). Reproduced from table 2 in Greenwood RJ (2002). Head injury for neurologists. *J Neurol Neurosurg Psychiatry* **73** (Suppl. 1): i8–16 with permission from the BMJ Publishing Group.[46]

Even with concussive injuries involving little or no period of loss of consciousness, injuries to the brain can occur with focal contusions and disruption of cerebral connections secondary to diffuse axonal injury. However, the physical signs of organic disease can be minimal, and accurate estimates of PTA may be confounded by a prolonged period of sedation during and after surgical interventions and intensive care. Diagnostic pointers include other features of high kinetic energy impact (high-speed collisions, craniofacial fractures, spinal or proximal long bone limb fractures, visceral rupture, etc.). Magnetic resonance imaging (MRI) can usually demonstrate brain injuries objectively long after the event provided that the correct sequences are requested and the films reported by an experienced neuroradiologist. Finally, formal neuropsychological assessment may help distinguish between focal cognitive impairments, general intellectual underfunctioning compared with estimated pre-morbid ability, deficits more in keeping with anxiety and depression that may require psychiatric intervention, or even deliberate exaggeration of difficulties.

Approving return to work after concussion and minor brain injury

In certain occupations, for example safety-critical jobs or professional athletes participating in rugby or horse racing, even a minor head injury requires careful assessment before allowing the person to resume their usual activities. The potentially fatal risks of so-called 'second impact syndrome' have undoubtedly been exaggerated but clearly carry enormous medico-legal complications. The national governing bodies of certain sports in many countries now insist upon a medical examination as part of a 'return to play' protocol. Indeed in the USA, a normal brain scan may be a mandatory pre-requisite even though it is not at all evidence-based.[48]

The basic requirement is that the person is fully recovered from whatever effects they may have suffered, but this is sometimes hard to confirm with certainty. After a minor head injury, there are three main areas for the physician to consider: symptoms; physical signs of abnormal neurological function; and cognitive functioning.[48]

Symptoms On the face of it, it should be extremely easy to be satisfied that someone has returned to their pre-injury asymptomatic state—just ask the patient! However, those doctors who manage elite sportsmen know only too well that their patients cannot be trusted to tell the truth. Perverse incentives exist for the competitive sportsman to conceal the truth if the consequences of not competing are likely to affect their prize money or chances of being picked for the national squad. Similar motives may influence other workers. For example, employees who are desperate to accompany their colleagues on a long-planned overseas deployment or prestigious project team may be reluctant to admit to ongoing headaches and memory difficulties.

Neurological signs Unfortunately, the clinical neurological examination is not sensitive enough to enable the identification of people who are still symptomatic. Minor abnormal neurological signs are uncommon even after moderately severe traumatic brain injury, and after milder injury findings such as unequal pupillary size are more likely to reflect pre-existing conditions. Perhaps one of the most sensitive signs of impaired recovery is subtle impairment of co-ordination and balance. Although not usually part of the standard neurological examination, stringent tests of high-level balance such as the sharpened Romberg and Unterberger tests, single-leg stance and walking along a low beam as well as standard heel-to-toe gait will be examined routinely by sports physicians and team physiotherapists. In practice, physical performance should be tested in a protected training or simulator environment before allowing, for example, fire fighters and pilots to return to work or professional athletes to return to competition.

Cognitive functioning Neuropsychological tests have long been thought to be the most sensitive and objective measure of recovery after minor head and brain injury. Simple tests of orientation, attention, and recall have been incorporated into a standardized concussion assessment tool (SCAT) by an international consensus group. This can be used for any contact sports on the sidelines during a match, or by the roadside after an accident and can be extended to evaluate satisfactory recovery.[48] More detailed pencil and paper tests can also be used to chart and confirm recovery, and do not necessarily require a trained clinical neuropsychologist. However, the selection of appropriate tests that can be administered repeatedly to the same subject while avoiding inevitable practice effects does require special expertise. A further limitation is the wide range of compounding factors, some of which are shown in Table 6.4.

For these reasons, computerized neuropsychological test batteries have been developed that claim to minimize practice effects while sensitive to significant slowing of information processing speed and other relevant impairments. By using such instruments in a comprehensive programme of pre-season baseline testing, governing bodies such as the English Rugby Football Union and the Jockey Club have established data bases for participants in their respective sports that cannot only be used to compare an individual's performance after a single head injury, but also theoretically be used to identify those with a trend of deteriorating performance that might provide evidence of cumulative harm from repetitive head injuries.[48]

Vocational rehabilitation after moderate–severe brain injury

Early liaison with relevant healthcare professionals is highly desirable. Psychometric testing will usually establish the extent of any organic impairment. In association with an occupational therapist's cognitive screening and other assessments and knowledge of the work requirement, it may be used to formulate appropriate goals for return to work as an integral part of a person's rehabilitation.[49] Participation in a brain injury education programme may be beneficial to increase insight into residual difficulties, anticipate specific areas of potential difficulty at work and identify compensatory strategies. They can often usefully communicate this information to colleagues and line managers to facilitate understanding and adjustment. Ideally this should be an integral part of a formalized managed process of vocational rehabilitation.[50,51]

Employees should be advised to do everything they can for themselves to help recovery from the outset. This means regular meals, going to bed at reasonable hours, and adjusting their life-style to improve performance. Alcohol should be avoided or minimized, both because of reduced tolerance to intoxication and increased adverse neurobehavioural effects. Alcohol-related problems are not uncommon in patients who have had head injuries, perversely in those who should most avoid alcohol, and physicians should be alert to this possibility.

As with other organic lesions of the brain, functional improvement does occur but takes time and may be incomplete. Shift work is best avoided and medication that might impair concentration or cognition should be stopped unless absolutely necessary. For many employees after prolonged absence, returning to work too abruptly can be counter-productive and a graduated return is preferable, taking on limited responsibilities at first and then adding to them. This is because of a combination of physical deconditioning, particularly if commuting involves long journeys, and mental fatigue induced by cognitive inefficiency and increased multitasking. Ideally this should all be done as an integral part of a formalized managed process of vocational rehabilitation.[50,51]

Meningitis and encephalitis

Most infections of the CNS begin acutely over the course of hours or a few days, and involve both the meninges and brain to some extent, hence the term meningo-encephalitis. Many different viral, bacterial, and even fungal pathogens can cause an identical acute neurological syndrome with intense headache, fever, malaise, and drowsiness that may progress to coma and seizures, depending on the extent of cerebral involvement. After the first few days and appropriate timely antimicrobial treatment, the course is mostly one of slowly progressive improvement over several days or weeks. The prognosis and influence on work ability vary according to the organism and extent of underlying cerebral damage. Herpes simplex encephalitis, the most common cause of severe sporadic encephalitis in the Western world, can cause considerable memory impairment and these patients may never get back to intellectually demanding occupations. Other, less severe infections usually result in full recovery.

Better treatment for opportunistic infections and the development of highly active antiretroviral therapies has greatly reduced morbidity and mortality in those infected with HIV, and a marked decrease in the incidence of HIV-associated dementia. Nevertheless, because of their high prevalence, a high index of suspicion must be kept for neurological disorders in the HIV or AIDS patient. The risk of AIDS-related disorders, particularly opportunistic infections, depends on several factors, including CD4 count, exposure to infectious agents, and the use of antibacterial prophylaxis. When CD4 cell counts drop below 500/µl, so-called 'minor cognitive and motor disorder' may arise associated with minor difficulties in motor function and complaints of poor short-term memory and concentration, behavioural problems, or personality changes, as well as psychiatric symptoms of depression and anxiety. This may pose difficult decisions for the occupational physician and precede by many years HIV-associated dementia (also termed 'AIDS dementia complex' or 'HIV encephalopathy,') that develops as the CD4 count drops further, typically below 200/µl.

Alzheimer's disease and other pre-senile dementias

Dementia usually develops insidiously, most often after retirement, but poses a major diagnostic and management problem when it does occur in someone of working age. If the employee has been at the same job for many years, cognitive failure may be less obvious. They can work relatively well in familiar surroundings at routine tasks but new tasks are difficult. Colleagues may become aware of deterioration in driving safety or other work performance.

Dementia from occupational neurotoxic exposure is considered earlier in this chapter. Psychosocial work factors have even been implicated in the aetiology of dementia.[52]

Unfortunately, reversible causes of dementia (e.g. metabolic, normal-pressure hydrocephalus, and certain drugs including alcohol) are uncommon. (HIV-associated dementia is dealt with in the section on meningitis and encephalitis). Degenerative dementias are progressive by definition, and decisions about continuing employment must be objectively based on competency. Any occupational driving should be prohibited, and administrative safeguards instituted at diagnosis if medical retirement is not effected immediately.

Sporadic Creutzfeldt–Jakob disease (sCJD) generally presents after age 50 years with much more rapid progression over weeks or months, although cases aged less than 40 have been described), and 10% of cases are familial with autosomal dominant inheritance. A new variant of the disease (vCJD) was first described in 1996 from the UK National CJD Surveillance Unit based in Edinburgh, which maintains a website with up to date research and advice.[53] There is now compelling evidence suggesting vCJD is acquired from transmission of bovine spongiform encephalopathy to humans and over 150 cases of vCJD have been identified, primarily in the UK. These patients have had a number of distinctive features compared with classical sCJD. The average age of onset was less than 30 years, and disease duration was prolonged over 1 or 2 years. Anxiety and depression were common early symptoms, and other early signs were ataxia and sensory disturbances. The transmissible agent is abnormal prion protein isoform first identified in scrapie (PrPSc) that aggregates to produce cerebral amyloid.

Cases of CJD attributable to iatrogenic exposure have also been identified, mainly in recipients of human-derived growth hormone. There is no good evidence of an increased risk of sCJD through occupation, dietary factors, or animal contact, and the current favoured hypothesis is that sporadic disease is caused by a spontaneous mutation of prion protein to an abnormal form.

Neurological disorders of childhood

Cerebral palsy includes a group of childhood syndromes (historically classified as either spastic or dystonic) resulting from genetic and acquired insults to the developing brain, causing abnormalities in tone, posture, and movement. It is important to appreciate cerebral palsy includes a wide range of infectious, hypoxic–ischaemic, endocrine, and genetic conditions. Other developmental disorders of the posterior fossa and spinal cord such as Chiari malformations and spina bifida may cause similar disabilities, not least because of their association with hydrocephalus. Although not strictly affecting the CNS at all, certain other conditions occurring in childhood such as poliomyelitis or Guillian–Barré syndrome should be approached in the same way.

At the start of employment it is advisable to have a full medical and functional assessment so that work can be adjusted to allow the employee to use their skills with optimum efficiency. A systematic approach to a prospective employee, often a young school leaver, allows accurate identification of the key occupational considerations and prognosis, and avoids the danger of stereotyping, as someone with severe physical disability may have no intellectual impairment at all and vice versa.

Employment prospects are usually established during good education and training, enabling a young person to develop their potential abilities and attain appropriate vocational qualifications. It is usually valuable to obtain previous statements of educational needs that document the subject's abilities systematically. Minor motor impairments rarely pose a problem except during highly skilled activities. Machinery, office equipment, and vehicles can usually be adapted. Even though the underlying condition may not be progressive, secondary problems can occur earlier than in the normal population; for example, arthritis in a hip is more likely if the gait is affected, but these changes do not develop quickly.

Spinal cord injury and disease

The commonest neurological disease affecting the spinal cord itself is MS (see below). Primary tumours arising within the spinal canal are rare and are usually benign, the commonest being neurofibroma. However, the commonest cause of acute myelopathy is trauma, which tends to affect younger adults engaging in risk-taking activities and a significant proportion occurs at work. The return to work rate after spinal cord injury (SCI) at any level is significantly lower in the UK than in many other countries, which probably reflects the inadequate resources for more holistic rehabilitation and community mobility. Even if the workplace is easily accessible, people often lack the financial support to purchase valuable items of equipment and the physical endurance to cope with a resumption of full-time work. Yet the SCI victim is often very motivated, and this quotation on the Spinal Injuries Association website emphasizes their central role in educating colleagues and the occupational physician:[54]

> Living with spinal cord injury is like being reborn, with a body which doesn't behave as it used to, into a world that wasn't designed for it. You have to learn how to live again, physically and spiritually. Every spinal injury is unique and if you are to be the best that you can be you need to become an expert on your case. It is a very steep learning curve.

The employee may require reasonable time and space to use a standing frame during the working day, or to self-catheterize intermittently. The risks of developing autonomic dysreflexia also need to be considered in those with higher thoracic injuries. Regular maintenance physiotherapy may prove very worthwhile.

There are generally two tracks to employment after SCI—a fast track where people return to their pre-injury job or profession, substantially shortening the interval to return to work, or a slower alternative track after further re-education and training. Overall, less than half return to gainful employment after SCI even to a physically less demanding job.[55]

Multiple sclerosis

MS is the commonest neurological disorder affecting young adults. The diagnosis traditionally requires two or more CNS lesions separated in time and space, not caused by other CNS disease. The manifestations vary enormously because lesions can occur anywhere in the CNS. Common presentations include a single episode, lasting only a few weeks, of visual impairment, ataxia or focal motor or sensory disturbance.

MRI and cerebrospinal fluid analysis are abnormal in more than 95% of definite cases. MRI has also become essential to rule out conditions that could mimic MS. Updated diagnostic criteria use new MRI lesions to define separation in time and space.[56] These criteria are helpful after a clinically isolated demyelinating syndrome such as optic neuritis or transverse myelitis, when the risk of later evolution into MS is far greater in those with abnormal brain scans at presentation.

The majority present with relapsing and remitting disease, but MS is progressive from onset ('primary progressive MS') in about 20% of cases, particularly with later age of onset. More typically, there are three phases; initially relapses with full recovery, then relapses with persisting deficits, and later secondary progression. There is cumulative loss of oligodendroglia and neurons, with increasing demands on compromised surviving cells. In the progressive phase clinical remissions disappear, but constant low-grade immune activation continues or worsens.

The time course is extremely variable, as some patients may spend years or even decades in each phase, whereas about 10% rapidly become severely disabled. About 25% of patients have a benign form of MS that is not disabling. The prognosis is relatively good when sensory or visual symptoms predominate and there is complete recovery from individual relapses, a pattern commonest in young females. Negative prognostic predictors include cerebellar or pyramidal symptoms; frequent early attacks, development of secondary progression, or a primary progressive course, and age over 40 years at onset. Later onset MS is more common in men and often primary progressive; even when it begins as relapsing-remitting disease, secondary progression occurs earlier.

MS usually starts during working age and therefore may develop after an employee has passed a medical examination at the time of initial employment. However, in the era of flexible working practices, pre-employment assessments are likely to increase.

After a single episode with full recovery an employee should be able to return to normal work. If recurrent attacks are infrequent with full recovery, the amount of time off work over a period of years could be small. In more chronic cases regular assessment will be required to decide about physiotherapy or other ongoing help. Most patients with established disease will have attended hospital and their diagnosis and management policy been determined. If this has not occurred, referral to a specialist should be made before the employee's future work situation is decided. Beta-interferon and other disease-modifying treatments have been used as prophylaxis, but their long-term value is uncertain.

The initiating event for the first attack is unknown, but genetics and environmental factors both interact. Epidemiological studies have found an association between MS and residential latitude in different parts of the world, but the significance of those factors remains unclear. Trauma and stress have been implicated anecdotally as causing MS or triggering exacerbations, but the occurrence of any specific exacerbation cannot yet be causally linked to any specific stressor.[57] However, if a patient has not made a full recovery it is possible that certain environments may make the symptoms greater or more obvious, although no particular work environment should affect prognosis. Fatigue is one of the most common complaints among patients with established and disabling MS, typically magnification of postexertion fatigue and with sensitivity to heat and humidity. High temperatures are not well tolerated and some patients like to work in slightly colder environments than is usually desired by other employees as this reduces their symptoms.[24] Poor sleep and irregular hours are other factors that may worsen symptoms.

Psychological problems of chronic illness also need to be considered by the employee's medical adviser, such as depression. Occasionally, if there is considerable demyelination of cerebral white matter, insidious intellectual deterioration occurs that may not interfere with their work ability but require careful monitoring of the employee.[58] Euphoria can be an early sign of frontal lobe dysfunction, causing pathological contentment with physical disability. This has advantages for the sufferer as a patient, but not as an employee, as increased commitment is needed to overcome the disability and to continue to cope. Motivation to work is a very important factor in deciding whether employment can continue.

There is an unnecessarily high rate of unemployment among those with MS, associated with lower quality of life.[59] The factors relating to remaining in work are mainly disease-related, such as balance and walking abilities affecting accessibility of public transport or driving to and from work. However, the employment environment itself and lack of social support may compound the difficulties that people with MS experience. In particular, they receive little help, formal and informal, with work retention. To remain in work people with MS need good healthcare management and vocational rehabilitation as well as work and environmental modifications. Healthcare professionals should aim to minimize the disability that impacts on the work capacity using appropriate therapy interventions.[60]

Flexible working arrangements should allow them to take time off where practicable if they are unwell, or adjust working hours. This dual approach may be the most effective in helping people with MS to remain employed. Occupational physicians must consider the benefits of interventions and the complexity and timing of decisions by people with MS to continue or leave employment before recommending either action.[61]

Miscellaneous genetic disorders

A small but significant proportion of neurological disease is determined by mutations of a single gene. As our knowledge advances further, it is likely that the polygenetic contribution will be better understood in more common neurological conditions such as epilepsy, stroke, PD, and MS. Fortunately, these single gene mutations are rare, and may never be encountered, but they can present at almost any working age and will require systematic assessment if they arise.

Neurocutaneous genetic syndromes share a dominantly inherited predisposition to developing tumours of the nervous system. Neurofibromatosis type 1 primarily affects the peripheral nerves, and type 2 the CNS and acoustic nerves in particular. Von Hippel–Lindau disease confers a predisposition to various forms of neoplasms and cysts, including haemangioblastomas of the CNS and retina, and other generally benign tumours of abdominal organs. Tuberous sclerosis complex is characterized by a wide phenotypic spectrum that may include skin lesions, renal dysfunction, and seizures and/or learning disabilities secondary to cerebral hamartomas. Its severity depends on the type, size, number, and the location of involved lesions and organs.

In all of these syndromes, the diagnosis itself may be perfectly compatible with full-time working, but the risk of developing complications is unpredictable and justifies some form of regular occupational screening programme.

Huntington's disease, certain cerebellar ataxias, primary torsion dystonia, familial essential tremor, myotonic and facioscapulohumeral muscular dystrophies are all autosomal dominant conditions, while most of the other muscular dystrophies are X-linked. The best-known neurological conditions with a recessive pattern of inheritance include metabolic storage disorders and Wilson's disease, Friedreich's ataxia and the spinal muscular atrophies. Hereditary neuropathies may show either dominant or recessive inheritance. A bewildering array of clinical phenotypes have been described in association with dysfunction of the mitochondrial respiratory chain, many of which involve mutations of mitochondrial DNA passed on through the ovum by maternal, as opposed to autosomal, inheritance.

Motor neurone diseases

The term 'motor neurone diseases' describes a family of rare disorders resulting from selective loss of function of lower and/or upper motor neurones controlling the voluntary muscles of the limbs or bulbar region. Although the term used to be synonymous with sporadic amyotrophic lateral sclerosis, one of the most serious of these conditions that progresses relentlessly causing death within a few years of diagnosis, there is an extensive differential diagnosis requiring precise clinical and electrophysiological assessment. Occasionally, a pure motor peripheral neuropathy or neuronopathy is identified that responds to immunosuppressive therapy, while some other motor neurone syndromes such as primary lateral sclerosis or hereditary spastic paraparesis may progress only very slowly and have almost normal life expectancy.

Although rare, motor neurone diseases are important in relation to work, as they tend to present before retirement age. They are usually incurable and only symptomatic treatment is available for the various types of disability. Management should aim towards leading as normal a life as possible, ideally including work. However, this has to be seen in the context of a realistic prognosis. The occupational adviser should seek consent to obtain this directly from the treating physicians, and then help the employee weigh up the many complex factors involved before reaching a decision about possible medical retirement. If the prognosis is grave, it may be better to give up work and go round the world while limited time permits.

Alternatively, good rehabilitation can help maintain function and maximize work potential for those with less aggressive pathologies, as the inspirational example of Professor Stephen Hawking reminds us. Mental ability is unimpaired and the patient may be able to control their environment and operate a telephone with communication aids and other assistive technology, as well as being able to use a personal computer for most ordinary tasks. Misguided excessive physiotherapy may be exhausting and counter-productive, but speech therapy and swallowing assessments can be very helpful. Tube feeding prevents malnutrition because of dysphagia, and non-invasive positive pressure ventilation given overnight via a facemask can correct carbon dioxide accumulation from respiratory muscle weakness. All these techniques can help to maintain someone in work as long as they are able to remain motivated and productive.

Peripheral neuropathy

Neuropathy is a common condition with a very broad differential diagnosis (Box 6.4), but typically insidious in onset and producing gradually increasing disability. Progress is usually slow and many cases are asymptomatic or have little disability. The main exception is acute idiopathic inflammatory polyneuropathy or Guillain–Barré syndrome, in which symptoms develop rapidly

Box 6.4 Causes of peripheral polyneuropathy

- Genetic: hereditary neuropathies, inherited neurometabolic diseases
- Nutritional deficiencies: vitamins B1, B6, B12, E, folate
- Toxins: acrylamide, arsenic, lead, mercury, thallium, triorthocresyl phosphate, organic solvents
- Drugs: mainly cytotoxic agents, isoniazid, amiodarone
- Alcohol abuse
- Metabolic and endocrine disorders: diabetes, uraemia, amyloid, myxoedema
- Paraproteinaemia: monoclonal gammopathies of undetermined significance
- Connective tissue disorders: polyarteritis nodosa, rheumatoid arthritis, etc.
- Neoplastic and paraneoplastic
- Infectious: HIV, hepatitis B, *Borrelia*, herpes zoster
- Inflammatory and postinfectious neuropathies: Guillain–Barré syndrome, critical illness polyneuropathy
- Chronic inflammatory demyelinating polyneuropathy, Lyme borreliosis, HIV infection, sarcoidosis
- Cryptogenic, undetermined

over days and then resolve, normally completely, within weeks or months. Return to work is usually possible as soon as the employee is fully ambulant, although occasionally residual muscle weakness may persist indefinitely.

About 15% of all patients with diabetes mellitus have significant peripheral neuropathy. Either symmetrical sensory and autonomic polyneuropathies can occur, or isolated peripheral nerve lesions or multifocal neuropathies. Mixed syndromes are common. The cause of diabetic neuropathy is unclear; although it tends to occur more often in poorly controlled diabetics, the correlation is not tight.

Hereditary neuropathies such as Charcot–Marie–Tooth disease usually affect both motor and sensory nerves present during school years with foot deformity or difficulty in walking. A family history makes the diagnosis easier, but sporadic cases may arise by recessive inheritance or new mutations.

Peripheral neuropathy is a recognized complication of many toxic chemicals and therefore the onset of a peripheral neuropathy should always alert the doctor to the possibility of toxic chemical exposure at work (see p121).

Regardless of the cause, neuropathies are seldom a reason to cease work and as progression is slow the patient can often continue at work for many years. Care of the feet is vitally important in any sensory neuropathies, to prevent minor injuries being left untreated, the development of chronic ulceration and possibly even amputation. Educational tools are now widely available for the care of the diabetic foot, and apply equally to other neuropathic conditions. In some severe cases, walking aids such as ankle foot orthoses may improve function. The occupational physician should consider various workplace factors in any employee with a peripheral polyneuropathy (Box 6.5).

Box 6.5 Causes of peripheral polyneuropathy

- ◆ Motor function: check walking ability and balance is adequate for the job.
- ◆ Proprioception: an important component of balance, particularly if employees are working at heights.
- ◆ Pain and temperature sensory impairment: all footwear must be fitted with extra care, and any restrictive footwear or protective garments avoided; employees should not be exposed to extremes of temperature.
- ◆ Avoid activities that are hard on the feet, such as running and jumping, and standing or walking for prolonged periods without adequate rests.
- ◆ Reinforce quit smoking advice to minimize concomitant peripheral vascular disease.

Neuromuscular junction disease

Neuromuscular junction diseases are rare and the only one likely to be encountered is myasthenia gravis, an autoimmune disorder in which circulating antibodies interfere with normal neuromuscular transmission. Repeated or sustained exercise induces focal weakness, usually affecting limb girdle muscles, so an employee may first complain of proximal weakness when asked to do more physical work than usual. Myasthenia is difficult to diagnose in its early stages, when it may be misdiagnosed as psychogenic because objective weakness varies from one day to the next. However, myasthenia does not cause continuous tiredness or generalized fatigue and weakness of the eye muscles affects the majority of cases, when the diagnosis is easier to make. If suspected, examination should be carried out before and after exercise, and positive serum acetylcholine receptor antibodies are diagnostic, but occasional seronegative cases require more specialist investigation.

Provided the correct diagnosis is made, few cases become gravely ill nowadays because most cases respond well to treatment with the anticholinesterase drug pyridostigmine and immunosuppressants, including steroids. The great majority then enter remission, but may require treatment indefinitely and adverse drug effects need to be monitored carefully. Certain other classes of drug aggravate myasthenic weakness and should be avoided, and muscle-strengthening exercises are inappropriate. A small proportion of cases require thymectomy, either because of an associated thymoma, or thymic hyperplasia in early-onset seropositive subjects.

Muscle diseases

Muscle disease is less common than neurological disease. Some acquired myopathies are associated with drug treatment (e.g. statins, corticosteroids), or some other endocrine or malignant disease, on which its prognosis will depend. Polymyositis appears to be a syndrome of diverse causes that often but not always occurs in association with systemic autoimmune diseases, viral infections, or connective tissue disorders such as lupus and rheumatoid arthritis. Chronic polymyositis can give rise to mainly proximal weakness with periodic flare-ups that may require increasing doses of steroids and other immunosuppressant therapy.

Persistent muscle weakness and fatigue may affect survivors of acute respiratory distress syndrome and other critical illnesses, who may encounter apparently unexplained difficulties upon returning to work apparently fully recovered. The possibility of myopathy and/or polyneuropathy secondary to critical illness should be considered in anyone who has had a prolonged stay on an intensive care unit (see Appendix 7).

Muscular dystrophies are progressive genetic disorders and rarely pose problems in occupational medicine. The commonest forms present early and are usually so severe that they preclude work. However, some dystrophies and certain metabolic myopathies can present later in adult life and cause slowly increasing disability over many years, yet are clinically heterogeneous and require individualized occupational assessment regardless of the exact label. Problems are usually confined to muscle weakness and cramps and therefore the subject can often work with appropriate mobility aids for travelling to, from and moving about the workplace. Employees doing sedentary work may have little or no difficulty apart from climbing stairs, rising from low seats and reaching files from high shelves. Associated complications that may need consideration include increasing scoliosis, ocular, respiratory and cardiac involvement depending on the exact diagnosis.

Chronic fatigue syndrome

The overall incidence of all fatigue diagnoses in the UK General Practice Research Database decreased from 87 per 100 000 patients in 1990 to 49 in 2001, a reduction of almost half. Postviral fatigue syndromes decreased but the incidence rates of the specific but variously defined diagnoses of chronic fatigue syndrome, myalgic encephalomyelitis or ME, and fibromyalgia have risen, against a background of little change in symptom reporting. This is likely to reflect fashions in diagnostic labelling rather than true changes in incidence.[62]

A degree of limiting fatigue has been reported by 27% of working adults[63] but the prevalence of chronic fatigue syndrome is 0.1–2.6% depending on the criteria used. The underlying mechanisms remain poorly understood. In this series[64] of 14 studies meeting strict entry criteria and published between 1991 and 2002, the median full recovery rate was 7% (range 0–48%) over a timeframe between 5 and 10 years. The median proportion of those who improved was 39.5% (range 8–63%). The sample size varied from 20 to 3201. Fatigue should be considered abnormal when the fatigued person views him or herself to be ill which usually implies a degree of functional impairment. More loosely defined chronic fatigue has a better prognosis, about 25% fully recovering and half improving. Prognosis depends on the patient's beliefs, information supplied by clinicians and others together with coping skills and not focusing on the symptoms.[65]

Chronic fatigue is strongly associated with psychological distress without evidence for genetic co-variance.[66]

Occupational aspects include the crucial area of liaison and even mediation between management and employee. Also the general practitioner or specialist therapist needs to be encouraged to persist with energetic treatment with the opportunity of graded return to work emphasized. Realistic and pragmatic advice along with regular review is crucial rather than letting things drift.[67]

Treatments for chronic fatigue syndrome that show promise are cognitive-behavioural therapy and graded exercise therapy, the latter being more than a simple recommendation to exercise but involving a specific graded programme. It is easier to return to work after shorter absence and therefore early treatment and rehabilitation is vital. Shorter illness duration is a significant predictor of sustained remission and thus within an occupational setting it is vital for professionals to have a good method of identification in place.[68] It is crucial to consider co-morbidity such as depression in all forms of fatigue. Medical retirement is rarely if ever justified particularly in the light of current knowledge if permanence is a required criterion.[69]

References

1 Langton Hewer R, Tennant A. The epidemiology of disabling neurological disorders. In: *Handbook of Neurological Rehabilitation* (2nd edn) (eds Greenwood RJ *et al.*), pp. 5–14. Hove: Psychology Press, 2003.

2 The Neurological Alliance. *Neuro numbers: a brief review of the numbers of people in the UK with a neurological condition.* London: Neurological Alliance, 2003. Available online at http://www.neural.org.uk

3 Fyfe NCM *et al.* Assistive technology: mobility aids, environmental control systems, and communication aids. *Handbook of Neurological Rehabilitation* (2nd edn) (eds Greenwood RJ *et al.*), pp. 231–44. Hove: Psychology Press, 2003.

4 Department of Health. *National service framework for long-term conditions.* London: Department of Health, 2005.

5 Drivers Medical Group. *At a glance guide to the current medical standards of fitness to drive.* Swansea: Driver and Vehicle Licensing Agency, 2005. Updated every 6 months at www.dvla.gov.uk/at_a_glance

6 Appelbaum PS. Ethical issues in psychiatric genetics. *J Psychiatr Pract* 2004; **10**: 343–51.

7 Almqvist EW *et al.* Psychological consequences and predictors of adverse events in the first 5 years after predictive testing for Huntington's disease. *Clin Genet* 2003; **64**: 300–9.

8 Simpson SA *et al.* Minor injuries, cognitive failures and accidents at work: incidence and associated features. *Occup Med* 2005; **55**: 99–108.

9 Wilson BA, Herbert CM, Shiel A. *Behavioural approaches in neuropsychological rehabilitation: optimising rehabilitation procedures.* Hove: Psychology Press, 2003.

10 Costa G. Shift work and occupational medicine: an overview. *Occup Med* 2003; **53**: 83–8.

11 Horne JA, Reyner LA, Barrett PR. Driving impairment due to sleepiness is exacerbated by low alcohol intake. *Occup Environ Med* 2003; **60**: 689–92.

12 Holbrook AM. Treating insomnia. *BMJ* 2004; **329**: 1198–9.

13 Differential diagnosis and management of daytime sleepiness and nighttime wakefulness. *Journal of Clinical Psychiatry* 2004; **65** (Suppl. 16): 1–48.

14 Molhotra A, White DP. Obstructive sleep apnoea. *Lancet* 2002; **360**: 237–45.

15 Ulfberg J. Excessive daytime sleepiness at work and subjective work performance in the general population among heavy snorers and obstructive sleep apnoea. *Chest* 1996; **110**: 659–63.

16 Pelletier-Fleury N, Meslier N, Gagnadoux F, Person C, Rakotonanahery D, Oukesel H, Fleaury B, Racineux JL. Economic arguments for the immediate management of moderate to severe obstructive apnoea syndrome. *Eur Respir J* 2004; **1**: 53–60.

17 Provision of health assessments under the working time regulations 1998. *A guidance for occupational physicians and nurses* pp. 1–8. London: FOM/SOM, 1999.

18 Herxheimer A, Waterhouse J. The prevention and treatment of jet lag: It's been ignored, but much can be done. *BMJ* 2004; **326**: 296–7.

19 Merrison AF, Fuller G. Treatment options for trigeminal neuralgia. *BMJ* 2003; **327**: 1360–1.

20 Hardie RJ. Muscle spasticity. In: *Patient care in neurology* (ed. Williams AC), pp. 345–54. Oxford: Oxford University Press, 1999.

21 Vaughan J, Hardie RJ. The differential diagnosis of Parkinson's disease. *Rev Clin Gerontol* 2002; **12**: 40–51.

22 Hardie RJ, Rothwell JC. The management of tremor and ataxia. In: *Handbook of neurological rehabilitation* (2nd edn) (eds Greenwood RJ *et al.*), pp. 171–8. Hove: Psychology Press, 2003.

23 van Dijk FJH, Swaen GMH. Fatigue at work. *Occup Environ Med* 2003; **60** (Suppl. 1): i1–2.

24 Krupp LB. Fatigue in multiple sclerosis: definition, pathophysiology and treatment. *CNS Drugs* 2003; **17**: 225–34.

25 Holdcroft A, Power L. Management of pain. *BMJ* 2003; **326**: 635–9.

26 Earl CJ. Neurological disease and driving. In: *Patient care in neurology* (ed. Williams AC), pp. 367–71. Oxford: Oxford University Press, 1999.

27 Blain PG, Harris JB. *Medical neurotoxicology.* London: Arnold, 1999.

28 Gamble JF. Low-level hydrocarbon solvent exposure and neurobehavioural effects. *Occup Med* 2000; **50**: 81–102.

29 Committee on Toxicity of Chemicals in Food, Consumer Products and the Environment. *Organophosphates*. London: Department of Health, 1999.

30 Coggon D. Work with pesticides and organophosphate sheep dips. *Occup Med* 2002; **52**: 467–70.

31 British Association for the Study of Headaches. *Guidelines for all doctors in the diagnosis and management of migraine and tension-type headache*. Exeter: British Association for the Study of Headaches, 2004. Available at www.bash.org.uk

32 Jones J R *et al*. *Self-reported work-related illness in 2001/02. Results from a household survey*. London: Health and Safety Executive, 2003. http://www.hse.gov.uk/statistics/causdis/swi0102.pdf

33 Stewart WF *et al*. Work-related disability: results from the American migraine study. *Cephalgia* 1996; **16**: 231–8.

34 Silberstein SD. Migraine. *Lancet* 2004; **363**: 381–91.

35 Magnussen JE Becker WJ. Migraine frequency and intensity: relationship with disability and psychological factors. *Headache* 2003; **43**: 1049–59.

36 Ohayon MM. Prevalence and risk factors of morning headaches in the general population. *Arch Intern Med* 2004; **164**: 97–102.

37 Marlowe N. Self-efficacy moderates the impact of stressful events on headache. *Headache* 1998; **38**: 662–7.

38 Lipton RB *et al*. Stratified care vs step care strategies for migraine. *JAMA* 2000; **294**: 2599–605.

39 Caples SM, Gami AS, Somers VK. Obstructive sleep apnea. *Ann Intern Med* 2005; **142**: 187–97.

40 Gurubhagavatula I *et al*.. Occupational screening for obstructive sleep apnoea in commercial drivers. *Am J Respir Crit Care Med* 2004; **170**: 371–6.

41 Warlow CP *et al*. (eds) Which arterial territory is involved? Developing a clinically-based method of subclassification. In: *Stroke: a practical guide to management*. Oxford: Blackwell, 2001.

42 Tuchsen F, Jensen AA. Agricultural work and the risk of Parkinson's disease in Denmark, 1981–1993. *Scand J Work Environ Health* 2000; **26**: 359–62.

43 Park J *et al*. Occupations and Parkinson's disease: a multi-center case-control study in South Korea. *Neurotoxicology* 2005; **26**: 99–105.

44 Huang CC *et al*. Long-term progression in chronic manganism: ten years of follow-up. *Neurology* 1998; **50**: 698–700.

45 Racette, B A. *et al*. Prevalence of parkinsonism and relationship to exposure in a large sample of Alabama welders. *Neurology* 2005; **64**: 230–5.

46 Greenwood RJ. Head injury for neurologists. *J Neurol Neurosurg Psychiatry* 2002; **73** (Suppl. 1): i8–16.

47 World Health Organisation. *International Classification of Functioning, Disability and Health*. Geneva: World Health Organisation, 2001. http://www3.who.int/icf

48 McCrory P, *et al*. Summary and agreement statement of the 2nd International Conference on Concussion in Sport, Prague 2004. *Br J Sports Med* 2005; **39**: 196–204.

49 British Society of Rehabilitation Medicine and Royal College of Physicians. *Rehabilitation following acquired brain injury: inter-agency guidelines*. London: Royal College of Physicians, 2003.

50 Department of Work and Pensions. *Building capacity for work: a UK framework for vocational rehabilitation*. London: Stationery Office, 2004.

51 British Society of Rehabilitation Medicine, Jobcentre Plus, and Royal College of Physicians. *Vocational assessment and rehabilitation after acquired brain injury: inter-agency guidelines*. London: Royal College of Physicians, 2004.

52 Seidler A *et al*. Psychosocial work factors and dementia. *Occup Environ Med* 2005; **61**: 962–71.

53 http://www.cjd.ed.ac.uk

54 Anon Lynn. *Personal view*. Quotation from Spinal Injuries Association website, 2005. http://www.spinal.co.uk/about/default.asp?step=2&id=14

55 Tomassen PC, Post MW, van Asbeck FW. Return to work after spinal cord injury. *Spinal Cord* 2000; **38**: 51–5.

56 McDonald WI *et al.* Recommended diagnostic criteria for multiple sclerosis: guidelines from the International Panel on the diagnosis of multiple sclerosis. *Ann Neurol* 2001; **50**: 121–7.

57 Mohr DC *et al.* Association between stressful life events and exacerbation in multiple sclerosis: a meta-analysis. *BMJ* 2004; **328**: 731–6.

58 Ruggieri RM, *et al.* Cognitive impairment in patients suffering from relapsing-remitting multiple sclerosis with EDSS < or = 3.5. *Acta Neurol Scand* 2003; **108**: 323–6.

59 Roessler RT, Rumrill PD. Multiple sclerosis and employment barriers: a systemic perspective on diagnosis and intervention. *Work* 2003; **21**: 17–23.

60 Gibson J, Frank A. Supporting individuals with disabling multiple sclerosis. *J R Soc Med* 2002; **95**, 580–6.

61 Johnson KL *et al.* The cost and benefits of employment: a qualitative study of experiences of persons with multiple sclerosis. *Arch Phys Med Rehab* 2004; **85**: 201–9.

62 Gallagher AM *et al.* Incidence of fatigue symptoms and diagnoses presenting in UK primary care from 1990 to 2001. *J R Soc Med* 2004; **97**: 571–5.

63 Singleton N, *et al. Psychiatric morbidity amongst adults living in private households.* London: Office of National Statistics, 2001.

64 Glozier N. Chronic fatigue syndrome: it's tiring not knowing much-an in-depth review for occupational health professionals. *Occup Med* 2005; **55**: 10–12.

65 Cairns R, Hotopf M. A systematic review describing the prognosis of chronic fatigue syndrome. *Occup Med* 2005; **55**: 20–31.

66 Roy-Bryne P, Afari N. Chronic fatigue and anxiety/depression: a twin study. *Br J Psychiatry* 2002; **180**: 29–34.

67 Wessely S, Hotopf M, Sharpe C. *Chronic fatigue and its syndromes.* Oxford: Oxford University Press, 1998.

68 Nisenbaum R *et al.* A population based study of the clinical course of chronic fatigue syndrome. *Health Qual Outcomes* 2003; **1**: 49.

69 Stattin M. Retirement on grounds of ill health. *Occup Environ Med* 2005; **62**: 135–40.

Further reading

Greenwood RJ, Barnes MP, McMillan TM, Ward CD (eds). *Handbook of neurological rehabilitation* (2nd edn). Hove: Psychology Press, 2003.

Donaghy M. Neurology. In *Oxford textbook of medicine,* 4th edn (eds Warrell DA *et al.*), pp. 1075–9. Oxford: Oxford University Press, 2004.

Neurological Alliance. *Getting the best from neurological services: a guide for people affected by conditions of the brain, spine and nervous system.* London: Neurological Alliance, 2003. Available online at http://www.neural.org.uk

Stone J, Carson A, Sharpe M. Functional symptoms in neurology: management. *J Neurol Neurosurg Psychiatry* 2005; **76** (Suppl. 1): i13–21.

Chapter 7

Mental health and psychiatric disorders

E. L. Teasdale and M. P. Deahl

What is 'health'? One group of managers attending a conference was asked, without referring to a dictionary, to come up with their own definitions. Their reflections make interesting reading: 'Health is having an empty medicine chest, well-used trainers and not knowing who your family doctor is'; another said that 'Health is a state of mind and body which permits happiness—without undue reliance on the healthcare professions'.

The World Health Organization (WHO) defines health as a state of complete physical, mental, social, and spiritual well-being. The spiritual angle has little do to with religion in this context, it relates more to the need we all have to be treated as individuals and to grow and develop during our adult life. Many of the 'physical' aspects of occupational health are now well understood, e.g. dermatitis, noise-induced hearing loss. Over the last 10–20 years the mental, social, and spiritual aspects of health have come more into focus and are probably more difficult to understand and manage.

In the occupational or industrial setting, the emphasis on maintaining *mental* (as well as physical and social) well-being is essential to success. Occasional serious cases of mental illness must be recognized and managed appropriately. This should include the care of the individual who has a problem of substance abuse (e.g. alcohol or drugs of addiction), and the patient with a psychotic condition where prompt admission to hospital is required. In practice, however, the more common mental health problems encompass stress, anxiety, and depression, and their manifestation in the workplace. The most frequent condition under the mental health umbrella is stress and much effort has been directed to this end.

Establishing the fitness for work of individuals suffering from mental health problems is one of the biggest challenges facing occupational medicine. The basic human right to work is enshrined in the United Nations Universal Declaration of Human Rights (Article 23). This states that *'everyone has the right to work, to free choice of employment, to just and favourable conditions of work and to protection against unemployment'.*[1] This 'motherhood and apple pie' sentiment, however, overlooks the stark realities facing the mentally ill. The Royal College of Psychiatry has stated that the workplace is a microcosm of society as a whole, and employers and occupational physicians as well as individual sufferers themselves must contend with fear, ignorance, and prejudice that can pose far greater barriers to employment than the direct effects of mental illness itself.

The consequences of stigma have significant implications for employer and employee alike. Patients with established psychiatric disorders, especially psychoses and schizophrenia, are more likely to experience difficulty in finding work when compared with their peers with broadly comparable physical disabilities.[2] If they are lucky enough to find a job they are less likely to be promoted to positions of responsibility and find themselves more likely to lose their job when problems arise. *Pari passu* employees already established in the workplace who develop mental health problems are more likely to conceal these from their employer or find other less stigmatizing excuses to take sickness leave. The consequences of concealment are considerable; underperformance at work, damaged relationships in the workplace, problems taken home damaging social lives, and making secondary victims of families and loved ones. Finally, in more demanding work environments (such as the emergency services) the job itself may cause or exacerbate mental health problems and in these circumstances a conspiracy of silence may develop between employer (unwilling or unable to create a psychologically less demanding environment) and employee (reluctant to admit to an inability to cope).

Uncomfortable or embarrassing as it may be, mental health, as well as mental illness in the workplace, cannot be ignored. There will occasionally be serious cases of mental illness that must be recognized and managed appropriately. In practice, the more common mental health problems encompass stress-related illness such as anxiety states and depression. Employers are required to conduct risk assessments and take reasonable steps to minimize workplace stress, often intangible and ill-defined factors that, nevertheless, can cause ill health and disability as great as that caused by any physical hazard.[3] When mental health problems arise as a result of occupational factors, employers have a clear duty of care to identify these and expedite access to treatment in a timely manner.[4] Assessing the employability of an individual with mental health problems, problems that are mostly unseen, and lacking objective markers of severity, requires considerable skill and experience. Disentangling the effects of illness from (work avoiding) abnormal illness behaviour and (occasionally) frank malingering can challenge the most experienced psychiatrist. Finally, actively promoting antidisability discrimination policies and facilitating the employment of individuals with established psychiatric disorders requires commitment and determination in a workplace where stigma and discrimination is invisible but pernicious as mental illness itself, is all too often the norm. Doctors should not be too quick to criticize employers, however, as ironically this stigma and discrimination is arguably at its worst among healthcare organizations and the medical and nursing professions themselves—the very people who should be acting as advocate and champion for the patient.

The extent of the problem

Mental illness is a massive and burgeoning public health problem. The prevalence of common psychiatric disorders is shown in Table 7.1.

It is thought that one family in four will have a member suffering from mental illness; even if employees themselves are in robust mental health they may still be significantly disturbed and their work performance significantly impaired by a mentally ill relative or friend.

The employment statistics among the mentally ill make grim reading. Patients with severe enduring mental health problems account for 8% of long-term disabled people of working age. Of these only 18% are in some form of employment (even though 30–40% are thought capable of holding down a job) compared with 52% of non-mentally long-term disabled.[6] Even the more minor and less severe mental disorders are associated with poor employment statistics. Adults with neurotic disorders are four to five times more likely to be permanently unemployed compared with the rest of the population: 61% of males and 58% of females with a single neurotic disorder are in work compared with 75% and 65% respectively in the general population. Co-morbidity is common in psychiatry and further reduces employment prospects. In patients with two concomitant neurotic disorders the proportions in work fell further to 46% of males and 33% of females. Patients with phobic disorders had the bleakest employment record: only 43% of males and 30% of females were working. This does not mean the mentally ill are 'work-shy' as despite these high rates of unemployment as many as 90% of patients state they would like to return to work

Table 7.1 Prevalence of common mental disorders in men and women (rates per 1000)[5]

	Men	Women	Total (averaged across the two sexes)
All neuroses	135	194	164
Mixed anxiety and depression	68	108	88
Generalized anxiety	43	46	44
Depression	23	28	26
Phobias	13	22	18
Obsessive-compulsive disorder	9	13	11
Panic disorder	7	7	7
Personality disorder	54	34	44
Obsessive compulsive	26	13	19
Avoidant	10	7	8
Schizoid	9	8	8
Paranoid	12	3	7
Borderline	10	4	7
Antisocial (psychopathic)	10	2	6
Dependant	2	0	1
Schizotypal	0	1	1
Histrionic	–	–	–
Narcissistic	–	–	–
Probable psychosis	6	5	5

if the opportunity presented itself. Among those with neurotic disorders who were unemployed and actively seeking work, 70% had been unemployed for more than 1 year (i.e. 7 % of all people with a neurotic disorder).[7]

The economic burden of mental illness

Approximately 80 million working days per year are lost in the UK as a result of mental illness with an estimated cost to employers of £1.2 billion. This figure is almost certainly an underestimate given that mental health problems are often undetected or misdiagnosed. On average approximately 3000 people in the UK per week move on to incapacity benefit; musculoskeletal disorders account for 28% of these with psychiatric disorders coming a close second at 20%. In a recent survey, one in five days of certified sickness absence was due to psychiatric illness, accounting for 92 million lost working days.

The overall direct costs of mental illness are believed to be about £32.1 billion: this comprises £11.8 billion in lost employment, £4.1 billion in costs to the NHS, and £7.6 billion in Social Security payments.[8] The indirect economic and human costs are massive.

How mental health problems might interfere with work?

A diagnostic label does little to assist the occupational physician regarding an individual's employment potential. The mentally ill, like the rest of us, have their individual strengths and weaknesses and a thorough appraisal of abilities, deficits, and functional capacity should be integral to any occupational assessment. Excluding an individual on the basis of diagnosis alone is not only discriminatory but also excludes a lot of potential talent from the workplace. On being asked whether a diagnosis of an eating disorder should be an automatic bar to entry into medical school, one of the authors (MD) was obliged to point out that a number of the most distinguished luminaries of the medical profession would never have qualified if such a prohibition was in force!

Psychiatrists often talk at cross-purposes with their occupational health colleagues, particularly when report writing and commenting on the employment prospects of an individual. Mental health professionals typically use an 'illness' model to describe their patients where the emphasis is on the relapsing nature of the disorder with the prospect of remission or 'cure' (with the right treatment). Although appropriate in acute psychiatric settings and in planning mental health services, this is often unhelpful in the occupational environment where a disability model, focusing on enduring problems, strengths, and weaknesses, is more useful. The 'disability' model informs the changes and adjustments that might be necessary in the workplace to enable the individual to successfully return to work. The expectation is that others will take steps to facilitate a return to work rather than passively waiting for an individual to simply 'get better'. Disability highlights the interaction between impairment (be it physical or sensory handicap or the lack of self-confidence found in depression) and the obstacles that might exist in the workplace including attitudes, working practices, policies, and the physical environment that may exclude an individual with that impairment from full participation. A social model of disability is not only consonant with government policy but helps establish a dialogue between mental health services, service users, and employers assisting employers in fulfilling their responsibilities under the Disability Discrimination Act (DDA) 1995. Understanding disability focuses on the discrimination and social exclusion perceived by many mental health service users and helps promote employment opportunities giving hope to the mentally ill and an opportunity for them to recover social role and status.[9]

Psychiatric disorders may impair one or more domains of psychological or social functioning and it is important to systematically assess each of these in turn.

Impaired concentration and attention

Any mental illness may significantly impair concentration and attention. This may be due to the distractibility and preoccupying worries associated with anxiety states or hypomania, the retarded slow thought processes seen in depressive disorders and states of relative malnourishment associated with eating disorders, or the poverty of thought or thought disorder associated with schizophrenia and other psychotic disorders. Many psychotropic drugs used in the treatment of these disorders are themselves associated with marked behavioural effects such as reduced concentration and attention span. Simple clinical tests of concentration and attention such as 'serial 7's' are crude indicators of actual performance and concentration and attentional deficits are best assessed by an occupational therapist using 'in vivo' tasks that resemble those required in the workplace.

Impaired motor skills

Abnormal involuntary movements as well as a paucity of movement may hamper work performance. Psychomotor slowing is seen in many depressive disorders and the tremor associated with anxiety may impair skilled motor tasks. Tardive dyskinesia and other involuntary movements associated with schizophrenia are not only disfiguring but also disturbing to others making individuals more isolated and making integration into a working environment more difficult. Antipsychotic drugs (including many of the newer atypical agents) may produce marked extra pyramidal symptoms, which themselves may become a cause of significant disability.

Impaired communication and social skills

The ability to communicate effectively and get on with colleagues is one of the most important predictors of success at work. The caricature of the typical job for patients with severe enduring mental illness (if they are fortunate enough to find work) is the lonely and isolated life of a security guard (typically on permanent night shifts). Doubtless this may be appropriate and what some individuals actually want but, equally, it may merely be a means for employers to discharge their obligations under disability legislation while keeping their mentally ill employees 'out of sight and mind' of the rest of the workforce. Many patients, especially with long-term disorders, have significant difficulties interacting with others. This may be due to the illness itself, for example, the lack of self-confidence associated with depression, or paranoid thinking seen in schizophrenia, other psychoses and personality disorders. Conversely, many of those who are mentally ill simply lack practice and the opportunity to maintain and refine normal social skills and do surprisingly well if they are gradually challenged.

Risk to self and others

A risk assessment is now an integral and explicit part of any psychiatric examination and a written statement regarding risk is part of the care plan of any service-user subject to the Care Programme Approach. Rates of suicide and self-injurious behaviour are not peculiar to depression and are elevated across the range of psychiatric disorders. This includes neurotic and so-called minor psychiatric disorders. There can be no doubt that the high suicide rates associated with certain occupations such as veterinary medicine and anaesthesia are at least, in part, attributable to the ready availability of lethal means to individuals employed in what can be an isolated, lonely yet demanding and stressful working environment.

The risk to others associated with mental illness is overstated and wickedly exaggerated by the media. The mentally ill are far more likely to harm themselves than others. Nevertheless, occupational physicians have a duty to reassure employers and expect a clear and unequivocal assessment of risk from the psychiatric team.

The effects of abnormal illness behaviour

Motivation, commitment, and willingness to work are perhaps the best predictors of success (or otherwise) in the workplace, irrespective of psychiatric diagnosis. Many individuals with significant psychopathology are punctual, reliable, and hard working employees who perform their duties to the satisfaction of all and without giving any hint that they may be suffering from significant disorder (illness denying abnormal illness behaviour). Conversely, others with a similar disorder but with a lesser degree of symptomology may be profoundly handicapped and incapable of work. Illness behaviour affects everybody one way or the other, it is unconsciously determined and must be clearly distinguished from malingering.

Why work matters: the psychosocial benefits

The protestant work ethic has left an indelible mark on our society. Work is integral to our sense of personal identity, self-esteem, and worth. A fulfilling job promotes mental well-being, and in the mentally ill, is an important long-term prognostic indicator.[10] Unemployment, conversely, is associated with despair, mental illness, and suicide.[11] Employment is a necessary condition for the well-being of both the individual and society as a whole. It brings profit or benefit to the employer or organization and increases (usually economic) output and productivity. It provides income to the individual and with it an improved standard of living to the employee as well as improving the economic productivity of society. It reduces the financial burden on the state, increases consumer spending, tax revenue, and economic output. These benefits are obvious. However, work brings with it a number of less tangible advantages to the individual such as social status and recognition, contact, support and an important forum for establishing social relationships, a daily routine and excuse to get out of bed in the morning as well as a sense of personal achievement.[12] Work tells us who we are and enables us to demonstrate this to others. Our identity (how we think of ourselves) is often determined by our job. The first two questions in most social encounters between strangers is typically 'Who are you and what do you do?'

Obstacles to employment

There is little evidence to demonstrate whether particular types of services or interventions are effective in getting the mentally ill back to work. The employment of disabled people in general depends on the state of the economy, including the rate of growth, overall employment rate, and extent of any labour shortages. The mentally ill, and individuals with significant learning disabilities, experience greater difficulty obtaining paid work than any other disabled group. Although a number of voluntary sector employment schemes exist that work in collaboration with mental health services, the poor employment statistics suggest that there is a clear gulf between these resources and the open labour market. Stigma and discrimination over and above that shown towards other disabled groups is the invisible barrier or glass ceiling that pervades society. The welfare system has clear disincentives to returning to work and many patients find themselves in an endless cycle of further education and voluntary work always mindful of the benefit trap and the need to limit any (poorly paid) work for fear of compromising their (usually more rewarding) state benefit entitlements. GPs, employers, and even mental health professionals have typically poor expectations of the capabilities of the mentally ill as well as overestimating the risk to employers of employing individuals with mental health problems.[13] Moreover, psychiatrists and other mental health professionals often have a very poor understanding of the workplace and seldom liaise directly with occupational physicians and almost never visit to see and discuss the specific job or range of tasks undertaken and overview the organization where their patient is employed.

Fit for work? Assessment for employment

Assessment requires skill and experience and can be an important intervention in its own right. People with mental health problems suffer from a mutual lack of understanding between occupational physicians and mental health professionals. The dichotomy between illness and disability models of illness has already been described. In practice this means that psychiatric reports are often unhelpful to occupational physicians and fail to provide the necessary information needed to determine whether an individual is employable in a given work environment. Past behaviour is often the best predictor of future performance and detailed work histories often give a better indication of an individual's employability than any diagnostic label or measure of psychopathology. Tests of IQ, temperament or aptitude have very poor predictive validity. Personal objectives, motivation, and confidence are far better predictors. The person most likely to succeed is the individual who *really* wants the job! Motivation predicts success in the workplace; however, getting a job itself can be a powerful motivating factor, particularly for individuals who have been repeatedly unsuccessful. It is important therefore to bear these factors in mind and give apparently unmotivated individuals (especially those who have had more than their fair share of rejection and setback), a chance and not prematurely exclude them from the workplace, unwittingly denying them the very thing they need to help them move on and escape the fetters of illness.

A comprehensive occupational assessment has three key ingredients: an appreciation of the individual and their strengths and weaknesses; the nature of the workplace and demands of the job; and the desired outcome for both individual and employer. Individual factors to be considered include past employment history, skills, and work performance, and individual factors including motivation, confidence, and personal aspirations. Finally, the workplace itself should be considered in terms of the expectations of peers and managers, opportunities for supervision, training, and development and links to other employee development programmes.

It should be realized, however, that there are circumstances in which some caution in job placement should be exercised. For example, fitness assessment must consider the risk to the public, third parties, and personal safety in safety-critical jobs (e.g. airline pilots, train drivers, lorry drivers, fire fighters, perhaps even electricians and engineers employed by railway companies). In the NHS there has been a lot of discussion about pre-employment screening of nurses for psychiatric illness; this has become a factor following patient deaths. The GMC has similar concerns about mental illness and poor performance in doctors; questions of fitness to practice should be asked in the early phases of treatment for florid psychoses, etc. However, blanket judgements should be resisted, provided that there are no legal considerations that apply.

Back to work: reintegration into the workplace

A successful return to paid work is perhaps one of the most meaningful yet least used measures of health outcome in addition to being an important positive prognostic indicator, irrespective of psychiatric diagnosis. Too many patients with mental health problems make a good clinical and functional recovery only to find themselves living in an impoverished parallel world of social exclusion, and become aimless, underoccupied and unfulfilled. This existence not only potentially undermines an already fragile self-esteem but is itself a harbinger of further mental health problems. Government policy promoting social inclusion has not adequately addressed the widely perceived gulf that exists between the provisions made by health, social services, and voluntary sector to prepare service users for the workplace, their final stage of recovery, and the demands of the employment market itself. Moreover, traditional mental health services themselves are focused on symptomatic improvement and pay too little attention to occupational outcome and success in the workplace.

While a variety of schemes are provided by both the statutory and voluntary sector to help reintroduce mental health service users to the workplace, there is little evidence to demonstrate their effectiveness. Anecdotally, it is far easier for service users with an established pre-morbid work record to secure employment compared with those who have never been in work and for whom opportunities remain poor. The effectiveness of any employment scheme provided by the statutory and voluntary sector designed to return service users to the labour market will be limited unless employers are more proactive in recognizing the special needs of those recovering from mental illness and doing more to accommodate these within the workplace.

Recovery and return to work

Individuals who have held down a job but have been on a period of (often lengthy) sick leave and are recovering from mental health problems face a number of particular difficulties when they consider returning to work. There is, however, much that an occupational health service can do to maximize the likelihood of a successful outcome. First, it is important to establish whether the mental health team anticipates a return to pre-morbid functioning and, if not, what residual disabilities there are? Would an early return to normal duties help or hinder recovery? In particular, would a period of part-time employment or restricted duties be helpful in enabling the individual to rebuild confidence and re-acclimatize themselves to the work routine? It is especially important to evaluate the extent to which the demands of the employee's job itself may have been contributory to the development of mental health problems, and a decision made on whether or not it is either safe or appropriate for the individual to return to their former job and working environment.

The DDA requires that 'reasonable adjustments' are made where an individual's health needs to be taken into consideration. The occupational physician can do a great deal to help with rehabilitation by putting the case for modified hours, working from home on a temporary basis or even as a permanent arrangement on some days. Occasionally, it helps employees settle back into work more efficiently if tasks can be selected initially, which are relatively simple in nature and reduce any pressures that might otherwise cause difficulty.

There are occasions, of course, where the employee may blame the organization, the system of working or their manager for their health problem. This is often the case following an absence related to stress with resulting anxiety and/or depression. There may be a need for the manager to sit down and discuss the circumstances, specific tasks, or event that seem to have precipitated the illness and any absence. On occasions, a different job or relocation may be a sensible solution.

Work schemes and sheltered employment

For those with more serious mental health problems or those never before employed, a variety of schemes exist intended to ease the transition into the workplace. Sheltered employment and occupational rehabilitation are not new concepts and were historically an integral part of the asylum regime. With the advent of community care and the closure of large mental hospitals, much of this activity sadly failed to move into the community with the patient. This resulted in the provision of employment schemes in community settings being increasingly provided by the voluntary sector and becoming haphazard and patchy, both geographically and in terms of quality and meeting local need. One of the few surveys conducted has shown a 40-fold variation in provision across health authority areas. Unfortunately, but not surprisingly, the highest levels of provision are generally found in the most affluent areas.[14] Across the UK more than 130 different organizations offer some form of sheltered employment, including 77 providing open employment and with approximately 50 set up as 'social firms'.[15,16]

Models

A variety of models exist to facilitate a return to work. Sheltered workshops and factories (e.g. Remploy) provide mostly unskilled manual work for individuals with severe enduring mental illness. They are useful in introducing individuals to the work situation in a safe environment and provide occupation for those who would otherwise be unable to cope with the demands of open employment. Very few individuals in these schemes, however, move into the open employment market and the organizations themselves often experience difficulty in maintaining profitability, which puts their viability at considerable risk. A more recent variant of sheltered employment is the 'social firm'. In this model a business is developed as a commercial enterprise with mental health service users employed throughout the organization and not simply as manual labour. Social firms are not primarily engaged in rehabilitation and employees are paid the going rate for their work. A further variation to this model seen more commonly in Europe is the

'Social Enterprise'; a semi-commercial concern that also has the clear objective of providing training and rehabilitation.

Pre-vocational training enables individuals to have a period of preparatory training and a gradual reintroduction to the workplace with the expectation of them moving into the open employment market. It is a means to an end and not an end in itself. Tailored to individual need, this may include specific skills training, a period in a sheltered work environment or in a job that is ring-fenced and sponsored by a rehabilitation agency.

'Supported employment' aims to place individuals directly into the workplace without lengthy preparation or training. Service users are expected to obtain work directly in the open employment market. The employee is hired competitively and employed on the same basis as other employees, with full company benefits, but with supervision and mentoring from the support organization to maximize the likelihood of a successful outcome.[17] Assessment is on the job and support is continued indefinitely. Perhaps this, more than any other model, most effectively bridges the gap between mental health services and the employment community.

User employment programmes

Many NHS Trusts now employ current or former (health) service users in jobs that demand a history of mental health problems as part of the personal specification for the post. Service users are employed on terms and conditions of service identical to other employees and additional support is made available for those who need it. Many of these posts involve patient advocacy where the insight and personal experiences of former service users can clearly be brought to bear for the benefit of patients. Service users are increasingly employed in major service development roles such as National Service Framework Local Implementation Teams and increasingly serve as members of senior medical staff Appointments Advisory Committees. Indeed, service user involvement has become a key performance indicator with which all Mental Health Trusts are required to comply. This active participation of service users in high profile positions of obvious importance within the NHS is of immense symbolic value, challenging stigma, prejudice and the widely held poor expectations about the employability of mentally ill people in positions of responsibility in the workplace.[18]

Common psychiatric disorders

Despite advances in the classification of different psychiatric disorders with the advent of the WHO International Classification of Disease (ICD), and the US psychiatry specific Diagnostic and Statistical Manual (DSM), psychiatric terminology is still used very loosely and imprecisely, both in primary and secondary care. A diagnostic label may be misleading and is no substitute for a clear description of the symptoms and signs in any particular case. Diagnostic codes described below are from the ICD (10th edition).

Prognosis in psychiatry is an inexact science as there are numerous psychosocial variables that influence the course of any particular case. In general, however (and somewhat paradoxically), the outcome of psychotic, bipolar, and other more severe mental disorders can often be predicted with greater accuracy than more minor disorders that are influenced to a greater extent by the vagaries of personality, illness behaviour, and the presence of psycho-social stressors (which include domestic/home, employment/work, and social/community factors).

Adjustment disorders (including acute stress reactions): F43.2

These are short- and medium-term reactions to stressful events and comprise extreme reactions to the event itself or preoccupying concerns about the event. Individuals typically feel overwhelmed or unable to cope and may experience marked anxiety or depression. Conversely they may present with a variety of somatic complaints including headaches, dizziness, abdominal pain, chest pain, and palpitations. They may misuse alcohol or illicit substances to self-medicate. Most of these reactions are self-limiting and resolve within weeks or a few months. Medication, including antidepressants and anxiolytics, may be used to alleviate the more severe symptoms and respite from continuing stressful circumstances (including the workplace) may be appropriate for a short period. However, a gradual return to normal functioning is itself generally therapeutic and the expectation should be one of full recovery. Adjustment disorders may evolve into more chronic illnesses such as major depression and other anxiety states; however, the absence of any past psychiatric history and the presence of a 'robust' pre-morbid personality generally predicts a good outcome.

Post-traumatic disorders (PTDs) including post-traumatic stress disorder (PTSD): F43.1

Following traumatic events, the symptoms of PTSD (i.e. intrusive memories, nightmares, flashbacks, hyper-arousal, and avoidance symptoms) are normal phenomena and the majority of cases, similar to the adjustment disorders described above, resolve spontaneously without medical intervention. In a minority these symptoms fail to improve or deteriorate and individuals may go on to develop a PTD. This diagnosis/label should not be considered until the symptoms have been present for at least 6 months. PTD is of particular interest to employers, not least because the traumatic event may have been the result of exposure to an occupational factor(s) and be the subject of litigation.

PTSD has become a popular subject and of great interest to the media. There has, however, been an overemphasis on PTSDs and a relative lack of interest in other, if not more common, PTDs such as major depressive disorders, phobic, and other anxiety states as well as enduring changes of personality. Classic PTSD is not the commonest PTD and when it does occur, it is frequently complicated by other psychiatric co-morbidity. Following accidents for example, the most common reaction is a simple phobia. Depressive disorders are the second commonest reaction and are more likely to be seen in individuals with a pre-morbid vulnerability to depression (i.e. family history of depression, poor quality parenting, poor self-esteem, and a lack of confiding relationships). PTSD is generally seen less frequently than these other PTDs. There is still debate regarding the extent to which a traumatic event *per se* can lead to PTSD or to what extent a vulnerable personality is necessary condition for PTSD to develop. Delayed PTSD can occasionally occur in which symptoms do not become manifest for several months following a traumatic event. However, the delayed presentation of PTSD is much more common when a symptomatic individual conceals their symptoms and avoids seeking help, as a consequence of wishing to avoid reminders of the traumatic event.

There has been much interest in the effectiveness of early interventions following traumatic events in the hope of reducing the incidence of subsequent long-term psychiatric morbidity, in particular, the provision of Critical Incident Stress Debriefing (CISD) or Psychological Debriefing (PD). Recent randomized controlled trials have failed to demonstrate any benefit for CISD and, indeed, some have even suggested that they might do harm, raising the issue of what, if anything, employers should offer to their workforce as part of their duty of care following exposure to traumatic events. Although this remains a subject of much debate, most authorities would agree that education on what to expect in the aftermath of traumatic events is appropriate. Victims of trauma are given information about the normal stress response, what symptoms and problems may present, at what point these should be considered abnormal, and where and when to seek help. Advice should also be given about the need to avoid dangerous coping strategies such as a reliance on alcohol and other substances of potential abuse. Practical support should be offered wherever possible to help individuals adjust and return to a normal life-style and work routine. Finally, a mechanism of simple health screening should be implemented at appropriate time intervals following a traumatic event to enable the early detection of an emerging PTD so that treatment can be instituted as early as possible, thereby maximizing the chances of a successful outcome.

The treatment of established PTDs depends on the symptom profile of the patient. Phobic, depressive, and other anxiety disorders should be treated accordingly. PTSD itself responds to cognitive-behavioural therapy (CBT) and medication—selective serotonin reuptake inhibitors (SSRIs). There is much less evidence to support the use of other psychotropic drugs in this condition. Benzodiazepines, in particular, are generally considered unhelpful. Eye movement desensitization and reprocessing is an effective psychological technique (albeit somewhat less so than conventional CBT) and is becoming more widely used and, in some cases, can be very successful. It is equally important to treat co-morbid disorders, particularly substance misuse as it is unlikely that any treatment will be effective while a patient continues to misuse alcohol or other substances of potential abuse.

The treatment of PTDs is frequently complicated by litigation and there can be no doubt that lengthy legal proceedings and repeated examinations for legal reports are unhelpful and can impede recovery. There is no evidence, however, to suggest that the successful resolution of legal proceedings for the claimant leads to any significant improvement in the course of chronic severe PTSD and the prognosis in such cases is often poor. The symptoms of PTSD typically fluctuate and may deteriorate on anniversaries and following reminders of traumatic events. An ex-serviceman who survived the sinking of the RFA Sir Galahad in the 1982 Falklands War had been successfully working for several years as a long-distance lorry driver until he was asked to drive goods by ferry to Ireland. His symptoms dramatically worsened and he was unable to work. His employer was unaware of his previous trauma exposure, and when briefed simply changed the routes on which he worked to avoid sea crossings. He rapidly improved without any medical intervention and now works and functions normally. Noteworthy in this case is the fact that this individual had significant baseline PTSD symptomatology but was nevertheless able to successfully hold down a job until faced with a reminder of his traumatic experience. In PTSD, perhaps more than any other psychiatric disorder, there is a very poor correlation between illness behaviour and the extent of any psychopathology. It is unclear why some individuals 'soldier on' with significant symptoms, whereas others with minor degrees of psychopathology become completely disabled and totally consumed by the quest for compensation and legal redress for the perceived wrongdoings of their employer. The long-term prognosis and occupational outcome is unpredictable and can be very variable. However, the earlier PTSD is detected and treatment instituted (particularly before maladaptive behaviours, such as substance misuse, have become established), the better the outcome.

Bipolar affective disorder: F31.#

These are characterized by episodes of depression, mania, or an admixture of both. Mixed affective states are common and mood, disordered thought (including flight of ideas), motor behaviour (overactivity or retardation), arousal (irritability or withdrawal), perceptual abnormalities (including mood congruous delusions or hallucinations), or behavioural disturbances (retardation or disinhibition) may fluctuate and vary independently of each other. Patients may manifest predominantly depressive or manic symptoms and no two individuals are entirely the same. Although full recovery from major mood swings is the norm, many patients display lesser degrees of emotional instability requiring treatment between episodes. Factors to be considered in assessing the employability of bipolar patients include frequency of relapse, functional capacity during periods of well-being and adherence to any long-term treatment plan, particularly their compliance with mood stabilizing medication. Co-morbid substance misuse during episodes is generally a poor prognostic sign. Disturbed sleep and sleep deprivation are important triggers for episodes of mania and shift work or work involving long distance air travel may be unsuitable for individuals with bipolar disorders.

Chronic fatigue syndrome (CFS or ME): G93.3

This describes a heterogeneous group of disorders of varying severity all characterized by reduced energy levels, varying degrees of fatigue, and a variety of other somatic and psychological symptoms. Fatigue is a common symptom and is a feature of a wide range of physical and psychiatric disorders. The incidence of CFS is 300–500 per 100 000 of the population per year. There are several definitions of CFS, all of them require an illness comprising substantial physical and mental fatigue that lasts at least 6 months, impairs daily activities in the absence of any abnormal physical examination findings and laboratory investigations. Postviral fatigue and (benign) myalgic encephalitis (ME) are frequently used when the onset of fatigue appears to follow a specific trigger such as a viral illness and when symptoms fail to meet diagnostic criteria for 'neurasthenia' (F48.0). The terminology employed by clinicians varies widely, however, and it is important to clarify the precise nature of any symptoms and disability in individual cases. In addition to lack of energy and fatigue, patients with chronic fatigue states commonly also complain of postexertional malaise, worsening fatigue following mental or physical activity, musculoskeletal aches and pains, sleep disturbance (typically hypersomnia and non-refreshing sleep quality), headaches, and other somatic symptoms. Co-morbid depression and other psychiatric disorders are common. It is also important to ensure that patients have been adequately investigated to exclude occult underlying physical pathology, particularly where there is associated weight loss, any other unexplained physical signs, a history of foreign travel and where there are myalgic symptoms only, unaccompanied by mental fatigability.

The aetiology is uncertain and is the subject of debate. It is important to appreciate that the symptoms of CFS are not 'all in the mind' and may be genuinely disabling. Contrary to stereotype, chronic fatigue often improves spontaneously and although there is no definitive management applicable in all cases, effective treatment does exist and the successful management of CFS with a good outcome is possible. Critically, the patient's attitude towards treatment is important in helping decide the most appropriate therapeutic approach in individual cases.

Graded exercise and cognitive behavioural psychotherapy are of proven efficacy in the treatment of CFS, equally it is important to treat any depression or other associated co-morbid disorders. When assessing future employability it is important to ensure that every patient has a clear management plan with the expectation of recovery. Lack of motivation can be a problem for the treating physician as well as the patient: therapeutic nihilism is all too common and many patients languish only to become further disabled, without any clear focus or direction to their treatment.

It is important to resist applications for ill health retirement for at least 2 years following a diagnosis of CFS/ME; not even hinting that this may be an option. Most employees will return to good health. If the possibility of there being an option of retiring on health grounds is voiced, this is likely to (subconsciously, perhaps) impair progress.

Chronic mixed anxiety and depression: F41.2

Low mood, sadness, and anxiety are features of normal life, experienced by everybody and are not in themselves pathological. Many individuals experience symptoms severe enough to impair normal daily activities but which are insufficient to meet diagnostic criteria for either a depressive episode or other anxiety disorders. They are described and classified in various ways but include dysthymia (a mood disorder characterized by feeling sad, 'blue', low, 'down in the dumps', and loss of interest or pleasure in one's usual activities), mixed anxiety, and depression. Characteristic features include one or more physical symptoms (fatigue, insomnia, pain, etc.) and an admixture of anxiety and depressive symptoms, each in varying degree, and present for more than 6 months. It is all too easy to 'medicalize' problems of living and there is little evidence that traditional medical approaches are effective. Medication is of uncertain value in these more minor disorders and a successful outcome is more likely when the patient is encouraged to adopt a healthier life-style, participate in formulating a recovery plan that identifies trigger factors and addresses any obvious psychosocial stressors. Supportive counselling may be useful in helping patients address these issues and take personal responsibility for their own recovery. Brief cognitive approaches challenging unfounded worries and challenging negative assumptions, problem-solving approaches, and relaxation techniques may all be useful. Once again the occupational health professional, physician, or nurse/occupational health adviser, can reasonably expect an employee to have devised a clear plan in collaboration with their GP, emphasizing recovery and return to normal functioning. Motivation and the willingness to accept responsibility for this is probably one of the best predictors of a successful outcome.

Depression: F32#

Depression is common, potentially disabling, but also eminently treatable in the majority of cases. Although the clinical features of major depression are well known, it is important to appreciate that patients may present with various physical complaints such as fatigue or pain or with related psychological problems such as anxiety. Depression may also be triggered by physical disorders where it may pass undetected, yet nevertheless can be a major obstacle to recovery. It may only be on direct questioning that the classic signs of depression such as generalized anhedonia (defined as 'a total loss of feeling of pleasure in acts that normally give pleasure') and morbid negative thoughts of guilt, worthlessness, etc. are elicited. The symptoms of depression often develop insidiously and it may only be with hindsight that an employee under-performing in the workplace is recognized as suffering from a depressive disorder. Predictors of long-term outcome include pre-morbid personality and the presence of co-morbid disorders, particularly substance misuse. Despite the effectiveness of antidepressant drugs and CBT, it is important not to rely exclusively on these. Many depressed patients require non-specific interventions, including supportive counselling, to help them to adjust their life-style and minimize the impact of any major psycho-social stressors. The prospect of work can be intimidating for many depressed patients who may lack confidence and motivation; moreover many perceive their employment (rightly or wrongly) as contributory to their disorder.

Acute psychotic disorders: F23.9

These include first episode psychosis, acute schizophrenia and schizoaffective-like psychoses, acute delusional disorders, and other transient psychoses including those brought about by elicit drugs. Patients may present with hallucinations, strange beliefs or fears, perceptual disturbances or apprehension and apparent confusion. Families, employers, and other agencies typically seek help for inexplicable behavioural changes such as withdrawal, suspiciousness, self-neglect, or threats. Not uncommonly first episode psychoses may present with a period of vague somatic complaints, anxiety, or other neurotic symptoms that may precede the development of frank psychotic symptoms, sometimes by months or even years. The course and eventual outcome of acute psychoses are unpredictable; however, one-third of cases make a full recovery and remain well thereafter. In general, the outcome is better when the onset of psychosis is more rapid and set against a background of a robust pre-morbid personality. Individuals who demonstrate a rapid response to antipsychotic medication also have a generally better outcome. The diagnosis of schizophrenia can only be confidently made with the passage of time and individuals with even the most severe psychotic symptoms may make a complete recovery. It is important to adopt a positive approach and keep an open mind towards the employee who develops a psychotic illness: one of the authors (MD) has a patient who has had three severe episodes of a schizophrenia-like psychosis but remains generally very well on small amounts of antipsychotic medication and who successfully holds down a job as a senior police officer with the full knowledge and support of his employer.

Stress, strain, and burnout

Life is busy for many people employed in the developed world; jobs are often complex. Organizations usually employ few people with serious mental health problems; however, they do employ many who have the potential to become stressed with the result that in addition to any anxiety, or worse, which may result, they be less productive and useful. More senior staff are particularly expected to contribute by being creative and innovative and come up with solutions to problems. It is precisely these attributes and skills that diminish when 'stress', 'strain', or 'burnout' become established.

Although not psychiatric disorders in their own right and not described in the ICD-10, these loosely defined lay terms are among the commonest mental health related causes of impaired work efficiency. They may themselves be harbingers of more serious mental health problems, conversely, they may be the manifestation of an undetected underlying psychiatric disorder. Unfortunately, the terms are used to describe various states of mind and, once again, it is important to establish the exact nature of any particular problems and the symptoms and signs in each individual case.

One observer described stress as 'a reality, like love or electricity—unmistakable in experience but hard to define'. Stress, of course, is not confined to (and often not caused solely by) the work-place but may be related to home life and the social scene. The UK's Health and Safety Executive defines stress as 'the adverse reaction people have to excessive pressure or other types of demands placed on them'. In the work environment, it arises when the demands of the work environment exceed the employee's ability to cope with or control them. This makes an important distinction between pressure, which can be positive (*pressure cannot be a state of mind*) if managed correctly, and stress, which can be detrimental to health.

All jobs involve some degree of pressure and often such pressures can be positive, improving performance and giving job satisfaction. Where the pressure reaches excessive levels, and continues for some time, it can lead to mental and physical ill health. More information is available from: www.hse.gov.uk/stress.

Strain is an alternative term (analogous to its use in engineering parlance) used to describe the consequences of pressure or the load placed on the individual. Stress is not necessarily undesirable, a degree of stress (or pressure) improves performance and it is only when the symptoms of stress become excessive either in intensity, frequency, or chronicity that the consequences become pathological.

Burnout can be considered as the end-point in the breakdown of the adaptational process that results from a long-term mismatch between the demands placed upon an individual and the emotional resources that can be brought to bear to cope with these. 'Burnout' therefore results from prolonged and excessive stress caused by work, home, or social factors or, as is often the case, a mixture of two or three of these. Burnout and depression share a number of common features and there is approximately 25% co-variance. The two, however, are not synonymous. Depression is more likely to be associated with fatigue, anergia (characterized by lack of energy) and morbid depressive cognitions, including ideas of guilt, worthlessness, and self-blame, whereas individuals with burnout are more likely to feel aggrieved and embittered towards their employer. In contrast to depression, the symptoms of burnout tend to be work specific and not pervasive, affecting every aspect of life, at least in the early stages.

Burnout is more frequently observed in younger, less experienced employees. Other vulnerability factors include an anxiety-prone personality prone to poor self-esteem and an avoidant, non-confronting coping style. Vulnerable individuals feel powerless to influence their work (and home) environment and perceive an external locus of control in which events and achievements are attributed to chance or to others who are more powerful. This should be compared with those with an internal locus who tend to ascribe events or achievements to their own efforts and abilities. They are usually good at influencing and negotiating such that they, themselves, remain in charge of all, or at least the important, aspects of their lives. Attitudes towards work, such as high or overambitious expectations, are also associated with burnout as well as certain work-related stressors such as time-pressure and an excessive workload.

Stress

As noted earlier, many of the cases of mental ill-health seen in the workplace are different manifestations of stress or, more exactly, stress-related illnesses.

All work puts some pressure on individuals; in general the more demanding the work the greater the pressure. This normally leads to higher output and satisfaction with work. However, a point of diminishing returns is reached beyond which increasing the load leads to reversed effects: lowered efficiency, job satisfaction, performance, and mental well-being. Stress itself is not an illness; rather it is a state. However, it is a very powerful cause of illness. Long-term excessive stress is known to lead to serious health problems.

Recent years have seen a bewildering array of books, magazine articles, television programmes, and training courses about stress. Some of these can help you find out what stress is, but they rarely give you much of an idea what you can do about it. Stress is best thought of as a series of physical and mental reflexes that exist because they have had a purpose. They are designed to put your body and mind into overdrive for short periods of time, and to help you to deal with short-term crises. It is presumably because they have a survival value that they have been bred into us in times long gone.

The problem in the modern world is that few of the pressures that produce stress, so-called 'stressors', can be dealt with by direct physical action—no matter how much we might be tempted by the idea. The aim of quickly getting rid of the stress is usually hard to achieve. As a result we are left with the physical and mental effects of stress over periods of weeks, months, or even years as the stressors do not go away.

Many people feel that experiencing unpleasant stress is a weakness or that they should be able to use their mind or their logic to switch stress off. That is unrealistic; most of us have had the experience of feeling jittery after a 'near miss' in the car, even though we know that the threat has passed and we are completely safe. The stress responses are a set of automatic reflexes that cannot be switched off.

The following graphic depicts the relationship between stress, or pressure/demands on the individual (along the horizontal axis), and performance or output (the vertical axis)—this is sometimes called the 'Human Function Curve' and provides an important model in aiding understanding of the negative effects of stress.

Pressure performance stages

This relationship can be demonstrated for physical responses to stress (e.g. the changes that can be observed in breathing rate and blood pressure) and psychological performance (e.g. performing mental arithmetic under time pressures), or in terms of group performance such as the productivity or efficiency of an organization.

Note that initially performance improves under pressure. This is why athletes often produce better results when competing than they do in practice sessions. The whole science of training and sports coaching is aimed at building competitors up to optimal performance for the day of the big event. However, this improvement does not go on forever. There comes a point where performance begins to deteriorate—an experience that all of us will have recognized in others, if not in ourselves. If the pressure is not reduced, then performance is suboptimal and may even lead to breakdown.

We all perform at our best when under the right amount of pressure. There comes a point when the pressure becomes too much and our performance suffers. It is important to be aware of the consequences and notice when our efficiency is beginning to fall off. Most people are unable to monitor their own stress levels but are better at seeing it in colleagues or in friends or family. Brief overload does nothing more than temporarily reduce performance, major overload can prolong serious illness. Stress, of course, is a normal part of life. The challenge is to manage the pressures so that life is productive and enjoyable.

In an organization (at the workplace), the spectrum of effects ranges from reduced productivity, an increase in errors, lack of creativity, poor decision-making, job dissatisfaction, disloyalty, an increase in sick leave, unpreparedness, requests for early retirement, absenteeism, accidents, theft, organizational breakdown, or even sabotage.

In many organizations, only quite serious consequences (in the second half of the list), are monitored or recognized.

The consequences of stress to the individual include anxiety, fatigue, insomnia, relationship problems, emotional instability, depression, psychosomatic diseases, excessive smoking, cardiovascular problems, increased alcohol consumption, drug abuse, eating disorders or even suicide.

The following case studies illustrate what may happen.

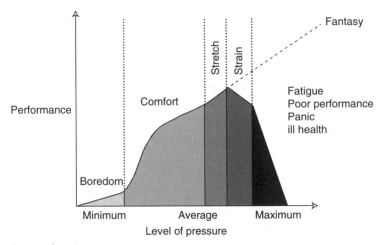

Fig. 7.1 The human function curve

A 42-year-old male scientist has to co-ordinate the development of a new product. He works night and day—co-ordinating the efforts of people from individual departments. He has been told—'the business depends on you'. His free time shrinks, his wife and family get the rough edge of his tongue over many months, he feels unsupported at work and unable to say he can't cope. At 9pm after a train journey he bursts into tears on the station platform. Six months later he still lacks confidence but is learning to work more effectively and still find time for himself and his family. Getting the balance across all areas of life is important—making time for each is essential for good health.

A 34-year-old female marketing manager is engaged in a number of negotiations with other companies. New projects and negotiations are initiated regularly and require concentration over long hours. The projects require managing—she plays a key role in supporting and advancing each one. Work starts at 8am and never seems to stop. Holidays and weekends don't exist. Hobbies are a thing of the past. She wishes headcount requirements to manage new projects were considered at the outset. On many occasions she has been seen leaving her office at 9pm. Eventually she is taken off her job for 2 weeks rest. She is lucky—her overwork was recognized as such and she is not considered to have failed. Others are branded as 'weak'.

A nurse, highly regarded by her peers, ceased to work to her usual high standards following a reorganized work schedule. She complained bitterly about the change and on one occasion appeared tearful while discussing it with a colleague. She resented attempts to get her to seek medical advice, feeling that she was being accused of professional incompetence. Eventually her employer persuaded her to see a psychiatrist in the hospital 'for an informal chat'. It transpired that she was coping with an elderly ill mother at home who required almost constant attention during her off-duty time and who complained of being ignored as a result of the reorganized work schedule. This conflict was too much to bear and she became depressed. The answer to this problem lay not in a changed work pattern, but in a restructuring of the support for the mother so that the patient could lead her own life without feeling guilty about neglecting her mother.

A 56-year-old civil engineer developed anxiety attacks, impaired concentration, and reduced sleep. These were prominent in the evenings and during weekends. He was a perfectionist and was regarded as a conscientious and reliable worker, with very little time off sick. He had a good marriage and plenty of support from his wife; there were no crises or difficulties in his personal life that could account for the recent onset of anxiety and depressive symptoms. His symptoms had started when he was given a new job. He had supervised projects when new motorways were built and had done this for many years. His new responsibilities moved him out of his 'comfort zone' into engineering informatics projects. While his managers were happy with his work, he did not believe that he was doing it to his own high standards. The resulting anxiety and depression were treated with antidepressants (which also had anxiolytic effects) and a prolonged period away from work on sick leave. While almost all patients with depression will improve over a 2-year period, even the consideration of a return to work in this man was accompanied by a relapse and he became tearful and fretful. After a period of more than 3 years of experiencing the symptoms of depression, an ill health retirement was granted.

A 27-year-old junior manager is well trained and capable. He works hard but is unable to prioritize his tasks and gives each one his full attention. No one asks him to outline his workload and allocate appropriate time to each task. He works 10 or 11 hours daily and is usually busy with work at weekends. In addition, his widowed mother is in hospital and he wants, and feels obliged, to visit her regularly. He becomes anxious, then feels desperate, panic-stricken, and eventually depressed. One month's intensive treatment, as an outpatient, restores his health, vigour, and enthusiasm. He needs training in managing his time. His manager should not only allocate work but check that all her staff are managing their work in a sensible way. They may need coaching on priority setting and the sensible allocation of time; and also updates on the ever changing business requirements, which govern when specific tasks need to be completed. These skills are an important element of training and development for individuals.

Psychiatric injury and stress

If asked, many employees will say that they are 'stressed'; perhaps it has become almost a 'badge of honour' meant to indicate that the individual has a very busy or important job.

However, the courts do recognize work-related stress and in one case, appealed to the House of Lords in 2004, a landmark ruling put the onus on employers to keep up-to-date with what causes occupational stress and the effectiveness of any precautions they may take.

The ruling, in the case of *Barber v Somerset County Council,* made it clear that being unsympathetic to complaints of occupational stress or having autocratic or bullying leadership could count against an employer.[20] The case centred on former schoolteacher Leon Barber, who suffered a mental breakdown in November 1996, after working long hours following a restructuring at his school the year before. He had spoken to the head teacher and two deputies but nothing had been done to assist him. The judge had taken the view that more should have been done for him and that the school had been in breach of its duty of care. The law lords agreed that, once an employer knew an employee was at risk of suffering injury from occupational stress, it was under a duty to act.[21] This duty continued until something reasonable was done. Certified sickness absence because of stress or depression needed to be taken seriously by employers, requiring an inquiry from the employer. They stated that employees should not be brushed off unsympathetically, or by sympathizing and simply telling them to prioritize their work without taking steps to improve or consider the situation further. Critically, a management culture that was sympathetic and supportive could make a real difference to the outcome of a case. Monitoring employees who are known to be suffering from occupational stress was recommended. The statutory duty to carry out risk assessments had also been recognized by the judgment.

The Court of Appeal ruled that information given in confidence to the Occupational Health Service/Team does not mean that the employer knew of a claimant's increased susceptibility to mental ill health—contrasting with the DDA employment code, which states that an employer is deemed to know what the occupational health professionals know. For stress-at-work cases to succeed, claimants must show not only that the job made them ill but also that they made the employer aware that it was causing actual or impending damage to health. An employer cannot argue that psychological injury is not foreseeable in more extreme cases—such as prison healthcare staff having to deal with suicides.[22]

The role of the employer in maximizing health and well-being

It is commonly believed that resources to deal with mental health should be directed at offering professional support to individuals with problems.

As with other areas of occupational health, there are a great many preventative actions which can be taken and, of course, the full spectrum of health should be promoted.

In order to ensure that people feel fulfilled and perform well for the organization for which they work, it is important that they are healthy and their well-being is considered. There should be a focus on optimizing performance, with proper attention being paid to the way work is organized in terms of appropriate role descriptions, correct resource allocation, and full consideration given to requests for flexible working—all contained within a supportive culture that encourages good management of all aspects of performance. All organizations want their staff to be effective at work and it is essential that personal development is encouraged and people are rewarded and

Table 7.2 Organizational success/individual well-being

ORGANIZATION	Poor performance	Improving performance	Excellent performance
INDIVIDUALS	*Progressively worsening* **"Health"** *state of health*	*Improving health & well-being*	**High energy levels**
	SUPPORT REQUIRED	**SKILLS**	**OPTIMIZING PERFORMANCE**

		– Task/project
		– Team
		– 'Life management'
			• **Work Organization**
			 -Role description
			  inc.content & dimensions
			 -Resource allocation
			 -Supportive culture
			 -Good performance
			  management
			 -Flexible working
			• **Employee Effectiveness**
			 -Personal development
			 -Reward and recognition
			 -Work/home balance

recognized for work done well. Key to long-term effectiveness is an appropriate balance between work and home life.

This should be backed up with appropriate training and education so that staff are, or become, confident and competent. This should primarily revolve around the tasks and skills required, e.g. assertiveness, team-building, leading a project, etc. Life management skills are important and training should be available (how to manage one's time, give presentations, learn to say 'no', etc.) If both organization and training/education are fully addressed then staff should be healthy and be able to perform effectively at their workplace. However, many people run into problems from time to time and advice and support services should be available—perhaps by way of an Employee Assistance Programme (EAP) or, if mental problems are more significant or require specialist help, referral to an occupational health professional, clinical psychologist or psychiatrist.

Much of this effort should be proactive to ensure that staff have the skills to manage the complexity that is part and parcel of everyday life.

Two light-hearted definitions of health were used to introduce this chapter. However, clarity on what we mean by 'health' and 'well-being' is critical if we wish to maximize the contribution that can be made by staff. As Robert Rosen made clear 'Healthy people make healthy companies (*and organizations*). And healthy companies are more likely, more often, and over a longer period of time, to make healthy profits (*maximize output*) and to make healthy returns on investments.'

One of the authors (ELT) has, with others in AstraZeneca—particularly the Global Well-being Manager, John Staley—tried to define 'Well-being', this is the conclusion:

> Promoting 'Well-being' is a sound business ideal. If we are to expect people's continued energy and commitment at work we must provide the right environment, in which people feel positive and enthusiastic about what they are doing, have a clear sense of purpose, confidence in their ability to meet the challenges, and pride in their individual contribution to the organization's success.
>
> Actions that effectively promote well-being lead to a more healthy, energised work environment and increased effectiveness. The dynamic and positive working environment this encourages helps us to attract, develop and retain top talent, and reduces the impact of ill-health.

There are perhaps two distinct elements—the *organizational response* and the *individual elements.*

Well-being: the organization

Well-being is a useful collective term for all measures and resources aimed at enhancing well-being and promoting health. It includes four organizational responses:

1. *Intelligent leadership*
   - respect for the individual and their diverse needs.
   - recognition and support for individuals and their wellness.
   - encouragement and role modelling of effective behaviours (wellness, health, and work/home balance).

2. *Positive environment*
   - well-designed roles with the opportunity to make a positive contribution and be recognized and rewarded.
   - a working environment that takes into account safety, security, and ergonomic considerations.
   - opportunities for social interaction at work.

3. *Focus on health*
   - occupational health programmes that promote health and wellness.
   - counselling and life management resources.
   - encouragement of healthy life-styles (including diet and exercise) beneficial to employees.
   - effective return to work procedures where illness impairs personal wellness.

4. *Optimum work/home balance*
   - opportunities to discuss and agree flexibility in working patterns, subject to business need (e.g. job-sharing, flexitime, term-time contracts, reduced hours, working from home).
   - family-friendly policies (e.g. business travel, e.g. no meetings on Mondays or Fridays when attendees have to travel long distances—unless business critical, maternity/paternity leave, childcare provision).

Well-being: the individual

Well-being is the positive outcome of a number of physical, social, mental, and emotional factors that, working together, help us live happily and creatively.

There are four platforms to individual well-being:

1. *Self-belief*
   - dignity, self-awareness, and self-confidence are essential if we are to respect ourselves and others.

2. *A balanced life—where there is harmony between:*
   - our physical health, assisted by a healthy life-style.
   - our relationships with family and friends.
   - our need to learn and develop.
   - our emotional stability.
   - our ethical values and the support they give for behaviour and direction in life.
   - our working life and the rewards it offers.

3. *Time and energy management*
  - having a life-style that gives us time for all the various activities that we are required, and wish, to do (these include home life, wider family, leisure, social activities, and time alone—as well as work!).

4. *A future we look forward to*
  - having ideas, hopes, and enthusiasm as we look ahead in our lives.

Conclusions

There should be a focus in the workplace on health and well-being. This should be an integral part of a comprehensive approach to managing a high-quality organization. A well thought through, proactive approach to mental health and an organized way of dealing with ill health cases is key.

Mental health problems are common in the workplace, where they impair performance and work efficiency as well as being frequent causes of absenteeism. They may cause or add to the burden of unemployment.

In addition to the direct effects of any psychopathology on occupational functioning, the stigma and discrimination that surrounds mental illness creates additional obstacles to the successful reintegration into the working environment for individuals who are all too often lacking in self-confidence and struggling to cope with a fragile self-esteem. Close liaison between occupational physicians, psychologists, psychiatrists, and GPs should be a part of any comprehensive occupational assessment that should focus on disability, not diagnosis. When permission to do so is given, managers can very usefully help in identifying where specific factors, (poor) working relationships, and/or working arrangements may have been contributory. They can often be key to arranging for individuals to be successfully reintroduced to work, and facilitate a modification to working hours, usually for a defined period and then reviewed.

Employers should expect a balanced view of future employability. An overoptimistic appraisal is not only damaging to a business but potentially sets the individual up to fail, leading to further mental health problems. Conversely, overpessimistic assessments deny hope and opportunity to a significant section of society, creating further social exclusion and increasing the financial burden on the state. Past work performance, motivation, and the enthusiasm of the employee are the best predictors of a successful return to work regardless of diagnosis. (It should be remembered that adjustments may have to be made to working arrangements.) Ironically, it is exactly those same qualities (i.e. a past history of employing individuals with mental health problems and the tolerance of employers towards mental illness, motivation and enthusiasm, reflecting a commitment to disabled minorities) that are required of the employer if individuals recovering from mental illness are to successfully take up their place in society as productive individuals, with the same rights and opportunities as their peers.

References

1 United Nations (1948) Universal Declaration of Human Rights. http://www.un.org/Overview/rights.html

2 Manning C, White P. Attitudes of employers to the mentally ill. *Psychiatr Bull* 1995; **19**: 541–3.

3 Cox T. *Stress Research and Stress Management: putting theory to work.* London: Health and Safety Executive, 1993.

4 *Walker* v. *Northumberland County Council.* Queens Bench Division. All ER, 1995.

5 Singleton N, Bumpstead R, O'Brien M *et al. Psychiatric morbidity among adults living in private households, 2000.* London: Office of National Statistics, National Statistics Office, 2001.

6 National Statistics Office. *Labour force survey.* London: National Statistics Office, 2000.

7 Meltzer H, Gill B, Petticrew M *et al. Economic activity and social functioning of adults with psychiatric disorders. OPCS surveys of psychiatric morbidity in Great Britain.* Report No. 3. London: HMSO, 1995.

8 Patel A, Knapp M. Costs of mental illness in England. *PSSRU Mental Health Res Rev*, 1998; **5**: 4–10.

9 Oliver M. *The politics of disablement.* Basingstoke: Macmillan, 1990.

10 Schneider J. Work interventions in mental care: some arguments and recent evidence. *J Ment Health* 1998; **7**: 81–94.

11 Bartley M. Unemployment and ill-health: understanding the relationships. *J Epidemiol Community Health* 1994; **48**: 333–7.

12 Warr P. *Work, unemployment and mental health.* Oxford: Oxford University Press, 1987.

13 Warner R. *Recovery from schizophrenia. Psychiatry and political economy* (2nd edn). London: Routledge, 1994.

14 Crowther RE, Marshall M. Employment rehabilitation schemes for people with mental health problems in the North West Region: service characteristics and utilisation. *J Ment Health*, 2001; **10**: 373–82.

15 Grove B, Drurie S. *Social firms—an instrument for economic improvement and inclusion.* Redhill: Social Firms UK, 1999.

16 Crowther RE, Marshall M, Bond GR *et al.* Helping people with severe mental illness to obtain work: systematic review. *BMJ* 2001; **322**: 204–8.

17 Becker DR, Drake RE, Concord NH. Individual placement and support: a community mental health centre approach to rehabilitation. *Community Ment Health J* 1994; **30**: 193–206.

18 Perkins RE, Buckfield R, Choy D. Access to employment. *J Ment Health* 1997; **6**: 307–18.

19 *WHO guide to mental and neurological health in primary care.* London: Royal Society of Medicine Press, 2004.

20 Lords' ruling means employer's need to look for signs of stress. *Occup Health* 2004; **5**.

21 Psychiatric injury and stress; the employer's duty of care. *Health Saf Bull* 2004; 332.

22 Stress and the law at work. *Occup Health* 2005;

Chapter 8

Epilepsy

I. Brown and M. C. Prevett

Introduction

Epilepsy is a common condition that affects large numbers of working people. In about one-third, epilepsy is the only handicap, and in others there are additional neurological, intellectual, or psychological problems. Uncontrolled epileptic seizures can lead to injury and may impact on education and employment, but antiepileptic drug (AED) treatment is effective in approximately 70% of people with epilepsy.

Definitions

Epileptic seizures

Epileptic seizures are the clinical manifestation of an abnormal and excessive discharge of cerebral neurons and may involve transient alteration of consciousness, motor, sensory, autonomic or psychic phenomena. Epileptic seizures are caused by a wide variety of cerebral and systemic disorders, and may be *provoked* (acute symptomatic seizures) or *unprovoked*.

- Provoked or acute symptomatic seizures occur during an acute cerebral or systemic illness and do not constitute a diagnosis of epilepsy.
- Unprovoked seizures may be the late consequence of an antecedent cerebral disorder such as meningitis, head injury, and stroke (remote symptomatic seizures), or there may be no clear antecedent aetiology (idiopathic and cryptogenic).

Epilepsy

Epilepsy is defined by a tendency to recurrent unprovoked epileptic seizures.

Classification of epilepsy

The international classification of epilepsies and epileptic syndromes[1] incorporates anatomical, aetiological and syndromic features, but includes many rare syndromes and can be difficult to apply in clinical practice. Another more commonly used approach is to classify epilepsy by seizure type (Table 8.1). Seizures are divided into two main categories, partial and generalized.[2]

Partial seizures

In partial (focal or localization-related) seizures the abnormal neuronal discharge starts in a localized area of brain. The clinical manifestations vary widely and are determined by the anatomical localization and spread of the neuronal discharge. Partial seizures are subdivided into three categories:

- Simple partial seizures in which there is no alteration of consciousness (also known as an aura)

Table 8.1 Classification by seizure type

I	Partial (focal) seizures
	(a) Simple partial seizures
	(b) Complex partial seizures
	(c) Secondarily generalized seizures
II	Generalized seizures
	(a) Generalized tonic–clonic seizures
	(b) Absence seizures
	(c) Myoclonic seizures
	(d) Atonic seizures
	(e) Tonic seizures
	(f) Clonic seizures
III	Unclassified epileptic seizures

Adapted from the International League Against Epilepsy classification
of seizure type, Commission on Classification and Terminology of the ILAE, 1981.

+ complex partial seizures in which consciousness is impaired or lost
+ secondarily generalized seizures in which the epileptic discharge starts focally and then
  spreads to the rest of the brain usually triggering a tonic–clonic seizure. Both simple and
  complex partial seizures can evolve into a secondarily generalized seizure.

Generalized seizures

In generalized seizures the abnormal neuronal discharge is widespread and involves both cerebral
hemispheres from the onset. Generalized tonic–clonic (*grand mal*), absence (*petit mal*), and
myoclonic seizures are the most common types of generalized seizure in people without other
neurological or intellectual problems. Tonic, atonic, and clonic seizures tend to occur in people
with diffuse cerebral disorders associated with learning disability. In all generalized seizures there
is abrupt onset with loss of awareness without any warning or aura.

Incidence and prevalence

A British study of treated epilepsy showed an incidence rate of 80.8 (95% confidence
interval 76.9–84.7) per 100 000 per year.[3] The incidence is higher in childhood and in the elderly.
Throughout working life, from the age of 16 to 65 years, first seizures occur at a rate of approximately 40 cases per 100 000 per year. The lifetime risk of having a seizure is estimated to
be 2–5%.

The prevalence of epilepsy in England and Wales in 1998 was estimated to be 7.7 cases per 1000
in men and 7.6 cases per 1000 in women. The National General Practice Study of Epilepsy showed
that 62% of patients had tonic–clonic seizures (either generalized or secondarily generalized),
11% complex partial seizures and 12% mixed partial seizure types; other seizure types were
uncommon.[4] Seizure frequency varies enormously between individuals with about a third
experiencing less than one seizure per year and about 20% more than one per week.

Causes of epilepsy

Studies have shown that a cause can be confidently established only in a minority of new cases of
epilepsy (20–40%). The most common causes of epileptic seizures in adults are listed in Table 8.2.

Table 8.2 Common causes of adult onset epileptic seizures

Cerebrovascular disease
Head injury (and neurosurgery)
Cerebral tumour
Vascular malformation (cavernoma, arteriovenous malformation)
Disorders of cortical development
Perinatal injury and hypoxia
CNS infection (meningitis, encephalitis, cerebral abscess)
Genetic
Degenerative disorders (e.g. Alzheimer's disease)

The proportion of patients in whom a cause is identified depends on the extent of investigation, particularly neuroimaging (computed tomography or magnetic resonance imaging). Advances in magnetic resonance imaging technology have allowed identification of more subtle structural causes such as disorders of cortical development. Among patients with drug-resistant epilepsy, detailed magnetic resonance imaging can detect a potential cause in up to 75%.[5]

The proportion of patients with symptomatic epilepsy increases with age. In the National General Practice Study of Epilepsy cerebrovascular disease was the most common aetiological factor in 15% (49% in patients over the age of 60 years), 6% of seizures were attributed to a cerebral tumour, 3% to trauma, 2% to infection, and 7% to other causes.[4]

Toxic causes of epilepsy are rare. Seizures may very occasionally occur as a result of lead encephalopathy, almost always in children. Seizures have occurred in employees overexposed during the manufacture of chlorinated hydrocarbons, and ingestion of or gross overexposure to organochlorine insecticides has resulted in status epilepticus.[6] Epileptiform abnormalities on EEG have been recorded in the absence of any clinical abnormality in workers exposed to methylene chloride, methyl bromide, carbon disulphide, benzene, and styrene, although the significance of these observations is uncertain.

Recurrence of seizures

Estimates of recurrence rates after a first seizure have varied from 27% up to 84%, the variation reflecting selection bias in the study population.[7] Aetiology has an important influence on the risk of recurrence. In the National General Practice Study of Epilepsy (NGPSE) seizures associated with neurological deficits presumed to be present from birth had a 100% rate of relapse within the first 12 months, whereas seizures associated with a lesion acquired postnatally carried a risk of relapse of 75% by 12 months.[8] The presence of generalized spike and wave activity on EEG also appears to increase the risk of recurrence.

Randomized studies have shown that the risk of recurrence after a first seizure is reduced by AED treatment.[9,10] Patients started on treatment after a first seizure are, however, no more likely to achieve remission than patients in whom treatment is delayed until after two or more seizures and the decision to treat should be based on individual factors and the estimated risk of recurrence.

The risk of recurrence decreases as time elapses after the first seizure, a fact that is often of great importance in resolving issues concerned with safety at work. In the NGPSE (in which only 15% of patients with a first seizure received treatment) the risk of recurrence after a seizure-free

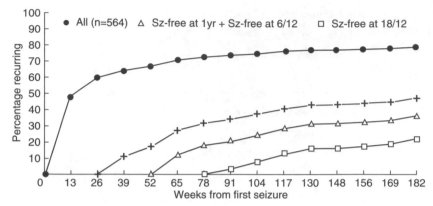

Fig. 8.1 Actuarial percentage recurrence rates after a first seizure for those still free of recurrence at 6, 12, and 18 months, and for all patients.[8] © 1990, reproduced with permission from Elsevier.

period of 6 months was 44%, after 12 months seizure-free the risk was 32% and after 18 months seizure-free the risk fell to 17% (Figure 8.1).

Chances of remission

Although there is a high risk of recurrence after a first seizure most people developing epilepsy become seizure-free. In the NGPSE, if patients with single or provoked seizures are excluded, 62% achieved a 5-year remission after 9 years of follow-up.[11] In another population based study the 5-year remission rates were 65% at 10 years and 76% at 15 years.[12] Most patients who go into remission do so within the first 2 years after diagnosis and, as time elapses without seizure control, the chances of subsequent remission decreases.

Age and seizure type do not appear to influence the chances of remission significantly but a syndromic classification can be useful prognostically. For example benign rolandic epilepsy (benign epilepsy with centrotemporal spikes) develops in childhood and spontaneous remission occurs in 98–99% of cases by the age of 14 years. Juvenile myoclonic epilepsy, however, develops in adolescence and although responsive to AEDs, is associated with a lifelong disposition to seizures and more than 90% of patients will relapse if treatment is withdrawn.

Twenty to 30% of patients continue to experience seizures despite AED treatment.[13] The introduction of eight new AEDs since 1990 has had little impact on this figure. There is no evidence that the newer drugs are any more effective than standard treatment and a poor response to initial treatment with any drug appropriate to the type of epilepsy, whether standard or new, seems to predict a poor response to other drugs. A recent prospective study found that among previously untreated patients 47% became seizure-free with their first AED and 14% became seizure-free during treatment with a second or third drug.[14] In only 3% was the epilepsy controlled by a combination of two drugs. AEDs licensed in the UK are listed in Table 8.3.

Prevention of epilepsy in the workplace

Primary and secondary prevention

The avoidance of head injuries is the most important preventive measure and is fundamental to safety at work, in the home, and on the road.

Table 8.3 Antiepileptic drugs available in the UK

Standard first-line drugs
Carbamazepine, sodium valproate

Other drugs licensed for first use monotherapy
Lamotrigine, oxcarbazepine, topiramate, phenytoin

Second-line and add-on drugs
Acetazolamide, clobazam, clonazepam, ethosuximide, gabapentin, levetiracetam, phenobarbitone, piracetam, pregabalin, primidone, tiagabine, vigabatrin, zonisamide

Epilepsy does not follow a trivial head injury; if the head injury is associated with a depressed fracture (especially if the dura is torn), an intracranial haematoma, or focal neurological signs, then there is a significant risk of later epilepsy.

A large community survey of a head-injured population[15] confirmed findings by previous workers that the risk of seizures early (within 7 days of the injury) and late seizures (after 7 days of the injury) can be determined by an assessment of the severity of the brain injury. Severe head injuries (loss of consciousness, amnesia lasting more than 24 hours, subdural haematoma, and brain contusion) are accompanied by a substantially increased risk of epilepsy over the next 10 years. (Standardized incidence ratio 17.0 (95% CI 12.3–23.6).) Because of this significantly increased risk, patients who have suffered a serious head injury should be treated in a similar way to those that have already suffered a convulsion including a 6–12-month ban on driving. The use of antiepileptic medication does not affect the risk of developing post-traumatic epilepsy but it does reduce the frequency of early seizures.[16]

The wearing of seatbelts by all motorists and the introduction of an approved safety helmet for cyclists and where appropriate in the workplace are the obvious first preventive measures. (Paradoxically, this reverses the usual order of safety steps in occupational health and makes personal protection top of the list.) Making the working environment safe should be the first step, but often, the unpredictability of events makes this impossible. It should be compulsory that safety helmets are worn at all times in areas specified by the works safety officer or safety committee. As a second step, the workforce should be made aware of areas where other employees are operating above, so that these can be avoided if possible. A safety helmet will not protect an individual from serious head injury if anything heavy is dropped from a great height. If work has to be performed underneath such a hazard, steel netting should be rigged to catch anything that falls. The other main preventive measure is the avoidance of precipitating factors. Some of these are described below.

Shift work

Seizures are common just before and just after waking, especially in idiopathic generalized epilepsy, and so it might be supposed that the introduction of a shift system into the work programme of a person with well-controlled epilepsy would predispose them to an increased frequency of seizures. Documentary evidence of a change in seizure frequency has not been established. This may be due to people with epilepsy electing to avoid shift work, as indicated by Dasgupta et al.[17] Many people with well-controlled epilepsy, however, can work on rotating shifts without problems.

Night work may be an exception. Patterns of sleep are disturbed by night work and to a lesser extent by other types of shift work. Night workers sleep for shorter periods during their working week and sleep longer on rest days, to make up the deficit.[18] Sleep deprivation is an important precipitant of seizures for some individuals and is best avoided by those with idiopathic generalized epilepsy.

Stress

An association between stress and seizure frequency has often been reported anecdotally. Changes in brain arousal lead to changes in excitability and this may affect neuronal discharges, particularly of those neurons that surround an epileptic focus. Is there any scientific evidence to support this association? Substantial numbers of patients report that the frequency of their seizures increase if they are exposed to stress, but stress itself may also be associated with other seizure-provoking factors such as alcohol and sleep deprivation and there may be reporting bias as people search for an explanation of the increased frequency of their seizures.

Paradoxically, inactivity and drowsiness may also be related to an increase in seizure frequency. The possibility that stress and its associated factors may affect seizure control should be considered when employees with epilepsy are moved to different areas of responsibility.

Photosensitivity and visual display equipment

Photosensitivity epilepsy is a form of reflex epilepsy and is rare in adults and usually associated with idiopathic generalized epilepsy. It may need to be considered where a light source flickers. The overall prevalence is 1 in 10 000 but it is twice as common in women; 90% of patients have suffered their first convulsion due to photosensitivity before the age of 25 years.[19–21] Photosensitivity may be increased following deprivation of sleep. Spontaneous seizures may occur in photosensitive subjects.

The diagnosis of photosensitive epilepsy is supported by performing an EEG recording with a photic stimulation and eliciting a photoconvulsive response. This is usually a generalized discharge of spike wave activity elicited by the flickering stimulus and persisting after the stimulus has ceased. False positive tests can also arise: some individuals have a paroxysmal EEG response to photic stimulation without any evidence of having had a seizure.[19–21] Television is a common precipitant of photosensitive epilepsy. The provocative stimulus is the pattern of interlacing lines formed by the flying spot from the electron gun.

Proximity to the screen appears to be an important factor, as this enables the viewer to discriminate the line pattern; most television sensitive patients reveal their sensitivity at a viewing distance of 1 metre or less. Background illumination is another factor. Flickering sunlight (e.g. through the leaves of a tree), faulty and flickering artificial lights and glare are also occasional precipitants. Swimming in bright sunlight may constitute some risk because of glare and flicker patterns on the water surface. Helicopter rotor blades and aeroplane propellers may also provoke episodes.

The use of visual display equipment (VDE) in employment constitutes a much smaller risk than that incurred when viewing television. The majority of VDE screens have relatively slow phosphors in the tubes to reduce apparent flicker and, in addition, they usually do not use an interlaced line pattern.

The probability of a first convulsion being induced by VDE is exceedingly small and, even in the established photosensitive subject, seizures are unlikely to occur. It is therefore essential that a known sufferer of epilepsy is not disadvantaged in any way when applying for work that involves the use of VDE. Regrettably this is still a common reason for job refusal, although it cannot be justified on the grounds of risk.

The Civil Aviation Authority (CAA) has recognized the special risks that may be associated with flying, especially from the slow flicker that is visible through helicopter blades. The CAA has always performed an EEG investigation as part of its routine medical screen on helicopter pilots applying for commercial licences. This is now required in the UK for professional fixed-wing aircraft pilots following the harmonization of aviation medical standards throughout the European Union and another 12 states (collectively known as the Joint Aviation Authorities, JAA). Introduced on 1 July 1999, it is now a mandatory investigation on all professional pilots on initial examination. No requirement exists for the investigation to be repeated routinely, and none is proposed, other than when indicated clinically.

Interestingly, medical assessors in the UK used to undertake EEG investigation as part of their routine medical screen on all applicants for professional fixed-wing aircraft pilots but, after many years of data collection, the risk and cost–benefit analyses showed that this was not helpful. Although the UK has largely influenced the European harmonization process it was unable to avoid the reintroduction of this test.

Other types of reflex epilepsy

Although reflex epilepsy may occasionally be induced by reading, concentrating, being suddenly startled, or hearing music or bells, this is rare.

Alcohol and drugs

Alcohol misuse increases the risk of epileptic seizures. Seizures may be caused by alcohol withdrawal, a direct toxic effect of alcohol, or associated metabolic disturbance (e.g. hypoglycaemia) and cerebral trauma. Seizures may also occur with chronic alcohol misuse in the absence of withdrawal or other identifiable cause. Alcohol misuse may complicate established epilepsy increasing the risk of seizures and other complications.

A number of drugs lower seizure threshold. Antidepressants, particularly tricyclics, are commonly incriminated. Others include isoniazid, penicillin, lignocaine, and antipsychotics such as chlorpromazine and haloperidol. Some of the newer antipsychotic drugs, notably olanzipine, are associated with epileptiform abnormalities on EEG.

Fluctuating serum levels of AEDs, which may arise from poor adherence to treatment or interactions with other drugs, increase the risk of seizures. Sudden withdrawal of AEDs, especially phenobarbitone and benzodiazepines, may also result in seizures.

What to do if a seizure occurs

If a seizure is likely to occur at work, supervisors and workplace colleagues should be warned and instructed in appropriate first-aid measures. Convulsive seizures are almost always short-lived and do not require immediate medical treatment. The person should be made as comfortable as possible preferably lying down (eased to the floor if seated); the head should be cushioned and any tight clothing or neckwear loosened. The patient should remain attended until recovery is complete. During the attack, the patient should not be moved, unless they are in a dangerous place—in a road, by a fire or hot radiator, at the top of stairs, or by the edge of water, for instance. No attempt should be made to open the mouth or force anything between the teeth. After the seizure has subsided the person should be rolled on to their side, making sure that the airways are cleared of any obstruction, such as dentures or vomit and that there are no injuries that may require medical attention. When the patient recovers consciousness there is often a short period of confusion and distress. The person should be comforted, reassured, and allowed to rest. An ambulance or hospital treatment is not required unless there is a serious injury, the seizure has lasted more than 5 minutes;[22] the person has had a series of seizures without recovering consciousness between them; or the seizure has features which differ significantly from the patient's usual form.

Responsibility of the physician in the workplace

The first task is to establish without doubt that a seizure has occurred. The employee should attend the occupational health department as soon as possible and remain off work in the interim period. A detailed history of the event should be obtained and information sought from the patient and any reliable witness to try to establish the nature of the attack. Interviewing work colleagues and relatives who witnessed the event can be extremely useful, as the subject usually remembers very little beyond the first few seconds; however, it is very unwise to rely solely on the patient's account, written reports from witnesses or second-hand anecdotal information.

The past medical history may reveal risk factors for the development of epilepsy such as febrile seizures in childhood, previous significant head injury, or previous stroke. Relevant points about the family history and consumption of drugs or alcohol should also be obtained. The patient should always be fully examined, as a seizure may occasionally be the first symptom of a serious systemic illness such as meningitis, or of a structural cerebral lesion: detailed medical assessment is always necessary

Permission to contact both the GP and any hospital consultant should be obtained from the patient. It is often useful to contact these physicians informally and discuss the situation that has arisen. This should be followed by a formal letter giving a concise account of events and the examination findings, and requesting any further relevant information.

Not all episodes of unconsciousness are epileptic seizures. The most common differential diagnoses are syncope (vasovagal or cardiac) and non-epileptic seizures (pseudoseizures) with an underlying psychological basis. Other possible diagnoses include transient ischaemic attacks (TIA) and migraine.

Prolonged cerebral anoxia due to syncope may produce some stiffening, twitching, and even incontinence, although a generalized seizure (secondary anoxic seizure) is unusual. The circumstances of the event, prodromal symptoms and rapidity of recovery will usually allow distinction between syncope and an epileptic seizure. Non-epileptic seizures can be very difficult to distinguish from epileptic seizures and specialist advice is usually required.

The focal ischaemia of a TIA does not usually involve loss of consciousness and often causes neurologically negative features, such as aphasia or paresis, and only rarely causes muscle jerking.

Once it has been established as far as possible that a single, unprovoked, seizure has occurred the following procedure should be adopted:

1. The medical notes must state clearly the course of events and that a seizure has taken place.

2. Management should be contacted and given clear and concise recommendations, in writing, regarding placement of the employee. Such written recommendations should be constructed with the agreement of the employee and should not breach codes of medical confidentiality. If epilepsy has been confirmed (not just a single seizure) some employees prefer to inform their immediate supervisor. It is worth discussing the possibility of such disclosure, with the patient.

3. The occupational physician and occupational health nurse must become familiar with any AED prescribed and have a sound knowledge of potential adverse effects.

4. Consideration should be given to sensible employment restrictions (see p 177).

Consideration of potential new employees

The most significant factor in recruiting a new employee is how well qualified that individual is for the job. It would be unrealistic to state that all jobs are suitable for a candidate with epilepsy, but it is reasonable to state that the majority of jobs are suitable. Individual cases should be considered on their merits and the reader is strongly recommended to consult the training manual prepared by the International Bureau of Epilepsy.[23] This gives some excellent practical advice, provides an assessment questionnaire and illustrates some typical cases with vocational scenarios.

In December 1996 the provisions of the Disability Discrimination Act 1995 (DDA) came into force. This legislation is intended to protect disabled people, and people who have been disabled, from discrimination in the field of employment. The impairment of epilepsy falls within the Act even if it is medically controlled. However, precedence is given to the Health and Safety at Work Act 1974 (HSAWA) when safety issues arise. In the case of epilepsy, the decision must be based on risk assessment and medical evidence, and never on prejudice or assumption (the decision may have to be defended in court). It is essential that sufficient thought is given to the possibility of making 'reasonable adjustments to the workplace'. With epilepsy, this is nearly always possible except where there is a statutory bar (e.g. the driving of large goods vehicles). Often a safe place of work can be found for any employee, unless the hazard and risk is an integral part of the job (e.g. working as a steeplejack or on an oil rig). Similarly, provided that driving is only a small component of the job (less than 15%), an employee should not be refused employment if they do not hold a valid driving licence.

In summary, therefore, when considering the placement of an applicant with epilepsy, the most important consideration is risk and methods of risk reduction or elimination. Every case will need to be assessed on its merits by a suitably qualified team after examination of the medical and occupational evidence. This action will protect both the applicant and the employer.

Sensible restrictions on the work of people with epilepsy

Proposed restrictions must be discussed fully with the employee and with management. Clear written instructions should be given to management regarding placement, responsibilities and review. Confidentiality must not be breached (see above). Restrictions should be no more than necessary on common-sense grounds, as would apply equally to any individual subject to sudden and unexpected lapses in consciousness or concentration, however infrequent.

In the USA it is illegal to deny employment to an otherwise qualified applicant because of disability, provided the disability does not impair health and safety standards at the workplace. The Epilepsy Foundation of America (EFA) has developed a comprehensive interview guide summarized by Masland.[24] The guide helps to define the important considerations and the success rate in placing people with epilepsy is far greater if they have fewer than six seizures per year.

In general, minor attacks are less disruptive than major ones, but periods of automatism (performance of acts without conscious will) may upset colleagues. Other particularly disadvantageous characteristics are prolonged periods of postictal confusion and atonic and tonic seizures where the possibility of serious injury is increased.

It is impossible to provide dogmatic advice as the circumstances in individuals and industries vary a great deal. Sensible restrictions, however, include avoidance of the following:

- climbing and working unprotected at heights
- driving or operating motorized machinery
- working around unguarded machinery
- working near fire or water
- working for long periods in an isolated situation.

Hand-held powered tools may be a hazard if they can be fixed in the 'on' position.

There are certain jobs with special hazards where the risk of even one seizure may give rise to catastrophic consequences. These jobs fall into two groups:

1. The first of these is mainly in transport, and includes vocational drivers, train drivers, drivers of large container-terminal vehicles, crane operators, aircraft pilots, seamen, and commercial divers.

2. The second group are jobs that include work at unprotected heights, e.g. scaffolders, steeplejacks, and firemen; work on mainline railways; with high-voltage electricity, hot metal or dangerous unguarded machinery or near open tanks of water or chemical fluids.

The working environment and any equipment to be used by the employee with epilepsy should always be inspected by the occupational physician. The safety officer and the employee's immediate supervisor should also be involved in any decisions.

It is important to remind the employee that contravention of agreed restrictions may endanger not only their own life, but also those of their colleagues and friends. The employee should also be reminded that it may be impossible to make any insurance claim for financial compensation for personal injuries should an accident occur as a result of evasion of agreed restrictions.

Lifting of restrictions

A policy should be established for terminating any restriction on work practices. This policy should be made known to the affected employee and not altered unless circumstances are exceptional. There is little place for partial lifting of restrictions: the employee is either considered safe or not. If a work restriction is removed after a period of freedom from seizures, the employee should be instructed to report any further attack to the occupational health staff or to a personnel officer or manager. If AED treatment is stopped or changed, consideration should be given to close monitoring at work for a period, or to the temporary reintroduction of restrictions.

It may be found that following the introduction of medication, control is still poor with an unacceptable rate of seizure recurrence. It is important that every effort is made to improve control before the individual is rejected or restrictions imposed for employment or promotion. Perhaps there are specific precipitating factors that can easily be avoided, e.g. alcohol or poor compliance with medication. It is important to consider whether or not an appropriate AED has been chosen, whether adequate blood levels have been achieved (see below) and perhaps most importantly, that the diagnosis is correct and the possibility of non-epileptic seizures (pseudoseizures) has been eliminated.

Perhaps the employee forgets to take their medication or decides not to take it? All these possibilities should be explored and the occupational physician or occupational health nurse should co-ordinate their efforts with the family doctor and hospital consultant.

There should be a planned time-scale for the review of restrictions. An explicit date should be offered, as this will confirm that the employee's future is considered to be important and that they are still a valuable member of the workforce. In this respect, it seems reasonable to follow, for employment purposes those guidelines issued by the Department of Transport for ordinary driving licences (see Chapter 28). An employee who is safe to drive a machine as dangerous as a car should be safe to undertake virtually all industrial duties. Jobs with special hazards are listed above. After an initial seizure, the Department of Transport advises that a subject may not drive a car for one year, and it seems reasonable to follow the same practice for restrictions relating to physical safety in industry.

Effect of antiepileptic drugs on work performance

The aim of AED treatment is control of seizures without significant adverse effects and in most patients this aim is achievable. For others, particularly those requiring combination therapy, a balance must be struck between seizure frequency and adverse effects.

Acute adverse effects, either idiosyncratic or dose-related toxicity, are usually rapidly reversible on drug withdrawal or dose reduction. The chronic adverse effects of AEDs are more difficult to control and can potentially impact on work performance but it is often difficult to separate the effects of AEDs from the effects of the underlying aetiology of the epilepsy and of the seizures themselves.[25]

In patients treated with a combination of AEDs, a reduction of drug intake leads to improvements in cognitive function. Although there is some uncertainty about the differential effects of individual AEDs on cognitive function, it is generally considered that adverse cognitive effects are greater with phenobarbitone and phenytoin than with carbamazepine and valproate. There is evidence to suggest that some of the newer AEDs are better tolerated. Lamotrigine, for example, has a generally favourable cognitive profile both in healthy volunteers and patients with epilepsy. Oxcarbazepine also seems to have little impact on cognitive function in healthy volunteers and in patients with newly diagnosed epilepsy. The wider range of AEDs now available increases the likelihood of achieving a treatment regimen without adverse effects.

Patients with epilepsy often complain of memory impairment. In some cases this is secondary to impaired attention and concentration that may be affected by AEDs. More often memory impairment is related to temporal lobe dysfunction related to the underlying cause of the seizures.

The occupational physician should work closely with the neurologist so that they both understand what is happening to the patient. The occupational physician must understand the clinical situation as well as the work situation. Close liaison is required to determine whether the patient's drug regimen is appropriate for their particular employment or whether it could be modified to better meet particular employment requirements. If made aware of these requirements by the occupational physician, the neurologist may be able to exploit new therapeutic opportunities.

Special work problems

Disclosure of epilepsy to employers

In an ideal world, individuals with epilepsy would freely disclose how their seizures affect them, and how often and when they occur, and information would exist on their medication and likely prognosis. The occupational physician could then, from their own knowledge of the work processes at the factory or office, advise employment in a sector which maximized the employee's potential and opportunities for promotion and minimized any risk to them or to their colleagues.

Only about a third of the working population have even a nominal contact with an occupational physician, however, so the situation is less than ideal. People with epilepsy are aware that they are at a competitive disadvantage and that their choice of vocation may be limited. Their opportunities for mobility and promotion within a company may also be perhaps unfairly restricted. They may suspect that they will not be allowed to join the pension fund. Finally, they may have to face the condescension and scrutiny of their fellow workers.

It is not surprising, therefore, that the presence of epilepsy is often concealed from employers. A survey of people in London with epilepsy showed that over half of those who had had two or more full-time jobs after the onset of epilepsy had never disclosed their epilepsy to their employer, and only 1 in 10 had always revealed it.[26] If seizures were infrequent, or usually nocturnal, such that the applicant considered that they had a good chance of getting away with concealment, then the employer was virtually never informed. Among those who declared their condition, two variables correlated with failure to gain employment: frequent seizures and lack of any special skills.

This state of affairs will be improved only slowly by educational programmes. Another possible way forward includes a clearer definition of jobs that can be undertaken by people with epilepsy. Such a definition has been considered and published by the International Bureau for Epilepsy,[27] which considered that the vast majority of jobs are suitable for people with epilepsy, especially where the person possessed the right qualifications and experience. Blanket prohibitions should be avoided and the organization of work practices should be examined to reduce potential risk to an acceptable level.

Accident and absence records of those with epilepsy

It is widely believed that people with epilepsy are more accident-prone and have worse attendance records than other workers. However, this view is not substantiated by the available literature. Many studies must be biased, as workers with epilepsy tend to get placed in inherently less risky work. The most significant study of work performance that attempted to eliminate this bias was conducted by the US Department of Labour[28] more than 45 years ago. A statistical comparison was made of 10 groups with different disabilities, including people with epilepsy, with matched unimpaired controls in the same jobs. Within the epilepsy group, no differences were found in absenteeism but their incidence of work injuries was slightly higher. The differences noted in accident rates were not, however, statistically significant. The general conclusion of this study was that people with epilepsy perform as well as matched unimpaired workers in the same jobs in the manufacturing industries.

In a small study in 1960,[29] Udell demonstrated that discriminatory practices against the recruitment of people with epilepsy are unwarranted, if based on the notion that as a group, they have high accident rates, poor absence records and low production efficiency. However, any applicant with epilepsy must be appraised individually with regard to the degree of seizure control and any other associated handicap. Employers should have a receptive policy for recruitment and job security. This may encourage employees to admit the problem and allow industry an opportunity to appraise their abilities and place them appropriately.

The more recent study of epilepsy in British Steel[17] generally supported these findings. There was no significant difference between epilepsy and control groups with regard to overall sickness absence, accident records, and five different aspects of job performance. Work performance, however, was significantly reduced in people with epilepsy who also had an associated personality disorder. The British Steel study emphasized that, although some degree of selection has to be applied when employing people with epilepsy, the overall performance of those with epilepsy compares well with that of their colleagues. The major task, however, is not to prove that performance at work is satisfactory, but to challenge and change the often firmly held and deeply entrenched prejudices of employers.

Current employment practices

An informal survey (Ian Brown, unpublished data 1996) of attitudes and practices with respect to epilepsy within the previously nationalized industries, armed forces, teaching profession, National Health Service (NHS), and Civil Service revealed an interesting dual approach adopted by most occupational health departments. There was often a carefully worded and apparently inflexible statement of corporate policy, yet many occupational physicians adopted a more sympathetic approach. This was usually only obvious, however, if the physician was contacted personally. Such practices were only found in doctors who worked in industries and services that had the flexibility to relocate affected workers and follow performance.

The Armed Forces were found to be the least flexible. In the case of new entrants, proven cases of epilepsy are not accepted for service and those who had suffered a single seizure less than 4 years before entry are also rejected. For serving personnel a single seizure after entry necessitates full examination of the individual, restricted activities, and observation for a period of 18 months. Full reinstatement is awarded only after assessment by a senior consultant. Aircrew who have suffered a single seizure after entry are grounded permanently and servicemen who suffer more than one seizure will be considered for discharge on grounds of disability. The Armed Forces also employ a large number of civilians but the policy for these individuals is more flexible than for servicemen. For civilians, the most significant factor is how well qualified an individual is for a particular job and if that job is safe or can be safely adapted to accommodate a person with a history of epilepsy.

Epilepsy is also a contraindication for employment in the Police Force. The police expect all their officers to be fit for all duties. Officers who develop epilepsy during service are usually retired, but only after careful individual assessment (personal communication to I.B.).

Many of the large and often previously nationalized industries follow similar codes of practice but are able to pursue a more sympathetic and accommodating approach. Epilepsy declared at the pre-employment stage may be a contraindication to employment but is rarely an absolute bar. The discretion of the examining physician may allow for some compromise if the applicant has a special skill or quality to offer and if the job is suitable. Epilepsy developing in service can often be accommodated if the employee is willing to be relocated but this may involve some loss of earnings and status. If unacceptable retirement on grounds of ill health is usually offered.

The Department of Education and Employment has a flexible policy for the employment of school teachers with epilepsy and allows its locally appointed part-time medical officers to use reasonable discretion. Difficult cases are referred to the Department's medical advisers and each is judged on its own merits.

The NHS has made considerable progress over the last decade but still has no national guidelines. This is by virtue of the numerous separate employers that collectively form the entity known as the NHS. Virtually all trusts and health authorities have an occupational health service and many have the benefit of a consultant adviser in the specialty. Guidelines on occupational health issues, as they may affect NHS employees, have been constructed by the Association of National Health Occupational Physicians (ANHOPS) and these include guidance on epilepsy. The guidelines state that all individuals must be assessed on their merits. They emphasize that the epilepsy should be well controlled and that the care of the patient must never be compromised.

The Civil Service has an open and documented policy on the recruitment and employment of people with epilepsy. The health standard for appointment in the Civil Service requires that a candidate's health is such as to qualify that person for the position sought and that the person is likely to give regular and efficient service for at least 5 years or for the period of any shorter appointment. The Civil Service Occupational Health Service stresses that epilepsy *per se* is not a bar to holding any established appointment apart from those posts with special hazards.

Getting employers to understand about epilepsy

Many of those with epilepsy are unemployed. Even if employed, many workers with epilepsy are still frequently denied promotion because of their disability or because of misconceptions about it.

In a survey of employers in the USA it was found that few would employ people known to them to have had a generalized seizure within the previous year. In this study,[30] Hicks and Hicks recorded the following consistent reason given for the failure to offer employment to people with epilepsy: 'they create safety problems for themselves and other workers'. Such reasoning has not varied for more than two decades. These authors pointed out that this assumption is misconceived and not supported by published data. An encouraging feature of this study was evidence of a positive change in attitude. Although the cause remains uncertain changes in the law in the USA and the continued efforts of public and private agencies may well be responsible.

To improve employers' understanding, regular informal health education seminars could take place at work. A well thought out programme that involves the personnel department, occupational health team, and interested union representatives may prevent some problems occurring. Topics such as epilepsy, stress, or alcohol abuse should be discussed openly with the benefit of expert advice being immediately available. The occupational physician or occupational health nurse can play a major part in informal health education and changing attitudes. Health education is concerned not only with the prevention of disease but in the understanding of disease in others. Problems such as epilepsy are often shrouded in mystery or considered as too unsavoury to discuss in detail. For such a common complaint, with a prevalence of about 5–10 per 1000 of the population, the ignorance still demonstrated is astonishing. Many employees, both on the shop floor and in management, consider that someone with epilepsy also has some degree of mental handicap combined with a lesser or greater physical infirmity. Certainly such problems may coexist but they are the exception. It is of paramount importance that health professionals should dispel myths and bring a sense of proportion to the issue.

The hard work of agencies such as Epilepsy Action, the National Society for Epilepsy (NSE), and the Employment Medical Advisory Service (EMAS) has done much to inform employers. Misconceptions about epilepsy are slowly disappearing and attitudes changing.

Medical services and opportunities for sheltered work

Most people with epilepsy are capable of normal employment without need for supervision or major restrictions. A minority will have additional handicaps and may only be able to work in a sheltered environment. Poorly controlled seizures, physical disability, low intelligence, and poor social adaptive skills will pose additional problems. The following specialized facilities are available in the UK for people with epilepsy.

Medical services

The NHS provides medical services for people with epilepsy through its general practitioner and hospital services. All patients with a suspected first seizure should be seen as soon as possible by a specialist in the management of epilepsy.[31] Most patients will be seen in neurology, paediatric, or learning disability psychiatry clinics. Those patients entering remission will usually be referred back to primary care within 12 months. The care of the 20–30% whose epilepsy proves difficult to control is usually shared between general practice and hospital clinics. Epilepsy nurse specialists attached to hospital services or based in primary care provide advice and support for people with epilepsy. Some regional neuroscience centres provide tertiary epilepsy services with facilities for specialist investigation and surgical treatment.

Residential care

Residential care is required for a small proportion of people with severe epilepsy and is usually provided by social services as part of their community care responsibilities. In addition, there are, however, epilepsy charities, residential centres, and special assessment centres that cater for the particular needs of patients with epilepsy, as outlined below.

Epilepsy charities

National Society for Epilepsy

The NSE, founded in 1892, is the UK's largest epilepsy charity. It provides residential care, medical services (in conjunction with the National Hospital for Neurology and Neurosurgery in London) and information, support, and training.

A wide range of written information is available including information for patients on epilepsy and work. The NSE is also committed to campaigning for improved services for people with epilepsy.

Epilepsy Action (British Epilepsy Association)

Epilepsy Action aims to raise awareness about epilepsy and modify regressive attitudes towards epilepsy. It also provides advice and information about epilepsy.

Residential centres and schools for people with epilepsy

In the UK, there are a number of special schools and centres for epilepsy, the largest of which are the Chalfont Centre for Epilepsy, the David Lewis Centre and the National Centre for Young People with Epilepsy (NCYPE). These provide residential care for people with epilepsy, usually associated with other handicaps, who are unable to live independently in the community. Some provide sheltered employment. Financial support is usually provided through the local authority, the health service or private or charitable funds.

Special medical assessment centres

There are several special assessment centres in the UK providing short-term and social in-patient assessment for people with severe or complicated epilepsy. The largest is the Chalfont Centre for Epilepsy. Others include the Park Hospital in Oxford for children and the David Lewis Centre in Cheshire.

Relationship between the occupational physician, consultant neurologist, and general practitioner

Recommendations received from the neurologist may differ from those acceptable to the occupational physician who must consider the best interests of the patient in their particular working environment. The family doctor, who may have cogent views and is likely to have closer knowledge of the patient, and their family can liaise with both these two specialists. It is advantageous if all the doctors involved work together to avoid conflicting advice. In companies with an occupational health service an employee with epilepsy should be encouraged to contact the nurse and discuss problems as they arise. The nursing service at work is often readily accessible to the employee and has a special role in counselling and health education. Confidential notes should be kept and the case discussed with the occupational physician at the earliest opportunity. Any employee with epilepsy should be reviewed regularly by the occupational health service and at least annually.

Existing legislation and guidelines for employment

For a more detailed discussion of legal aspects, see Chapter 2 and also Carter.[32] The Health and Safety At Work Act (HSAWA) makes no reference to the disabled and applies to all employees regardless of their health. The dual responsibility of employer and employee to safeguard health and safety is entirely reasonable but may create problems. Many people with epilepsy do not disclose it to an employer for fear of losing their job or not being offered one. Under these circumstances the employee with epilepsy may contravene Section 7 of the HSAWA, if they knowingly accept a job that poses unacceptable risks. An employer may legally refuse to employ an applicant for a job on any grounds except those of sex and race without necessarily giving reasons for the decisions. The law relating to discrimination does protect disabled applicants (see below and Chapter 3) and became law in 1995 as the DDA. Part II of the Act introduces a general principle of non-discrimination into employment. A special legal duty is imposed on the employer to make reasonable adjustments to working arrangements to accommodate safely the disabled person. It may be genuinely impossible for employers to make such arrangements, or the costs to do so may be prohibitive. Under these circumstances and quite uniquely (as compared with other discrimination legislation), the Act allows the employer to discriminate where the discrimination can be justified by reasons that are 'material to the circumstances of the particular case and substantial'.

Someone who suffers from epilepsy will benefit from the provisions of the DDA because they suffer from a substantial, long-term impairment, which may affect day to day activities. Furthermore, the fact that epilepsy is controlled by medication does not deny the person protection. Employers, therefore, must be prepared to make reasonable adjustments to accommodate a person with epilepsy. A typical and common example might be an applicant for a job who is unable to presently hold a Group I driving licence because of a recent convulsion. The job applied for requires the applicant to hold a Group I driving licence but the driving component of the job is only about 10% of the duties. Under these circumstances, it would be reasonable for the employer to provide an alternative means of transport for the employee. If the driving component was a substantial part of the job, then it would not be reasonable for the employer to provide an alternative means of transport.

What are the legal implications if a worker develops epilepsy while in service? The DDA applies equally to employees in service with the same provisions as stated above. All employees are also covered by the Employment Protection (Consolidation) Act 1978; as amended, this Act protects against unfair dismissal and protection is conferred after 1 year's continuous employment. It is possible to avoid its provisions by offering a temporary or probationary contract but this can only be for a limited period.

Is dismissal on medical grounds unfair? The Employment Relations Act 1999 has increased the maximum compensation for unfair dismissal from £12 000 to £50 000. This is more likely to be a deterrent to the unscrupulous employer. The employer may be obliged to justify their decision to an industrial tribunal on at least one of five fair reasons for dismissal. Three of these are pertinent to this chapter:

- Is the employee capable of performing their duties safely and efficiently?
- Has it become impossible for the employee to continue to work without contravening a statutory duty or restriction?
- Is it extremely difficult or financially prohibitive for the employer to make reasonable adjustment to working arrangements that would allow the employee to be accommodated safely (DDA 1995)?

The third reason was upheld in an industrial tribunal and is a good example of the employer justifying impracticability (*Smith* v. *Carpets International UK plc*, 11 September 1997, case no. 1800507/97). Mr Smith, an employee with a history of epilepsy, was employed as a warehouseman in 1994. He had not suffered a seizure for 9 years and the company's occupational physician considered his condition to be well controlled. No restrictions were therefore imposed. Mr Smith regrettably suffered further convulsions and the doctor therefore considered it was dangerous for him to work in the warehouse because of the heavy machinery and forklift truck work. Following a risk assessment it was concluded that no adjustments could be made to the job. An offer of alternative work was not accepted by Mr Smith as it would have been less well paid. The case went to an industrial tribunal and the employer's case was upheld as the circumstances had been appropriately assessed and reasonable investigations had taken place to examine what adjustments could be made to accommodate Mr Smith. Alternative work was offered and the employer was not expected to reorganize totally the way in which the warehouse work was carried out.

Incapability, illegality (contravention of a statutory duty or restriction), and impracticability are all fair grounds for dismissal. The Industrial Tribunal makes the final decision, subject to an appeal to the Employment Appeal Tribunal but it will require that the employee has discussed their state of health with the employer (if possible), made absolutely sure that the employee is incapable of doing the job in question, that an alternative job is not available and the present job cannot be suitably adapted or adjusted.

Some employers are under the misconception that an applicant with a history of epilepsy will not be accepted into the pension fund. This is generally untrue but the pension scheme assessors will consider all cases on their merits and very occasionally certain restrictions are placed on individuals joining with specific medical problems. Life cover or ill health retirement provision may be reduced if the risk is considered very significant but this will only be in relation to an accident or disability occurring in direct relation to the specific disability described. In the majority of cases, there is no restriction and occupational pension schemes are far more liberal than independent life assurance schemes.

No special insurance arrangements are necessary for a worker with epilepsy. The employer's liability insurance covers everyone in the workplace—provided the employer has taken the disability into account when allocating the individual to a particular job. Failure to disclose epilepsy will render the employer's insurance invalid and should an accident occur as a direct result of the condition it is unlikely that a claim for compensation will be met.

To summarize the legal position, the employee with epilepsy is protected by the same legislation and should enjoy the same pension rights as any other employee. They can be dismissed from employment if the disability seriously interferes with their capability to perform their duties satisfactorily or safely. Dismissal can also take place if the employee's medical condition contravenes statutory regulations governing the job.

The Driving Licence Regulations and their effects

The licensing for driving is one of the few areas in which there is legislation related to epilepsy (see also Chapter 28). Regulation is deemed necessary because seizures are undoubtedly a potential cause of road traffic accidents in drivers suffering from epilepsy. Although the overall incidence of road traffic accidents may not be higher in people with epilepsy, the risk of serious accidents and fatal accidents is increased.[33] Ideally legislation should balance the excess risks of driving against the social and psychological disadvantage to the individual of prohibiting driving. In the UK, it is the licensing authority (DVLA) and not the sufferer's personal medical advisers, which makes the decision to allow or bar licensing. The regulations are based, where possible, on research into the risks of seizure recurrence in different clinical circumstances. Licensing is divided into two groups, with more stringent conditions applied to Group 2 licences because more time is spent driving and the consequences of accidents are often more serious.

- ◆ **Group 1 licences** (those for motorcars and motorcycles). An applicant for a licence who suffers from epilepsy shall satisfy the following conditions:
  - he shall have been free of any epileptic attack during the period of 1 year immediately preceding the date when the licence is granted; or
  - in the case of an applicant who has epileptic attack(s) only while asleep, shall have demonstrated a sleep-only pattern for 3 years or more, without attacks while awake.
  - the driving of a vehicle will not be likely to endanger the public.
- ◆ **Group 2 licences** those for large goods vehicles and passenger carrying vehicles, i.e. vehicles over 7.5 tonnes, or nine seats or more for hire or reward). An applicant for a licence shall satisfy the following conditions:
  - no epileptic attacks have occurred in the preceding 10 years.
  - the applicant shall have taken no AED treatment in the preceding 10 years.
  - there will be no continuing liability to epileptic seizures.

The purpose of the third condition is to exclude people from driving (whether or not epileptic seizures have actually occurred in the past) who have a potentially epileptogenic cerebral lesion, or who have had a craniotomy or complicated head injury, for example. With all driver licensing, single seizures and mild seizures are subject to the same regulation. If a seizure is considered to be 'provoked' by an exceptional condition which will not recur, driving may be allowed once the provoking factor has been successfully or appropriately treated or removed and provided that a 'continuing liability' to seizures is not also present. For Group 1 licence holders, treatment status is not a legal consideration but it is recommended that driving be suspended from the commencement of drug reduction and for 6 months after drug withdrawal.

Van, crane, and minibus drivers will need to be found alternative employment within the company, as with those whose job also involves driving. The safety of forklift truck drivers will depend on individual circumstances.

For advice on driving with other neurological disorders and after head injuries, see Chapter 28.

Conclusions and recommendations

Many people do not disclose a past or present medical history of epileptic seizures when applying for a job or during a routine examination at the workplace. This may well cause major problems for the individual and the employer and, on occasions, inadvertently contravene HSAWA or invalidate insurance cover. However, the DDA now confers some protection on those with epilepsy. The unenlightened attitudes of some employers have led to secrecy or denial by those affected. The possibility of dangerous situations arising at work or dismissal without recourse to appeal may be the outcome. A competent occupational health service, trusted by both shop-floor and management, can be invaluable in resolving conflicts and giving advice.

Responsibility for the employment and placement of a person with epilepsy rests with the employer and they should take appropriate medical advice. Each case must be judged on its merits in the light of all the available information. Any attempt to advise managers without a sound and complete understanding of the requirements of the job is unfair to both the employee and the employer. Every employee with epilepsy must be regularly reviewed. The development of good rapport and mutual trust will encourage employees to report any changes in their condition or medication and discuss anxieties that have arisen.

A sensible approach by managers, with access to medical advice, should help the individual to come to terms with their condition, appreciate the reasons for any restrictions and understand that decisions taken on the basis of such medical advice are in their best interests. The employer should drop old prejudices in favour of current knowledge about epilepsy. This will only occur when all those concerned with epilepsy undertake the responsibility of educating employers, the general public and perhaps some members of the medical profession.

References

1 Commission on Classification and Terminology of the International League Against Epilepsy. Proposal for revised classification of epilepsies and epileptic syndromes. *Epilepsia* 1989; **30**: 389–99.

2 Commission on Classification and Terminology of the International League Against Epilepsy. Proposal for revised clinical and electroencephalographic classification of epileptic seizures. *Epilepsia* 1981; **22**: 489–501.

3 Wallace H, Shorvon S, Tallis R. Age-specific incidence and prevalence rates of treated epilepsy in an unselected population of 2 052 922 and age-specific fertility rates of women with epilepsy. *Lancet* 1998; **352**: 1970–3.

4 Sander JWAS *et al.* National General Practice Study of Epilepsy: newly diagnosed epileptic seizures in a general population. *Lancet* 1990; **336**: 1267–71.

5 Li LM *et al.* High resolution magnetic resonance imaging in adults with partial or secondary generalised epilepsy attending a tertiary referral unit. *J Neurol Neurosurg Psychiatry* 1995; **59**: 384–7.

6 Davies JE *et al.* Lindane poisonings. *Arch Dermatol* 1983; **119**: 142–4.

7 Chadwick D. Epilepsy after first seizures: risks and implications. *J Neurol Neurosurg Psychiatry* 1991; **54**: 385–7.

8 Hart YM *et al.* National general practice study of epilepsy: recurrence after a first seizure. *Lancet* 1990; **336**: 1271–4.

9 First Seizure Trial Group. Randomized clinical trial on the efficacy of antiepileptic drugs in reducing the risk of relapse after a first unprovoked tonic-clonic seizure. *Neurology* 1993; **43**: 478–83.

10 Marson A *et al.* Immediate versus deferred antiepileptic drug treatment for early epilepsy and single seizures: a randomised controlled trial. *Lancet* 2005; **365**: 2007–13.

11 Cockerell OC *et al.* Remission of epilepsy: results from the National General Practice Study of Epilepsy. *Lancet* 1995; **346**: 140–4.

12 Annegers JF, Hauser WA, Elveback LR. Remission of seizures and relapse in patients with epilepsy. *Epilepsia* 1979; **20**: 729–37.

13 Sander JWAS. Some aspects of prognosis in the epilepsies: a review. *Epilepsia* 1993; **34**: 1007–16.

14 Kwan P, Brodie MJ. Early identification of refractory epilepsy. *N Engl J Med* 2000; **342**: 314–19.

15 Annegers JF, Hauser WA, Coan SP, Rocca WA. A population based study of seizures after traumatic brain injuries. *N Engl J Med* 1998; **338**: 20–4.

16 Temkin NR, Dikmen SS, Wilensky AJ, Reikm J, Chabal S, Winn HR. A randomised double blind study of phenytoin for the prevention of post-traumatic seizures. *N Engl J Med* 1990; **323**(8): 497–502.

17 Dasgupta AK, Saunders M. Dick DJ. Epilepsy in the British Steel Corporation: an evaluation of sickness, accident and work records. *Br J Ind Med* 1982; **39**: 146–8.

18 Wilkinson RT. Hours of work and the 24 hour cycle of rest and activity. In: *Psychology at work* (ed. Warr PB), pp. 31–54. Harmondsworth: Penguin, 1971.

19 Kasteleijn-Nolst Trenite DGA. Photosensitivity in epilepsy: electrophysiological and clinical correlates. *Acta Neurol Scand* 1989; **125**: 3–149.

20 Wolf P, Goosses R. Relation of photosensitivity to epileptic syndromes. *J Neurol Neurosurg Psychiatry* 1986; **49**: 1386–91.

21 Jeavons PM, Harding GFA. *Photosensitivity epilepsy*. London: Heinemann, 1975.

22 Lowenstein DH, Bleck T, Macdonald RL. It's time to revise the definition of status epilepticus. *Epilepsia* 1999; **40**: 120–2.

23 Troxell J, Thorbecke R. *Vocational scenarios: a training manual on epilepsy and employment*. Second Employment Commission of the International Bureau for Epilepsy. Heemstede, The Netherlands: International Bureau for Epilepsy, April 1992.

24 Masland, RL. Employability, Part V111. Social aspects. In: *Research progress in epilepsy* (ed. Rose C), pp. 527–32. London: Pitman, 1983.

25 Kwan P, Brodie MJ. Neuropsychological effects of epilepsy and antiepileptic drugs. *Lancet* 2001; **357**: 216–22.

26 Scambler G, Hopkins AP. Social class, epileptic activity and disadvantage at work. *J Epidemiol Community Health* 1980; **34:** 129–133.

27 Employment Commission of the International Bureau for Epilepsy. Employing people with epilepsy. Principles for good practice. *Epilepsia* 1989; **30**: 411–412.

28 US Department of Labor. *The performance of physically impaired workers in manufacturing industries.* US Department of Labor Bulletin No. 293, Washington, DC: US Government Printing Office, 1948.

29 Udell MM. The work performance of epileptics in industry. *Arch Environ Health* 1960; **6**: 257–64.

30 Hicks RA, Hicks MJ. The attitudes of major companies towards the employment of epileptics: an assessment of 2 decades of change. *Am Correct Ther J* 1978: **32:** 180–2.

31 NICE (National Institute for Clinical Excellence). The epilepsies: diagnosis and management of the epilepsies in adults in primary and secondary care (Clinical Guideline 20). London: NICE, 2004.

32 Carter T. Health and safety at work: implications of current legislation. In *Epilepsy and employment* (eds Edwards F, Espir M, Oxley J), pp. 9–17. London: Royal Society of Medicine, 1986.

33 Taylor J, Chadwick D, Johnson T. Risk of accidents in drivers with epilepsy. *J Neurol Neurosurg Psychiatry* 1996; **60**: 621–7.

Chapter 9

Vision and eye disorders

R. V. Johnston and J. Pitts

Introduction

When considering the interaction of the visual system and the working environment, consideration should be given to the effect of vision on work and the effect of work on the eyes.

Vision can affect work by influencing the ease with which information is gathered and decisions made, and by affecting the feedback available for task completion. It therefore has an influence on safety (for example, in transport) and quality control (for example, in manufacturing). Visual ergonomics, such as the use of optical correction and displays, should be optimized to visual physiology and psychology, and the task at hand. This holds true whether the worker has normal vision or is visually impaired.

Diseases of the eye or nervous system result in varying degrees of visual disability that can be compensated for by neural and psychological adaptation, such as learning to use contrast instead of colour, and using non-visual cues to gather information. Personal training and ergonomic support will allow people who are visually impaired to function safely in the workplace in appropriate roles.

Work can have an influence on vision, which may be transient or permanent. Visual fatigue, and alteration in the relative intensity of different colours, for example, can occur in an environment of glare. Hazards in the workplace include gases, dust, light, heat, and risk of impact injuries. Permanent disability may occur, for example, via an intraocular foreign body due to projectiles, and visual ergonomics should take account of eye protection.

Vision, perception, and error

The visual system consists of the eyes, the oculomotor system, the afferent visual pathways and the visual processing areas of the brain.

The anterior part of the eyes consists of the cornea and the lens, which refract light to produce a focused retinal image. The pupil of the iris varies in diameter according to ambient light levels and this has a secondary effect on depth of field, optical aberration, and the subjective sensations of glare and comfort. The lens can accommodate and the eyes can converge to bring close objects into view.

The anterior segment of the eye produces a real, inverted image of the outside world on the retina, which lies in the fundus of the eye. Photoreceptors (rods and cones) transduce light energy into altered membrane potentials. The processing of visual information begins in the retina, whose ganglion cells send action potentials to the brain.

The oculomotor system aligns the eyes on an object, so that a stereoscopic (3-dimensional) image of the world can be obtained. When an object is moving, the eyes can track it by pursuit movements. When an object enters our peripheral vision, the eyes can move rapidly towards it by saccadic movement. When the head moves, the vestibulo-ocular reflex produces compensatory eye movements in the opposite direction, which stabilize the retinal image. When an object is brought near, the eyes converge. These reflexes are mediated in the brainstem, and their efferent pathways are the third, fourth, and sixth cranial nerves.

The afferent visual pathways consist of the optic nerves, the optic chiasm, the optic tract, and the optic radiations. There are two main functional systems, the central visual system and the ambient visual system. The central visual system (parvocellular system) is concerned with detailed scrutiny of form and colour. It starts with the cone photoreceptors, which are concentrated in the macula, the central part of the retina, and are sensitive to colour. It is assessed clinically by measuring visual acuity (VA) and colour vision.

The ambient visual system (magnocellular system) is concerned with movement, orientation, and navigation. It starts with the rod photoreceptors, which are concentrated in the more peripheral retina, and are sensitive to small amounts of light and movement. It is measured clinically by various methods of visual field testing, and lesions at various points in the system produce characteristic visual field defects. Defects also produce problems with balance.

The visual processing areas of the brain consist of the occipital, parietal, and temporal lobes. The occipital poles process the visual information and relay information regarding orientation to the visual association areas in the temporal and parietal lobes. There are functionally separate systems for pattern recognition and localization.

Perception is more than vision, and is affected by neural processing, as well as attitudes and experience. Not only can errors occur because there is a primary defect in the visual system (for example in colour matching tasks), but also, even with perfect sight, the visual system can be fooled by a number of well-known illusions that work on central information processing mechanisms. Error rates are greater under the stresses of fatigue and high workload.

Ergonomics is the science relating the interaction between man and machine, and concerns information (display ergonomics) and inputs (control ergonomics). Good displays present information in a legible, coherent manner, without crowding, and with intelligent use of icons and colours to convey meaning. They respect the physiological and psychological limitations of the human visual system.

Control ergonomics, in addition to respecting anthropometry and posture, should use labelling, icons and colours with respect to human visual performance, to convey accurately the function of levers, knobs, and switches.

Assessment of vision

Visual acuity

Central visual function is measured using VA. The subject is positioned 6 m from the test chart. This distance gives the numerator of the VA. The line on the chart which can be read gives the denominator. At 6 m, if the eye can distinguish five seconds of arc, the subject will be able to see the line labelled 6. Thus, 6/6 vision means the subject can see at 6 m what he ought to be able to see at 6 m. 6/60 vision means the subject can see at 6 m what he ought to be able to see at 60 m.

Near VA is measured by using standard printer's font sizes at 33 cm. It is important to realize that the actual working distance may be greater, such as 50 or 100 cm, in which case near VA should be measured at that distance as well.

These methods assess static VA. Specialized tests of dynamic VA may be better at predicting performance at certain tasks. In occupational health settings, optometers are often used to screen employees. While these may be better at assessing function in certain industrial tasks such as inspection of mechanical parts, the Snellen test of VA is more reproducible.

Visual fields

Visual fields are measured using dynamic or static techniques. The simplest example of a dynamic technique is the confrontation method, where the examiner's face is used as a fixation target and the subject indicates when he can see the examiner's hands as they are moved in from the periphery. This can be documented more accurately using machines such as the Goldman perimeter.

The problem with dynamic techniques is that they are labour-intensive and require expert operators, and so the emphasis nowadays is on static techniques, where the target does not move but instead blinks on and off. Such machines can be automated to present targets of varying intensity and construct an accurate map of the subject's field of vision.

Colour vision

Colour vision can be assessed by a variety of techniques. The commonest in use for screening purposes is the Ishihara test plate, which was designed to detect the commonest form of inherited colour deficiency, red/green confusion. Various lanterns have been developed and applied in an effort to assess the ability of, for example, recruits to the Navy to distinguish coloured lights at sea.

More detailed methods can also detect acquired colour vision defects, such as the blue/yellow defects, which occur in optic nerve disease or as a side-effect of drugs such as amiodarone or ethambutol. These include matching tests, such as the Farnsworth–Munsell 100 Hue test, which was developed for the textiles industry, and scores the subject on their ability to match colours, which are very close to one another.

Recent research at City University has produced a new technique that isolates the use of colour signals and quantifies the severity of blue–yellow and red–green loss (http://www.city.ac.uk/arvc). This is particularly useful in occupational fields where some degree of colour deficiency may be tolerated without significantly affecting visual performance.

A recent review of the 1958 British birth cohort has shown no increase with colour deficiency in the rate of unintentional injuries in driving or in the workplace.

Stereoscopic vision

Stereoscopic vision is one of the mechanisms of depth perception, and enables us to see in three dimensions. It depends on the brain's ability to reconstruct a 3-dimensional image using the slight disparity in the image between the eyes.

Stereoscopic vision is stated in seconds of arc. Stereopsis of 120 seconds of arc gives a stereoscopic range of 120 m, 60 seconds gives 240 m, and 30 seconds gives 480 m. Stereopsis is much more important for visual tasks relatively near, and in certain occupations such as crane operators and forklift drivers.

Beyond approximately 0.5 km, the use of monocular (psychological) cues is of greater importance in judging depth. These are relative size, perspective, overlapping, position in field, washout due to atmospheric scattering of light (Rayleigh scattering), and parallax. Monocular workers use these psychological clues to depth perception at all distances.

Four per cent of the population are amblyopic, and12% of the population lack stereoscopic vision. Childhood disturbances in vision may prevent it from developing, and age reduces stereopsis; by age 65 it is absent in 33%, and reduced in a further 33% of the population.

Common eye disorders and their effects on visual function

It is important to avoid making assumptions on an individual's ability based on a disease label. One diagnosis may have a vast range of functional effects depending on individual factors such as disease severity, personality, and the level of support in the home and work environment.

Refractive errors

In myopia (**short-sightedness**), the eye is relatively long, and the rays of light are brought into focus short of the retina. A corrective lens will be concave (minus). Myopia is associated with degeneration of the vitreous and peripheral retina, and an increased risk of retinal detachment. People with myopia are also prone to early onset macular degeneration.

In hyperopia (**long-sightedness**), the eye is relatively short, and the rays of light have a virtual focus behind the retina. A corrective lens will be a convex or positive. Hyperopia is associated with an increased risk of squint and amblyopia in childhood, and with angle closure glaucoma in later life.

In astigmatism, the cornea has different radii of curvature in different axes. This is often described as being shaped like a spoon or a rugby ball. Astigmatism may be myopic, hyperopic, or be a mixture of both. Astigmatism is notorious for causing symptoms of eye strain, as the ciliary muscle has to go through continuous gymnastics trying to produce a focused retinal image between two competing meridians.

There is a distribution of refractive errors in the population depending on the gene pool. In Celtic areas there is a greater incidence of long-sightedness and in South-east Asia there is a greater incidence of myopia.

Myopia, hyperopia, and astigmatism are all correctable with spectacles, contact lenses, and laser eye surgery. Spectacles can be manufactured in materials that afford some eye protection, or a spectacle prescription can be incorporated in protective eyewear.

Contact lenses have the advantage of producing a more physiological retinal image, but at the cost of a reduced oxygen supply to the cornea, which can result in the growth of peripheral vessels in the normally avascular cornea. Contact lenses also require regular maintenance, and if hygiene is compromised or the corneal epithelium is scratched, there is an increased risk of infection. Corneal bacterial ulcers can be sight-threatening. There are some environments, for example the very dry or the dusty, which are just not suitable for contact lens wear, and there are certain people who cannot tolerate contact lenses either due to hypersensitivity or to personality factors.

Modern techniques of refractive eye surgery, including laser, are becoming more popular, but these techniques are not without risk.

Radial keratotomy, uses cuts through 95% of the thickness of the peripheral cornea in a spoke distribution to weaken the globe. This produces a long-sighted shift. Its disadvantages include a diurnal variation in refractive error. Glare disability is common. This procedure was first introduced in the early 1970s but is rarely performed nowadays, although patients may be seen who have previously had it carried out.

Photorefractive keratectomy has been used since 1988, and uses an excimer laser to mould the shape of the cornea. In low myopia it typically removes some 10% of the corneal thickness, and does not alter the structural strength of the globe. A subepithelial haze peaks at 2–3 months and then gradually disappears at 12 months, after which there may be no visible signs of surgery on slit-lamp examination. The refraction stabilizes at 3 months. For myopia under 6.00 D, about 50% reach 6/6 or better at 1 year, and for over 6.00 D, the figure is 25%. Significant regression is more apparent in these higher myopes. Glare sensitivity is increased in the first month, and visual function under dilated pupil conditions may remain compromised for a year or more. Haloes occur when the pupil diameter exceeds the ablation zone, which rarely exceeds 6 mm now, and is more of a problem with previously treated patients and some high myopes and younger patients, who tend to have larger pupils.

Laser-assisted *in-situ* keratomilieusis (LASIK) was developed in 1990. It uses a micro-keratome mounted in a suction ring to raise a uniform flap of corneal surface tissue, and the excimer laser to mould the underlying stroma to the desired shape. The flap is then repositioned over the newly shaped cornea. Haze, scar formation, and pain is minimal due to the intact epithelial surface. Postoperatively, there is a C-ring visible at the slit-lamp, but this fades with time. Seventy per cent of myopes under 12 D and 50% over 12 D get 6/12 unaided or better at 6 months. Over 3 million procedures have been performed worldwide.

Astigmatism is more difficult to treat, and the treatment of hyperopia is in its infancy. Some occupational groups, for example the military, prohibit refractive eye surgery and some, such as civil aviation, demand careful postoperative monitoring.

Presbyopia describes the reduction in accommodation that accompanies age. It occurs earlier in hyperopes, and later in myopes. It is easily corrected with a plus lens in spectacles or contact lenses, but accurate correction critically depends on determination of the individual's working distance. Recent UK guidelines on surgical scleral expansion techniques for presbyopia point out that the evidence for efficacy is sparse.

External eye diseases

Allergy

Allergies are becoming more common in the population. The atopic triad of asthma, eczema and hay fever also causes allergic conjunctivitis, with subtarsal papillae. The condition may be worse in spring, or be present all year round, and can be controlled with the long-term use of mast cell stabilizing agents. Use of long-term steroids should be avoided, as these produce cataract and glaucoma.

Allergic contact dermatitis can occur on the lids, particularly due to secondary contact with sensitizing agents on the hands. Occasionally, one can identify a discrete substance in the working environment which the employee is sensitive to. An example is wheat germ protein.

Conjunctivitis

Infection Infective conjunctivitis can be bacterial, viral, or chlamydial. Viral conjunctivitis can result in an epidemic that can decimate a workforce ('shipyard eye'), and it is recommended that affected subjects be sent home promptly until the conjunctivitis has recovered.

Keratitis is infection of the cornea, commonly in the form of a corneal ulcer. Infection may spread into the eye, causing hypopyon (pus in the anterior chamber), and the condition can rapidly result in blindness. Soft contact lens wear is a risk factor for keratitis.

Fungal keratitis is seen in agricultural workers, and is seriously sight threatening. Any such worker must be referred urgently for an eye opinion when they complain of red eye with blurred vision. The key predisposing factor is trauma, with implantation of spores into a corneal abrasion by vegetation or an animal's tail. Eye protection for agricultural workers should not be neglected.

Dry eye

Reduction in the amount or degradation in the quality of tears causes discomfort and predisposes to infection. The condition is due to an autoimmune attack on the lacrimal glands, and is also seen with poor nutrition and recent emotional upset.

Some working environments exacerbate the symptoms of dry eye. When a worker complains of dry eye symptoms, it is important to measure the relative humidity in the workplace. Some workplaces cannot be humidified, and the worker will need to be placed elsewhere if simple lubricant eye drops do not solve the problem.

Cataract

This term describes an opacification of the lens. This is a normal ageing phenomenon, and visible lens changes are apparent almost universally from the age of 40. Cataract can be accelerated by a number of factors including diabetes, trauma and steroids.

There are number of common misconceptions around this condition. Cataract can now be treated at any stage. It used to be that the cataract had to 'ripen' before it could be removed. Nowadays, surgery can be performed at any point where the vision deteriorates to the extent that the patient is unable to carry out the desired visual tasks. Modern phaco-emulsification surgery is carried out as a day case through a small incision under local anaesthesia and heals very rapidly, with a minimum of astigmatism, and a minimum amount of time off work.

The glaucomas

In this family of diseases, one sees a triad of raised intraocular pressure, optic nerve damage, and visual field loss.

Intraocular pressure is maintained by the balance of production and drainage of aqueous humour. As the pressure rises, perfusion of the optic nerve head falls, which results in ischaemic and direct pressure damage to the fibres serving the visual field. Clinically, this appears as cupping. The normal cup/disc ratio is widely quoted at 0.3, but recent work has shown that this depends on the optic disc diameter, so that larger ratios may be normal in individuals or races with larger discs. A useful nomogram has now been produced.

In primary open angle glaucoma, the rise in intraocular pressure is insidious, intermittent, and asymptomatic. Pressure spikes occur in the early morning, so that the raised pressure may be missed. It is now possible to carry out 24-hour pressure monitoring to detect these spikes. The visual loss starts from the physiological blind spot, and will not be noticed by the patient. Detection of primary open angle glaucoma depends on screening. Traditionally, this form of glaucoma was treated with eye drops, and surgery was offered later in the disease. This gave rise to poor results and a bad reputation for glaucoma surgery. Nowadays, surgery is offered earlier in the disease and the results are much better. Primary open angle glaucoma is more common in myopes.

In normal tension glaucoma, the features are identical but the pressure is low or normal. This must be distinguished carefully from primary open angle glaucoma with pressure sampling during a diurnal low. The cause is thought to be impaired perfusion in the optic nerve head or primary neural degeneration. The disease is more difficult to treat and this has given rise to the concept of target intraocular pressure, which states that one should aim for the pressure reduction of 30% of the pressure at diagnosis.

In angle closure glaucoma, the outflow of aqueous is blocked by contact between the iris root and the peripheral cornea. This is an extremely painful condition, which produces blurred vision, red eye, headache, and vomiting. Sometimes it occurs in a more insidious, chronic form, which is a cause of recurrent headaches. Angle closure is more common when the eye is short, as in hyperopia, or when the lens swells, as in cataract. Treatment consists of making a small hole in the periphery of the iris (a peripheral iridectomy) using surgery or the YAG laser.

Squint

In this family of conditions, the visual axes of the eyes are not aligned. This may produce double vision if the squint is of recent onset and occurs in an adult whereas, if this squint is of gradual onset, particularly in a child, the brain learns to suppress the image from the squinting eye to avoid diplopia. In these circumstances, binocular vision is impossible and stereopsis is absent.

Childhood squints result in amblyopia (lazy eye) if they are undetected before the age of 5 years. There are many adults who have amblyopia as a result of undiagnosed squint in childhood, and they do not all have obvious squints. If stereopsis is important occupationally, it must be positively measured.

Adult squints are more commonly due to muscular or neurological disorders and must be investigated. Double vision is disabling and can cause serious danger if, for example, the employee is involved in transport or in working at a height. Emergency treatment involves occluding the squinting eye, but this leaves the subject without binocular vision or temporal field.

Double vision occurs in the direction of action of the weak muscle and, in the chronic situation, this may be occupationally relevant. For example, diplopia, which occurs only in upgaze, due to weakness of an elevator muscle, would be disabling to a forklift driver but not to an office worker.

Squint can often be treated with surgery to lengthen or shorten the extra-ocular muscles. Modern techniques include adjustable suture surgery and botulinum toxin injection.

Retinal vascular disorders

Diabetes

Diabetes mellitus causes a spectrum of eye problems, the root cause of which is capillary closure and ischaemia. These problems are seen in both Type 1 and Type 2 diabetes.

In background retinopathy, one sees dots and blots, due to capillary microangiography. In pre-proliferative retinopathy, one sees variation in venous calibre, deep cluster haemorrhages and cotton wool spots (also called soft exudates), which are in fact retinal infarcts. In proliferative retinopathy, one sees new vessels, which grow from the venous side of the circulation, commonly at the disc or from the major vascular arcades, and which are fragile and prone to bleed. Bleeding causes vitreous haemorrhage, and subsequent organization can cause tractional retinal detachment (retinitis proliferans).

The development of retinopathy is related to diabetic control. Significant retinopathy rarely occurs in the absence of proteinuria. Good control reduces the incidence of these diabetic complications. The National Service Framework for diabetes gives the frequency with which patients should be screened for the complications of diabetes.

Central retinal vein occlusion

Venous occlusion is commonly idiopathic, but may be caused by systemic hypertension, ocular hypertension and hyperviscosity. These conditions must be excluded, and the patient watched for ischaemic complications.

Central retinal artery occlusion

Central retinal artery occlusion may be due to emboli from the heart wall, the cardiac valves and the great vessels. Some patients have prodromal episodes of amaurosis fugax. The patient must be adequately investigated, as some of these causes will predispose to stroke. They should have ECG, echocardiography, carotid Doppler and blood tests for polycythaemia, excess white cells and platelets, hyperproteinaemia, hyperviscosity, and abnormal coagulation.

Posterior ciliary artery occlusion

This gives rise to anterior ischaemic optic neuropathy, producing a clinical triad of reduced acuity, afferent pupillary defect and milky swelling of the optic disc ('pale papilloedema'). It is most commonly due to giant cell arteritis, associated with polymyalgia rheumatica, which is sometimes associated with a raised erythrocyte sedimentation rate and C-reactive protein, and a positive temporal artery biopsy.

Sickle cell retinopathy

Sickling in the retinal circulation causes peripheral retinal ischaemia and new vessel formation. Exposure to cold will necessitate that some occupational groups have to be screened for sickle cell disease.

Retinal detachment

Tractional retinal detachment, where the retina is pulled off by organizing scar tissue, has already been covered in the context of diabetes. Another example would be the late scarring resulting from an intraocular foreign body.

The more common variety of retinal detachment is caused by thinning and degeneration in the peripheral retina. This is combined with degenerative changes in the vitreous. The vitreous jelly liquefies and becomes mobile. In other areas the vitreous forms degenerate fibres, which contract. Where abnormal adhesions exist between the vitreous and the retina, the vitreous pulls on the retina as it contracts, tearing it and completing the formation of holes in the degenerate area. The fluid vitreous passes through the holes, allowing the retina to peel from the underlying tissue like freshly stripped wallpaper.

The retina obtains its nutrition from the underlying retinal pigment epithelium (RPE); if it is separated from the RPE by fluid for long, the photoreceptors die. A macula-on detachment is, therefore, regarded as a surgical emergency because there is still potential for preserving central vision.

Treatment of retinal detachment is surgical. Fresh holes can be spot-welded with the Argon laser. Very peripheral small detachments can sometimes be treated by injecting gas into the vitreous. Larger detachments require an operation to push the sclera on to the hole in the retina to obtain a seal, in combination with localized freezing to cause an adhesive scar.

Modern techniques of vitreo-retinal surgery allow the vitreous to be removed and replaced with gas, fluid or oil, and these techniques have dramatically improved the success rate of retinal detachment repair. These techniques must be carried out by a subspecialist in vitreo-retinal surgery.

Macular degeneration

Throughout life, the photoreceptor cells are serviced and maintained by specialized phagocytes in the retinal pigment epithelial layer. These can reach a point where they can no longer effectively dispose of the toxic by-products of photoreceptor cell metabolism, and this is hastened by cumulative exposure to high-energy wavelengths of light, e.g. in outdoor occupations or in long-haul aircrew.

There is some evidence that adequate nutrition and nutritional supplements, by supporting the body's ability to handle toxic metabolites, can delay the onset and the progression of early macular degeneration.

The early sign of macular degeneration is a build-up of hyaline deposits known as drusen. These are associated with RPE atrophy and thinning of Bruch's membrane, which separates the capillary layer of the choroid from the retina. This is known as 'dry' macular degeneration, and is often associated with normal vision.

In some patients, new vessels grow from the capillary layer of the choroid, break through Bruch's membrane, and come to lie directly under the RPE, where they proliferate and can leak or bleed. This known as 'wet' macular degeneration, and it is associated with a severe reduction in central vision.

Any recent onset maculopathy should be urgently assessed in the eye clinic. There is a therapeutic interval of less than 3 months, but some patients will benefit from laser or newer approaches which involve injecting a substance (verteporforin) intravenously, and activating it with light to destroy the proliferating vessels. Retinal translocation surgery and gene therapy are possible areas for improvement in the treatment of macular degeneration in the future.

If all else fails, it is important to remember that these patients do not lose peripheral vision and so are never blind in the total sense, although the central vision is severely reduced and they may not be able to read or recognize faces.

The condition generally starts in one eye and becomes bilateral. Age related macular degeneration is the commonest cause of blindness in the developed world, and can occur well before retirement age. Young patients may develop macular problems early if they have high myopia. It is important to assess both the patient and their workplace with a view to improved lighting or relocation.

Working conditions, luminance, and visual fatigue at work

Lighting and visibility

Visibility is affected by lighting and other factors including atmospheric conditions (often reduced in foundries and mining), and glare from reflective surfaces. Lighting is extremely important to the health and safety of all employees. The more rapidly a hazard is seen, the more easily it can be avoided. The types of hazard and the degree of risk in the working environment will determine the lighting requirements for safety.

Poor lighting can result in significant costs to a business in terms of:

- time off work due to injury or accidents
- reduced efficiency and productivity.

Lighting in the workplace

Regulation 8 of the Management of Health and Safety at Work Regulations (MHSW) 1992 requires employers to have lighting which is suitable and adequate to meet the requirements of the workplace. Ideally, the lighting should be natural, and there is a requirement to provide emergency lighting where people may be exposed to danger.

Measurement of available light should be made using an appropriate light meter. Owing to the different frequencies of light sources that are commonly found in the workplace, a light meter with variable light source settings should be used.

Typical light source settings include daylight, fluorescent, mercury, and tungsten. The luminance should be task related and depends on a number of factors including the size of the detail, the contrast with its background, the speed and accuracy of the task required, and the age of the employee. The older employee may require higher levels of luminance to achieve the same levels of visual efficiency, due to age-related miosis and lens opacity.

In addition to general diffuse lighting, therefore, the level of illumination may need to be increased by the provision of local lighting at each workstation, under the control of the employee. Care must be taken, however, to ensure that this does not become the source of glare for other employees working in the vicinity. More diffuse light sources tend to be a lesser source of glare. Detailed recommendations are given in the Charted Institution of Building Services Engineers (CIBSE) Code for Interior Lighting.

In any working environment, under the MHSW Regulations, there is a requirement to assess possible risks in the workplace. This includes considering whether the lighting arrangements are satisfactory and whether they pose any significant risk to staff.

Display screen equipment (DSE)

Despite many articles in the lay press, there is no evidence that working with computer screens can harm eyesight. Temporary effects result from the following factors:

- DSE images are inherently blurred, and as blur is a stimulus to the accommodation reflex, the eyes undergo a constant focussing search, which is tiring. Focus may also be less accurate.

- Ciliary spasm produces a measurable increase in the resting point of accommodation after DSE use. After 4 hours this produces approximately 0.11 D of myopia which can take 15 minutes to resolve.

- Concentrating on a VDU also produces a reduction in blink rate due to concentration, and this can produce dry eye symptoms.

Frequent work breaks are advised to avoid these temporary effects, particularly with visually demanding or repetitive work. This is written into the Health and Safety (Display Screen) Regulations 1992.

Headaches attributed to eyestrain may be due to ergonomic problems, which result in poor posture and muscular strain. The Display Screen Regulations emphasize the importance of correct seating at workstations.

Equipment should be properly maintained to avoid flicker, glare, and reflection. There should also be flexibility in positioning of the screen, keyboard, and source material to allow the operator to adjust the workstation to meet their visual requirements.

Presbyopic individuals may have difficulty because their reading spectacle correction does not correct their sight for the distance required for DSE work. The Association of Optometrists suggests that operators be able to read N6 throughout the range 75–33 cm and have any phorias at working distances corrected, unless they are well-compensated or suppression is present. The near point of convergence should be normal and any convergence insufficiency should be treated.

The EC Directive entitles 'users' to be tested periodically. These are people who:

1. normally use DSE for continuous or near-continuous spells of an hour or more at a time; and

2. use DSE in this way more or less daily; and

3. have to transfer information quickly to or from the DSE

This can be achieved by software tests used on the DSE, and the results can be collated on the computer. The Directive makes the employer responsible for the provision of an optical correction necessary for the DSE task at the appropriate working distance.

Matching visual capability to the task required

There any many varied and complex types of work in industry today. Ramazzini, the father of occupational medicine, stressed in 1700 the importance of knowledge of the workplace. It is still as important today that any professional advising on visual performance visits the place of work to gain a full understanding of the task and obtains precise knowledge of its demands on the employee.

In addition, an assessment of the individual is required to determine whether the visual abilities on testing match the visual requirements of the job. If there is a mismatch there are two possible courses of action:

- The task can be adjusted if possible. The Disability Discrimination Act (1995) may apply, and requires an employer to make a 'reasonable adjustment' (see below).

- The visual capabilities of the individual can be enhanced by spectacles or other visual aids.

Unfortunately, many occupations have prescribed visual standards that are not task related. This may change in the future if the philosophy of evidence-based medicine begins to involve regulatory medicine. In aviation, for example, there is an opportunity to relate the standards to the tasks by the use of the simulator, and such studies are being carried out to assess the real importance of colour vision.

In driving, studies have failed to relate poor vision to accident rates. This may be partly due to the fact that accidents do not generally have a single cause, and often result from a combination of events. It remains true, however, that the standards used for driving are not based on an evidential link between them and driving performance. Where vision is borderline for driving legally, driving simulators and a functional test of driving in an assessment centre would be of value.

Visual fatigue

To avoid fatigue, it is essential to ensure the working environment is optimum in terms of lighting and ergonomic considerations. Uncorrected astigmatism, and defects in accommodation and convergence are notorious for causing asthenopia; it should be noted that these are treatable. Personality factors and motivation also play a part.

Spectacle correction and the type of lens (single vision, executive, i.e. bifocals with a reading segment horizontally across the full width of the lens, bifocal, trifocal, varifocal) must be optimal for the working distance(s) of the task. For example, one employee may prefer a single vision correction at 66 cm for a VDU screen with a document holder at the same distance, and another might prefer a bifocal with a 66 cm distance correction for the screen and a 33 cm near correction for documents at a conventional reading distance.

Employment of people with visual impairment: the possible

Under the National Assistance Act 1948, blind certification is defined in occupational terms. A person is legally blind if they cannot do any work for which eyesight is essential. The Act is careful to say 'any work for which eyesight is essential' rather than just the person's normal job, or one particular job. Generally, those with VA less than 3/60 can be certified blind. If the vision is better than 3/60, blind registration is possible if there is a contracted field of vision, particularly inferiorly.

There is no legal definition of partial sight. The guideline is that a person can be certified as partially sighted if they are substantially and permanently handicapped by defective vision caused by congenital defect or illness or injury.

Partial sight registration entitles the same help from the local authority department of Social Services as blind registration, but without the financial benefits and tax concessions.

It is more difficult to adapt to visual loss if you are older, or if the onset is sudden or very recent. Patients may require help with the bereavement reaction associated with sight loss as well as with skills re-training. Depression associated with sight loss is compounded by job loss and the feeling of uselessness that goes along with this. It is therefore vital that the occupational physician assist with job replacement as soon as possible.

Confusion exists between partial sight and monocularity. Monocularity gives rise to problems with awareness in the temporal visual field until the affected person learns compensatory head movements. Depth perception for near and middle distances are problematic until he learns to use monocular cues and other behaviours to judge depth. A person who loses an eye (due to trauma or tumour, for example) does not become partially sighted. Advice on coping with monocularity is given in the book *A Singular View: the art of seeing with one eye* by Frank Brady.

Employment of people with visual impairment

'Getting my first job was the most important event of my life. Everything else good rested on that.'

These are the words of Dr Fred Reid, Chair of RNIB's Education and Employment Committee. Fred worked as a University Lecturer. He is totally blind.

RNIB estimates only one in four of blind and partially sighted people of working age are actually in work. This figure of 27% is not only below that of the employment rate of the non-disabled population of the UK, which, in spring 2002 stood at 80.7%, but is also significantly below that for the general disabled population, which, at the same time, was 47.6%. Obviously, blind and partially sighted people are at a serious disadvantage in the labour market.

Part II of the Disability Discrimination Act (DDA) makes it unlawful for all employers except the armed forces to discriminate against workers or job applicants on the basis of their disability. Employers are required to make what are known as 'reasonable adjustments' in order to accommodate existing workers who become disabled and to make the recruitment and selection process accessible to disabled jobseekers. However recent government research found that more than one in three employers (37%) were unaware of Part II of the DDA, or of any other legislation relating to disabled people and employment. The same report shows that in a survey of 2,000 employers, a massive 92% said that they thought it would be either 'difficult' or 'impossible' to employ someone with impaired vision. Indeed, people with impaired vision are, according to this research, the most difficult to employ of a wide range of disabled people.

Yet visual impairment need not be a barrier to employment; blind and partially sighted people succeed in a wide variety of jobs. Care assistant, futures trader, PR consultant, sheet metal worker, script reader, child physiotherapist, solicitors, stonemason, test rig operator, chef, security guard—these are but a few of the jobs we know that blind and partially sighted people are undertaking. This list should explode the myths about what blind and partially sighted people can do, and stands as a challenge to others to move away from practices that limit blind and partially sighted people's expectations and towards practices that explore their abilities. For example screen magnification, and/or synthetic speech can give a person with sight loss access to a PC and enable them to email, surf the Net, word process and use spreadsheets. Or perhaps low vision aids and task lighting will suffice.

Employers who have experience of employing disabled people feel that they are no different to other employees and provided as good a service as their peers. Like the rest of the workforce blind and partially sighted staff can be set targets and employers can expect them to deliver as the best person for the job.

'Brian was just the best person for the job'—Jackie May, Manager of a day centre and employer of Brian Fitzpatrick a partially sighted day Centre Officer.

'When we interviewed Kate she was the best person for the job at the time, irrespective of her disability'—Elaine Russell, Bolton at Home and employer of Kate Howard, a Community Support officer who is blind.

Government schemes

The Government's Welfare to Work programme includes a number of different interventions designed to assist disabled people into employment. Jobcentre Plus is the agency responsible for providing employment-related services to all disabled people of working age, through Disability Employment Advisors (DEAs). DEAs act as referring agents to specific employment-related programmes aimed at disabled jobseekers. These programmes are provided by contracted agencies (including RNIB). For more information about government welfare to work programmes see the Jobcentre Plus website at http://www.jobcentreplus.gov.uk.

Employers worry about the financial costs of employing blind and partially sighted people. Unfortunately many remain unaware of Access to Work, a Government scheme that provides practical and financial support to disabled people in work. It can cover up to one hundred per cent of the additional costs associated with employing a blind or partially sighted person including funding for a work based assessment, adaptation of premises and equipment, special aids, support workers and travel to and from work. An application for Access to Work support needs to be made by the disabled individual and details can be found on the Jobcentre Plus website.

Staying in work

Like many newly disabled employees people who develop sight loss often give up their work unnecessarily because they believe difficulties that have arisen cannot be overcome. This is also true of those whose condition worsens. A process of disability leave may be necessary to allow these people time away from work to adjust and learn new working methods and for the employer to make the adaptations needed to enable the employee to resume work. An example of disability leave is given in the DDA code of practice (available to download from the DRC website at http://www.drc-gb.org.uk).

Disability leave begins with an initial assessment involving the individual, their employer and where necessary, a specialist adviser. This results in an action plan, designed to bring about the changes they have agreed. If a period off work is needed to carry out the plan, this will be regarded as a period of disability leave when the employee's job is protected though their income may come from their regular salary, as paid leave, or from state benefits.

Ocular hazards and toxicology

Heat

Direct thermal burns to the ocular surface occur with sparks and molten metal injuries. Infra-red radiation can cause damage to the anterior lens capsule, and is implicated in a form of occupational cataract in glassblowers.

Light

Light is hazardous to the eyes and the skin. Photons impacting in tissues produce direct damage to cells, and produce free radicals, which cause further damage. Chronic exposure to sunlight causes skin damage in the form of solar elastosis and keratosis, basal cell carcinomas, and squamous carcinomas. These conditions are more common in outdoor workers.

Sunlight can cause an acute keratitis, particularly when it is reflected from sea or snow (Labrador keratopathy), intensifying its effect. The harmful wavelengths are ultraviolet (UV) B (295–315 nm). Chronic surface exposure causes conjunctival elastosis and pterygium formation. Sunlight also causes damage within the lens, and is cataractogenic; the harmful wavelengths are UVA (315–380 nm). Phototoxic damage to the retina by high energy blue light of 400–500 nm is also thought to be a risk factor for macular degeneration.

Light causes glare. Discomfort glare does not degrade VA but causes distraction, aversion, and fatigue. Disability glare causes a reduction in VA due to veiling, dazzle, and scotomatic glare.

In veiling, for example due to windscreen reflections, a diffuse light source is superimposed on a retinal image, thus reducing contrast. In dazzle, for example, the headlights of oncoming vehicles, a bright light source is scattered within the eye, thus reducing contrast at the fovea. In scotomatic glare, for example flashes from arc welding, a brilliant light source temporarily bleaches the photoreceptors. The recovery time increases with age.

Good quality sunglasses protect the eyes from the toxic effect of light, by filtering out harmful wavelengths, and there is some evidence that antioxidants in the diet and in supplements may also be protective.

Throughout life, the photoreceptor cells are serviced and maintained by specialized phagocytes in the retinal pigment epithelial layer. These can reach a point where they can no longer effectively dispose of the toxic by-products of photoreceptor cell metabolism, and this is hastened by cumulative exposure to high-energy wavelengths of light.

There is some evidence that adequate nutrition and nutritional supplements, by supporting the body's ability to handle toxic metabolites, can delay the onset and the progression of cataract and macular degeneration. Vitamins A (beta-carotene), C (ascorbic acid), and E (tocopherol) are protective due to an anti-oxidant effect. The development of cataract is known to be due to oxidative damage to lens and photoreceptor proteins and lipids. Vitamin C is secreted into the aqueous humour in response to increased blood levels. The antioxidant vitamins are found in green leaves, where they evolved to protect the plants themselves from the stresses of UV exposure and the generation of oxygen from photosynthesis.

Zinc plays a part in retinal metabolism and may be protective. Zinc is present in the enzyme superoxide dismutase. The choroid and retina have the highest concentration of zinc in the body, and night blindness occurs in zinc deficiency, even in the presence of normal levels of vitamin A. Zinc is found naturally in meat, whole grains, and pulses. Zinc supplementation decreases copper levels, so co-supplementation with copper is recommended.

Selenium also has an antioxidant function. It is found in seafood, meat, and cereals. It is the metal element in the enzyme glutathione peroxidase. Carotenoids are yellow pigments found in coloured vegetables, and which have an anti-oxidant role. The maize carotenoid zeanthin and the melon/spinach carotenoid lutein are concentrated at the human macula.

A reduced risk of macular degeneration is found in relation to a high serum level of carotenoids. The essential fatty acid GLA (found in oil of evening primrose) may protect against dry eye. Omega-3 fatty acids such as docosohexaenoic acid (DHA) are found in oily fish such as mackerel and herring. They have a role in preventing cardiovascular disease and are found in high concentrations in the photoreceptor outer segment. It must be noted that some vitamins can be toxic, particularly in smokers, and that a safe upper limit must be applied to supplementation.

It is likely that vitamin supplementation will prove to be of benefit in populations exposed to high levels of UV stress such as outdoor workers. It is possible that, in addition to a direct protective effect on the tissues of the eyes, micronutrients preserve visual function by a protective effect on general health.

The light intensity passing through the filters in sunglasses should have a transmittance of 15%, reducing luminance at the ocular surface to 1000 cd/m^2. The transmittance of harmful wavelengths such as UVA/UVB and blue should be 1%. This can be achieved using a combination of reflective coatings and absorbing pigments in lenses.

UV radiation is a cause of acute keratitis (welder's flash), retinal damage and maculopathy in arc welding. This has been reported even with short duration exposure or when wearing eye protection, and has also been reported to be potentiated by photosensitizing drugs such as fluphenazine. Welding UV exposure has been implicated as a risk factor for skin and ocular malignancy.

Laser

Laser is an acronym for Light Amplification by Stimulated Emission of Radiation. Laser is a monochromatic (single wavelength), collimated (parallel), and coherent (in-phase) beam of light, which delivers high energy over a small area. Applications of laser include cutting and shaping materials, measurement, recording, displays, communications, holography, remote sensing, surveying, uranium enrichment, medical uses, and as weapons.

Lasers are classified according to their energy levels and the risk of injury. In general, laser bio-effects can be photochemical, thermal, or acoustic. Photochemical effects are generally transient and are a form of scotomatic disability glare. Thermal effects are retinal burns, which cause permanent scotomas.

The site of laser damage is in the posterior segment, where the light is converted to heat by absorption within the pigments of the RPE and retina, to produce a burn. The burn has more functional effect if it is at the fovea, which occurs when the patient was looking directly at the laser source at the moment of discharge. Acute eye injuries occur in medical and industrial settings with inadequate eye protection, but there is evidence of more chronic damage in the form of diminished colour vision in workers using lasers over long periods.

Laser hazards can be significantly reduced by proper safety procedures. Multiple types of filter exist to protect against beam-related injuries, and these are not always easy to distinguish, particularly in a dark work environment. It is imperative that the eye protection worn contains a filter appropriate to the wavelength of the laser being used.

Non-beam hazards associated with laser include thermal injury, fire, smoke plume, and electrical hazards. There should be a qualified laser safety officer whose responsibilities include regular inspection ad maintenance and training of staff in risk reduction.

An evidence-based protocol should be established for the diagnosis and management of laser injuries. Retinal laser lesions that cause serious visual problems are readily apparent on ophthalmological examination, and do not cause chronic pain without physical signs. Alleged laser injuries can result in lengthy medico-legal claims.

Radiation

Ionizing radiation causes damage to both the lens of the eye (cataract) and the posterior segment (radiation retinopathy). Radiation retinopathy presents clinically as degenerative and proliferative vascular changes, mainly affecting the macula. It is more pronounced in diabetes and is thought to result from oxygen-derived free radical damage and be influenced by endothelial cell antioxidant status.

Microwave injury has been documented as causing lens and retinal damage.

Electrical shock

High voltage shock has been documented to produce cataract, which is amenable to standard surgical treatment.

Chemicals, particles, fibres, allergens, and irritants

Caustic chemicals (acids and alkalis), solvents (alcohols such as n-butanol, aldehydes, and ethers), anionic or cationic surfactants, methylating agents such as dimethyl sulphate, aniline dyes, and toxic vegetable products such as Euphorbia saps can all cause damage to the corneal and conjunctival epithelium, which can result in late scarring and opacification.

Exposure may be in the form of a splash, but the conjunctiva of the eye is a mucous membrane and is affected by the same gases (e.g. ammonia) that cause respiratory embarrassment. The pathogenesis of ocular toxic reactions varies with the agent, but for example, surfactants cause emulsification of the cell membrane lipid layer. A superb resource for particular toxins is the excellent textbook, *Ophthalmic Toxicology* by George Chiou.

Fibres and dust in the atmosphere also cause irritation. Part of the response to atmospheric irritants is lacrimation, and this reduces VA by a surface effect, as well as being distracting. This may compromise safety in situations such as mining and work at heights.

Allergic reactions have been reported to a vast number of challenges across a wide array of occupational groups. Allergic reactions may be acute or chronic, and can occur as allergic contact dermatitis in the eyelids with chemicals commonly spread from the hands, or as allergic conjunctivitis due to aerosols, pollens, animal dander, and proteins in food manufacture. Adequate ventilation is more effective than eye protection in these situations.

Glass fibres occasionally lodge under the lids or in the lacrimal puncta, where they can be very difficult to visualize due to their virtual transparency.

One study of chemical industry workers in South Africa showed an increased prevalence of ocular disorders including tear film disorders, dry eye conditions, allergic conjunctivitis, and conjunctival melanosis. Forty-one per cent of the ocular disorders in this study were thought to have resulted from occupational exposure.

In veterinary nurses, a prevalence of allergic disorders of 39% was found in one study of attendees at an international conference in Australia. In animal handlers (vets, vet nurses, breeders, trainers, laboratory animal handlers, researchers) who develop allergic symptoms, 80% will report rhino-conjunctivitis (compared with 40% with skin symptoms, and 30% with occupational asthma). One prospective study showed the mean time to first symptoms in newly appointed lab workers exposed to rats as 7 months for eye and nose, 11 months for skin, and 12 months for chest. Ocular bites have been reported as another hazard in this occupational group.

ASHRAE (The American Society of Heating, Refrigeration and Air conditioning Engineers) have recommended environmental controls for animal rooms at 10–15 air changes per hour with 100% outdoor air, relative humidity of 30–60%, and a temperature of 61–84 F. Good workplace hygiene aims to reduce exposure to hair, dander, urine, and saliva, as does the wearing of lab coats, gloves, face shields, and respirators. Emergency procedures should be in place for managing anaphylaxis, including staff training in CPR and availability of adrenaline.

Occupational injuries and eye protection

Recent statistics from the USA show eye injuries at work accounting for 13% of all eye injuries, compared with 40% at home, 13% on the street, 13% playing a sport, 12% other, and 9% unknown.

MacEwan studied all eye injuries over a 1-year period in Glasgow, and found that 60.9% were due to work, that the majority of work-related eye injuries were due to buffing and grinding, and that in 83% the required eye protection was not being worn.

A recent study in Hong Kong showed that in 85% of eye injuries in the construction industry, no eye protection had been worn. The following were associated with lower risk:

- longer duration in the current job;
- job safety training before employment;
- regular repair and maintenance of machinery or equipment;
- wearing safety glasses regularly;
- a requirement for wearing eye protection.

Injuries to the eyes can occur in isolation, but the more severe injuries occur in the setting of more widespread trauma, in which case the ATLS principles of rapid primary survey and detailed secondary survey apply.

ATLS (Advanced Trauma Life Support) comprises the rapid initial assessment (primary survey) and simultaneous treatment of life-threatening conditions in the sequence of ABCDE:

- Airways maintenance with cervical spine immobilization
- Breathing and ventilation
- Circulatory support with control of haemorrhage
- (Disability)—neurological status
- (Exposure)—examine completely undressed while preventing hypothermia.

Once the patient is stable, a systematic secondary survey is carried out to identify definitive injuries to the brain, head and eyes, face, neck, thorax, abdomen, pelvis, and extremities, so that appropriate specialist care can be instituted.

In an industrial setting, the common eye injuries seen are corneal abrasion, corneal and sub-tarsal foreign bodies, superficial burns, and chemical burns. Severe blunt injury, penetrating eye injury, intraocular foreign body, and compressed air injuries are rare, and their management is essentially to provide rapid first aid and then protect the eye while the patient is transferred to a specialist unit.

Corneal abrasion

In this condition the corneal epithelium is damaged by a scratch. The abrasion can be highlighted with fluorescein drops and blue light. The treatment is antibiotic ointment and padding of the eye. Healing is rapid and complications are rare, but these do include infection and impaired healing with recurrent spontaneous breakdown of the epithelium (recurrent corneal erosion syndrome).

Corneal foreign bodies

These are commonly seen where workers are under a raised platform, or in grinding incidents. The metal is embedded in the epithelium and superficial stroma of the cornea. It is easily removed, but this is best done at the slit-lamp. Metal ions pass into the cornea and oxidize, forming a semi-solid rust ring. This is best removed with a corneal burr, again at the slit-lamp. Removal of the rust ring is sometimes best deferred until the day after the primary foreign body is removed, and several sessions are sometimes necessary to allow the cornea, which is only 0.5 mm thick, to heal. After each session the treatment is as for a corneal abrasion.

Subtarsal foreign bodies

There is a longitudinal ridge under the upper eyelid where loose foreign bodies become trapped, abrading the cornea with each blink. These are easily removed with a cotton bud after everting the lid. The vertical corneal abrasions on the upper cornea are managed as above.

Superficial burns

These are common in welders, who know them as arc eye or flash. The injury is caused by UV light, but the symptoms of surface cell death are delayed for several hours, and include lid swelling, blepharospasm, ocular pain, photophobia, and profuse lacrimation. Treatment is with topical analgesia, antibiotic ointment and padding.

Chemical burns

Chemical injury causes direct cell death and ischaemic necrosis, followed by ingress of leucocytes and release of inflammatory mediators such as prostaglandins, cytokines, superoxide radicals, and lysosomal enzymes.

Acids tend to cause superficial effects; due to surface coagulation, the acid does not penetrate the eye. These tend to cause stromal haze and ischaemia affecting less than one-third of the corneal limbus. They are associated with a good visual prognosis.

Alkalis tend to cause deeper effects; the alkali penetrates the eye and the pH in the anterior chamber rises rapidly, damaging intra-ocular structures such as the iris, the drainage angle, and the lens. These cause stromal opacity and ischaemia affecting more than one-half of the corneal limbus. They are associated with a poor visual prognosis.

Immediate irrigation is the priority, using water, saline, Ringers lactate, balanced salt solution or, in reality, whatever is available and safe. Ideally, irrigation is continued using an intravenous infusion set while holding the lids open with a speculum if necessary. Following transfer of the casualty to a specialist centre, medical treatment includes steroids, antibiotics, and ascorbic acid, and late surgery may be necessary to deal with scar tissue. Secondary glaucoma is a real risk.

Blunt injury

Haematoma (black eye) may hide a severe eye injury until the swelling subsides.

Orbital apex fractures are associated with high velocity injuries and result in damage to the optic nerve, which can only withstand ischaemia for 2 hours, or pressure-induced disturbance of axoplasmic flow for 8 hours. If such an injury is suspected, the consensus favours systemic steroids and early neurosurgical decompression.

Orbital blowout fracture describes a situation where the eye is propelled backwards and the walls of the orbit fracture outwards into the ethmoid and maxillary sinuses, leaving the eye and the orbital rim intact. This injury was first described in the New York Police Department in 1957. Clinical features are enophthalmos, diplopia, surgical emphysema, and infra-orbital nerve anaesthesia. Radiology shows the hanging drop sign in the maxillary antrum, and a computed tomography scan may help quantify the bony defect. Management is controversial, with equally vociferous proponents of early surgery and conservative management, and no clinical trial evidence. In terms of first aid, antibiotics are useful because asymptomatic sinus infection is common, and the patient should be instructed not to blow their nose as this can spread infection to the soft tissues of the orbit and because surgical emphysema can compress the optic nerve.

Contusion injuries of the globe cause damage at the point of impact and contre-coup injuries. These include hyphaema, iris damage, angle damage, lens damage, vitreous haemorrhage, retinal oedema (commotion retinae), retinal breaks and detachment, and traumatic optic neuropathy. Their management is best left to specialist centres, with first aid during transfer consisting of adequate analgesia and anti-emesis and a Cartella eye shield to protect the eye.

Penetrating injury

These are often painless. Signs include a visible laceration, prolapse of intra-ocular contents (iris appearing as a dark knot of tissue, vitreous as a blob of jelly) and a collapsed anterior chamber. Extreme caution should be exercised in examining the eye to avoid prolapsing the ocular contents. One of the authors has met a patient whose iris was removed by a well-meaning first-aider, thinking that a knuckle of prolapsed iris was a foreign body at the limbus. The eye should be covered with a Cartella shield and anti-emetics or sedation given as necessary while preparing for transfer. Some injured eyes do well with primary repair and secondary reconstruction, but an eye damaged beyond repair should be removed within 2 weeks to prevent the development of sight-threatening autoimmune inflammatory disease in the fellow eye (sympathetic ophthalmitis).

Intra-ocular foreign body (IOFB)

This is a special type of penetrating eye injury, where a small metallic body lodges in the eye, leaving a tiny entry wound that may not be apparent on casual inspection. The diagnosis depends on accurate history-taking, with the patient usually hammering metal on metal without eye protection. The diagnosis must be made early to prevent metal ions diffusing into the eye tissues causing late toxicity and blindness. A missed IOFB is a frequent cause of clinical negligence claims, and a negative orbital X-ray does not exclude the diagnosis.

Compressed air injuries

Surgical emphysema can compress the optic nerve and in situations where the vision is deteriorating, emergency decompression of the orbit can be performed with an intravenous cannula or by dis-inserting the lateral margin of the lower eyelid (emergency cantholysis).

Eye protection

This is an element of visual ergonomics that follows on from task analysis, and must be part of a programme of continuous staff training within a culture of safety consciousness.

Generally, products should comply with the EU Personal Protective Equipment Directive, bear the CE mark and be appropriate to the actual hazards of the work undertaken with regard to dimensions, lens quality, optical power, prescription, field of vision, transmittance of infra-red and UV, luminous transmittance, signal recognition, frame requirements, mechanical strength, impact resistance, abrasion resistance, resistance to molten metal, and resistance to dust and gas.

Standards exist for different forms of protection, for example, BS EN 166 for personal eye protection, BS EN 169 for personal eye protection used in welding. One supplier offers over 200 different products for eye protection! The following criteria should be used in selection, and employers should consult the legislation and the Health and Safety Executive guidance available from HMSO.

1. Type of hazard
   (a) mechanical (flying debris, dust, or molten metal)
   (b) chemical (fumes, gas, or liquid splash)
   (c) radiation (heat, UV or glare)
   (d) laser (over a wide spectrum of wavelengths).

2. Type of protector
   (a) a safety face shield protects face and eyes but does not keep out dust or gas. It can be comfortably worn for long period
   (b) safety goggles provide protection for all hazards and may be worn over spectacles
   (c) safety spectacles are comfortable but will not keep out dust, gas or molten metal. Prescriptions are easily incorporated.

3. Type and shade of lens.
   (a) toughened and laminated glass is less impact resistant but more resistant to abrasion
   (b) polymethylmethacrylate and polycarbonate offer high impact resistance but are easily scratched.

First aid at work

Planning

Risk assessment should include the possibility of chemical splashes to the eyes, the number of employees likely to be affected, and the optimum sites for positioning of emergency eye wash stations. Training should be given to staff in the actions to be taken if they or their colleagues are injured. Training must be updated regularly.

In remote workplaces, a prearranged telemedicine service provides an invaluable source of information for the care of casualties including eye injuries.

Assessment

An adequate light with magnification and fluorescein eye drops are necessary to examine eye casualties. Local anaesthetic drops are invaluable in calming the situation down and enabling adequate examination. Proxymetacaine does not sting, but has to be stored refrigerated.

A vision chart should be at hand. The number of the local eye unit should be available with printed and laminated protocols for injury management at the first aid station, and an emergency management slate for record keeping.

Irrigation

Immediate irrigation is the priority, using water, saline, Ringers lactate, balanced salt solution or, in reality, whatever is available and safe. Ideally irrigation is continued using an intravenous infusion set while holding the lids open with a speculum if necessary.

Eye shields

In suspected eye injury, a transparent Cartella shield can be taped over the eye while arranging transfer. Shields should be secured with suitable tape, and Friar's balsam is useful to keep the skin sticky for long transfers in patients who may be sweating profusely.

Medications

Prior to transfer of the casualty to a specialist centre, emergency medical treatment may include antibiotic drops as directed by the telemedicine service. A preparation such as chloramphenicol Minims should be at hand. Ointment should not be used in eye injury as it may enter the eye in penetrating injuries. Preservative-free drops will not cause problems in this situation.

Acknowledgement

The authors of this chapter would like to thank Dr Philippa Simkiss and the Royal National Institute of the Blind for co-authoring the section on the employment of visually impaired people.

Further reading

Vision, perception, and error

Cumberland P, Rahi JS, Peckham CS. Impact of congenital colour vision deficiency on education and unintentional injuries: findings from the 1958 British birth cohort. *BMJ* 2004; **329**: 1074–5.

Dutton GN. Cognitive vision, its disorders and differential diagnosis in adults and children: knowing where and what things are. *Eye* 2003; **17**: 289–304.

Ernsting J. *Aviation medicine* (3rd edn). London: Butterworth Heinemann, 1999.

Examples of bad design ergonomics are given at http://www.baddesign.com

Assessment of vision

Barbur JL, Harlow AJ, Plant GT. Insights into the different exploits of colour in the visual cortex. *Proc R Soc Lond* 1994; **258**: 327–34.

Blais BR, Tredici T Sr. Keep your eye on the individual's visual function. *Occup Health Saf* 2003; **72**(10): 30–8.

Cumberland P, Rahi JS, Peckham CS. Impact of congenital colour vision deficiency on education and unintentional injuries: findings from the 1958 British birth cohort. *BMJ* 2004; **329**: 1074–5.

Common eye disorders and their effects on visual function.

Civil Aviation Authority. The effects of laser refractive surgery on visual performance and its implications for commercial aviation. CAA Paper 2001/4, London, 2001.

European Glaucoma Society. Terminology and guidelines for glaucoma, 2nd edition. Savona: Dogma srl; 2003.

Jawetz E. The story of shipyard eye. *BMJ* 1959; **5126**: 873–6.

National Institute for Clinical Excellence (2004). Scleral expansion surgery for presbyopia. London: National Institute for Clinical Excellence, 2004.

Thomas PA. Fungal infections of the cornea. *Eye* 2003; **17**: 852–62.

Working conditions, luminance, and visual fatigue at work

Association of Optometrists. Guidance on Visual Standards for VDU/DSE users. AOP Members Handbook. London: Association of Optometrists, 2002.

Chartered Institute of Building Services Engineers. Code for Interior Lighting. Chartered Institute of Building Services Engineers, London, 1994.

College of Ophthalmologists. *Vision and display screen equipment*. London: College of Ophthalmologists, 1993.

Commission of the European Communities. *Council directive on the minimum safety and health requirement for working with display screen equipment*. Commission of the European Communities 90/270 EEC, 1990.

Health and Safety Executive (1992). *Visual display units*. London: HMSO, 1992.

North RV. *Work and the eye* (2nd edn). London: Butterworth Heinemann, 2001.

Occupational Optometry Online at: www.college–optometrists.org/college/releases/2004/08_09_2004.htm

Smith NA. *Lighting for occupational optometry*. Handbook No. 23. Leeds: H and H Scientific Consultants Ltd, 1999.

The Health and Safety (Display Screen Equipment) Regulations 1992. London: HMSO, 1992.

The Management of Health and Safety at Work Regulations 1992 (SI No 2051).

Software tests include:

City University Vision Screener, City Visual Systems Ltd, Woodford Green, Essex IG8 7LJ

Vue Test, Keeler Ltd, Clewer Hill Road, Windsor, Berks SL4 4AA

Employment of people with visual impairment: the possible

Aston J et al. *Employers and the New Deal for disabled people: qualitative research: first wave*. Department of Work and Pensions Report No. 145. London: The Institute for Employment Studies, 2003.

Baker M, Simkiss P. *Beyond the stereotypes: blind and partially sighted people and work*. London: Royal National Institute for the Blind, 2004.

Brady F. A singular view: the art of seeing with one eye pp. 1–139. Toronto: Edgemore Enterprises Ltd 1992.

Bruce I, Baker M. *Employment and unemployment amongst people with sight problems in the UK*. London: Royal National Institute for the Blind, 2003.

Office for National Statistics. *Labour force survey*. London: Office for National Statistics, 2002.

Roberts S et al. *Disability in the workplace: employers' and service providers' responses to the Disability Discrimination Act in 2003 and preparation for 2004 changes*. Report No. 202. London: Department of Work and Pensions, 2004.

Royal National Institute for the Blind. *Work matters* (DVD). London: Royal National Institute for the Blind, 2004 (Available from Royal National Institute for the Blind customer services 0845 702 3153).

Ocular hazards and toxicology

Archer DB, Gardiner TA, Ionising radiation and the retina. *Curr Opin Ophthalmol* 1994; **5**(3): 59–65.

Barkana Y, Belkin M. Laser eye injuries. *Surv Ophthalmol* 2000; **44**(6): 459–78.

Cellini M et al. Photic maculopathy by arc welding. A case report. *Int Ophthalmol* 1987; **10**(3): 157–9.

Chiou GCY. *Ophthalmic toxicology*. New York: Raven Press, 1992.

Jones N (ed.) *Craniofacial trauma*. London: Oxford University Press, 1997.

Kozielec GF, Smith CW. Welding arc-like injury with secondary subretinal neovascularisation. *Retina* 1997; **17**(6): 558–9.

Magnavita N. Photoretinitis: an underestimated occupational injury? *Occup Med* 2002; **52**(4): 223–5.

Mainster MA, Stuck BE, Brown J Jr. Assessment of alleged laser injuries. *Arch Ophthalmol* 2004; **122**(8): 1210–17.

Phelps Brown NA et al. Nutrition supplements and the eye. *Eye* 1998; **12**: 127–33.

Pitts J. Manchineel keratoconjunctivitis. *Br J Ophthalmol* 1993; **77**: 284–8.

Pitts J. Orbital blow-out fractures. *Eye News* 1996; **3**: 12–14.

Power WJ et al. Welding arc maculopathy and fluphenazine. *Br J Ophthalmol* 1991; **75**(7), 433–5.

van Soest EM, Fritschi L. Occupational health risks in veterinary nursing. *Aust Vet J* 2004; **82**(6): 346–50.

Taylor HR *et al.* The long-term effects of visible light on the eye. *Arch Ophthalmol* 1992; **110**: 99–104.

Zamir E, Chowers I. Concerns about laser pointers and macular damage. *Arch Ophthalmol* 2001; **119**(11): 1731–2.

Occupational injuries and eye protection

Caesar R, Gajus M, Davies R. Compressed air injury of the orbit in the absence of external trauma. *Eye* 2003; **17**: 661–2.

Details of eye hazards, protection and selection guides at www.bunzlsafety.ie/selectionguides/ppe/eyewear.html

Details of eye protection testing from a company specialising in this area at www.bsi-global.com/Testing+Certification/Products/eyewear.xalter

MacEwan CJ. Eye injuries: a prospective survey of 5671 cases. *Br J Ophthalmol* 1989; **73**: 888–94.

Pitts J. Principles of eyelid repair. In: *Fundamentals of clinical ophthalmology* (eds Collin JRO, Rose GE) pp. 7–14. London: BMJ Publishing, 2002.

Perry M *et al.* Emergency care in facial trauma—a maxillofacial and ophthalmic perspective. *Int J. Care Injured* 2005; **36**: 875–96.

Yu TS, Liu H, Hui K. A case-control study of eye injuries in the workplace in Hong Kong. *Ophthalmology* 2004; **111**: 70–4.

First aid at work

Beaudoin A. Comparing eyewash systems. *Occup Health Saf* 2003; **72**(10): 50–6.

Kunimoto DY *et al. The Wills Eye Manual: Office and Emergency Room Treatment of Eye Disease*, fourth edition. Philadelphia: Lippincott, Williams and Wilkins, 2004.

Eagling EA, Roper-Hall MJ. *Eye injuries: an illustrated guide*. London: Butterworths, 1986.

Mortland KK, Mortland DB. Designing for laboratory safety: emergency shower and eyewash stations. *Clin Leadership Manage Rev* 2003; **17**(4): 233–4.

Chapter 10

Hearing and vestibular disorders

B. P. Ludlow and K. B. Hughes

Hearing

The ear comprises the pinna, ear canal, middle ear, and inner ear together with central auditory connections. Disease can affect one or more parts. A comprehensive assessment is required in order to evaluate the suitability of applicants for employment in different environments. The occupational physician needs to understand how different employment environments will create, aggravate, or predispose to the development of disease in the healthy or diseased ear. Only then will employees be fairly and sensibly engaged for work that does not prejudice their health and does not put at risk the employer or other members of the workforce.

Occupational health assessment

A comprehensive health questionnaire will cover previous medical conditions, including treatments, together with any ongoing treatment. Particular account needs to be taken of skin disease both general and local to the ear and previous ear disease, especially where surgery has taken place.

Head injury associated with a loss of consciousness can cause sensorineural deafness with a pattern of loss indistinguishable from that associated with noise damage. Such injuries should be recorded and audiometry carried out.

General medical conditions also need to be considered, particularly those that may affect balance. Questions also need to cover familial diseases such as atopy and the early development of deafness, which may indicate a familial trait that at a later date may be misinterpreted as damage occurring from occupational noise exposure. Particular note should be taken of previous employments and hobbies where noise exposure has been a factor.

A detailed examination will cover the skin, the shape and the size of the ear canal, presence of excessive hair, presence or absence of wax together with canal pathology (skin diseases or osteoma). The condition of the tympanic membrane needs to be recorded, together with evidence of surgical scars both postaural and endaural (between the tragus and the root of the helix). Tuning fork assessment (512 cps), both Weber and Rinne, should be recorded and pure tone audiometry conducted in a certified sound-proofed environment if there is a risk of the employee being subjected to excessive levels of noise. Self-recording audiometry or manual audiometry can be carried out. The greater sensitivity of self-recording audiometry must be understood (thresholds are approximately 3 dB more sensitive than those found by manual audiometry).

Hearing difficulty

Hearing 'impairment' can be measured. A hearing 'disability' arises out of the impairment and is the problem the individual experiences. 'Handicap' results from the impairment or disability that limits the person. Pure tone manual or self-recording audiometry is not a measure of 'hearing' but is the accepted surrogate. Individuals with the same measured impairment will vary in the degree of disability or handicap that they experience.

Much will depend on their motivation and the attitude of employers and fellow workers. The hard of hearing and deaf need only be excluded from a minority of jobs and the Disability Discrimination Act (1995) requires that employers make reasonable adjustments to the workplace so that the number of jobs that cannot be done by the hearing impaired is minimized. There are, however, tasks where hearing impairment is not compatible with employment, where the safety of the individual or others could be compromised, particularly where there are high levels of responsibility such as in civil airline pilots. Consideration should also be given to the risk of aggravating an existing impairment.

Defective hearing, however, is a hidden disability and 'communication' difficulties can be interpreted as stupidity or behavioural faults. Even when acknowledged, the difficulties in communication may not be addressed because of other pressures within the workplace. Hearing aids are assumed to restore hearing to normal, which they rarely do, and an understanding of the need for people with impaired hearing to require additional help from visual cues needs to be understood.

The inner ear's response to the damaging effect of noise varies. There are, undoubtedly, people with a genetic susceptibility to the effects of noise[1] and those who have will lose more hearing than others for a given degree of noise exposure.[2] Women are thought to be slightly less susceptible than men, melanization is protective, fair haired, blue eyed people are more sensitive and Caucasians more sensitive than those of African descent.

Synergism also occurs: current opinions suggest that presbyacusis and noise-induced hearing loss are additive. However, noise damage is more important in early life while presbyacusis may be the dominant factor later. Previous damage from congenital loss, head injuries, ototoxic drug treatment, or even concurrent chemical exposure (toluene in the printing industry) may predispose to the development of sensorineural loss.

Finally, conductive loss should not be assumed to protect the inner ear from the damaging effects of noise.[3,4] Various studies have indicated that it does not, although one study has suggested that it does.[5] The behaviour of the pathological ear in a noisy environment is not wholly predictable.

Prevalence of hearing impairment

A survey of the adult population in the UK[6] found that 20% had a hearing impairment of 25 dB or greater in the better hearing ear (average threshold: 0.5, 1, 2, and 4 kHz). The prevalence of degrees of hearing loss as a function of age is given in Table 10.1. It should be noted that a 25 dB

Table 10.1 Percentage of people in six age groups whose hearing threshold levels (averaged over 0.5, 1, 2, and 4 kHz) were at or over 25, 45, and 65 dB HL in the better ear

Age group	% at or exceeding		
	25 dB HL	45 dB HL	65 dB HL
17–30	1.8	0.2	<0.1
31–40	2.8	1.1	0.7
41–50	8.2	1.7	0.3
51–60	18.9	4.0	0.9
61–70	36.8	7.4	2.3
71–80	60.2	17.6	4.0
Overall	16.1	3.9	1.1

Box 10.1 Some definitions

Pure tone audiometry measures the hearing threshold level (HTL) at each of a range of test frequencies in each ear. The physical unit of measurement is decibels (hearing level), abbreviated to 'dB HL', except that the 'HL' should be omitted when the statement refers to HTL. The reference zero for dB HL is based on a standardized biological baseline of normal hearing in young persons, which varies with test frequency and with type of earphone and measuring coupler used for calibration and is covered by an ISO standard.

The unit 'dB SPL' (sound pressure level) or 'dB(lin)' relates to an absolute physical measure of sound pressure of 20 mPa (milli-pascals). The unit 'dB(A)' refers to the SPL after application of standardized A-weighting filters to reduce the influence of low-frequency and very high-frequency components of a sound, thus giving a better representation of its potential to cause hearing damage, speech interference, reduced work performance, and annoyance.

average hearing threshold (HTL) in the better ear is only just outside what is conventionally regarded as the normal range of hearing. Many with this degree of loss however will have some hearing difficulties in adverse auditory conditions. A HTL of 35 dB is the usual level at which audiologists would consider hearing amplification and a HTL of 45 dB can definitely be considered to produce a handicap.

Data on the proportions of people who experience various degrees of hearing difficulty and ear discharge are available from the National Study of Hearing (NSH) and are shown in Table 10.2. Difficulties are common and need to be taken into account in assessing an individual's fitness for work.

Tinnitus

Estimates of the prevalence of tinnitus in industrialized countries are based on the NSH. Approximately 15% have or have experienced tinnitus lasting over 5 minutes in duration. At least 8% experience tinnitus causing difficulties getting off to sleep and/or moderate annoyance and 0.5% have tinnitus, which has a severe effect on their normal life.

The incidence rises with age and increasing hearing loss. It can be exacerbated by exposure to noise at work, stress, or intercurrent illness. Early counselling is essential to avoid permanently disabling tinnitus. Workers who get embroiled in legal arguments with their employer over the development of tinnitus are often in the legal system for a year or two and by this time the tinnitus tends to become established and extremely problematic. Early referral to tinnitus counsellors offers the best prospect for resolution.

Ear discharge

Bacterial or fungal infections of the ear canal skin are frequently associated with ear discharge. Fitness for work can be affected by personal hygiene or ability to use hearing protectors. A predisposition to eczematous skin reactions can aggravate or even initiate a problem, and may lead to a person who is otherwise fit to move from that particular environment.

Barometric problems

Eustachian tube dysfunction, in particular where there is already evidence of middle ear damage, may bar workers from certain occupations, notably in flying or diving or working in compressed

Table 10.2 Frequency of hearing difficulty and of ear disorder by age and sex (percentages with sizes of samples shown in brackets)

| | Age group (years) and sex | | | | | |
| | 17–24 | | 25–44 | | 45–64 | |
	M	**F**	**M**	**F**	**M**	**F**
Difficulty in hearing (better ear)						
	(1980)	(2157)	(4038)	(4300)	(3734)	(4161)
None	97	98	96	97	86	92
Slight	2	2	4	2	11	5
Moderate	0.4	0.1	0.5	0.4	2	2
Great	0.1	0.2	0.1	0.2	0.6	0.7
Cannot hear at all	0.1	0.0	0.1	0.2	0.2	0.5
Difficult to hear in a quiet room						
Normal voice	(1674) 1	(1881) 2	(3291) 2	(3512) 2	(2937) 7	(3178) 5
Loud voice	(1664) 1	(1842) 1	(3457) 1	(3255) 1	(2837) 3	(3051)
Very difficult to hear in noise						
	(2859) 12	(3052) 15	(6030) 20	(6430) 19	(5709) 36	(6346) 27
Discharging ear (ever)						
	(2584) 13	(2761) 15	(5347) 15	(5762) 17	(5043) 18	(5617) 16
Hearing aid (ever)						
	(2603) 0.6	(2774) 0.6	(5327) 0.7	(5827) 1	(5113) 3	(5722) 3
Significant hearing impairment						
	(295) 0.3	(341) 0.3	(748) 0.0	(778) 0.3	(778) 0.6	(894) 0.3

air (see also Appendices 1 and 4). A well healed mastoid cavity is not in itself a bar to flying but any recurrence of disease activity would result in a need to change employment.

Clinical aspects of work capacity

Loss of hearing alone seldom leads to a period off work. The associated effect, however, on the psychology of the individual, the strain of communication, and its effects on safety and efficiency need to be considered by the employer with the interests of the worker foremost. Tinnitus can be disabling, particularly if the work environment aggravates it or if it leads to tiredness from loss of sleep. Ear infections, particularly where aggravated by working conditions, should be taken seriously. Workers may need to be redeployed promptly in order to allow resolution of the underlying condition.

Working efficiency and safety

There are few jobs where perfect hearing is essential. For the majority it is sufficient that the applicant (wearing a hearing aid if appropriate) can communicate in the normal working environment. Consideration should, however, be given to the consequences of hearing aid failure and its potential effect on safety.

Where auditory requirements are more stringent, particularly in respect of safety, then careful assessment is necessary, including audiometry. Simple tests of hearing, including voice tests, can be conducted in a reproducible form but audiometric assessment has largely supplanted them and has the advantage of providing an objective record.

Conductive hearing losses due to middle ear disorders usually result in the loss of auditory sensitivity, whereas sensorineural losses from cochlear damage can impair both frequency and temporal resolution as well as sensitivity. Workers with conductive losses therefore tend to have less disability than those with cochlear losses.

Hearing aids

Hearing aids improve hearing sensitivity provided that there is some usable residual hearing. Digital aids have now largely superseded analogue ones but the benefits in individual cases are still uncertain and often a matter of trial and error with different models. Binaural fittings have theoretical advantages. Only 25–33% of patients use them at present, although this figure is rising.

Most occupations are compatible with the wearing of a hearing aid but there are certain environments (for example, coal mines and flammable atmospheres) where models have to be chosen with care for their electrical safety. The manufacturer's data sheet or the Medical Devices Agencies can provide information on the suitability of particular aids.

Special work problems, restrictions, or needs

Defective hearing and accidents

It seems likely that noise sometimes contributes to accidents from failure to hear warning signals.[7,8] Nevertheless, serious accidents due to deafness or noise interference appear to be uncommon. In a life-style survey conducted by the Trent Regional Health Authority in 1992, there were over 6000 respondents to a postal questionnaire who were under the age of 50 years. Fifty-one of these possessed hearing aids: these people report a sixfold increase in odds for accidental injury at work, but no increase in the home or on the road, as compared with those without hearing aids.

Unsuitable work for people with hearing defects

Questions of capability arise particularly in jobs in which the actual task is an auditory one and where accurate hearing of speech and/or of other auditory signals is important. Exceptions can be made, particularly where the hearing-impaired person is already trained and experienced, or where there is some special connection with defective hearing, e.g. teachers of the deaf, and social workers for the deaf. Major factors in defining acceptability include the degree of expected responsibility for others and the extent to which the impairment may undermine the public's confidence. These factors cannot be quantified readily. Each employer should consider carefully, in each case, whether or not it is essential to exclude people with defective hearing from certain jobs. For further information on the impact of defective hearing on employability and the means of reducing its effect at work the reader should consult Kettle and Massie[9] and the *Deaf and hearing impaired* booklet (EPWD 20) issued by the Employment Service.[10]

Legislation and guidelines for employment

The main employment problem related to hearing and the ear is that of noise-induced permanent threshold shift, i.e. irreversible hearing damage. However, noise *per se* also has recognized nuisance effects that can impair health and safety, e.g. annoyance, interference with communication and extra-auditory symptoms. There have been reports of adverse effects on general health. Sound may directly stimulate the autonomic nervous system. There is some evidence relating noise exposure to increased risk of heart disease.[11]

Background

HSE estimates that about 80 000 establishments have noise levels in excess of 85 dB(A), thereby exposing 1.3 million workers to potentially harmful noise levels. These figures may be conservative as many sole-trader and agricultural operations are unlikely to have been counted.[12] HSE further estimates that 170 000 people in the UK suffer from deafness, tinnitus, or other ear problems as a result of excessive noise exposure in the workplace. On average at 'noisy' sites one in four workers is exposed to levels over 85 dB(A).

The 1989 Noise at Work Regulations aim to protect the workforce from harmful noise exposures. These Regulations require employers to issue hearing defenders on request to employees who are potentially exposed to noise at a continuous equivalent 8-hour exposure of 85 dB(A) and to ensure that all workers are protected when the noise level exceeds 90 dB(A). Many employers have opted to introduce mandatory use of hearing defenders at 85 dB(A), anticipating further more stringent standards in the future.

Implementation of the EU Physical Agents Directive

The Noise at Work Regulations came into effect on 1 January 1990 and were amended in February 2006. Directive 2003/10/EC set minimum health and safety requirements regarding exposure of workers to the risks arising from physical agents, including noise. The Directive lowered the action levels from 85 dB(A) and 90 dB(A) to 80 and 85 dB(A) respectively. Under the old regulations a peak sound pressure exposure of 200 Pa* was set. The new rules fix a peak level for each action level of 112 Pa and 140 Pa respectively. Additionally, a limit value of 87 dB(A) and 200 Pa. peak has been set in the UK.[13] Table 10.3 compares some key provisions of the old and new rules.

Table 10.3 A comparison of the 1986 and 2003 Directives on Control of Noise at Work

Provision	1986 Directive	2003 Directive
Reduce risk	To lowest level reasonably practicable	Eliminate at source or reduce to minimum
Assess and/or measure exposure	Where noise is experienced	Where people are, or are likely to be exposed to noise
Assessment period	8 hours	Exposed at or above 80 dB(A)
Workers entitled to a hearing test	Exposures at or above 85 dB(A)	Exposed at or above 80 dB(A) and/or 112 Pa.
Health surveillance	No duty	Appropriate surveillance required when indicated by risk
Issue hearing protection on request	85 dB(A) and 200 Pa	80 dB(A) and 112 Pa
Mandatory wearing of hearing protection	90 dB(A) and 200 Pa	85 dB(A) and 140 Pa
Limit on exposure	–	87 dB(A) and 200 Pa at ear
Warning signs and control access	90 dB and 200 Pa where reasonably practicable	85 dB(A) and 140 Pa where technically feasible
Exemptions	Sea and air transport	Conflict with public service activities

*Pascals (SI unit of pressure; 1Pa-1 newton per square metre).

HSE Guidance

HSE published *A Guide to Audiometric Testing Programmes* in 1995. This gives advice of a general nature that remains relevant today. The guidance raises several pertinent questions:

- Is the hearing condition stable or unstable?
- Will it be aggravated by further exposure to noise?
- What is the extent of the established hearing loss?
- Will the person use a hearing aid and will it be safe to do so at work?
- Are there any specific hearing requirements for the job in question?

The guide further advises that, in view of the stability of noise-induced hearing loss, continuing exposure 'will usually be acceptable where adequate hearing protection is used and where residual hearing ability is not so poor as to make the risk of further hearing loss unacceptable'. According to the guidance, even if a doctor advises against continuing employment, if there is no risk to others, then employees should be permitted to continue in the same job with the employer's agreement. (It would be prudent to record this agreement in writing.)

The guidance recognizes that there will be a 'few employees who have responsibility for the safety of others and who need to communicate easily and to hear auditory warning signals where "severe hearing loss" will cause difficulties'. It is good practice for this requirement to be made clear at the time of recruitment. Moreover, advisers should consider devising a trade specific test based on checking the individual's ability to hear at the specific frequencies of the warnings, possibly against a background of speech to simulate the workplace. Such a test can be used as objective evidence to support a recommendation of fitness or lack of fitness for a given type of work.

The need to carry out audiometric testing is not explicitly required by statute but it is inferred by the Management of Health and Safety at Work Regulations 1992, which require the provision of appropriate health surveillance in relation to any risk to health and safety. The new Noise at Work Regulations require surveillance, and audiometry forms a useful part of a surveillance programme. Therefore a prudent employer would include audiometric screening in his hearing conservation programme, for all workers exposed to noise above an action level requiring use of hearing defenders. Many companies now institute a programme in which hearing defenders should be issued on request above the first action level.

Hearing damage was considered unlikely below 80 dB(A) when the original work to delineate the relationship between noise exposure and HTL was conducted in the 1960s. More recently it has been accepted that damage is unlikely to occur at continuous exposure levels below 75 dB(A),[14] hence even adopting a policy to invoke a hearing conservation programme based on the lower exposure limit set in law will leave some workers who may be exposed above that level still within the 'legal' limits. Screening audiometry as part of a well run hearing conservation programme will help to identify those workers who are developing threshold shift in order to consider appropriate action.

Principles of a hearing conservation programme

Although the 1990 Regulations did not make hearing conservation mandatory, the requirement for health surveillance imposed by the new Directive might best be met by instigating a hearing conservation programme. As with other areas of occupational health practice, personal protective equipment—hearing defenders—should only be used as a last resort.

Any hearing conservation programme depends first of all on the identification of hazardous areas and noise sources, reduction of noise at source, and then education of managers and the workforce. The best way of monitoring the success of the programme is by audiometric screening in the exposed population.

Medico-legal considerations

One of the arguments sometimes advanced for pre-employment audiometry is that it may safeguard against civil claims in cases where damage actually pre-dates the employment. A question then arises regarding the wisdom, in medico-legal terms, of employment in noisy surroundings of the considerable number of people who have some degree of hearing impairment. However, the medico-legal risk is slight provided that the assessment is followed by appropriate and properly conducted hearing conservation measures, including a documented explanation to the employee about the hazards to hearing, the implications of hearing loss and the means of preventing it. The presence of pre-existing hearing impairment *per se*, or ear disease, is not a valid bar to employment. Similar considerations apply to the use of serial monitoring audiometry and the action to be taken when hearing deterioration is detected.[15]

Assessment of fitness for work

Many employers, particularly small firms, recruit staff without any medical screening. Conversely, there are some employers who reject applicants if their pre-employment audiogram demonstrates a dip at or about 4 kHz. This policy is very difficult to justify now that the DDA and the Noise at Work Regulations are in force. This is particularly relevant as many employees with hearing damage are bringing particular skills to a noisy occupation and are otherwise well qualified for the job in question. The majority of employers who perform audiometry do so for three purposes:

- to establish a baseline for the individual, particularly if they are to work in a noisy environment
- as a means of monitoring change in their employees' hearing so that appropriate steps can be taken to prevent any further deterioration
- as part of an ongoing process of education.

In practice, very few cases are identified in industry where the hearing loss causes a severe enough disability to preclude employment.

Serial audiometry

Periodic audiometric testing is generally considered a necessary ingredient of a comprehensive hearing conservation programme. It should be conducted annually for 2 years after the baseline pre-employment audiogram, to detect those particularly vulnerable to noise-induced hearing loss, and thereafter every 3 years.

The main use of serial audiometry is to detect deterioration in the hearing status of individuals or groups; also as an aid to their effective counselling. Safety indications for redeployment are restricted to those situations where hearing impairment puts the individual, the working group, or the plant at risk. Such instances are rarely encountered in general industry. Each case has to be assessed in the light of the particular job content and working conditions in order to reach an equitable decision.

Arguably, conducting a screening audiogram on an employee within their last few days of employment could provide evidence to defend a subsequent personal injury claim for unrelated subsequent hearing loss. However, it might also identify a problem hitherto not recognized.[16] HSE's Guidance Note MS 26, *A guide to audiometric testing programmes* (1995) provides reference information.

Identification

It can be challenging to assess personal noise exposures in environments where noise levels fluctuate widely. Nevertheless, workers must wear hearing protection when the levels are calculated to reach or exceed 85 dB(A). Help may be sought from occupational hygienists to map noise hazardous areas in the workplace and to assess workers' exposures. Personal dosimeters are commercially available.

It is worth noting that on the equal energy principle an unprotected exposure of 115 dB(A) for just 28 seconds equates to an 8-hour equivalent exposure at 85 dB(A). Unfortunately, in very high noise areas it is common to see workers lift the edge of their ear muff in order to hear what somebody next to them is shouting. In such a brief exposure the worker may have exceeded their whole day's predicted safe maximum dose.

Reduction at source

Elimination of the hazard is the ideal standard. For example, when plant machinery is replaced, the noise output should be considered in the contract specifications. With machinery and equipment that cannot be substituted the maintenance schedule should be considered—poorly maintained equipment tends to be noisy. Either the machine or the operator may be enclosed within a sound-attenuating enclosure. Some muffling can be retro-fitted to existing equipment, although this tends to be expensive. Secondary glazing and acoustic baffles may be used inside buildings to reduce noise from outside.

As propagated noise follows the inverse square law, simply doubling the distance between the source and the person reduces the potential noise exposure by 6 dB. Thus noise factors should always be considered when designing new buildings or plant layouts.

Education

It is vital that all employees are educated adequately during their induction training and that this instruction is periodically refreshed. Training should be directed at all levels. The point should be made that many leisure activities lead to noise exposure exceeding workplace action levels. Potentially damaging levels of noise from personal stereos may affect the hearing of the present generation, particularly as it ages.

Hearing protection

If all else fails then hearing protection should be considered. In certain conditions specialist active noise reduction equipment may be considered but for the most part the choice lies between ear muffs, deformable ear plugs, or a combination of both. The choice needs to be pragmatic or the worker will not wear it. It also needs to take into account the attenuation offered, bearing in mind that the real attenuation obtained in the workplace may be up to 10 dB less than the level stated by the manufacturer based on laboratory testing. Poorly maintained equipment will reduce the attenuation as will spectacle frames: these break the ear muff seal and can reduce attenuation by several dB. Likewise, helmet mounted muffs offer a lower protection factor than free standing muffs mounted on a sprung headband.

It is often said that wearing hearing protection in noise reduces the ability to communicate. This is not true; those with normal hearing are in fact better able to hear speech effectively in noise if they are wearing some form of hearing protection. The problem is that those who already have some hearing damage are worse off.

Clearly, within a workforce there will already be a number of workers who have impaired hearing. Accordingly, when introducing or revising hearing protection policies, employers should consider the need for visual alarm warnings as a supplement to acoustic warnings. Such systems are simple to implement using similar technology to that used at supermarket checkouts where the auditory 'supervisor call' is supported by a flashing light to indicate which till instigated the help request.

In the same way, as long as hearing is normal, the use of deformable ear plugs beneath a communications headset can be beneficial. Musicians often complain that they cannot play properly while wearing hearing defenders. However, it is feasible for them to learn new or different auditory cues to compensate for the different tonal qualities that they will hear when the sound is attenuated. In any case, although there is a transitional arrangement from implementation of the Directive for the music and entertainment sector, by 2008 musicians will have to comply fully with the Regulations.

Considerations when choosing hearing protectors

If the concept of protecting workers by use of PPE is accepted, then one might assume that hearing defenders with the highest available level of attenuation would be the best choice. Unfortunately this assumption is flawed. There is growing evidence that overprotection can lead to degradation of performance by reducing aural stimuli too far. Psychologically this can lead to a sense of isolation in the worker. Physically it can also compromise communication by attenuating important speech sounds below the wearer's HTL.[17] Therefore, it is important to balance the level of attenuation against other factors when deciding which type of protective equipment to provide. It is unlikely that a single device will prove suitable for all noisy workplaces, even within the same factory and even before the individual differences of the potential wearers are taken into account.

The European Guidance Document EN 458, available from the British Standards Institute as BS-EN 458 2004 *Hearing Protectors: Recommendations for Selection, Use, Care and Maintenance* provides sound advice on selection of hearing protective equipment and remains the only document that provides guidance on hearing protection that maximizes the ability to communicate in noisy environments. It implies that hearing protection should be selected on the basis that noise at the ear is attenuated to between 70 and 85 dB(A). (The new Noise at Work regulations require that exposure levels are below the action level as measured at the ear canal, unlike the 1989 rules where exposure in the free field was taken.)

Another factor that needs to be considered when recommending hearing protection includes the amount of attenuation that will really be achieved when the devices are worn in the workplace rather than when tested in the laboratory. Several factors come into play here: the comfort of the device (which could discourage the user to wear it correctly), the ease of use, breaches of the device's seal round the pinna caused by items like spectacle frames, the standard of maintenance of the equipment and general integration with other items of personal protective equipment. If the wearer has already suffered a degree of permanent threshold shift from ageing or previous noise damage, they are more likely to override their protection to communicate. The attenuation achieved in the real world may only be half or less than that claimed from laboratory testing. For example, where 30 dB of attenuation is expected only 8 dB may be obtained.[17–19] Thus, when selecting hearing protectors as part of a noise management programme, the adviser should strive for three key factors: sufficient attenuation, maximum comfort and maximum communication.

Audiometry

Baseline audiometry should be conducted on all workers who are employed to work in a noise hazardous area. Some people are more susceptible to noise-induced hearing loss than others, hence the need to repeat initial audiometry within the first year of employment to detect such cases and to offer them the early opportunity of job relocation. Thereafter, audiometry should be performed periodically for as long as the individual is exposed to a noise hazard. There is no hard and fast rule specifying the intervals between tests. Some programmes are planned around an annual audiometry test, others every second year, and yet others three yearly.

The main use of serial audiometry is to detect the deterioration of hearing status in individuals or groups. Results may be used as an aid to their effective education or counselling. It is rare in general industry to have to exclude a worker from their job because of developing threshold shift, although it is important to assess each case on its individual merits. In doing so it is important to recognize that audiometry, particularly the type of screening audiometry conducted in industry, is not an exact measure. Differences in reading of several dB can arise from day to day in the same individual, even with the same equipment and the same operator.

It is usually said that audiometry should only be carried out on workers after they have been away from the workplace, ostensibly in quiet conditions, for 14–16 hours. This is so that temporary threshold shift does not lead to false positive results. However, there is an increasingly popular view that testing the worker during the working day is a more valid screening assessment.[16] If their audiogram is normal when they have come to the test straight from the production area the findings can be reassuring; if hearing is impaired, they may be more likely to comply with a request to avoid leisure noise for 16 hours or so and to undergo a repeat tests. If the initial test shows threshold shift but the subsequent one is normal, the worker is getting an excessive noise exposure in the workplace. Consideration should be given to referring those who fail audiometry again at a subsequent repeat audiogram to an ENT consultant for a specialist opinion.

Performing the test

Screening audiometers are widely available and have superseded voice recognition tests as the primary means to assess hearing ability in pre-employment tests, as well as the best way to undertake serial screening tests. Audiometry can be undertaken using a simple manual pure-tone audiometer and headphones in a quiet room. Companies with occupational health facilities now tend to use automated computerized audiometers and place the subject in sound attenuating booths. This helps to increase the accuracy of the results and also reduces the likelihood of false readings. Subjects of manual audiometry in open rooms were often able to hear or sense the operator pressing the test button and could indicate hearing the tone when in fact they could not.

Test subjects are exposed to pure tone sounds at different sound pressures across a range of frequencies. The worker indicates or presses a button at the point where they first detect the sound and this is recorded as the threshold of hearing for that sound. The results are often recorded both as a table of figures and as a graph. They allow comparison year on year as well as comparison with population norms. Typically, screening tests will be conducted at frequencies of 500 Hz, 1 kHz, 2 kHz, 3 kHz, 4 kHz, and 6 kHz. Many people will now also screen at 8 kHz. Use of higher frequencies as an aid to early identification of noise-susceptible people has been suggested, but it is error prone and should not be used.

Once the audiometric results are recorded a number of different methods may be adopted to assess disability, for compensation or to decide fitness for a particular job. Some employers have specific standards for their workforce. In particular, in the early stages of noise-induced permanent threshold shift the frequencies most affected are those about 4 kHz; this is often called 'the 4 kHz dip'. Noise, however, is not the only cause of 4 kHz dips.

Specific employment regulations and standards

Armed services

Medical fitness is assessed in terms of a PULHHEEMS score (see Table 10.4), in which H relates to the auditory acuity for each ear. The quality of hearing is judged on an eight-point scale where 1 indicates exceptionally good and 8 indicates unfit for service. Application of the grade when determining fitness for a specific job tends to be more rigidly used for new recruits than to existing

Table 10.4 Audiometric standards in the armed services

| PULHEEMS H grade | Sum of HTLs (dB) | | General description |
	0.5, 1, and 2 kHz	3, 4, and 6 kHz	
H1	Not >45	Not >45	Good hearing
H2	Not >84	Not >123	Acceptable hearing for most purposes
H3	Not >150	Not >210	Impaired hearing. Unfit for entry
H4–H8	>150	>210	Very poor hearing. Restrict duties or redeploy existing service personnel

Service personnel. This is in keeping with HSE's guidance. The general standard for entry to any ground appointment is H2; for aircrew and other specialist duties H1 is required. The PULH-HEEMS grade for hearing is assessed by summing the HTL levels of the three lower frequencies (500 Hz, 1 kHz, and 2 kHz) and of the three higher frequencies (3 kHz, 4 kHz, and 6 kHz). To be classed H1 hearing levels must be better than the summed level standard in both higher and lower frequency ranges. (See Table 10.4.)

Civilian flying

The detailed requirements of commercial aviation staff are given at Appendix 1. Civil aircrew rarely lose their licence due to hearing problems but a history of vertigo would debar further flying. The CAA standards for professional pilots are given in Table 10.5 and are common across the 29 states comprising the Joint Aviation Authority (JAA). Instrument rated private pilots must also meet the same standard of hearing. JAA regulations require audiometry to be conducted at eight frequencies, the six used by the Armed Services PULHHEEMS and at 250 Hz and 8 kHz. However, fitness assessment is judged by hearing acuity at four frequencies as shown in the table. Pilots undergo audiometry every 5 years up to the age of 40 and 2-yearly thereafter.

Police

The tests performed and their interpretation vary from one police force to another. Some forces set an aggregate hearing loss entry standard based on pure tone audiometry, but that standard is set for guidance and subject to ENT advice. The level may be relaxed in certain cases, particularly for older recruits who have worked in noisy occupations. Additionally, some forces adopt a formal hearing conservation programme covering specialist officers such as armed response units and traffic police.

Table 10.5 Hearing standards of the UK CAA for pilot licences: class 1 (professional pilot) medical certification

Hz	Initial dB(A)	Renewal dB(A)
500	20	35
1000	20	35
2000	20	35
3000	35	50

Fire Services

Entry and in-service standards can vary between different forces and brigades, but most require good hearing. In 1989 the Report of the Joint Working Party of the Home Office on Medical Standards and Firefighters said:

> It is essential that firefighters should be able to hear instructions and signals, and good hearing is necessary. The whisper test combined with otoscopic examination and tuning fork tests can be used but audiometry is more accurate. A portable audiometer with ear muffs, used in a quiet room would give sufficiently accurate readings capable of detecting significant hearing loss which could then be more fully assessed at an audiological clinic.

Merchant Navy

The required standard of audiometric fitness varies between companies (see Appendix 2). Impaired hearing sufficient to interfere with conversation may lead to classification as 'permanently unfit'. A unilateral hearing defect is considered in relation to a specific job. Hearing aids are allowed in some jobs but not for engine-room, electrical, or radio personnel.

Railways

For train drivers a practical hearing test may be conducted under operational conditions according to a defined protocol. When pure tone audiometry is used there are stricter standards for new entrants than for periodic review of employees. For example, for entry into train crew and safety grades the HTL loss must not exceed 20 dB averaged over 500 Hz, 1 kHz, and 2 kHz frequencies or 25 dB at 4 kHz, while the standard is relaxed to 30 dB for existing employees. Hearing aid users are deemed unfit for footplate duty on main line services or for any tasks working on operational track.

Driving

Although defective hearing may lead a driver to miss a warning sound, hearing loss *per se* does not debar an individual from driving. The profoundly deaf must notify the DVLA when they reach the age of 70 but are unlikely to lose their licence unless they are considered totally unable to communicate in an emergency. The same criteria are applied to Goods Vehicle and Public Service vehicle drivers. Defective hearing need only be notified to the DVLA if it indicates an underlying pathology, which is likely to affect fitness to drive.

Infrasound and Low frequency sound

Low frequency sound is normally defined as that below 100 Hz while infrasound is that below 20 Hz. Natural sources such as thunder and wind have large low-frequency components. Gunfire, diesel engines, jet engines, and driving on motorways with a partially open car window can also generate significant levels. The ear is not particularly sensitive at these low frequencies.

Concern has been expressed that as most damage from exposure to high levels of low-frequency sound may occur in the speech-range frequencies, 'A' weighting may under-represent the risk to hearing and that energy—time trade-offs may not apply to hearing protection calculations. Moreover, hearing protectors are least effective at low frequencies and low frequency sound is very hard to attenuate by other means. Fortunately, there is no evidence to suggest that low frequency sound actually produces damage to hearing.

Noise exposure at these frequencies can cause recognized extra-auditory symptoms, but fortunately due to the impedance mismatch between airborne acoustic energy and the body, symptoms do not start until about 130 dB.

Nuisance and other extra-auditory effects of noise

In the legal sense a nuisance is defined as something that interferes with an individual's reasonable enjoyment of their property. Noise can degrade quality of life, affect an individual's performance and cause annoyance. It is distracting and can interfere with sleep. Annoyance due to noise depends on many factors including the characteristics of the noise itself, the hearer and group or population dynamics.

In 1994 the Netherlands Health Council published a report that considered the health risks potentially linked with noise and the exposure levels at which such effects were thought to arise (Table 10.6).

Conclusions

Normal hearing is difficult to define, as the definition is essentially arbitrary and age-dependent. Notwithstanding the work in the 1960s of Burns, Robinson, and others to define population normal hearing ranges and predicted effects of noise exposure, wide individual variation exists in the degree of perceived handicap from a given measurable hearing disability. Moreover the effect of a disability on the individual's fitness to work depends greatly on the particular job requirement and working environment. These difficulties have to be seen in the context of quite high prevalences of measurable hearing impairment (Table 10.1) and reported hearing difficulties (Table 10.2) in the general population. Fortunately, 'normal' hearing—in audiometric terms—is required in only a few jobs.

For the most part tests of hearing are unnecessary, other perhaps than a simple record of the applicant's hearing ability during interview. Where a job requires a test of ability to hear, although audiometric standards are often applied, it may be better to use an objective test and observation of the individual's ability to work in (simulated) operational conditions. Audiometry is not a good test of someone's ability to communicate, but it is a useful tool in a hearing conservation programme to identify individuals whose HTL is changing, and particularly for identifying those with a noise-related threshold shift.

Balance

A study of the mechanisms of balance is a delight to physiologists who appreciate the sophistication of the systems involved. To physicians facing patients, often anxious and unsure, the complaint

Table 10.6 Levels of noise exposure linked with health effects. Extract from a Report by the Health Council of the Netherlands[14]

Effect	Exposure type	Dose (dB(A))
Hearing loss	8-hour occupational	75
	24-hour environmental	70
Hypertension	Occupational	<85
Ischaemic heart disease	Environmental road noise between 06:00 and 22:00 hours	70
Annoyance	Occupational office	<55
	Occupational industrial	<85
Disturbed sleep pattern		40
Awakening from sleep		60
Adverse effect on mood next day		<60

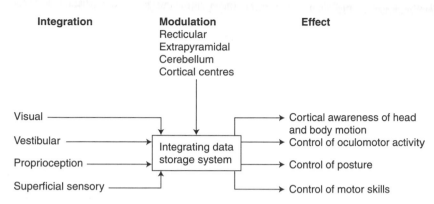

Fig. 10.1 Maintainance of equilibrium

of 'dizziness' induces a feeling of dismay as they grapple with imprecisions in the history and try to relate it to pathology. Often their own lack of knowledge transmits itself and destroys the confidence between patient and doctor which is so important.

Gowers, in 1893, defined vertigo as 'any sense of movement either in the individual himself or in external objects that involves a defect, real or seeming, in the equilibrium of the body'. More succinctly, vertigo is an hallucination of movement.

The sophisticated system developed in humans to maintain equilibrium involves integration of sensory information from the visual senses, the vestibular apparatus and the proprioceptive systems, especially those in the neck and limbs. This information is integrated with activity arising in the cortex, cerebellum, and extrapyramidal systems. Output is via the cortical awareness of position and movement, control of oculomotor activity and control of posture and motor skills (see Figure 10.1).

Pathology affecting any of these systems, together with the pervasive influences of cardiovascular, endocrine, and intrinsic neurological disease can affect this integrated system and lead to disequilibrium. In attempting to understand the pathology, physicians must focus on the symptom complex and history, for investigations are rarely definitive and often, at best, only a guide.

The difficulty is compounded by any psychological reaction on the patient's part, and the possibility that the patient may intentionally or unintentionally influence their environment. It is important that the occupational physician understands the physiology of balance and the patho-physiology of imbalance in order to make a proper judgement on the employment role. The first concern is to ensure the safety of the individual and other workers; but the occupational health adviser will also need to consider the risk and effects of future sickness absence, particularly where the employee is part of a team.

Principal disorders

'Dizziness' and 'giddiness' are terms that describe a wide variety of experiences. They may result from disorders of the vestibular, neurological, ophthalmic, cardiovascular, or musculoskeletal systems, or they may be of psychological origin, or some combination of these. Their cause, and even the likely system of origin, is often difficult or impossible to define. Distinction between central vascular and general neurological (including psychological and vasovagal) disorders is often arbitrary, or unwarranted when both forms of disorder are present (as quite often occurs). On the other hand, differentiation between peripheral (end-organ and eighth cranial nerve) and central neural origin is usually possible and helps to define the type of disorder, its likely prognosis, and appropriate management.

Two important aspects of vestibular physiology explain most of the features of peripheral vestibular disorders.

- The vestibular end-organs have a basal rate of nerve discharge and can be stimulated to increase or decrease their rate of firing. The end-organs of the semicircular canals on the two sides of the head are paired, and the afferent inputs to the central nervous system from each side act in opposition. Most but probably not all, disorders of the peripheral vestibular system cause a reduction in the resting rate in the corresponding part of the eighth cranial nerve. In such cases, the left–right imbalance so caused results in the eyes and body being reflexly deviated towards the side of the lesion. This is often reported as a sense of falling, or imbalance, to that side. The slow phase of nystagmus is also observed in this direction. The vertigo (or sense of rotation) and the fast phase of nystagmus localize to the opposite direction (the unaffected side) in such a case.

- The central vestibular system has a marked ability to compensate for chronic imbalance in the neural tonus between the two sides, and to habituate or adapt to frequently repeated or constant stimulation. Such habituation enables the acute disturbance of a severe unilateral vestibular failure to become self-limiting, especially in young patients. Over a few weeks, the sufferer passes from a state of intolerable vertigo with nausea and vomiting at rest, through to vertigo only on movement and, finally to momentary vertigo on major rotational movement of the head or body. If symptoms of dizziness last continuously for longer than 2–3 weeks, the cause is rarely vestibular.

Compensation for chronic imbalance in neural tonus is achieved more easily in the younger patient. Labyrinthine sedatives are useful in the acute phase, to overcome the unpleasantness of the initial nausea and vomiting, but thereafter the key to rehabilitation is active provocational exercises such as those devised by Cawthorne and Cooksey.[21] Overprotection should be avoided. A confident and positive attitude in the attending physician will aid recovery and dispel ideas of early retirement on medical grounds.

Stimulation by sound

The cochlea responds readily to faint acoustic stimuli and yet it is susceptible to damage by sustained excessive noise levels. In contrast, the vestibular apparatus, whose perilymph and endolymph are in direct continuity with the corresponding fluids in the cochlea, is less liable to injury. The explanation lies in the cochlea's microstructure which is so uniquely responsive to mechano-acoustic stimulation. On the other hand, the organization of the vestibular labyrinth is such that the cupulae or maculae are much less likely to respond to rapid to-and-fro stimulation arising from sound at ordinary levels. Nevertheless, the human vestibular system does respond to acoustic stimulation to some extent.

Even in health, very high noise levels—at and above 135 dB sound pressure level (SPL), e.g. those very close to powerful jet engines running at high power—can cause vertigo, nausea, and other unpleasant symptoms, such as fluttering of the cheeks, chest, and abdomen, and heating of hairy surfaces and skin folds. The saccule may also function as a receptor for low-frequency acoustic signals.

When a pathological disorder of the internal ear is present, however, levels of sound in the region of 110–120 dB SPL may cause a form of vertigo. This is known clinically as the Tullio effect. The 'sono-ocular' test takes advantage of this: if such stimuli cause nystagmus in the absence of visual fixation, this is taken as evidence of internal-ear pathology. The mechanism is uncertain. Its importance in the industrial context is that industrial noise seldom stimulates giddiness unless there is some pre-existing disorder of the internal ear.

The potentially damaging effects of noise exposure on the cochlea are now well recognized. Noise-induced damage to the vestibular part of the internal ear is less well documented, although evidence relating to this is accumulating.[22] Noise-induced vestibular disorders exist, but further epidemiological and clinical research is required to determine whether or not these (apart from the Tullio phenomenon) can be produced by the noise levels in industry. However, it should not be assumed automatically, even when vestibular and cochlear disorders coexist, that the occurrence of the former implies disease of constitutional origin. Not only is it perfectly possible for coincident vestibular and cochlear disorders to have different aetiologies, it seems possible that the vestibular disorder itself might sometimes be due to damage by noise.

Understandably, employers are anxious about employing people who suffer from dizziness. Their prejudice is often heightened by the inherent difficulty of ruling out psychological illness and uncertainties about prognosis.

Prevalence

Two community surveys conducted in the 1950s in the Vale of Glamorgan and in Annandale (Dumfries and Galloway) reported that dizziness and giddiness were common: 23% of a random sample of men and women had experienced the symptom at some time (Table 10.7). Episodes were mostly transient but, in 3%, vertigo symptoms lasted for a year or longer.

Patients who complain of a loss of balance are referred to a variety of specialists and it is, to an extent, a lottery as to whether or not they end up with an ENT surgeon, a neurologist or in a cardiology or general medical clinic.

This haphazard approach can result in patients waiting many months for a diagnosis and appropriate management. Minor pathology can result because of the delays in assessing significant persisting disabilities with a consequent loss of employment and many treatable conditions go untreated resulting in persistent incapacity.

Clinical aspects affecting work capacity

Relation to fitness for particular types of work

There are two main concerns in fitness assessment:

- that acute disorienting episodes that come on without warning may cause a danger to the worker or to others;
- that recurrent attacks may result in unpredictable absences from work.

Table 10.7 Prevalence of history (past or present) of dizziness or giddiness according to age (after Hinchcliffe[23])

Age group	History of dizziness or giddiness %
18–24	17
25–34	20
35–44	19
45–54	23
55–64	35
65–74	29

Disorders of balance may sometimes lead to premature retirement, especially when the effects are recurrent or prolonged and there seems no reasonable prospect of an acceptable degree of recovery of rehabilitation. Only rarely does the acute, unexpected disorientation lead to serious accidental injury of death.

In some cases, however, dizziness is a manifestation of a more serious underlying disorder, such as cardiovascular disease, cerebral tumour, or multiple sclerosis, which itself may have serious implications for work ability and life expectancy.

Treatment and rehabilitation

In the acute phase, the management of vestibular symptoms should be based on vestibular suppressive drugs; in the chronic phase Cawthorne and Cooksey's[21] head and balance exercises are more effective. Dizziness may nevertheless lead to prolonged or frequent absences from work. Additionally, sedative side-effects may occur with many of the vestibular suppressive drugs, such as cinnarizine and prochlorperazine. This is especially true of drugs used to prevent motion sickness, such as hyoscine, and those with antihistamine-like properties, e.g. meclozine, dimenhydrinate, and promethazine. Treatment with these drugs may impair work efficiency and safety, and especially safety to drive. They also interact with alcohol. Treatment of unsteadiness in older people with phenothiazines, such as prochlorperazine, tends to aggravate postural hypotension and to cause parkinsonism. Because of these side-effects, vestibular suppressive drugs should be phased out as soon as possible and replaced by a programme of vestibular rehabilitation.

Special work problems, restrictions, or needs

The problems of recurrent or prolonged periods of illness and the side-effects of treatment have been mentioned above. They are not specific to any particular job, but there are certain work tasks in which an acute attack of vertigo or imbalance could prove extremely dangerous. These are outlined below.

Work on or near potentially hazardous machinery

The risk will depend on the size, nature, and power of the machine, and the extent to which its dangerous parts are shielded. Each case has to be assessed individually. Factors to be considered include the ways in which the disorder affects the person and whether they are likely to experience warning symptoms of an impending attack and to be able to take appropriate avoiding action.

Other potentially dangerous situations

Working with molten metal, caustic acids, or alkalis, and working in isolation or near deep water, is also potentially dangerous. Much the same considerations apply as with work near moving machinery. Some patients' attacks may be related to, or induced by work at heights.

Work in moving environments

The likelihood of motion sickness is increased by most forms of vestibular disorder. Preventative drugs may be used, but due consideration must be given to the risk of side-effects that undermine work safety and efficiency. Probably the best solution, if possible, is to give the affected worker a conditional trial in the environment in question.

Diving

Chronic or recurrent vestibular disturbances are usually a bar to diving, especially scuba diving (see Appendix 4). This is because spatial orientation depends on three main factors: vestibular function, pressure sense, and visual cues. Underwater surroundings may be dark or murky, reducing or removing the visual input; there is also a much reduced pressure sense even when the diver is on the bottom, as the human being then has a similar specific gravity to that of the environment. Orientation thus depends heavily on the vestibular system; if this is deficient a very dangerous situation can easily arise.

Jobs with high levels of responsibility for the safety of others

Sudden onset of acute vestibular impairment while in control of a vehicle can give the operator a false impression that the vehicle has veered from its correct direction. This may lead to unnecessary corrective action and cause an accident. Acute vertigo may also cause a reflex response that causes the driver to misdirect the vehicle. People subject to vestibular or similar disturbances should not drive vehicles, boats, or planes until they are fully recovered and have been free of attacks for at least a year.

Existing legislation and guidelines for employment

Medical assessment

Unlike hearing, vestibular function cannot be measured quickly and easily. Therefore, vestibular function tests have not been standardized for use in occupational assessments. Testing is generally limited to simple clinical manoeuvres such as the Romberg test or heel–toe walking in a straight line and an inspection of the eyes for nystagmus. These procedures can only detect substantial disturbances of balance, or nystagmus due to central, or to recent and severe peripheral, vestibular disorders. Usually most reliance is placed on the history of severity, duration, frequency, nature, and effects of vestibular episodes.

Special restrictions

Driving The DVLA must be informed by a licence holder or applicant with this disability (see also Chapter 28). People who are liable to sudden disabling attacks of giddiness or fainting are banned from holding a motor vehicle driving licence. In the case of attacks of vertebrobasilar artery insufficiency, a person is advised to stop driving and report the condition. After a first episode, the ordinary driving licence is usually revoked for at least 3 months. Recurrent cases may be reviewed when satisfactory control of symptoms is achieved. A licence may be restored for 1, 2, or 3 years, and permanently if there have been no symptoms for 4 years. The same policy is adopted for Menière's disorder, vestibulopathies, and positional vertigo. Normally, any person with a persisting vestibular disorder, Menière's disease, positional vertigo, or a single transient ischaemic episode is regarded as unfit to drive vocationally (passenger carrying vehicles, large goods vehicles and taxis).

Flying The determining factors in fitness assessment are whether the licence holder may become incapacitated while in control of an aircraft and whether they can function effectively. Clearly, vertigo or imbalance arising from Menière's disorder, vestibulopathies, or positional vertigo would not be compatible with flying. More borderline or uncertain conditions do occur, and in these cases, fitness decisions are made by the Civil Aviation Authority following an examination by a doctor specially qualified in aviation medicine (see also Appendix 1).

Merchant navy Menière's disease is the only vestibular disorder specified in the Department of Transport regulations on medical fitness of seafarers: it implies permanent unfitness, as do transient ischaemic attacks, which often present as episodes of dizziness (see also Appendix 2).

Diving Fitness to dive is covered by statutory medical standards. With few exceptions, disorders of balance constitute an absolute bar to working as a commercial diver (see also Appendix 4).

Armed forces The degree to which a vestibular disorder will affect the physical (P) assessment in the PULHEEMS system depends on its nature, severity, and effects. The interpretation of the P assessment in terms of fitness for service depends on the particular branch of service and is closely related to the actual requirements of the job and the limitations that physical disorders would place on its performance.

Police, fire, and other public services In general there are no specific regulations. Certification of fitness depends on a non-specialist medical opinion on the likelihood of incapacity during operational duties. For firefighters, who may work up ladders or in conditions of minimal visibility, a more stringent criterion needs to be applied. The Home Office guidelines of 1970 specified that 'evidence of labyrinthine disturbance, a history of vertigo or any condition which would impair a candidate's sense of balance' would render a recruit unsuitable for employment in fire fighting.

General industry Where pre-employment screening is performed, unless there is a specialized need, enquiry tends to be limited to the general question: 'Do you suffer from fits, faints, blackouts, or dizzy attacks?' The data from the NSH referred to earlier imply that such symptoms rarely interfere with work. Where the severity is sufficient to cause problems, the potential employer tends to err on the side of caution, sometimes to the detriment of the individual. Occupational physicians tend to be more liberal. This unsatisfactory situation arises from the difficulties in diagnosis and uncertainties in prognosis mentioned earlier.

Similar problems are encountered during employment. If an employee develops disabling vertigo, the employer must review the safety of the individual and the group with whom they work. Restrictions on driving, work at heights, or near moving machinery are commonly imposed. These, and the uncertainties regarding regular attendance at work, raise questions of employability. In such cases, as much information as possible should be obtained on the aetiology, treatment, and prognosis and weighed against the job requirements before taking any final decision.

Conclusions and recommendations

Disturbances of equilibrium are common in men and women of all ages. Mostly these are transient and inconsequential. Confidence in the attending physician, sympathy from the occupational medical services, and a positive attitude to rehabilitation, using provocational exercises rather than trying to sedate the vestibular system with drugs, are the key to a successful and early return to work.

Few causes of disequilibrium have substantial implications for fitness at work, although absences from work can arise and can be recurrent. Except in classical cases these disorders are difficult to diagnose and to assess.

Real work limitations may arise if there is a liability to acute episodes of vertigo or imbalance, especially if these are unpredictable. Restrictions have to be imposed where the work is near unguarded, moving machinery or at heights, involving driving or exposure to motion (as in ships), or where the job has a high level of responsibility, or where there is a potential risk of injury to others. Episodes like these are incompatible with diving, flying, or work in safety-critical situations.

References

1 Carter NL. Eye colour and susceptibility to noise induced permanent threshold to shift. *Audiology* 1980; **19**: 86–93.

2 Henderson D, Subramanian M, Boettcher FA. Individual susceptibility to noise induced hearing loss: an old topic revisited. *Ear Hearing* 1993; **14**: 153–68.

3   Meshang DP, Hyde ML, Flukelstein DM, Alberti PW. Unilateral otosclerosis in noise induced hearing loss. *Clin Otolaryngol* 1991; **16**: 70–5.

4   Simpson DC, O'Reilly BF. The protective effect of a conductive hearing loss in workers exposed to industrial noise. *Clin Otolaryngol* 1991; **16**: 274–7.

5   Nillson R, Bore E. Noise induced hearing loss in shipyard workers with unilateral hearing loss. *Scand Audiol* 1983; **12**: 125–40.

6   Davis AC. The prevalence of hearing impairment and reported hearing disability in Great Britain. *Int J Epidemiol* 1989; **18**: 911–17.

7   Acton WI, Wilkins PA. Can noise cause accidents? *Occup Health Saf* 1982; **12**: 14–16.

8   Wilkins PA. The role of acoustical characteristics in the perception of warning sounds and the effects of wearing hearing protection. *J Sound Vibration* 1982; **100**: 181–90.

9   Kettle M, Massie B (eds) *Employers' guide to disabilities*, (2nd edn), pp. 19–23. Cambridge: Woodhead-Falkner, 1986.

10   Employment Service: *Deaf and Hearing Impairment Booklet*, EPWP 20. Sheffield: ES, 1988.

11   Babisch W, Elwood PC, Ising H. Road traffic noise and heart disease risk: results of the epidemiological studies in Caerphilly, Speedwell and Berlin. In: *Noise as a public health hazard*, Vol. 3 (ed. Vallet M), pp. 260–7. Bron: INTRETS, 1994.

12   Honey J *et al*. The costs and benefits of the noise at work regulations. *HSE Contract Res Rep* 1989; No. 116.

13   HSE Website http://www.hse.gov.uk/noise/issues.htm.

14   Noise and Health. Report of a Committee of the Health Council of the Netherlands (1994) No1994/15E. The Hague, 1994.

15   *A guide to audiometric testing programmes*. Guidance note. Sheffield: Health and Safety Executive, 1995.

16   Jones CM, Hughes KB. Hearing and vestibular disorders. In: *Fitness for work, the medical aspects* (3rd edn) (eds Cox RA, with Edwards FC, Palmer K), pp. 182–209. Oxford: Oxford University Press, 2000.

17   Dobie RA. *Medical-legal evaluation of hearing loss*, p. 190. New York: Van Nostrand, 1993.

18   Berg G. Attenuation and protection: we can achieve both. *Proceedings of the 7th International Congress on Noise as a Public Health Problem*, pp. 187–90. 1998. Sydney, Australia: Noise Effects '98 Pty.

19   Abel SM, Alberti PW, Rokas D. Gender differences in real-world hearing protector attenuation. *J Otolaryngol* 1988; **17**(2): 86–92.

20   Abel SM, Alberti PW, Haythornthwaite CA, Riko K. Speech intelligibility in noise with and without ear protectors. In: *Personal hearing protection in industry* (ed. Alberti PW). New York: Raven Press, 1981.

21   Cooksey FS. Rehabilitation in vestibular injuries. *Proc R Soc Med* 1946; **39**: 273–8.

22   Hinchcliffe R, Coles RRA, King PF. Occupational noise induced hearing vestibular malfunction? *Br J Ind Med* 1992; **49**: 63–5.

23   Hinchcliffe, R. Prevalence of the commoner ear, nose and throat conditions in the adult rural population of Great Britain: a study by direct examination of two random samples. *Br J Prev Soc Med* 1961; **15**: 128–40.

Chapter 11

Spinal disorders

K. T. Palmer and C. G. Greenough

Introduction

Non-specific low-back pain (LBP) is one of the commonest conditions afflicting adults of working age. It represents a leading cause of short- and sometimes long-term disability and a major cause of sickness absence. The problem posed in assessing fitness for work in back pain sufferers is one that all occupational physicians frequently face. Neck pain and its associated disability are scarcely less common, as judged by population surveys. Collectively, therefore, axial pains affecting the spine pose a major challenge to the decision-maker.

Commonly, a number of placement and fitness questions arise. In assessing the absent worker with a current episode of spinal pain, it is reasonable to ask:

◆ When will symptoms improve or resolve? Is this a short- or a long-term problem?

◆ Are any further investigations required to exclude serious pathology signifying long-term incapacity? Who (among the many with spinal pain) should be referred for such an assessment?

◆ At what point should the occupational physician intervene to hasten rehabilitation? And by what means?

◆ Has work contributed to the onset of symptoms? Might it worsen or prolong them?

◆ Is it safe and appropriate to return of the worker to the same job or does the work need to be modified, initially or in the long-term?

◆ When is chronic spinal pain serious enough to declare a person permanently unfit for work? How does this vary according to the nature of the job? Could more be done to avoid or control the typical demands of work before the point is reached?

◆ Following spinal surgery, when will the patient be fit for work? Should special restrictions be considered and if so under what circumstances?

At the pre-employment stage the issues are different but no less difficult:

◆ Are there any specific inquiries (questions, examination findings and investigations) predictive of future spinal pain, including spinal pain leading to serious disability or sickness absence?

◆ How should these be employed in assessing fitness for job placement? In particular, how should a past history of spinal pain be regarded? Are any characteristics sufficiently predictive to warrant work restrictions?

And more generally:

◆ What active steps can be taken to promote fitness for work and to prevent spinal pain?

◆ What obligations exist under the health and safety legislation and under the Disability Discrimination Act?

◆ Do current policies on back pain promote well-being and avoid needless work restrictions?

In attempting to answer these taxing questions it is necessary to appreciate the frequency and natural history of low back and neck pain, the markers of serious spinal pathology, and the research evidence on fitness assessment and preventing disability from spinal pain.

It is also important, for simple mechanical LBP, to be aware of recent evidence-based advances in management and rehabilitation. Adoption of modern consensus guidelines has led in the community setting to better coping and faster recovery. Specific guidelines have also been developed for the management of workers and these address, in part, some of the questions posed above.

In this chapter we review these initiatives and the problem of assessing fitness for work in those with spinal pain. Emphasis is given mainly to simple non-specific axial spinal pain as this is the commonest. Only rarely does the clinician make a more specific diagnosis; but occasionally serious pathology underlies symptoms and different responses are needed in clinical management and job placement. Some account is also provided of more specific spinal pathologies including prolapsed intervertebral disc (PID), spinal stenosis, fusion surgery, ankylosing spondylitis (AS), Scheuermann's disease, fractures, and spinal cord injury.

Non-specific low back pain

Prevalence and natural history

According to UK surveys, LBP has a point prevalence of 17–31%, a 2-week to 3-month prevalence of 19–43% and a lifetime prevalence of 60–80%.[1] A similar picture exists internationally.

Leg pain of the sciatic type has a lifetime prevalence of 14–40%, although by the strictest clinical criteria only about 3–5% of adults have true sciatica.[1]

Many episodes of LBP are short-lived and go unobserved by doctors. But the picture of development, persistence, recovery and relapse is a complicated one, especially when related to a person's life course. Young adults entering first employment already report a past history of back pain, as do school children, and the prevalence of symptoms rises only modestly with age thereafter.[1,2]

In the Manchester Back Pain Study[3] a majority of those with back pain had consulted their general practitioner (GP) about symptoms. Some 70% of presentations represented fresh episodes, 20% were acute-on-chronic exacerbations, and 10% a continuation of chronic background discomfort. Three months later, 27% of cases had resolved fully and 28% had improved, but in the remainder symptoms were either static (30%) or worsened (14%).

Among improved cases a high relapse rate ensues. For example, in the occupational setting Troup et al. found that approaching 50% of incident cases received further treatment and incurred work loss in the first year of follow-up.[4]

The likelihood of further attacks is greatest among those with recent symptoms and falls off as the latest episode recedes in time (Table 11.1).[5] In one prospective study,[6] of nurses initially free

Table 11.1 Likelihood of further back pain according to time from the last episode.[5] Reproduced under the terms of the click-use licence.

Time since last episode	Likelihood of attack in the next year
<1 week	76%
1–4 weeks	63%
1–12 months	52%
1–5 years	43%
>5 years	28%

of LBP for at least 1 month at baseline, some reported a more distant previous episode: their odds of having a recurrence during 18 months of follow-up were greater in comparison with those who did not. When the most recent episode lasted less than week and occurred more than a year before, the odds ratio (OR) for recurrence was 2.7. At the other extreme, when symptoms had lasted more than a month and occurred within the preceding year, the OR rose to 7.3.

Overall it has been estimated that 20% of people with LBP will continue to have symptoms of some degree over long periods of their life, while 5–7% will report these as chronic illness.[1]

Disability and sickness absence

There is only an approximate agreement between the severity of reported symptoms and disability, and likelihood of loosing work time or seeking healthcare. Thus, in general, patients who consult a GP have a similar pattern of symptoms to non-consulters;[3] and the best predictor of future work loss is the past history of this behaviour.[5,6]

Economically, the impact of LBP is considerable. It has been estimated that each year 150 million days of work incapacity occur from this cause; 3.7 million back pain sufferers (7% of the adult population) consult their GP about their back pain; 1.6 million attend a hospital outpatient department; 100 000 are admitted to hospital; and 24 000 have surgery on the back.[1]

Figure 11.1 provides a current best estimate of the distribution of work loss among workers with back pain and makes plain that there are two essential patterns: (1) a large majority of sufferers take a little time off work, and (2) a small minority take many days off. Some 67% of workers with LBP episodes return to work within a week, 75% within a fortnight, and 84% within a month; but 10% exceed 60 days and at 6 months about 4% are still absent.

The probability of returning to work is a function of time, as shown in Figure 11.2. The longer a person is off the lower their chance of an eventual return, and at six months this probability falls to 50%. In addition, the curve for those in a recurrent episode of back pain is displaced unfavourably relative to those in their first illness episode.

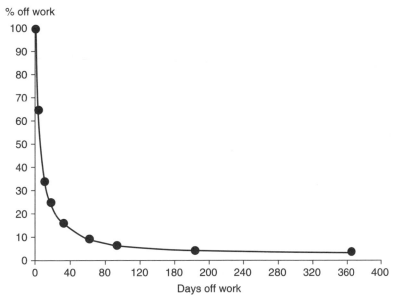

Fig. 11.1 Duration of work loss with back pain (adapted from reference 1 and reproduced under the terms of the click-use licence).

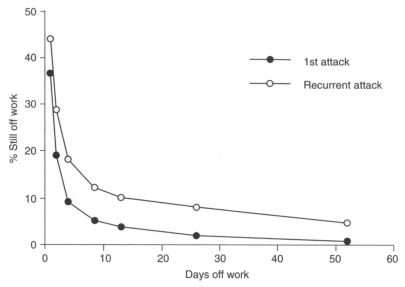

Fig. 11.2 Return to work after a first or recurrent back pain attack (adapted from references 7 and 11).

Possibly Figure 11.2 reflects a natural sorting of people according to the severity of their initial illness; but another widely held interpretation is that lack of work hardiness becomes self-fulfilling. Reduced mobility, lethargy and passivity may have effects on muscle strength and tone that raise the physical effort of work; while long term escape from the responsibilities of work may foster a dependent attitude or erode self-confidence for work. Whatever the reason, these figures and the two-group absence pattern provide a rationale for encouraging an early return to work, with special effort directed towards those in transition from the short-term to the long-term stages. Active intervention at 4–12 weeks is often advocated, as described below.

Time trends

The time trends for disability from LBP in the UK are striking. Between 1978 and 1992 inflation-adjusted expenditure on Sickness and Invalidity Benefits rose 208% (as compared with a rise of 55% for all incapacities) and outpatient attendances for back pain increased fivefold.[1] These changes occurred at a time when the physical demands of work were likely if anything to have lessened. A comparison of two large population surveys a decade apart (1988–1998) found only a small rise in LBP overall with no corresponding rise in functional disability.[8]

These and other observations suggest that experience of disability may be influenced importantly by culture and by prevailing societal beliefs and expectations about health. This idea, which is formalized in the biopsychosocial model of LBP,[7] has been incorporated into management strategies to rehabilitate the affected sufferer, as described below.

Risk factors

Many factors, both occupational and personal, can contribute to the onset and severity of LBP, including age, gender, smoking status, physical fitness, anthropometry and lumbar mobility, strength, psyche and mental well-being, other aspects of medical history, pre-existing spinal abnormalities, and physical demands of work. A complete account of risk factors is beyond the

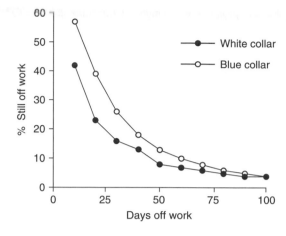

Fig. 11.3 Return to work times in blue- and white-collar workers (adapted from reference 7 with permission from Elsevier © 1998).

scope of this chapter. Moreover, evidence on these is not always consistent and compelling. Interested readers are referred to comprehensive reviews published elsewhere;[9,10] here only a brief overview is given, with focus on aspects that matter in assessing fitness for work.

Rates of back pain vary substantially by industry, occupation and by job title. In general back pain is reported somewhat more often in people with heavy manual occupations, and workers in these jobs tend to lose significantly more time from work during back pain episodes (Figure 11.3).[11]

Certain physical exposures carry a consistently higher risk of reported back pain. These include lifting, forceful movements, exposure to whole-body vibration, and awkward working postures (Table 11.2).[10] In several studies, the combination of adverse physical exposures, like lifting and awkward posture, carries an even higher risk (Table 11.3).[12] However, back pain is common even in white-collar settings and some authorities consider that physical risk factors only account for a small proportion of the observed overall effect.

Psychosocial factors may be important in many cases. In a longitudinal study conducted within the Boeing Company, psychological distress and dissatisfaction with work were the best predictors of new onset LBP over a 4-year follow-up.[13] They proved to be more important than any of the physical risk factors studied, although still not highly predictive. In the Manchester Back Pain Study, people free of back pain but more distressed at baseline were more likely to report a new episode over the next 12 months and more likely to see a doctor;[14] those who were dissatisfied with their work were also more likely to report a new episode. Psychological factors, including

Table 11.2 Evidence for a causal relationship between physical work factors and back pain (adapted from reference[10], p xiii)

Risk factor	Strong evidence (+++)	Evidence (++)	Insufficient evidence (+/0)	Evidence of no affect (–)
Lifting/forceful movement	✓			
Awkward posture		✓		
Heavy physical work		✓		
Whole-body vibration	✓			
Static work posture			✓	

Table 11.3 Estimated relative risk of lumbar disc prolapse according to the posture and method of lifting (Adapted from reference 12 with permission from Elsevier and Kelsey JL *et al*, J Orthop Rse 1984; **2**: 61 with permission from John Wiley & Sons)

Lifting method	Relative risk	95% confidence interval
Avoids lifting with twisted body	1.0	(reference group)
Lifts while twisting body, knees bent	2.7	(0.9–7.9)
Lifts while twisting body, knees straight	6.1	(1.3–27.9)

fear-avoidance beliefs and behaviours, have also been associated with delayed recovery among established cases[15]—these represent risk factors for chronicity and disability.

Assessing back pain and disability

Pain, by definition, is a subjective personal experience. Therefore, assessing its severity against objective benchmarks is an imprecise process. Several formalized clinical and research approaches have been employed.

Simplest is the use of the visual analogue scale. The pain sufferer is asked to make a mark on a line, drawn on a recording sheet and anchored at each end by descriptors such as 'I have no pain at all' and 'my pain is as bad as it could be'. The distance of the mark along the line is measured, and provides a proportionate measure of pain severity, relative to the maximum scale value. This does not circumvent the problem that people's perceptions of pain may differ, but it does offer the opportunity to measure change over time within the same individual.

Other approaches, such as the McGill questionnaire, classify pain by its intensity and a set of adjectives that incorporate the emotional response to pain (throbbing, gnawing, sickening, etc.).

Disability from back pain can be gauged clinically by its interference with activities of daily living–such as sitting, walking, sleeping, and dressing together with more energetic activities. The Low Back Outcome Score is simple to use and is well validated (Table 11.4).[16]

Other well-recognized assessments, such as the Oswestry and Rowland and Morris questionnaires are also, quick, simple, and as robust as more complex approaches to assessing disabling pain.[17]

Another well used, extensively tested, and helpful scale in the occupational health setting is that proposed by Von Korff *et al.*[18] (Table 11.5). This combines elements of intensity, disability, and persistence in one simple grading scale. Some 4.7% of the Canadian adult population report back symptoms that place them at grade IV and 7.2% at grade III.

One *disadvantage* common to all these approaches is their subjective reliance on the patient's own account of affairs. 'Functional Capacity Evaluation (FCE)' aims to provide independent corroboration of impaired performance. Waddell describes several simple, standardized, quick clinical tests that can be used (such as the shuttle walk test, the 'five minutes of walking' test and the 'one minute of stand up' tests); but he cautions that FCEs are only semi-objective. Some, however, have been found in pain management programmes to be good markers of clinical change, which is a useful attraction. More sophisticated machine-based assessments have been used and can produce useful data. But none of these tests is reliable in detecting malingering.

Assessing the worker who presents with low-back pain

As work limitation from LBP is frequent across all groups, most occupational physicians will evaluate patients with current back-associated sickness absence and will need to assess their prognosis and fitness for work. Guidelines from the Faculty of Occupational Medicine emphasize

Table 11.4 The Low Back Outcome Score (maximum score 75) (reprinted from reference 16 with permission from Lippincott, Williams and Wilkins)

Current pain (visual analogue)	0–2	scores	9
	3–4	scores	6
	5–6	scores	3
	7–10	scores	0
Employment	full-time original work		9
	full-time lighter work		6
	part-time		3
	not working—disability		0
Domestic chores/'odd jobs'	normally		9
	most, or all but more slowly		6
	a few but not many		3
	none		0
Sport/active social (dancing)	back to previous level		9
	almost as much as before		6
	some—much less than before		3
	none		0
Resting	no need to rest		6
	little needed, occasionally		4
	about half each day		2
	more than half the day		0
Treatment/consultation	never		6
	rarely		4
	about once a month		2
	more than once a month		0
Analgesia	never		6
	occasionally		4
	almost every day		2
	several times each day		0
Sex life	unaffected		6
	mildly affected		4
	moderately affected/difficult		2
	severely affected/impossible		0
Sleeping	unaffected		3
Walking	mildly affected		2
Sitting	moderately affected/difficult		1
Travelling/dressing	severely affected/impossible		0

Table 11.5 Grading of chronic back pain and disability (after Von Korff et al.[18])

Grade	Degree of disability	Intensity
I	Low	Low
II	Low	High
III	High	Moderately limiting
IV	High	Severely limiting

that occupational physicians have 'a professional duty to support the worker with LBP and should do so whether or not occupational factors play any part in causation'.[19]

Triage assessment and investigation

One aspect of this duty concerns appropriate investigation. Back pain is a symptom and not a diagnosis. However, in an estimated 85% of presentations no underlying pathology can be identified and serious causes are rare. In recent years this has prompted a pragmatic approach to assessment, endorsed in a number of well-respected reports and based on the principles of triage.

Cases of LBP should be classified on the basis of a few simple clinical criteria (Box 11.1)[7] into one of three groups:

1. simple backache; or
2. nerve root compression or irritation; or
3. possible serious spinal pathology (less than 1% of all back pain).

The aim is to identify, among the many, the few requiring urgent investigation; and for the rest to follow a conservative management plan bolstered, if recovery is stalled, by early active rehabilitation. Urgent specialist referral is required only in exceptional circumstances.

Box 11.1 Diagnostic triage in patients presenting with low back pain, with or without sciatica (adapted from reference 7)

Simple backache (90% recover within 6 weeks)

- Presents age 20–55 years
- Lumbosacral area, buttocks, thighs
- Mechanical in nature: varying with activity and with time
- Patient well

Nerve root pain (50% recover within 6 weeks)

- Unilateral leg pain >LBP
- Dermatomal distribution

> **Box 11.1 Diagnostic triage in patients presenting with low back pain, with or without sciatica (adapted from reference 7)** *(continued)*
>
> ## Nerve root pain (50% recover within 6 weeks)—cont'd
>
> - Sensory symptoms in same distribution
> - Straight leg raising reproduces the pain
> - Motor/sensory/reflex change only in one nerve root
>
> ## Red flags: possible serious spinal pathology
>
> - Age at onset <20 or >55 years
> - Violent trauma
> - Constant progressive pain
> - Thoracic pain
> - History of carcinoma, steroid use, drug abuse, or HIV
> - Unwell, weight loss
> - Widespread neurological features
> - Structural deformity
> - Features of cauda equina syndrome (problems of micturition/faecal incontinence; saddle anaesthesia—anus, perineum, genitalia; progressive motor weakness; gait disturbance; sensory level)

The role of investigation is limited. In the presence of so-called 'red flags' (Box 11.1), plain spinal X-rays, a measurement of the erythrocyte sedimentation rate, or a limited series magnetic resonance imaging (MRI) in suspected metastatic disease or infection are indicated. In the absence of worrying features investigation is rarely indicated and in particular, the use of computed tomography and MRI is unwarranted and inadvisable in most situations. Usually the prior probability of serious spinal pathology will be low, and in this situation the positive predictive value of the test will be low, i.e. many image positive findings will give a false indication of serious pathology, with needless attendant costs in resources, distress, and exposure to radiation.

Other issues in assessment

More generally, a review commissioned by the UK Faculty of Occupational Medicine[19] has prompted several specific recommendations for occupational physicians assessing workers with back pain (Box 11.2). This advice follows research evidence highlighting:

- the limited value of examination findings, including height, weight, and lumbar flexibility in predicting the prognosis of non-specific LBP;
- the poor correlation of symptoms and work capacity with X-ray and MRI findings;
- the important role of personal and work-associated psychosocial factors in persistence of symptoms, disability, and response to treatment; and
- the importance of workers' own beliefs and expectations in their capacity for work.

Box 11.2 Guidance from the Faculty of Occupational Medicine on assessing the worker who presents with back pain (adapted from reference 19)

- Screen for red flags and nerve root problems (see Box 11.1)
- Clinical examination otherwise limited in OH management and predicting vocational outcome
- Clinical, disability, and occupational history important, focusing on impact on work and occupational obstacles to recovery and return to work
- Screen for 'yellow flags' (Box 11.3) as markers of developing chronic pain and disability; use this assessment to instigate active case management at an early stage
- X-rays and scans not needed for occupational health management
- Incident LBP that may be work-related should be investigated and advice given on remedial action and the risk assessment

---

The evidence-based review identified several relevant prognostic indicators, including age (over 50 years) and a history of:

- prolonged and severe symptoms;
- radiating leg pain; and
- a poor response to previous therapy.

It recommended that an adequate clinical history should cover these aspects of the history, and collect information about the job—to appreciate its physical demands, the scope for job modification, and the attitudes and concerns of the worker and manager.

Psychosocial 'yellow flags' (Box 11.3), should also be sought. Although imperfect indicators, these denote a higher risk of chronicity and disability, and so their presence may suggest the need for early active case management.

Managing the worker with a fresh episode of low-back pain

The Faculty's review stresses the importance of following current clinical management guidelines. Several such evidence-based guidelines now exist; from these the Faculty selected the model of the Royal College of General Practitioners (RCGP) UK[20] to align occupational health practice with that of primary care. (A comparison with other guidelines is offered below.)

Box 11.3 Psychosocial ('yellow flag') risk factors

Factors that consistently predict poor outcomes:
- Belief that back pain is harmful or severely disabling
- Fear-avoidance behaviour and reduced activities
- Low mood and withdrawal from social interaction
- Passive expectation of help (rather than a belief in self-participation)

Keeping active

A central component of the RCGP guidelines is advice to continue ordinary activities of daily living as normally as possible 'despite the pain'. Many trials indicate that this approach can give equivalent or faster symptomatic recovery from acute symptoms, and leads to shorter periods of work loss, fewer occurrences, and less sickness absence over the following year than advice to rest until completely pain free.[19]

This advice is captured in a user-friendly way in *The Back Book*,[21] an evidence-based booklet developed in conjunction with the RCGP clinical guidelines (Box 11.4). This is a valuable hand-out to patients. Details on its availability are provided at the end of the chapter.

Keeping active at work

Continuation of ordinary activities implies encouraging the worker to remain in his or her job, or to return to it at an early stage, *even if this still results in some LBP*. Direct evidence that this hastens rehabilitation is limited for the occupational setting (in contrast to primary care and community research), but the same general principles are thought to apply.

Box 11.4 Extracts from *The Back Book*,[21]* which aims to promote self-coping in sufferers through positive evidence-based messages

Back facts:

◆ … back pain need **not** cripple you unless you let it!
  Causes of back pain:

◆ … it is surprisingly difficult to damage your spine

◆ … back pain is usually not due to anything serious

Rest vs. active exercise:

◆ … bed rest is bad for backs

◆ … exercise is good for you–use it or lose it

Copers suffer less [than avoiders] at the time and they are healthier in the long run. To be a coper and prevent unnecessary suffering:

◆ Live life as normally as possible …

◆ Keep up daily activities …

◆ Try to stay fit …

◆ Start gradually and do a little more each day …

◆ Either stay at work or go back to work as soon as possible …

◆ Be patient …

◆ Don't worry …

◆ Don't listen to other people's horror stories …

◆ Don't get gloomy on down days …

*The Back Book is available from The Stationery Office, St Crispins, Duke Street, Norwich NR3 1PD or bookshops (ISBN 0–11–702078–8).

Most workers are able to follow this advice and remain at work or return to it within a few days or weeks. In some situations a return to full normal duties may not be possible—as when work requires exceptional levels of physical fitness (e.g. emergency rescue or military combat duties) or unavoidable manual handling of heavy loads. But such circumstances should be unusual. The Manual Handling Regulations require heavy physical tasks to be avoided or minimized, generally, by adaptation of the work and the provision of lifting aids. Guidance that accompanies the Manual Handling Regulations suggests ways in which lighter duties can be constructed.[22,23]

Any prolonged period off work raises the chance that symptoms will become chronic. It is preferable to find or devise temporary light duties or an adapted pattern of work to encourage uninterrupted employment, and the earliest possible resumption of normal duties should be encouraged.

Doctors and managers commonly employ work restrictions in returning patients with LBP to the occupational environment. Evidence for their effectiveness is, however, rather poor. In 2003, Hiebert *et al.* reported a retrospective cohort study of patients who experienced some absence from work because of LBP.[24] In this group 43% were provided with work restrictions. For a fifth of these workers restrictions were never lifted. Restricted duties did not reduce the incidence or duration of sickness absence and no significant reduction was observed in injury recurrence.

The advice given by health professionals is of critical importance. A recommendation to stay off work is often made on the basis of little or no evidence, but can seriously impair the prognosis.[25] In 1994 Hall *et al.* reported the results of a conservative treatment programme for LBP.[25]

Proper communication between the affected worker, the occupational health team and line managers, and a shared understanding of the rehabilitation goal are 'fundamental for improvement in clinical and occupational health outcomes'.[19] An organizational culture that secures high stakeholder commitment may also reduce absenteeism and duration of work loss.

Managing the worker who still has problems after 1–3 months

A worker with LBP who is still having difficulty in returning to normal occupational duties at 1–3 months has a 10–40% risk of still being absent at 1 year. By the time 6 months has passed, the risk is higher still. Thus a need exists to identify workers off work with LBP before chronicity sets in. Intervention after 4 weeks is more effective than treatment received much later, and a surveillance system should be established to identify and assess absence of this degree.

Active rehabilitation

At the subacute stage an active rehabilitation programme is needed. There is strong empirical evidence that intervention works and is cost-effective.[26,27] The optimum content of such a programme is not so clearly defined by research evidence, although certain premises are largely established:[19]

- the most effective rehabilitation programmes include a progressive increase in the amount of exercise to build physical fitness (the precise *type* of exercise seems less critical);
- they are based on behavioural principles of pain management;
- education on back care that uses the biomedical injury model is less effective than advice aimed at overcoming fear-avoidance and dependency behaviours. Further guidance is given elsewhere.

Pre-placement assessment

A past history of symptoms should not be regarded as a reason for denying employment in most circumstances.

Caution should be exercised in placing individuals with a history of severely disabling LBP in physically demanding jobs; but the correct course of action involves a value judgement. Intuitively it may seem obvious that individuals at higher recurrence risk should not be placed in jobs of high physical demand. Unfortunately, this logic has two problems—that of predicting future risk accurately enough, and that of distinguishing recurrence risk in a specific job from recurrence risk in any job (or no job). According to the HSE, the evidence base for matching individual susceptibility to a job-specific risk assessment is insufficient at present to achieve reliable health-base selection. Waddell *et al.* warn that such judgements carry 'substantial personal, societal, legal, and political implications'.[19]

Investigations and clinical tests

Traditional clinical investigations do little to inform the decision of job placement. The Faculty's evidence review[19] highlighted that future disability from LBP among job applicants is not predicted at all well by:

- examination findings (e.g. height, weight, lumbar flexibility, straight leg raising)
- general cardiorespiratory fitness
- isometric, isokinetic, or isoinertial measurements of back function
- X-ray and MRI findings.

Symptom-free applicants with single 'yellow flag' histories (Box 11.3) are at a somewhat greater risk of incident LBP, but not to an extent that justifies exclusion.

Collectively these observations suggest a limited role for pre-placement health screening—perhaps just to avoiding the very worst of mismatches between physical demands and back pain history.

Other guidelines

Emphasis has been given in this account on the Faculty's occupational health management guidelines for LBP, but it is instructive to compare these with other sources of advice. Several have been published, including a Canadian version from the Quebec Task Force,[28] an Australian one by the Victorian Workcover Authority,[29] and also reports from the ACC/National Advisory Committee on Health Disability, New Zealand;[30] and a working group of occupational physicians in the Netherlands.[31] Other statements have been prepared by the Agency for Healthcare Policy and Research,[32] the Institute for Clinical Systems Integration,[33] and the Preventive Services Task Force[34] in the USA; and the CSAG in the UK.[35]

Generally these agree on:

- the need for diagnostic triage, screening for red flags and neurological complications;
- the identification of potential psychosocial and workplace barriers to recovery; and
- advice to remain at work or to return to work at an early stage, with modified duties as necessary.

Within this broad framework some variations exist, as reviewed by Staal *et al.*[36] In particular, a few guidelines are more aggressive in their advice on referral, investigation and early intervention. Thus, according to the Quebec Task Force, a referral to a musculoskeletal specialist should occur after 6 weeks of absence; the US guidelines advocate X-ray examination if symptoms fail to improve over 4 weeks; and the US and Dutch guidelines both propose a graded activity programme after 2 weeks of work absence.

None of the guidelines provide a blueprint for implementation. But one clear message that has emerged from public health campaigns in Scotland and Australia is that patient views can be beneficially changed when a single consistent message, along the lines of *The Back Book*, is given by the media and healthcare professionals.

Prevention and risk management

Success in preventing spinal disorders depends upon an informed assessment of risk, and a package of risk reduction measures, underpinned by suitable management systems for monitoring and enforcement. A similar approach can help the affected worker to return to work.

A number of preventive measures may have value:

1. Training, to ensure a higher risk awareness and better working practices.

2. An induction period, to allow workers in unfamiliar roles to start out at a slower pace.

3. Job rotation and rest breaks, to avoid repetitive monotonous use of the same muscles, tendons and joints.

4. A programme of phased reintroduction to normal work, with temporarily lighter duties or shortened working hours, after sickness absence with LBP.

5. Task optimization, e.g. work reorganization to minimize the carrying load, improve the height from which loads are lifted, avoid awkward lifting and twisting, and replace manual handling by employing lifting aids instead.

Some excellent guidelines and nice case studies from the HSE illustrate this last approach.[22,23]

The case that such job modifications prevent back problems is intuitive and firmly rooted in ergonomic theory. It is also suggested by the research that identifies materials handling as a risk factor for LBP. But the evidence that well-designed workplace and job changes prevent LBP in practice is less clear-cut. Some interventions have not proved successful. In part this could reflect the difficulty of conducting well controlled randomized trials in the occupational health setting, or of implementing change effectively; but another view, favoured by some academics, is that the scope for preventing disability from LBP is limited, as it has other major non-physical explanations.

However, some well conducted studies have shown a clear benefit. For example, Evanoff *et al.* examined injury and lost workday rates before and after the introduction of mechanical lifts in acute care hospitals and long-term care facilities.[37] In the postintervention period rates of musculoskeletal injuries, mainly LBP, decreased by 28%, lost workday injuries by 44%, and total lost days due to injury 58%.

In practice, ergonomic theory is likely to hold, at least to the extent that some tasks will aggravate pre-existing and current LBP and hinder the goal of remaining at work. Also in practice, there is a legal mandate to assess risks from manual handling and to minimize unnecessary exposures within reasonable bounds; and simple ergonomic adjustments are likely to be construed as 'reasonable adjustments' within the scope of the Disability Discrimination Act for workers with serious back problems.

Neck pain

Prevalence and natural history

By any measure, neck pain is also common in the general population. Depending on precise definition, its lifetime prevalence in adults ranges from 26% to 71%,[38–40] the prevalence of symptoms in the past year varies from 12% to 34%, and the point prevalence (frequency of current pain) lies between 10% and 22%. In a British population survey involving nearly 13 000 adults of working age, 34% recounted neck pain in the past 12 months, 11% reported neck pain that had interfered with their normal activities over this period, and 20% had had symptoms in the past 7 days.[41]

Like back pain, neck pain is often persistent as some 14–19% of subjects report symptoms lasting longer than 6 months in the previous year. Also like back pain, it is commonly recurrent and a source of disability.

Occupational and personal risk factors

Occupational activities are sometimes blamed as a cause of neck pain. One systematic review concluded there was 'some evidence' for a relation with neck flexion, arm force, arm posture, duration of sitting, twisting or bending, hand–arm vibration, and workplace design.[42] In a second authoritative review, the US National Institute of Occupational Health concluded that there was 'strong evidence' for an association with static loading of the neck–shoulder musculature at work, and 'suggestive evidence' of risks from continuous arm and hand movements and forceful work involving the same muscle groups.[10] A recent longitudinal survey that made detailed video recordings of posture found a quantitative relation between having a bent and flexed neck for much of the working day and neck pain.[43]

This evidence has accrued from industry, among rather few occupations. In community samples the findings have been less consistent. For example, in Finland, the risk of chronic neck pain was higher in agricultural and industrial workers than in professionals[38] but the opposite was true in a survey of Hong Kong Chinese;[39] in another Finnish study, blue-collar and white-collar workers showed no clear-cut differences;[40] and in a UK population survey, no strong associations were found between occupational physical risk factors and neck pain.[41]

Psychosocial factors show a consistent relation to neck pain—in workplaces, in populations, and in patient clinics. Personal feelings of stress and tiredness, and occupational psychosocial stressors, like high work pressures and low job control, are both relevant. In many respects the situation parallels that of LBP, especially when symptoms are non-specific and unrelated to trauma or serious local pathology.

Assessing and managing the patient with neck pain

Several clinical features predict sickness absence among workers consulting medical services with neck pain. These include short duration, high intensity of pain, report of continuous pain, and certain physical signs (pain in the upper limb during rotation of head and pain in the shoulder during abduction of arm).[44] As might be expected, previous sickness absence attributed to neck pain is also predictive of future absence spells from this cause.[45]

Further investigations (e.g. radiology and MRI) are not indicated, except in rare circumstances. Changes of osteoarthritis will often be found, but the correlation between symptoms and X-ray appearance is inconsistent, and the predictive performance of such tests for future incapacity is generally low.

Guidelines on managing neck pain are at a less developed stage than those on managing LBP. In principle, and by analogy, the optimal approach should be similar to that for LBP: initial assessment by triage, followed for simple mechanical neck pain by advice to maintain activity and coping within the limits of pain. However, direct evidence on this is limited.

Complex versions of such advice have been embedded in programmes of multidisciplinary biopsychosocial rehabilitation; but a recent systematic Cochrane review found no good evidence to justify the effort. Specific exercise programmes, involving strength and endurance training, muscle training, stretching, and relaxation are also of uncertain benefit. Thus, strength and endurance training decreased pain and disability in women with chronic neck problems in one high profile trial, where stretching did not;[46] but in another major randomized trial, dynamic muscle and relaxation training did not lead to better relief or recovery than continuation of ordinary activity.[47]

Perhaps the best that can be said at present is that most neck pain, like most LBP, does not have a serious underlying cause; that triage is a means of identifying the few cases needing further investigation; that such investigations will rarely aid fitness assessment in the occupational health setting; and that simple symptomatic relief and advice to remain active is a sensible pragmatic approach, likely in most cases to be followed by an early return to work. Jobs that require workers to crane and twist their necks to an unusual degree (for example to inspect overhead electrical equipment in a confined space) and those that require full neck movements to ensure unrestricted field of view in safety critical situations may be ones in which a temporary fitness restriction will be required.

Spinal surgery

Although back and neck pain episodes are frequent, few patients require surgery. None the less, a small minority undergo such procedures. In this chapter it is not possible to consider every conceivable surgical procedure to the spine, but the most common ones will be addressed.

Surgery for lumbar nerve root compression

The commonest indication for surgery in the lumbar spine is neurological compression, which has two common causes—prolapsed intervertebral disc (PID) and spinal stenosis.

The management of the patient with lumbar neurological compression starts with a clear definition of sciatica. Pain radiating into the leg and foot cannot be considered sciatica unless evidence of neurological dysfunction is also present. It is almost 70 years since Kellgren, working in University College, London, elegantly demonstrated that referred pain from the back can produce a typical dermatomal pattern in the leg.[48] He injected hypertonic saline into the supraspinous ligament and described referral patterns exactly mimicking dermatomal distribution. It is clear, therefore, that *the commonly held belief that referred pain from the back does not radiate below the knee is false.* To diagnose sciatica, in addition to pain radiating in a dermatomal distribution, some corresponding sensory or motor symptoms and signs must be present.

Asymptomatic disc prolapse can be found in some 20–30% of subjects of working age on MRI scans.[49,50] The unfortunate patient with a referred pain into the leg and a coincidental asymptomatic disc prolapse on an ill advised MRI scan is obviously at risk of unnecessary and ineffective surgical treatment.

Prolapsed lumbar intervertebral disc

The commonest cause of nerve root compression in patients of working age is PID. Although the lifetime prevalence of sciatica from any aetiology is high, at some 40%, the lifetime prevalence of symptomatic lumbar disc herniation is considerably smaller, at 3–4% and only 1% of patients with acute LBP have nerve root symptoms. The one-year incidence of symptomatic PID lies between 0.1% and 0.5%.[51] Most cases occur at about 40 years of age. Symptoms are equally common in men and women, although men come to surgery 1.5–2 times more often.

So far as aetiology is concerned genetic issues appear to be of greater importance than mechanical loading.[52] Physical factors, flexion, rotation and whole-body vibration appear to play some role but the effect is not large.

Conservative management

As for LBP as a whole, most cases of PID resolve spontaneously. Initial back pain is usually followed by a dominating leg pain together with some neurological symptoms and signs. Leg pain will then tend to improve and approximately 90% of sufferers will experience spontaneous resolution.

In his seminal paper Weber[53] found that in patients with radiologically proven disc prolapse, during initial conservative management 70% reported decreased pain and 60% had returned to work within 4 weeks. Further, on long-term (10 years) follow-up they were able to show that patients with good long-term results with conservative therapy had demonstrated significant improvement within 3 months of onset. A Danish Study reported similarly that 75% of patients were able to resume activities within 28 days. Between 50 and 70% of conservatively treated cases will resolve completely.[54,55] The natural history of PID is favourable, irrespective of the size or location of the prolapse radiologically. Thus, conservative management is usually appropriate.

Following a first attack of sciatica, some 5% of subjects will experience a recurrence. Following a second attack, the incidence of recurrence rises further to some 20–30%, and following the third or subsequent attack recurrences occur in some 70% of patients (G Findlay, Personal Communication).

Conservative management still requires an active plan. The acute effects of prolapse and the enforced rest lead to significant muscular atrophy. Thus, it is important that normal activity is resumed or increased as soon as pain allows and not left until the pain settles completely. *The Back Book*,[21] although principally directed at mechanical back pain, is a valuable resource for patients with acute disc prolapse.

As pain settles, *in addition to* resumption of normal activities patients should be advised to undertake progressive maintenance exercises to promote muscle endurance and strength (Figure 11.4).[56]

In the management of the acute phase effective relief of pain is a vital consideration, as this will allow mobilization and resumption of activities at an earlier stage. There is little evidence available concerning the return to work following an acute disc prolapse.

There is no evidence that resumption of work activities is harmful or capable of precipitating a relapse of symptoms, any more than other normal activities. An analogy can be drawn with post-operative cases where Carragee *et al.* found that 97% of cases had returned to work by 8 weeks without any increased risk of recurrent disc prolapse or other complications.[57]

Most patients who avoid activity do so because of pain, fear, and negative advice. The key messages, as with simple LBP in the absence PID, are first that the more rapid the resumption of normal activities the better the overall prognosis and secondly that each incremental increase in

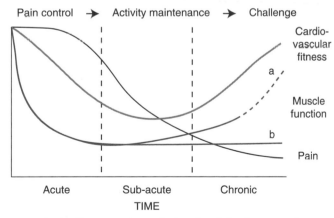

Fig. 11.4 Time course of pain, fitness, and muscle function following acute intervertebral disc prolapse. Failure to rehabilitate after the acute stage will result in ongoing decompensation (b) instead of return to normal back function (a).

Table 11.6 The 'Rule of Five' Modified from McCulloch and Macnab,[58] with permission from Lippincott, Williams and Wilkins

2 Symptoms	1 Leg pain, greater than back pain
	2 Specific neurological symptoms (paraesthesia)
2 Signs	3 Straight leg raising < 50% of normal and/or positive crossover test and/or positive bowstring test
	4 Two of four neurological signs (altered reflex, wasting, weakness, sensory loss)
1 Investigation	5 Positive concordant imaging

activity may cause a temporary increase in discomfort. The patient can be reassured that this is not dangerous. If the patient has not had any active management by 6 weeks, then involvement of an occupational health physiotherapist for advice, encouragement, and gentle mobilization is probably indicated. Occupational health services may promote such activities.

Surgical management

The major certain indication for surgery is worsening neurological deficit. In the absence of profound motor deficit, there is little indication for operative intervention within the first 6 weeks of symptoms. Even in patients with neurological deficit, improvement of sensory loss is unusual following surgery; so the main benefit is in pain relief where present.

Disc excision surgery is normally planned at a more considered pace. The criteria of Macnab or 'the Rule of Five'[58] have withstood the test of time as indications for such surgery (Table 11.6).

Surgery is more successful in relieving leg pain than back pain. Careful examination is required to confirm the presence of neurological deficit and sciatic tension signs according to Macnab's criteria. Muscle spasm and spinal tilt are less informative.

There has been a trend to admit surgical cases for shorter and shorter periods. Some surgeons now undertake microdiscectomy and fenestration and discectomy without a microscope on a day case basis. In a prospective randomized controlled trial[59] this led to a satisfactory outcome in terms of mobility, day time hours spent in bed on the first postoperative day and walking distance at 2 weeks; patients' views on the length of stay were good, and no increase in complications was noted, suggesting that such conventional procedures can be safely and beneficially undertaken as daycare cases.

The postoperative management of patients undergoing surgical treatment for PID is also changing. Fear of recurrence, re-injury or instability lead in the past to postoperative protocols that restricted activity. However, a study by Carragee et al.[57] has indicated that such restrictions may not be necessary. In this study patients were allowed to determine their own levels of activity postoperatively; or were urged to return to full activity as soon as possible. The mean time from surgery to return to work was 1.7 weeks and 25% of patients returned to work the following day; 97% of those working at the time of surgery returned to full duty by 8 weeks. At 2 years no patient had changed employment because of back or leg pain. Recurrent disc prolapse occurred in 6% (three patients) of whom one required surgical intervention. Thus when freed from restrictions imposed by healthcare professionals, patients returned to activities and work much more rapidly and in apparent safety. Magnusson et al.[60] have found no rational basis for lifting (manual handling) restrictions after lumbar spine surgery. In a recent review of rehabilitation after lumbar disc surgery, Ostelo et al.[61] found strong evidence that intensive exercise programmes commencing 4–6 weeks following surgery were more effective in improving functional status and produced a faster return to work as compared with mild exercise programmes.

Lumbar spinal stenosis

Spinal stenosis is usually a result of degenerative change, and as such occurs more often in older people. It is unusual before the age of 50. The commonest symptom is neurogenic claudication. Patients report pain in the legs which comes on and becomes worse during walking. This may be accompanied by symptoms of paraesthesia in the leg or even in the perineum. Eventually the patient is forced to stop both by pain and feelings of weakness in the legs. The cause of symptoms appears to be a restriction of blood flow to the cauda equina and nerve roots owing to venous obstruction by canal narrowing either centrally or in the intervertebral canal. Forward flexion of the lumbar region opens up the intervertebral canals and central canal and explains the typical simian gait these patients adopt being increasingly flexed on walking. After stopping, the symptoms gradually settle and settle more rapidly for a patient able to sit and flex the lumbar spine. Resolution of symptoms may take 5 minutes or so, and clinically this is a key discriminator from arterial claudication (where the recovery time is substantially less).

Clinical examination at rest may reveal no neurological abnormalities, although evidence of subtle weakness is present in some 50%. The diminution of ankle jerks is reported in a similar proportion of patients.

Because walking up an incline induces some lumbar flexion, total walking time on an upward incline is longer than walking on the flat. Similarly patients perform better on bicycle testing than on walking.

Conservative management

Non-surgical treatments include the use of non-steroidal anti-inflammatory drugs, prescribed to reduce swelling and inflammatory changes in degenerative joints, and also for their analgesic effect. However, clear evidence of effectiveness in neurogenic claudication is not available. Calcitonin, which demonstrated some effect in some studies,[62,63] may operate by a central analgesic effect, through improvement of the cauda equina blood flow, or through an anti-inflammatory effect. Calcitonin is more effective in patients with spinal Paget's disease. Recently, a randomized controlled trial of nasal calcitonin has demonstrated no effect over placebo.[64] Calcitonin in parenteral administration has not gained widespread use in neurogenic claudication. Epidural steroid injections have been used with positive results.[65] Such injections may provide relief for up to 10 months.

Surgical management

Onset of urinary or faecal incontinence is an indication for urgent assessment and operation. Otherwise, surgery for spinal stenosis is dictated by the severity of symptoms.

In 1992 Turner et al.[66] undertook a review of 74 articles reporting the outcome of surgery of spinal stenosis. Some two-thirds of patients had good to excellent results (although some were worse at follow-up). A similar proportion returned to their normal work and a further 12% were able to undertake work of some type. Allowing for those not in the workforce, some 80% of patients in work at presentation were able to resume working following surgery.

There is little agreement on the optimum postoperative regimen, or indeed on the optimum time for return to work duties. However, it would seem reasonable to plan a graduated return to work as a integral part of postoperative rehabilitation.

Surgery for low back pain

A number of procedures exist for the surgical management of LBP, of which the most common is spinal fusion. More recently there has been great interest in total disc replacement.

Spinal fusion

Spinal fusion is the gold standard against which other surgical procedures for managing of LBP are judged. However, it is important to appreciate that only a tiny fraction of patients presenting with LBP require surgery. Spinal fusion is a major operation, with success critically dependent on good patient selection. It may be appropriate in patients with chronic symptoms and significant disability, but the patient should already have undergone and failed a formal multidisciplinary intensive functional restoration programme (and not simply physiotherapy). Psychological distress and compensation claims are recognized predictors of inferior results.

Recently, a number of randomized controlled studies have enabled the utility of spinal fusion to be placed in context. In Sweden a prospective randomized controlled trial demonstrated significant improvement in pain reduction, disability and return to work in surgical patients compared with conservatively treated controls. The net return to work of surgical patients was 36% compared with 13% for conservatively managed patients.[67] In the UK a prospective randomized study of almost 350 patients found that an intensive multidisciplinary programme was equally as effective as spinal surgical stabilization, although both groups achieved a mean reduction in Oswestry Score of 11 points, identical to that of the surgically treated patients in the Swedish Study.[68] Similarly, a Norwegian study[69] demonstrated no significant difference between fusion surgery and an intense multidisciplinary programme based on cognitive principles. Again, the Oswestry reduction was between 12 and 15 points. Greenough et al.[70] demonstrated that anterior fusion was more successful in returning patients to work than instrumented posterolateral fusion (50% vs. 25%).

It is clear, therefore, that some chronic back pain patients in whom work restoration is unlikely with conservative treatment may be returned to work by fusion surgery and, moreover, that fusion surgery itself is not a contraindication to employment.

Most surgeons prefer to restrict vigorous activities until bony fusion has been achieved radiologically, a process taking 3–6 months. However, postoperative regimens vary considerably without apparent justification.

Total disc replacement

The indications for total disc replacement are similar to those for spinal fusion. Disc replacement has several advantages, including immediate stability (which allows early mobilization), preservation of motion (which may reduce degeneration at adjacent levels), and the avoidance of bone harvesting from donor sites. Potential disadvantages include displacement, long-term wear of the prosthesis, and the difficulties and complications of revision.

In 2003, de Kleuver et al.[71] noted in a review of nine case series comprising 564 disc replacements that good or excellent results were reported in between 50% and 81% of patients. The criteria for assessment of 'good' or 'excellent' varied from study to study and no overall comment was made on work capacity. But one study of 93 patients found that 31% of patients not working prior to surgery were able to return to work, whereas 20% of those working prior to surgery were not working at follow-up.

In 1999, Zeegers[72] reported on 50 patients of whom 43% returned to their usual occupation and 81% returned to some form of work.

Policies on postoperative rehabilitation vary considerably, and there is no consensus on optimum care. However, vigorous mobilization may be permitted at an earlier stage than for spinal fusion, as the fixation of the prosthesis is completed at the time of surgery. Return to work may thus be accelerated.

The cervical spine

Surgery to the cervical spine, like the lumbar and thoracic spine, may be indicated for neurological compression or, more rarely, for cervical pain.

Radicular compression by cervical disc herniation will produce pain and neurological dysfunction in the distribution of the affected nerve root. Like sciatica, neurological compression may be differentiated from referred cervical pain by finding a specific nerve dysfunction. The natural history of cervical disc prolapse is reported as being less benign than for the lumbar region. Up to half of patients treated conservatively continue to experience some radicular pain between 2 and 19 years follow-up.[73] For those patients with insufficient relief from conservative measures, surgery may be considered. Various techniques exist for surgical management of cervical disc prolapse, including anterior discectomy alone, to anterior discectomy with fusion, anterior discectomy with fusion and instrumentation, and more recently, discectomy with total cervical disc replacement. About 70% of patients have a good functional result following discectomy, whether or not fusion is employed. Postoperatively if no instrumentation is employed, a hard collar is worn for some 2 months, until radiological fusion is observed. The patient is mobilized thereafter.

As in the lumbar spine, postoperative management varies considerably between surgeons and there are no evidence-based reports to guide rehabilitation. It is possible the trend of shortened rehabilitation times and less time off work that has been observed following lumbar surgery, will be mirrored in future among patients undergoing cervical surgery.

Other spinal conditions

Ankylosing spondylitis (AS)

AS classically presents with an inflammatory onset and involves the sacroiliac and spinal joints. Most commonly, symptoms present in the fourth decade; they are unusual after 40 and rare after 50 years of age. Clinically, the pain is relieved by exercise and not relieved by rest, lumbar spine movement is limited and chest expansion is decreased. Early morning stiffness taking some time to wear off is frequently observed. Of the peripheral joints, the hip and the shoulder are most commonly affected.

Management relies on analgesics, non-steroidal anti-inflammatory drugs and disease-modifying antirheumatic drugs. Physiotherapy, particularly hydrotherapy, is clinically effective, although no well-controlled studies have proven its benefit. In the later stages of the disease, where ankylosis is established, pain is a less significant feature.

The National Ankylosing Spondylitis Society (NASS) comments that 'most people with AS are motivated and reported to have less time off work than average, mostly remaining in full time employment'[74] and evidence exists of this. None the less, AS has an impact on functional work capacity. A study by Boonen et al.[75] found that work disability and incapacity increased steadily with duration of disease. Sick leave was found to vary from 12 to 46 days per year. Work disability was noted to increase from 3% at 5 years of disease duration up to 50% at 45 years. After 5 years, 96% of patients retained employment, but at 45 years only 45% remained in work.

Possibly, the difficulties are greater for manual workers. The same research team found that among those with manual jobs there was a higher risk of quitting work with disability (relative risk 2.3, 95% confidence interval 1.5–3.4) than those with a non-manual job.[76] When compared with the general population the risk was 4.9 (3.5–5.9) for manual workers against 2.2 (1.6–2.7) for non-manual workers.

When at work, sufferers are advised by NASS[74] to avoid needless forward bending and to regularly change position. Prolonged car driving may increase pain and stiffness. Patients with rigid or stiff necks may be at greater risk in the event of driving accidents, and the car should be fitted with correctly adjusted head-restraints. Disease of mild severity will not preclude vocational driving, although this may not represent the best career choice in the longer-term. Workers with a rigid neck or severe peripheral joint involvement may be unfit to drive vocationally and need to inform the DVLA of their functional limitations.

Patients with AS are at risk of fracture following minor trauma. Failure to recognize such a fracture may lead to a progressive deformity, and on occasion to paralysis. Persistent localized pain in a patient with AS following trauma should be investigated with MRI scanning. In the ankylosed spine surgical fixation is frequently required to obtain satisfactory union.

About 6% of patients with AS require a hip replacement, which normally restores mobility and relieves pain. The work restrictions that ensue do not differ from those described elsewhere (see Chapter 12), although patients tend to be younger than normal for this surgical procedure.

Rarely, in poorly managed and advanced cases of AS, extreme spinal curvature may occur, limiting normal mobility, posture, and vision. In rare cases surgery is employed to straighten the spine and improve the posture.

Other peripheral complications of AS arise sometimes, the most common being uveitis. Further comments on work limitations can be found in the Chapter 13.

Scheuermann's disease

Scheuermann's disease is a kyphotic deformity developing in early adolescence. Estimates of its prevalence vary from 0.4% to 8% in the general population. The kyphosis is usually noticed clinically, but the diagnosis is radiological with the observation of end plate irregularities, disc space narrowing, and wedging of a minimum of three adjacent vertebrae. These definitions are important as irregularities of the vertebral end plates are common. For example, Fredenhagen[77] found abnormalities in 25–40% of Swiss Army Recruits, and Baud found some end plate irregularities in 60% of school children aged 14 years. There is evidence of a familial tendency. The process is an abnormality of the growth plate and the active process is terminated at the completion of growth.

Scheuermann's disease can produce a significant kyphosis, normally in the thoracic and thoracolumbar region of the spine. This is associated with a compensatory lumbar lordosis. Although it does have an impact on long-term pain and activity, this is perhaps less than has been generally supposed.

In general a history of Scheuermann's disease does not suggest the need for job restrictions or adapted work.

In 1993 Murray et al.[78] published long-term follow-up of 67 patients with a mean kyphosis of 71°. At an average of 32 years following diagnosis, back pain was more common and, in general, patients had taken up work with lower physical demands. However, the number of days absent from work because of back pain, the interference of pain with activities of daily living, self-consciousness, social limitations, level of recreational activities or the use of medication for back pain were not different from the normal population. The magnitude of the spinal curvature had an association with pain, but not with loss of time from work.

Osteochondritis of the spine resulting in end plate irregularities but not meeting the strict definition of Scheuermann's disease is now more commonly recognized and, represents a spectrum, with careful examination of plain radiographs revealing some abnormalities in up to 60% of the population. It is unlikely that such lesions will cause greater absence from work than for Scheuermann's disease, or impose any special fitness dilemmas.

Fractures

The thoracolumbar spine

Fractures in the thoracolumbar spine have been classified in several ways. For the current discussion a simple classification according to the method of Denis is probably the most helpful. Denis divided the spine into three conceptual columns: anterior (anterior body wall and vertebral body), middle (essentially the posterior body wall) and posterior (the posterior elements). Fractures of the anterior column are principally wedge compression fractures and are generally stable. Fractures of both anterior and middle column are often referred to as burst fractures.

Most single column and some two-column injuries are treated conservatively. In general the outcome is very satisfactory. Aglietti et al.[79] have published outcome data on the largest series of conservatively treated fractures. Two hundred and twenty patients were included. Two-thirds were men and half were employed in heavy manual labour. Forty per cent were treated in hyper-extension brace and the remainder in plaster jackets. At follow-up (which occurred about 9 years later) one-third were pain free, 8.5% were restricted at work because of pain, and 82% had returned to their previous employment (at an average of 6 months postinjury). Fifteen per cent had changed jobs and 3% had become chronic invalids. Job retention was poorer in those claiming compensation.

Burst fractures treated conservatively also have good results. A follow-up by Weinstein et al.[80] found that 90% of patients were able to return to their pre-injury occupation. Only 10% were completely pain-free, but the others reported only minimal or mild back pain. Burst fractures may also be treated surgically with the provision of internal fixation. Patients with some neurological deficit are more likely to undergo surgery, although a recent meta-analysis[81] demonstrated that there was no evidence that decompression of the neural elements improved neurological outcome.

Overall the long-term outcome of burst fractures treated surgically does not appear to be substantially different to those treated conservatively, although provision of immediate stabilization reduces immediate pain.

Vertebral fractures occur in cancellous bone and may be expected to heal within 3–4 months. After this period more vigorous activities should be encouraged and work return considered. Surgically treated patients with bone grafting take longer to consolidate but return with restrictions on lifting may be contemplated.

The cervical spine

The recovery from a cervical fracture is most heavily influenced by the occurrence of any concomitant spinal cord injury. If any significant cord deficit is present then the prognosis is that of the cord injury, the cervical fracture itself will normally unite and any long-term local sequelae are overshadowed by cord deficit itself. The following consideration applies to cervical injuries without neurological deficit.

Atlanto-axial injuries are normally treated conservatively with halo jacket or occasionally by surgical fixation. Satisfactory union is usual and the results of management are good. Approximately 12% of patients will report long-term pain.

In the subaxial region fractures are commonly managed conservatively with a halo vest and union rates of 90–95% are recorded. Long-term symptoms are more prominent with residual kyphosis of more than 20°. Fracture dislocations may be reduced by traction, or in some cases surgically. Following reduction, management may be continued with a halo vest but surgery is often undertaken to add stability and to promote fusion of the injured motion segment, especially for the mid-cervical region. Reduction of the fracture–dislocation is important. Seven of 10 patients with untreated dislocation have disabling pain. In reduced cases long-term symptoms are more common in conservatively managed patients. Following fracture mobilization may be vigorously commenced once bony union has been obtained, after 8–12 weeks. Again postoperative management and recommendations to return to work vary quite a lot from surgeon to surgeon.

Spinal cord injury

Injury to the spinal cord, including major injury to the cauda equina, is fortunately rare with an incidence of 20–30 per million per year in the UK. In the past paraplegia predominated but tetraplegia and paraplegia are now equally common. The age of injured patients is also increasing.

Functional independence is principally determined by the level of neurological injury. In addition to the motor function, the other main determinants of work capacity are the effects of the cord injury on bladder and bowel function, and the patient's vulnerability to pressure sores.

In general the UK has a poor record of returning patients with spinal cord injuries to work. Overall just 14% are in employment, as compared with a European average of 38% and almost 50% in the USA. This substantial underperformance is likely to be a combination of poor expectations, set up in the spinal cord injury centres, poor expectations in the field of occupational health, and inadequate response from employers.

The Disability Discrimination Act requires reasonable adjustments by employers to accommodate those with spinal cord injuries—including proper, and sometimes adapted, access to the place of work (e.g. ramps, widened doorways, a ground floor work station or access to a lift, special parking rights) and other reasonable assistance (e.g. choosing a job and work schedule to suit the worker's capability, reasonable time off for medical care, adjustments to the work station). Other than access, the most significant practical factor in returning to work is a toilet facility that has enough space and privacy for bladder and bowel management. Indwelling catheters are now used much less often than in the past, so facilities are needed to allow self-catheterization.

Many cord-injured patients will require some degree of retraining to re-enter the workforce. Advisors from the Spinal Cord Injuries Centre, the Disability Employment Advisors, together with employers and other training services and educational institutions will be involved and these efforts must be co-ordinated. The best predictors of return to work are, however, related to the individual, and include: previous employment, previous attitudes to work, job mobility, maturity, and verbal ability.

Despite the provisions of the Disability Discrimination Act spinal cord injury remains an area where patients in the UK are being significantly failed at present by the work rehabilitation process.

References

1 Clinical Standards Advisory Group. *Epidemiology review: the epidemiology and cost of back pain.* London: HMSO, 1994.

2 Walsh K *et al.* Low back pain in eight areas of Britain. *J Epidemiol Community Health* 1992; **46**: 227–30.

3 Croft P *et al. Low back pain in the community and in hospitals.* A report to the Clinical Standards Advisory Group of the Department of Health. Prepared by the Arthritis & Rheumatism Council, Epidemiology Unit, Manchester, 1994.

4 Troup JDG *et al.* Back pain in industry. A prospective study. *Spine* 1981; **6**: 61–9.

5 Biering-Sorensen F. A prospective study of low back pain in a general population. I—occurrence, recurrence and aetiology. *Scand J Rehabil Med* 1983; **15**: 71–80.

6 Smedley J, Egger P, Cooper C, Coggon D. Prospective cohort study of predictors of incident low back pain in nurses. *BMJ* 1997; **314**: 1225–8.

7 Waddell G. *The back pain revolution*. Edinburgh: Churchill Livingstone, 1998.

8 Palmer KT, Walsh K, Bendall H, Cooper C, Coggon D. Back pain in Britain: comparison of two prevalence surveys at an interval of 10 years. *BMJ* 2000; **320**: 1577–8.

9 Riihimaki H. Back and limb disorders. In: *Epidemiology of work-related diseases* (ed. McDonald C). London: BMJ Publishing Group, 1995.

10 Bernard et al. *Musculoskeletal disorders and workplace factors. A critical review of epidemiologic evidence for work-related musculoskeletal disorders of the neck, upper extremity, and low back* (Publication no. 97–141). Cincinnati, OH: US Department of Health and Human Sciences/NIOSH, 1997.

11 Watson P, Main C, Waddell G, Gales TE, Purcell-Jones G. Medically certified work loss, recurrence and costs of wage compensation for back pain: a follow-up study of the working population of Jersey. *Br J Rheumatol* 1998; **37**: 82–6.

12 Kelsey JL, Golden A, Mundt D. Low back pain/prolapsed lumbar intervertebral disc. *Rheumatic Dis Clin North Am* 1990; **16**: 699–716.

13 Bigos SJ, Battie MC, Spengler DM et al. A prospective study of work perceptions and psychological factors affecting the report of back injury. *Spine* 1991; **16**: 1–6.

14 Croft PR, Papageorgiou AC, Ferry S, Thomas E, Jason MIV, Silman AJ. Psychological distress and low back pain: evidence from a prospective study in the general population. *Spine* 1995; **20**: 2731–7.

15 Burton AK, Tillotson KM, Main CJ, Hollis S. Psychological predictors of outcome in acute and subacute low-back trouble. *Spine* 1995; **20**: 722–8.

16 Greenough CG, Fraser RD. Assessment of patients with low-back pain. *Spine* 1992; **17**: 36–41.

17 Roland M, Morris R. A study of the natural history of back pain. Part 1: Development of a reliable and sensitive measure of disability in low back pain. *Spine* 1983; 141–4.

18 Von Korff M, Ormel J, Keefe F, Dworkin SF. Grading the severity of chronic pain. *Pain* 1992; **50**: 133–49.

19 Faculty of Occupational Medicine. *Occupational health guidelines for the management of low-back pain at work. Evidence review and recommendations*. London: Faculty of Occupational Medicine, 2000.

20 Royal College of General Practitioners. *Clinical guidelines for the management of acute low back pain*. London: Royal College of General Practitioners, 1999 (www.regp.org.uk).

21 Royal College of General Practitioners. *The back book*. London: Stationery Office Books, 2002.

22 Health & Safety Executive. *Manual handling: solutions you can handle*. HSG115. Sudbury: HSE Books, 1994.

23 Health & Safety Executive. *Are you making the best use of lifting aids?* INDG398. Sudbury: HSE Books, 2004.

24 Hiebert FR, Skovron ML, Nordin M. Work restrictions and outcome of non-specific low back pain. *Spine* 2003; **28**: 722–8.

25 Hall-H, McIntosh-G, Melles-T et al. Effect of discharge recommendations on outcome. *Spine* 1994; **19**: 2033–7.

26 Scheer SJ, Watanabe KA, Radack KL. Randomised controlled trials in industrial low back pain. Part III. Subacute/chronic pain interventions. *Arch Phys Med Rehab* 1997; **78**: 414–23.

27 Van Tulber MW, Ostelo R, Vlaeyen J W et al, Behavioural treatment for chronic low back pain: a systematic review within the Cochrane back review group. *Spine* 2000; **25**: 2688–99.

28 Nachemson A, Spitzer WO et al. Scientific approach to the assessment and management of activity-related spinal disorders. A monograph for clinicians. Report of the Quebec task force on spinal disorders. *Spine* 1987; **12**(7S) (Suppl. 1): S1–59.

29 Victorian Workcover Authority. *Guidelines for the management of employees with compensable low back pain*. Melbourne: Victorian Workcover Authority, 1996.

30 ACC and the National Health Committee 1997. *New Zealand acute low back pain guide*. Wellington, NZ: Ministry of Health (www.nhc.govt.nz).

31 van der Weidw WE, Verbeek JHAM, van Dijk FJH, Doef F. An audit of occupational health care for employees with low-back pain. *Occup Med* 1997; **47**: 294–300.

32 Agency for Health Care Policy and Research. *Acute low back problems in adults*. Clinical Practice Guideline No. 14. Washington DC: US Government Printing Office, 1994.

33 ICSI. *Health care guideline: adult low back pain*. Internet, Institute for Clinical Systems Integration, 1998 (www.icsi.org/guide).

34 US Preventive Services Task Force. *Counselling to prevent low back pain*. Internet, National Guidelines Clearing House, 1996 (www.guideline.gov).

35 Clinical Standards Advisory Group. *Back pain*. Report of a CSAG committee on back pain. London: HMSO, 1994.

36 Staal JB, Hlobil H, van Tulder MW, Waddell G, Burton AK, Koes BW, van Mechelen W. Occupational health guidelines for the management of low back pain: an international comparison. *Occup Environ Med* 2003; **60**: 618–26.

37 Evanoff B, Wolf L, Aton E, Canos J, Collins J. Reduction in injury rates in nursing personnel through introduction of mechanical lifts in the workplace. *Am J Ind Med* 2003; **44**: 451–7.

38 Mäkelä M, Heliövaara M, Sievers K, Impivaara O, Knekt P, Aromaa A. Prevalence, determinants, and consequences of chronic neck pain in Finland. *Am J Epidemiol* 1991; **134**: 1356–67.

39 Lau EMC, Sham A, Wong KC. The prevalence of and risk factors for neck pain in Hong Kong Chinese. *J Public Health Med* 1996; **18**: 396–9.

40 Takala J, Sievers K, Klaukka T. Rheumatic symptoms in the middle-aged population in southwestern Finland. *Scand J Rheumatology* 1982; **47**: 15–29.

41 Palmer KT, Walker-Bone K, Griffin MJ, Syddall H, Pannett B, Coggon D, Cooper C. Prevalence and occupational associations of neck pain in the British population. *Scand J Work Environ Health* 2001; **27**: 49–56.

42 Ariens GAM, van Mechelen WV, Bongers PM, Bouter LM, van der Wal G. Physical risk factors for neck pain. *Scand J Work Environ Health* 2000; **26**: 7–19.

43 Ariëns GAM, Bongers PM, Douwes M, Miedema MC, Hoogendoorn WE, van der Wal G, Bouter LM, van Mechelen W. Are neck flexion, neck rotation, and sitting at work risk factors for neck pain? Results of a prospective cohort study. *Occup Environ Med* 2001; **58**: 200–7.

44 Viikari-Juntura E, Takala E, Riihimaki H, Martikainen R, Jappinen P. Predictive validity of symptoms and signs in the neck and shoulders. *J Clin Epidemiol* 2000; **53**: 800–8.

45 Smedley J, Inskip H, Trevelyan F, Buckle P, Cooper C, Coggon D. Risk factors for incident neck and shoulder pain in hospital nurses. *Occup Environ Med* 2003; **60**: 864–9.

46 Ylinen J, Takala EP, Nykanen M. Hakkinen A, Malkia E, Pohjolainen T *et al*. Active neck muscle training in the treatment of chronic neck pain in women: a randomized controlled trial. *JAMA* 2003; **289**: 2509–16.

47 Viljanen M, Malmivaara A, Uitti J, Rinne M, Palmroos P, Laippala P. Effectiveness of dynamic muscle training, relaxation training, or ordinary activity for chronic neck pain: randomised controlled trial. *BMJ* 2003; **327**: 475.

48 Kellgren JH. On the distribution of pain arising from deep somatic structures with charts of segmental pain areas. *Clin Sci Mol Med* 1939; **4**: 35–46.

49 Boden SD, McCowin PR, Davis DO, Dina TS, Mark AS, Wiesel S. Abnormal magnetic-resonance scans of the cervical spine in asymptomatic subjects. A prospective investigation. *J Bone Joint Surg* 1990; **72A**: 1178–84.

50 Jensen MC, Brant-Zawadzki MN, Obuchowski N, Modic MT, Malkasian D, Ross JS. Magnetic resonance imaging of the lumbar spine in people without back pain. *N Engl J Med* 1994; **331**: 69–73.

51 Kelsey J, White A. Epidemiology and impact of low back pain. *Spine* 1980; **5**: 133–42.

52 Battie M, Fideman T, Gibbons L, *et al*. Determinants of lumbar disc degeneration—the study of life time exposure and magnetic resonance imaging findings in identical twins. *Spine* 1995; **20**: 2601–12.

53 Weber H. Lumbar disc herniation. A controlled, prospective study with ten years of observation. *Spine* 1983; **8**: 131–40.

54 Weber H. The natural course of disc herniation. *Acta Orthop Scand Suppl* 1993; **251**: 19–20.

55 Hasenbring M, Marienfleld G, Kuhlendahl D et al. Risk factors of chronicity in lumbar disc patients, a prospective investigation of biologic, psychologic and social predictors of therapy outcome. *Spine* 1994; **19**: 2759–65.

56 Herkowitz H, Dvorak J, Bell G et al. (eds) *The lumbar spine*, p. 431. Lippincott Williams and Wilkins, 2004. ISBN 0781742978.

57 Carragee EJ, Han MY, Yang B, Kim DH, Kraemer H, Billys J. Activity restrictions after posterior lumbar discectomy. A prospective study of outcomes in 152 cases with no postoperative restrictions. *Spine*, 1999; **24**: 2346–51.

58 McCulloch J, Macnab I. *Sciatica and chymopapain*. Baltimore, MD: Williams and Wilkins, 1983.

59 Gonzalez-Castro A, Shetty A, Nagendar K et al. Day case conventional discectomy—a randomised controlled trial. *Eur Spine J* 2002; **11**: 67–70.

60 Magnusson ML, Pope MH, Wilder DG, Szpalski M, Spratt K. Is there a rational basis for post-surgical lifting restrictions? 1. Current understanding. *Eur Spine J* 1999; **8**: 170–8.

61 Ostelo RWJG, de Vet HCW, Waddell G, Kerckhoffs MR, Leffers P, van Tulder MW. Rehabilitation after lumbar disc surgery (Cochrane Review). In: *The Cochrane Library*, Issue 2. Oxford: Update Software, 2002.

62 Eskola A, Pohjolainen A, Alaranta et al. Calcitonin treatment in lumbar spinal stenosis: a randomised placebo controlled double blind cross over study with one year follow-up. *Calcified Tissue Int* 1992; **50**: 400–83.

63 Porter RW, Hibbert C. Calcitonin treatment for neurogenic claudication. *Spine* 1983; **8**: 585–92.

64 Podichetty VK, Segal AM, Lieber M et al. Effectiveness of salmon calcitonin nasal spray in the treatment of lumbar canal stenosis. *Spine* 2004; **29**: 2343–9.

65 Ciocon, G, Amaranath L et al. Caudal epidural blocks for elderly patients with lumbar spinal stenosis. *J Am Geriatr Soc* 1994; **42**: 593–6.

66 Turner JA, Ersek M, Herron L, et al. Surgery for lumbar spinal stenosis: attempted meta analysis of the literature. *Spine* 1992; **17**: 1.

67 Fritzell P, Hägg O, Wessberg P. Lumbar fusion versus nonsurgical treatment for chronic low back pain: a multicenter randomized controlled trial from the Swedish Lumbar Spine Study Group. *Spine* 2001; **26**: 2521–32.

68 Fairbank J et al. Preliminary results of the UK Spinal Stabilisation Trial. Presented at The British Orthopaedic Association, Birmingham, September 2003.

69 Brox J, S¨rensen R, Friis A, et al. Randomised clinical trial of lumbar instrumented fusion and cognitive intervention and exercises in patients with chronic low back pain and disc degeneration. *Spine* 2003; **28**: 1913–21.

70 Greenough CG, Taylor LJ, Fraser R. Anterior lumbar fusion: results, assessment techniques and prognostic factors. *Eur Spine J* 1994; **3**: 225–30.

71 de-Kleuver M, Oner F, Jacobs W. Total disc replacement for chronic low back pain: background and a systematic review of the literature. *Eur Spine J* 2003; **12**: 108–16.

72 Zeegers WS, Bohnen LM, Laaper M et al. Artificial disc replacement with the modular type SB Charité III: 2-year results in 50 prospectively studied patients. *Eur Spine J* 1999; **8**: 210–17.

73 Gore DR, Sepic SB, Gardner GM et al. Neck pain: a long term follow-up of 205 patients. *Spine* 1987; **12**: 1–5.

74 National Ankylosing Spondylitis Society. Leading a Normal Life. http://www.nass.co.uk/life.htm (accessed 21/1/05)

75 Boonen A, De-Vet H, van-der-Heijde D et al, Work status and its determinants amongst patients with ankylosing spondylitis. A systemic literature review. *J Rheumatol* 2001; **28**: 1056–62.

76 Boonen A, Chorus AM, Miedema HS, Heijde D van der, Landewé R, Schouten H, van-der-Temple H, van-der-Linden S. Withdrawal from labour force due to work disability in patients with ankylosing spondylitis. *Ann Rheum Dis* 2001; **60**: 1033–9.

77 Fredenhagen H, Untersuchungen bei Rekruten. *Schweiz Med Wochenschr* 1965; **95**: 675.

78 Murray PM, Weinstein SL, Spratt KF. The natural history and long-term follow-up of Scheuermann's kyphosis. *J Bone Joint Surg* 1993; **75A**: 236–48.

79 Aglietti P, Di-Muria, Taylor TKF *et al*. Conservative treatment of thoracic and lumbar vertebral fractures. *Ital J Orthop Traumatol* 1984; Suppl.: 83–105.

80 Weinstein JN, Collalto P, Lehmann ER. Thoraco-lumbar burst fractures treated conservatively, a long-term follow-up. *Spine* 1988; **13**: 33–8.

81 Boerger TO, Limb D, Dickson RA. Does canal clearance affect neurological outcome after thoraco-lumbar burst fractures? Review articles. *J Bone Joint Surg* 2000; **82B**: 629–35.

Chapter 12

Orthopaedics and trauma of the limbs

R. A. F. Cox and I. M. Nugent

Musculoskeletal disorders are among the commonest reasons for attendance at general practitioner and accident and emergency services. These disorders can have a significant impact on the workplace, employment, and productivity but their correct diagnosis and early treatment can reduce morbidity and facilitate an early return to work. The commoner musculoskeletal disorders and trauma of the limbs are discussed in this chapter, along with guidelines on their diagnosis, management, and prognosis.

Most morbidity in the working population arises from acute soft tissue or bony injury, but, with age, joint problems contribute increasingly. Congenital limb anomalies and acquired limb deficiencies are also discussed as well as genetic abnormalities and inherited conditions that affect the musculoskeletal system. As professional sport and leisure activities become more popular, a bigger population is seeking rapid access to diagnostic and treatment services. The demands on physicians and surgeons to return athletes to the arena quickly without compromising future health and performance are increasing.

The Disability Discrimination Act 1995 (DDA) places a responsibility on employees and employers to evaluate the impact of physical health on safety and performance at work. Some occupations, such as the rescue services and commercial divers require high levels of physical fitness for safe working practices. The role of the occupational physician is to assess the nature of the disability and how it affects functional activity in the occupation in question and to give advice on possible adaptations. Management will then need to decide if such adaptations are feasible. They may also need encouragement to employ those with unsightly deformities. Advice should also be given on how financial assistance can be obtained from the Department for Work and Pensions (DWP) for adaptations to the workplace, or to provide additional equipment to help a disabled person cope with the job successfully. Some of the conditions considered in this chapter are also referred to in Chapter 13 (Rheumatology).

Arthritis

Osteoarthritis

By the age of 50, 80% of the population have radiographic evidence of osteoarthritis (OA) in the hip, knee, or elbow. The overall prevalence in the working age population is 9.5%.[1] General 'wear and tear' is still considered an important aetiological factor. The knee and hip joints are most commonly affected and there appears to be a genetic predisposition to arthritis affecting the fingers, posterior spinal facet joints, and knees. Generally, OA deteriorates with time, but the rate at which this happens is variable. Stiffness and deformity follow insidiously, with swelling that may be due to synovitis, effusion, or osteophyte formation. Radiological changes often lag behind pathological features and there is little correlation between the clinical status and the radiological appearance. The characteristic radiological features are narrowing of the joint space, formation of osteophytes at the articular margins, sclerosis, and cyst formation. Simple analgesics are appropriate for mild disease, with the addition of non-steroidal anti-inflammatory drugs (NSAIDs) as necessary. NSAIDs inhibit prostaglandin synthesis and 70% of patients will respond to them in the early stages of disease. Femoral head collapse has been reported with the use of NSAIDs but appears to be a rare idiosyncratic reaction. Intra-articular injection of local anaesthetic and steroid tends to provide short-term relief and physiotherapy, including heat, cold, short-wave diathermy, and ultrasound may lead to symptomatic improvement. Surgery is required when restoration of function and the relief of pain cannot be achieved by these measures.

Adaptations to the workplace such as using powered appliances or high stools to relieve the need for prolonged standing may be necessary. Pain, commonly occurring 24–36 hours after excessive exertion, may be the limiting factor especially in physically demanding occupations. Following a minor injury, persisting symptoms may suggest the presence of underlying arthritis and the occupational physician may have to decide whether it is reasonable for an employee to continue working if his job is physically demanding. An employee who is severely restricted due to arthritis may be able to continue in their occupation after a joint replacement. If an employee is to make a satisfactory return to work after joint replacement surgery the occupational physician will need to maintain close liaison between the orthopaedic surgeon, general practitioner, physiotherapist, and employer.

Rheumatoid arthritis

Rheumatoid arthritis (RA) is the commonest form of chronic inflammatory joint disease. Typically it is a symmetrical, erosive, deforming, polyarthritis affecting both small and large peripheral joints. The course of the disease is often prolonged with exacerbations and remissions. The prevalence is approximately 1% and it is commoner in women (3:1), typically beginning in the third to fifth decade. The cause of RA is obscure, but there appears to be a multifactorial genetic predisposition. The onset is usually insidious with joint pain, stiffness, and symmetrical swelling of peripheral joints. Typically, the small joints of the fingers and toes are the first to be affected. The articular manifestations of RA are described in detail in Chapter 13. In many occupations employment is still entirely possible despite this condition; in others, modifications can be made to allow the employee to stay at work. However, heavy manual jobs and those requiring repetitive movements of affected joints are best avoided.

Juvenile chronic arthritis

Juvenile chronic arthritis (JCA) is a heterogeneous group of inflammatory joint diseases in young people characterized by chronic joint inflammation resulting in muscle weakness and osteoporosis. Partial involvement of the epiphysis may cause asymmetrical overgrowth and deformity and may cause limb length inequality. Pauciarticular onset (involvement of up to four joints) is the commonest presentation (70%), and this has a good prognosis (70% will be in remission with little functional disability after 15 years follow-up.[2] Resulting minor disability rarely requires surgery but occasionally major joint replacement is needed in the young adult. Polyarticular disease (five or more joints within the first 3 months of onset) occurs in 20% of cases. The majority of patients are seronegative for IgM rheumatoid factor and these patients respond well to early treatment. Seropositive disease resembles adult RA and commonly presents in girls approaching the menarche. It affects the hands and feet initially and later involves the larger joints. It tends to persist into adult life and is often referred to as juvenile RA (JRA, Still's disease). This variety often causes growth impairment and major joint destruction requiring multiple surgical procedures in late adolescent years and young adult life. Children who have suffered from this condition need careful career advice. It is important that they work within their strengths and capabilities and do not enter employment that would further stress already compromised joints. There are specific clinical problems related to each joint. These are principally due to growth disturbance, contracture, and joint destruction, and will be considered in later sections.

Arthritis of the hip

Pain from an arthritic hip is normally felt in the groin or in the region of the greater trochanter and radiates down the front of the thigh to the knee. Excessive physical activity is related to the development of OA of the hip. Retired footballers,[3] farmers and farm workers have more OA of the hip than age- and weight-matched controls. Arthritis of the hip, knee, and spine are by far the commonest clinical presentations. In RA the hip is involved radiographically in 33% within 5 years of onset, rising to 50% at 8 years). Problems in the hip joint in adolescence and young adulthood also follow congenital dysplasia or dislocation, Perthes' disease, slipped upper femoral epiphysis, or infection. Occupational causes of arthritis of the hip include aseptic bone necrosis in divers and compressed air workers. The onset of symptoms may be sudden with the collapse of the articular surface.

Hip arthroplasty is indicated in patients with incapacitating pain, which is refractory to conservative treatment. In most hip replacements both components are cemented to bone but sometimes, in younger individuals, uncemented prostheses are used. The latter facilitate future revision operations and require a postoperative period of non-weight-bearing and so have a longer initial recovery time. The improved success rate of total hip replacement as a result of advances in surgical techniques and materials has increased the frequency of joint replacement in the younger patient. Men and women of working age now regularly have hip replacements, and this has greatly improved their ability to continue at work in a wider variety of jobs.

Total hip replacement significantly relieves pain and increases mobility. Recovery from surgery depends on the original severity of the symptoms and the aetiology of the arthritis. Typically 6–8 weeks will elapse before driving can be recommenced and 3–4 months before any manual work can be resumed. Total hip replacement allows an otherwise active healthy individual to return to a light manual job. Heavy, arduous work is likely to cause premature failure of the prosthesis and individuals need to be counselled to avoid this. Working where safety could be jeopardized if a hip replacement subluxes or dislocates (such as working at heights, in the offshore industry, at sea or working alone in remote situations) may be inappropriate, and placement should be considered carefully. Some firefighters have been able to return to operational duties after total hip replacements. Of 10 firefighters who had recently undergone total hip replacement, seven had reached retirement age and left the service or left early on ill-health retirement while the three remaining had yet to serve 5 years postsurgery. Of five hip resurfacing operations (Birmingham) four were still surviving within 5 years of surgery.[4] Hip resurfacing appears to be a promising technique for younger patients (under 60) whose OA is uncomplicated by disabling inflammatory joint disease or osteoporosis. It is less invasive (i.e. requires the removal of less normal bone), which means faster recovery from surgery and potentially an earlier revision operation should it be necessary. However, long-term survival results are not yet available in everyday practice.

The occupational physician should carry out a risk assessment, taking account of the demands of the job and the mobility of the employee. It is important that any restriction of mobility should not compromise the safety of the worker or his colleagues. It is also important that employees with joint replacements are not allowed to undertake roles that may put a strain on the joint and disadvantage them in later life, but this may be hard to accept when a successful joint replacement has relieved their symptoms.

In many posts return to work will be possible, but in those where mobility and agility are essential the occupational physician should defer final assessment until full functional recovery is apparent. Premature risk assessment may compromise the employee's chance of returning to his job or prescribing appropriate adaptations. If neither is possible relocation or retirement may be necessary.

Complications of joint replacement are infrequent. Failure due to aseptic loosening occurs at a rate of 1–2% per year. Infection occurs in 1–2% of arthroplasties and is particularly associated with diabetes, RA, immunosuppression, and alcoholism. Deep venous thrombosis (DVT) after hip replacement occurs in 40–70% of people, pulmonary embolism (PE) in 1–10%, and fatal PE in 1% if preventive measures are not used. If DVT prophylaxis is employed the incidence can be reduced to less than 0.5%.[5] Flying for longer than 3 hours after hip replacement is not advised for at least 3 months. Well fitting, surgical support stockings should always be worn on any flight.

Arthritis of the knee

OA of the knee is commoner in heavy manual workers. Normal physical activity does not cause OA and runners are not more prone to it. Any severe physical activity will accelerate the degeneration of OA of the knee so the work of most sufferers from this condition may require to be significantly modified or even terminated.

Arthritis of the knee commonly presents with pain on weight-bearing, which radiates from the knee down the anterior aspect of the tibia. Night pain is less common than in hip disease. Examination reveals a limping gait, swelling, and a restricted range of movement. Genu varum deformity is commoner in OA and genu valgum in RA. Symptoms from early disease may be controlled by NSAIDs, quadriceps exercises, ultrasound, and ice. Knee bracing may control instability. Arthroscopic washout, resection of unstable meniscal fragments, and debridement of the knee may produce improvement in symptoms for up to 5 years in 60% of cases.

Total knee replacement is less common in the working population than is hip replacement, but its frequency is increasing. Total knee replacement has a 10-year success rate of over 90% in osteoarthritic patients over 60 years of age. The revision rate by 10 years is 3%. Rates for the survival of total knee replacements of 90% at 15 years and 97% at 10 years have been reported.[6,7] The initial recovery time from surgery tends to be slightly longer than for hips, but the later restrictions and limitations are similar. Employees should not be expected to engage in manual lifting and demanding physical activities particularly those involving kneeling or heavy impact on the knees. Working on uneven surfaces may be difficult, as will be prolonged standing.

Arthritis of the shoulder

The arthritic shoulder is much rarer than the arthritic hip or knee and is usually secondary to chronic destructive inflammatory disease or local trauma. Unilateral shoulder arthritis can often be managed symptomatically. Profound functional disability occurs when the condition becomes bilateral. Primary OA of the glenohumeral joint is rare but does occur. Degenerative arthritis is usually secondary to trauma (e.g. following intra-articular fracture), or to a long-standing rotator cuff injury. It is most common in those engaged in heavy manual work and in divers and compressed air workers who suffer aseptic bone necrosis. It presents most commonly between the ages of 50 and 60 with a history of painful arc syndrome and a decreased global range of movement. The glenohumeral joint is commonly involved in RA usually bilaterally. Synovitis of the rotator cuff may produce impingement, and tenosynovitis around the long head of the biceps may lead to its rupture. Most shoulder arthritis can be controlled with simple analgesics and NSAIDs. Physiotherapy may maintain or restore the range of movement.

In RA, aspiration of a tense joint effusion and intra-articular corticosteroid injection may control the symptoms. Arthroscopy with joint debridement, shoulder decompression, removal of loose bodies, or limited synovectomy may all give symptomatic relief. In young patients, excision of osteophytes and acromioplasty (partial excision of the acromion to reduce impingement with the humerus) may defer more radical surgery. When symptoms persist despite this, total shoulder arthroplasty (replacement of the humeral head and glenoid) may be necessary. The best functional results of total shoulder replacement are obtained in patients with OA, as the rotator cuff is usually intact and bone quality is good. These patients may regain a good range of movement as well as obtaining relief of pain.

Arthritis of the shoulder causes problems in occupations that require full mobility of the upper limbs. Carers often present with injuries with delayed recovery by the presence of arthritis. Occupations that involve work above shoulder height, especially if lifting is involved, will be affected by loss of mobility and pain in the shoulder. Driving, especially driving HGVs, may be difficult even with power steering, and chronic problems are a contra-indication to holding such a licence. The occupational physician will have to carry out risk assessments when lifting is inevitable, e.g. in mechanics and paramedics, but such posts are likely to be considered unsafe in those with arthritis of the shoulder. Adaptations required by the DDA may be very difficult if not impossible to recommend unless mechanical aids can be introduced.

Arthritis of the ankle

Primary OA of the ankle is rare. Secondary OA occurs most commonly after ankle fracture, ligamentous instability, or inflammatory arthritis. Despite being the most frequently injured weight-bearing joint, the ankle is least likely to suffer degenerative joint disease. OA after displaced ankle fractures occurs in 20–40% of patients, the frequency depending on the severity of the injury and the accuracy of its reduction. Physiotherapy is likely to give only temporary relief in established arthritis but may improve the stability. Shoe inserts and insoles can correct minor varus and valgus deformities, and boots with ankle supports may improve stability. Degenerative arthritis accompanied by lateral instability may be improved by lateral ligament reconstruction. Arthrodesis is indicated in isolated ankle joint OA or in RA with unilateral ankle involvement. Arthroscopy is effective for the removal of loose bodies, but its efficacy in the symptomatic relief of arthritis is less clear. Ankle joint replacement is not commonly performed, but is indicated in a few specific circumstances. Ankle arthrodesis provides good pain relief and little effect on physical mobility or agility, and is often the preferred procedure. Arthrodesis of the ankle joint itself produces minimal loss of function and limitations are likely to be minor. However, triple arthrodesis of the hindfoot is different and leads to a degree of loss of inversion and eversion that will affect balance. People who have had a triple arthrodesis may therefore have difficulty walking over rough ground, so farmers, foresters, and construction workers may not be able to work satisfactorily. Those who need to climb ladders may jeopardize their safety. Occupations that demand mobility or involve long hours of standing are likely to be difficult in people with arthritis of the ankles. Adaptations to the job may be possible, but where agility and pain-free movement are needed relocation or retirement may be the only practical solution.

Driving need not be affected as adaptations such as automatic transmission or hand controls can be provided. The Disability Employment Adviser (DEA) may well be able to help with a grant for such alterations in a car that is essential for employment.

Arthritis of the elbow

The elbow joint is involved in approximately half those with RA, in whom it is often disabling. OA of the elbow is usually the result of trauma. Arthroscopy may aid diagnosis and allows the removal of loose bodies. Joint replacement may produce satisfactory results in 90% of rheumatoid patients at 5 years, but only 75% in young patients with OA. Occupations requiring full mobility of the upper limbs especially those involving lifting are not suitable for those with this condition. Work involving long hours on keyboards is also likely to be difficult unless the keyboard can be placed well back on the desk so that the elbows can be supported in a relaxed position. Heavy fire doors in the working environment are problematic to those with arthritis of the elbow and other upper limb joints.

Arthritis of the wrist

Arthritis of the wrist may be primary (idiopathic) or secondary to fractures of the scaphoid or distal radius, or scapholunate dissociation (severe wrist ligament injury). A trial of non-surgical treatment is indicated in most patients. Steroid injections, NSAIDs, and splintage may be beneficial. Arthroscopy may be indicated to assess the state of the joint surfaces, to remove loose bodies, or to biopsy the synovium. Proximal row carpectomy relieves pain in approximately 90% of patients. It must be undertaken before degenerative change occurs in the midcarpal joints. It is indicated in those for whom residual mobility is important, but in manual labourers an arthrodesis is a better option. If surgical treatment is not possible any occupations requiring repetitive movements at the wrist, especially lifting or forced pronation or supination, may be impossible. Milder forms of arthritis may be helped by splints, especially before operative treatment becomes necessary. A voice-activated computer may help keyboard operators with chronic wrist problems. Occupations requiring a powerful grip, e.g. firemen, are very likely to be adversely affected if pain is a prominent feature.

Arthroscopy

Arthroscopy has revolutionized the management of many joint conditions. Advances in technology have allowed clear visualization of joints and manipulation of intra-articular structures. Surgery can be performed with minimal morbidity, usually as a day-case procedure and often under local anaesthesia. The techniques pioneered in the knee are now employed in many joints. Certain procedures that were previously impossible or technically demanding can now be undertaken (e.g. repair of a posterior meniscal tear). Indications for arthroscopy include synovial biopsy, removal of loose bodies, excision of osteophytes, irrigation of septic arthritis, drilling, or shaving within the joint (e.g. osteochondritis dissecans, chondromalacia patellae), and synovectomy.

The knee is the joint most commonly arthroscoped. Procedures include meniscectomy, meniscal repair, loose body removal, and cruciate ligament repair. The commonest arthroscopic procedure is meniscectomy. Postoperatively patients describe the knee as sore for a few days but it is not normally a painful procedure. Simple analgesia for 2–3 days is generally sufficient. Patients should be encouraged to walk as soon as recovery from the anaesthetic allows. Prolonged sitting on long car or air journeys is discouraged for the first 2 weeks to reduce the risk of DVT. Regular specific exercises must be performed to maintain muscle strength and range of motion. Patients may drive when able to walk comfortably unaided or using a single stick: generally 5–6 days after surgery. Long journeys within 2 weeks of the arthroscopy should be discouraged. Most people should be advised to return to work after about 2 weeks provided that short car or rail journeys are possible and the job does not require more than simple desk work. If a job involves heavy activity or repetitive climbing (including stairs) then 3 weeks may be required. For heavy manual labour, working at heights, using ladders, or kneeling or squatting, 4 weeks may be needed. Sports should be avoided for at least a month after surgery. Individual adjustments may be required, depending on the specific details of any injury and its duration. Generally speaking sport should not be restarted until the joint is free of swelling, the wounds have healed, and the leg is strong enough to exercise on comfortably.

Ankle arthroscopy is used for the treatment of articular and ligamentous pathology. Acute or recurrent ankle sprains may produce osteochondral fractures, loose bodies, or adhesions that can all be managed by arthroscopy. Ankle arthritis and bony spurs caused by repetitive injury are amenable to arthroscopic debridement. Ankle arthrodesis is now being performed arthroscopically.

Shoulder surgery is becoming increasingly amenable to arthroscopy. The use of lasers to perform shoulder stabilization and intra-articular burrs for subacromial decompression have reduced morbidity and allowed such operations to be done as day cases. Elbow and wrist arthroscopy is being used increasingly for treating arthritic and traumatic conditions.

There is now such a wide range of arthroscopic procedures being performed on different joints that advice on returning to work must depend on the complexity of the procedure, and the necessity for non-weightbearing, the presence of postoperative splints and the need to avoid DVT rather than on simple wound healing. Each case must be assessed on an individual basis.

Complications of arthroscopy are rare (about 1%) and are usually minor but can include haemarthrosis, infection, and thrombo-embolic disease.

Shoulder

Impingement syndromes

Shoulder impingement can be diagnosed when a patient has a positive impingement sign (pain on passive elevation) and a positive impingement test (disappearance of the pain following intrabursal injection of local anaesthetic). Subacromial impingement results in a painful arc of movement in active and passive forward flexion and abduction. Classically, the rotator cuff is impinged between 60° and 120° of abduction. Acute primary injury in young athletic individuals causes oedema and haemorrhage. There is diffuse pain located over the deltoid, local tenderness over the greater tuberosity, muscle spasm, and limitation of movement in addition to a positive impingement sign and test. A chronic impingement syndrome may occur in persons over 40 years of age with progressive persistent disability. In addition, symptoms often include locking and pain at night. Frequently, there is either a rotator cuff tear or biceps tendon rupture and secondary bone changes.

Subcoracoid impingement occurs in younger patients with an intact rotator cuff. The symptoms are more anterior and impingement occurs with the arm in flexion and internal rotation. Soft tissue impingement occurs between the lesser tuberosity and the coracoid/coracohumeral ligament complex. This presents in gymnasts, javelin throwers, swimmers, and tennis players. It may also occur after fractures of the greater tuberosity of the humerus or scarring after an anterior dislocation.

Non-surgical treatment of impingement syndromes consists of steroid or NSAID injection with local anaesthetic into the subacromial bursa, physiotherapy, and occasionally splintage. Surgical treatment may involve repair of the rotator cuff tear, excision of calcific deposits, decompression acromioplasty or arthroscopic decompression. Chronic impingement may lead to rotator cuff rupture, adhesive fibrosis (frozen shoulder), or degenerative arthrosis.

Rotator cuff injuries

The rotator cuff consists of the tendons of supraspinatus, infraspinatus, teres minor, and subscapularis blended with the fibrous capsule to form a hood over the glenohumeral joint. The actions of these muscles combine during elevation of the arm to draw the humeral head inwards and downwards, thereby stabilizing it in the glenoid fossa. The rotator cuff mechanism is susceptible to degenerative disease, trauma, and inflammation, which, singly or in combination, may cause it to rupture. Rotator cuff rupture occurs more commonly in men (10:1) and more often in the dominant shoulder. Rupture can be complete or partial. When the patient elevates the arm there is a characteristic reversal of the scapulohumeral rhythm, seen as a hunching of the shoulder at the start of the abduction. There is an inability to hold the arm in mid abduction, but there is retention of a good range of passive movement. Ninety per cent of patients with rotator cuff tears recover without surgery. Non-operative treatment is directed towards the relief of pain, stiffness, muscle spasm, and muscle atrophy. Physiotherapy, NSAIDs, and subacromial injections of local anaesthetic and steroids can all be used to good effect. The acute episode usually settles within 2–3 months after appropriate treatment. Operative treatment is indicated early for acute injuries in active individuals.

The extent of limitation of function depends on whether the rupture is partial or complete. Both will result in a degree of pain and loss of power in the arm with considerable functional impairment. Lifting of any load, especially above shoulder height, is likely to be very limited.

Shoulder instability

Acute anterior dislocation (see also p 287) is the commonest shoulder dislocation and accounts for 98% of all cases. The humeral head usually dislocates in response to forced external rotation in an abducted, extended position. Recurrent dislocations occur in 90% of patients who have their first traumatic dislocation under the age of 20 years; in 60% who dislocate for the first time between the ages of 20 and 40; and in only 10% who dislocate over the age of 40 years. Men are four times more likely to redislocate than women. All patients presenting with a recurrent dislocation should undergo a supervised rehabilitation programme with a physiotherapist to retrain the shoulder girdle muscles. No further treatment may be needed if modification of work or recreational activities can be achieved. A full assessment should be undertaken before anyone with a history of shoulder instability is employed in an occupation that involves lifting, straining, or pulling.

In the shoulder, disorders of the periarticular soft tissues are more common than arthritic conditions, and account for up to 95% of all shoulder pain. Abnormalities of the rotator cuff tendons are the commonest and most important intrinsic cause of painful shoulder syndromes. They are often associated with mechanical derangement related to degenerative change, or with an inflammatory arthropathy. Extrinsic causes of shoulder pain such as cervical nerve root or diaphragmatic irritation, myocardial disease, and thoracic outlet syndrome should be excluded.

Calcific tendinitis may present in two ways. The acute syndrome occurs as a sudden attack, often at night without any precipitating factor and is resistant to analgesics. Early aspiration of the calcific liquid deposit with infiltration of local anaesthetic and steroid may be the only way to relieve symptoms. The subacute syndrome comes on over several months with features of impingement but with an overlying element of pain at rest. Calcification occurs 1–2 cm medial to the insertion of the supraspinatus on the humerus and can be identified on a plain shoulder radiograph. Open surgical incision of chronic calcinosis is sometimes indicated.

Frozen shoulder is a relatively common problem, first described by Codman in 1934; it exists in the presence of a normal radiograph. Its cause is unknown and it can only be diagnosed when other intrinsic and extrinsic causes of pain have been excluded. Symptoms include diffuse pain (often at rest), which is worse at night. There is progressive restriction of active and passive movement, particularly external rotation (adhesive capsulitis). Initial treatment is with analgesics and frequent physiotherapy. With intractable cases manipulation under anaesthetic with steroid injection or rarely shoulder arthroscopy is necessary to divide adhesions. Frozen shoulder can cause considerable problems in occupations where full use of the upper limbs is essential. Most cases respond eventually to treatment, but employees may be unable to carry out their full duties for some 12–18 months and employers will need to be persuaded that in most cases there is likely to be a good outcome. If the patient is involved in repetitive work, in particular involving lifting, it is usually possible for the employee to return to full duties after clinical recovery. Once the problem has resolved it is unlikely to recur at the same site.

Biceps tenosynovitis is most commonly a secondary phenomenon but is primary in 5–10%. It is usually due to overuse or direct injury sustained at work or sport. Occasionally, it is due to a congenitally shallow bicipital groove or to a tight transverse humeral ligament. Treatment with an injection of anti-inflammatory drug is helpful but direct injection of steroid into the tendon must be avoided as this can cause later rupture. Arthroscopic decompression is sometimes required.

Subacromial bursitis is commonly secondary to a degenerative or inflammatory process but can occur primarily after acute or repetitive trauma. It presents as a subacromial 'painful arc syndrome' between 60° and 120° abduction. Treatment with physiotherapy, management of any primary inflammatory condition, and local injections are often successful, but surgical decompression may be necessary.

Careful evaluation of the working process is essential to make sure that work is not the cause of these problems. Repetitive movements of the upper arm or handling or lifting of patients, as carried out by nurses or other carers, can result in biceps tenosynovitis or subacromial bursitis. Recurrent attacks in such employees may mean that alternative roles will have to be considered. Working with arms at, or above shoulder height, especially lifting even small objects, may exacerbate the problems and adaptations to the work may have to be made if recurrence is to be avoided even after successful treatment.

Wrist pain

Wrist pain may arise from the joint itself or from any of the structures around it. The pain is usually the result of trauma, inflammation, or degeneration, i.e. tenosynovitis, carpal instability, RA, or wrist OA.

Persistent pain following an injury may be due to ligamentous instability or secondary arthritis after an intra-articular fracture. Scaphoid fracture, which is the second commonest 'wrist fracture' after the distal radius, may lead to chronic pain if non-union occurs. Fractures occur most often in young adult men and a proportion remain undetected. Un-united fractures may initially become asymptomatic but most will develop wrist arthritis within 10 years. Symptomatic arthritis causes stiffness and weakness and in an occupation where this becomes restrictive some form of wrist arthrodesis may be necessary.

Other causes of wrist symptoms with medically definable signs and symptoms may require surgical treatment. Ganglia are prominent swellings, which may appear alarming but are rarely painful or cause functional limitation.

The commonest problems arise from ganglia, which present as swellings at the wrist. On the palmar aspect they usually lie lateral to the flexor carpi radialis tendon and close to the radial artery. On the dorsum they arise either from the scapho-lunate joint or from the midcarpal joint. Many remain asymptomatic and require no treatment but others may require excision. There is a 10% recurrence rate following surgery.

Hand

Dupuytren's disease is a common condition characterized by contractures of the palmar and digital fascia. It is twice as common in men, and the incidence rises with age. It is usually an isolated finding but has a familial tendency and may have an association with diabetes, alcoholism, and epilepsy treated with phenytoin or phenobarbitone. It is no more common among smokers.

A history of trauma is not infrequently elicited, but it is uncertain whether blunt trauma or manual work are causative. It is likely that genetic predisposition is important and that the other factors determine the age of onset. The digits most frequently involved are the ring and little fingers, followed by the middle finger and thumb. The earliest sign of palmar disease is nodule formation when overlying skin blanches on full extension of the hand. Splintage may delay progression of the disease but will not reverse it. Surgery should be considered when deformities become fixed and the hand can no longer be placed flat on a table. In employees whose work requires fine dexterity, early treatment of Dupuytren's disease may be essential. Surgery is performed under general or regional anaesthetic and the involved fascia is excised from the palm and fingers. With more severe contractures skin grafting may be necessary. After correction of digital contractures, splintage in plaster for at least a week is recommended. Thereafter, a thermoplastic splint may be worn between periods of exercise, and later only at night. In severe disease long-term dexterity may be compromised following surgery, and following skin grafting manual workers may need to protect the palm by wearing gloves.

Lower limb

Knee

Chronic knee instability may occur as a result of undiagnosed acute injury, inadequate treatment, or repeated trauma. Stability depends on the cruciate ligaments and collateral ligaments and the extrinsic muscles.

The incidence of anterior cruciate ligament (ACL) rupture is 20 per 100 000 per annum in the UK. One-third of these will have symptoms of disabling instability sufficient to warrant reconstruction, one-third will have other symptoms but no reconstruction, and one-third are asymptomatic. A ruptured ACL may predispose to OA and an unstable knee predisposes to damage to the menisci. Following anterior cruciate rupture, only 17% are able to return to competitive sports while 50% can return to active work, including forestry and construction and recreational sports such as tennis, basketball, and downhill skiing.[8]

Clinical examination, often under general anaesthetic, is necessary to fully assess the injury. Arthroscopy can assess the state of the articular surfaces and menisci and may confirm cruciate ligament injuries. Magnetic resonance imaging (MRI) can be used as a non-invasive method for assessing these structures. Physiotherapy and exercises to strengthen the quadriceps, hamstrings, and gastrocnemius muscles may overcome a functional instability. If the knee recovers dynamic stability, surgery may be unnecessary. Instability associated with sport or certain occupations may be controlled by bracing.

Surgical reconstruction may be undertaken in intractable cases, in those involved in high-level sport, or when extreme physical fitness is required in the occupation, e.g. fire service or armed forces. Intra-articular procedures using bone-tendon or bone patellar tendon graft are currently popular. After reconstruction physical work may not be possible for 3–6 months and return to sport or full work for 6–9 months. The occupational physician will, therefore, have to anticipate a prolonged period of rehabilitation. Although results are likely to be favourable they cannot be guaranteed. Untreated chronic knee instability may progress and cause meniscal degeneration, meniscal tears, and subsequent early degenerative change. It is not currently known whether reconstruction will interrupt this cycle.

Meniscal tears can either be traumatic or degenerative in nature.

Degeneration of the menisci is a normal consequence of ageing and is frequently seen on MRI. Degenerative tears have been found in up to 60% of people over the age of 65. Joint line tenderness is the most accurate clinical sign. MRI is the gold standard for assessment of meniscal disorders.

Symptomatic meniscal tears are usually treated by arthroscopic partial resection. Isolated meniscal tears are very common, and after surgery have a good outcome. Manual workers should be able to return to work in 4–6 weeks office workers in 1–2 weeks. The prognosis is not as good in patients with associated chronic ACL tears and osteoarthritic changes. Recovery and return to sports is quicker in those with isolated meniscal tears as opposed to those with associated degenerative articular changes. Greater long-term arthritic changes are also noted in those who demonstrate varus malalignment after medial meniscectomy and valgus malalignment after lateral meniscectomy.[9]

Open meniscectomy is no longer performed because after open full meniscectomy 27% will have symptoms of arthritis within 20 years. Meniscal repair as opposed to resection is a relatively new technique, and as such there is limited long-term follow-up information. The overall success rate is 60–85%. Patients are often braced and knee flexion and squatting should be limited for several weeks to protect the repair.

There is no evidence that manual labour increases the process of degeneration in the knee. However, the presence of early signs of degeneration or damage should be taken into account when advising on employment.

Ankle

The commonest ankle complaint is pain following ankle sprain. Recurrent instability of the ankle usually occurs after repeated acute inversion injuries. The three parts of the lateral collateral ligament are partially or completely torn and heal in a lengthened position, resulting in lateral joint laxity. This commonly affects the anterior talo-fibular and calcaneo-fibular parts, allowing anterior subluxation of the talus in the ankle mortice (anterior draw sign of the ankle). It has been suggested that repeated 'going over on the ankle' may be due to proprioceptor damage in the ligament rather than laxity. Isolated injuries of the medial collateral ligament are much less common and chronic instability is rare. Medial ligament injuries tend to occur in conjunction with ankle fractures. There is no reliable information about the incidence of ankle ligament injuries, the incidence of instability or the risk of developing arthritis after ligamentous injury. The risk of developing instability is related to the severity of the initial injury and to the method and duration of treatment. Risk assessment of the situation after a full examination of the employee is the only way forward after such injuries. Any occupation demanding stability of the ankles may be affected by such injuries. Climbing ladders and working at heights, as well as lifting and carrying, especially over uneven surfaces, are likely to be difficult and possibly unsafe for anyone with an unstable ankle.

MRI is increasingly used to diagnose the extent and precise location of ligamentous disruption. Minor degrees of laxity without subluxation may be treated with ice, ultrasound, and 'wobble-board' exercises, which are thought to improve proprioception. Shoes with a lateral float on the heel may be helpful. If disability is related only to certain sporting activities, a lateral supporting ankle brace should be worn for sport but chronic conditions causing weakness, paralysis, or arthritis may require a permanent orthosis. Operative repair of acutely torn ligaments may be advisable in athletes. After early immobilization in plaster, mobilization in supportive orthoses is recommended. Adhesions are common after acute injury and may cause continuing disability unless appropriate rehabilitation is undertaken. Surgical reconstruction may be appropriate for chronic instability with disabling symptoms and positive MRI evidence. Surgical reconstruction may achieve stability at the expense of reduced inversion range and eversion power but this does not significantly affect normal function.

The occupational implications of such surgery will depend on the exact nature of the operation and the subsequent restriction in movement. In some cases driving and in other cases prolonged standing may be impaired.

Achilles tendon

Achilles tendinitis is a common condition often related to trauma or sporting injury. Spontaneous onset may be due to poor foot posture or systemic inflammatory conditions like gout or rheumatoid disease. Treatment consists of treating the primary cause as well as including orthotics and appropriate physiotherapy. Steroid injection should be avoided as this may cause subsequent rupture. In chronic resistant tendinitis an MRI scan may indicate an underlying degenerate cyst or tear, or constrictive peritendinitis. This may require surgical repair or decompression.

Achilles tendon ruptures occur as acute events but are classified as 'acute or chronic type' ruptures, depending on the history. 'Acute type' ruptures occur usually under 40 years of age during exercise without previous symptoms. 'Chronic type' tears occur in an older age group often with previous symptoms of tendinitis. Either type may be treated non-surgically, i.e. serial equinous casting (progressive plasters starting in full plantar flexion up to plantigrade over a 2-month period) but often the acute type in a younger patient is repaired surgically. Each treatment requires a minimum of 2 months in a cast followed by physiotherapy rehabilitation. Return to physical labour is usually possible at 3–4 months and sport at 4–6 months.

Tibialis posterior tendon

Tibialis posterior tendon dysfunction is a common condition. The muscle originates in the deep posterior compartment of the calf muscle group and inserts into the medial and plantar aspect of the foot. The tendon passes around the medial malleolus supporting the instep and stabilizing the midfoot. Dysfunction due to tendinitis, a split or a rupture, causes medial collapse of the midfoot, i.e. acquired pes planus or 'fallen arch'.[10] This can be diagnosed clinically by the inability to perform a 'single stance toe raise' and the presence of the 'too many toes' sign when viewed from behind (see Figure 12.1). This can be confirmed by ultrasound or MRI scan. Tendinitis will respond to rest and physiotherapy but a split or a tear will require surgery. Surgery may need 6 weeks protection in a plaster and long-term protection from orthotics. Full recovery is usual with return to normal function.

Foot

Painful afflictions of the foot frequently cause morbidity in the general population. Although some conditions can be attributed to particular professions, such as ballet dancers, they may be exacerbated by many activities. Considering the frequency of foot disorders, there are surprisingly few medico-legal claims for 'lower limb repetitive strain' or 'work-related lower limb disorder'.

Hallux rigidus is a painful limitation of movement of the metatarsophalangeal joint (MTPJ) of the big toe. The condition probably starts with repeated trauma to the big toe in adolescence. This produces a chondral defect on the metatarsal head between the apex of the dome and the dorsal margin of the articular surface. As the hallux is extended, abutment of the proximal phalanx against the defect causes pain. Later, osteophytes appear on the dorsal articular margin and form a mechanical block to extension. Further progression results in the characteristic radiographic appearances of OA.

Hallux rigidus presents in early to middle adult life when patients are physically active. Exercise exacerbates the symptoms and the desire to exercise must be taken into consideration when planning treatment. The ridge of the dorsal osteophyte can be a source of irritation in footwear. High heels and flexible-soled shoes also increase pain. NSAIDs and a change to rigid-soled footwear may alleviate the symptoms.

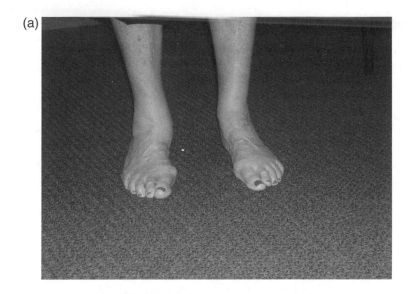

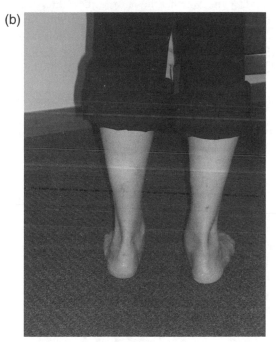

Fig. 12.1 'Rolling in' of the ankle and flat foot as seen from in front (a) with tibialis posterior dysfunction of the right foot and the 'too many toes' sign as seen from behind (b).

Excision of the dorsal osteophyte (cheilectomy) sufficient to allow 70° of passive dorsiflexion at surgery produces good results, unless OA of the joint is advanced. Arthrodesis is recommended in active younger individuals who do not wish to wear high-heeled shoes. After 10 years, 90% of patients report excellent results. The toe should be arthrodesed in approximately 15–20° of valgus and in 10–15° extension. Replacement of the first MTP joint with a prosthetic replacement produces satisfactory results in 80% of cases when fusion is inappropriate.

Hallux valgus is a very common condition consisting of excessive lateral deviation of the big toe at the first MTPJ and medial deviation of the first metatarsal. There is resultant prominence of the bone and soft tissues on the medial side of the first metatarsal head. The first MTP joint may be subluxated or dislocated. The treatment of hallux valgus is controversial. In younger people with relatively normal anatomy but a prominent bunion, existing footwear should be modified. If symptoms persist, a simple bunionectomy may be indicated. In more severe deformity a realignment osteotomy of the first metatarsal bone and soft tissue correction may be indicated. Following surgery 6–8 weeks will be necessary before return to work if this involves a great deal of standing or walking, and up to 3 months if heavy manual labour is involved. In older individuals or those with degenerative change, a Keller's procedure (excision of the basal one-third of the proximal phalanx with trimming of the medial osteophyte) may be the procedure of choice. Overall, the results in 90% of these operations are satisfactory.

Problems of the lesser toes are common and in the majority of cases the aetiology is unknown. A hammer toe occurs with hyperextension of the MTP joint accompanied by flexion at the proximal interphalangeal (PIP) joint with the distal interphalangeal (DIP) joint in neutral alignment. Callosities develop on the dorsum of the PIP joint and on the weight-bearing tip of the toe just distal to the nail. A claw toe occurs where there is hyperextension of the MTP joint accompanied by flexion deformity of both the PIP and DIP joints. Both claw and hammer toe deformities may follow a synovitis of the MTP joint whether the cause is idiopathic, traumatic, or arthritic. Dorsal subluxation of the proximal phalanx occurs first and may be influenced by crowding of the toes in the shoe. The severity of the patient's symptoms determines the need for treatment. Examination of the foot will indicate whether the deformity is flexible or fixed. Any underlying neurological cause should be identified. If foot ulceration or a mallet deformity is present, the patient should be investigated for the presence of diabetes.

In cases of mild deformity, the patient may only require advice about footwear and stretching of the shoes to prevent areas of pressure. Strapping deformities is no longer recommended, but chiropody may be helpful. Surgery is sometimes needed: the options include proximal hemiphalangectomy, arthrodesis, or excision arthroplasty of the PIP joint if there is troublesome contracture.

In deciding whether operative treatment of these conditions is indicated it should be borne in mind that the patient's safety may be compromised if they have difficulty in walking over uneven surfaces or wearing safety boots.

Metatarsalgia is pain arising from the metatarsal heads. Any condition that causes dorsal subluxation and clawing of the toes may cause the transfer of load from the toes to the metatarsal heads and consequent pain. Painful metatarsal heads may also occur from Freiberg's infraction, which is a condition most commonly occurring in the second and third decades. It is an example of an osteochondrosis in which avascular necrosis of the second, or rarely the third, metatarsal head occurs. The characteristic clinical features are pain on weight-bearing, swelling due to synovitis, and limitation of extension of the toe. Rarefaction is seen on the dorsal side of the head on early radiographs. Later, fragmentation and broadening of the head occur with thickening of the metatarsal shaft due to increased metatarsal load-bearing. These must be differentiated from a stress (march) fracture or Morton's metatarsalgia caused by an interdigital neuroma. Morton's metatarsalgia mainly affects middle-aged women and the condition is usually unilateral (85%). Patients complain of intermittent shooting pains or a constant ache in the region of the metatarsal heads, which is worsened by walking and relieved by rest or removal of their footwear. There is frequently tenderness in the third web space and a palpable click on squeezing the metatarsal heads. If the neuroma is large the toes may be spread. Subjective numbness in the distribution of the common digital nerve is a frequent complaint but there is often no objective sensory loss. Dorsal or plantar excision is usually followed by good relief of symptoms. Metatarsalgia can be a significant disability in workers who stand or walk for long periods.

Deformities of the feet may mean that the protective footwear now mandatory in many occupations cannot be worn comfortably. Equally so, it is often difficult to wear rigid footwear immediately after foot operations and adaptations may have to be allowed on a temporary basis after a suitable risk assessment.

In employees experiencing foot pain, the use of a high stool or chair may relieve the need for excessive standing, but work patterns may need temporary reorganization to reduce excessive walking. After operations feet are often painful because of the weight-bearing function and mobility of these areas. Adequate analgesia is important and both employees and employers will need reassuring encouragement as recovery proceeds after such operations.

Neuromuscular disorders

Neuromuscular disorders and their orthopaedic sequelae may be caused by disease of the upper motor neurone (e.g. cerebral palsy), the lower motor neurone (e.g. poliomyelitis), or muscle. Problems arise because of instability from muscle weakness or joint abnormality and from deformity due to relative shortening of soft tissues, muscle imbalance, and impairment of co-ordination.

Poliomyelitis is a very common cause of disability worldwide, but it is relatively uncommon in western Europe. There is an enormous variation in the extent and severity of weakness or deformity and, as with cerebral palsy, surgical and non-surgical treatments have to be tailored to individual problems. Surgery is sometimes needed to correct deformity (e.g. release of contractures, tendon transfer, arthrodesis) or to manage secondary complications of paralysis (e.g. arthritis). Although many people with limbs that have been markedly affected by polio are able to work for many years, premature retirement may have to be considered, especially from jobs that have been physically demanding. The requirement of the DDA will prevail and relocation, or job adaptations, must be considered before putting up a case for retirement.

Arthrogryposis multiplex congenita is a rare condition and is probably an intrauterine neuropathy. This causes fibrous contractures of joints and muscle and is characterized by severe joint stiffness and weakness. Knee deformities, clubfoot, and hip dislocation are common in early childhood. In severe cases life expectancy is reduced but in those surviving to working age there will be a major limitation in mobility although intelligence is normal. Often individuals require multiple surgical procedures to reduce contracture and to improve posture.

Peripheral nerve entrapment (see also p. 277)

Peripheral nerve entrapment may result from compression, distraction, angulation, or friction-producing symptoms and/or signs in a specific nerve distribution.

Median and ulnar nerve: conditions and entrapment

The commonest is **median nerve compression—carpal tunnel syndrome** (see Chapter 13). **Ulnar nerve entrapment** at the elbow is the second commonest site for nerve entrapment in the upper limb. The patient describes numbness and tingling in the ulnar nerve distribution, followed by pain in the elbow and forearm, which may disturb sleep. Motor signs include weakness of pinch with a positive Froment's sign (flexion of the terminal phalanx of the thumb occurs when adduction is attempted), weakness of grip due to paresis of flexor digitorum profundus to the ring and little fingers, small muscle wasting, and varying degrees of ulnar claw hand.

Ulnar nerve entrapment can also occur more distally where the nerve enters the hand through Guyon's canal. The commonest causes are a ganglion from one of the carpal joints or an occupational injury.

Radial nerve entrapment is rare. **Radial tunnel syndrome** (resistant tennis elbow) causes pain over the interosseous nerve, which should be distinguished from the lateral epicondylar pain of tennis elbow.

Peripheral nerve entrapment in the lower limb is rare. Idiopathic entrapment of the common peroneal nerve may occur in the fibular tunnel. Most are neuropraxias from acute trauma or compression, which result in a foot drop with inversion. Tarsal tunnel syndrome is due to entrapment of the distal part of the posterior tibial nerve at the level of the medial malleolus. Patients complain of pain in the foot in one or more distributions of the three terminal branches of the posterior tibial nerve. It may wake them from sleep and is worse after activity. There is local tenderness and a positive Tinel sign (distal paraesthesia on tapping directly on the nerve) behind the medial malleolus.

Surgical decompression relieves the pressure on the nerve by removing the anatomical structure causing the compression.

Peripheral nerve injuries

The axillary nerve, which innervates the important deltoid muscle, is vulnerable to traction injury during dislocation of the shoulder. This injury is usually relatively benign enabling regeneration and reasonably good functional recovery. It is best treated conservatively.

Brachial plexus lesions may be traumatic lesions, either from injury at birth or later by traction, penetration, irradiation, compression (including thoracic outlet syndrome), or neoplasia. The brachial plexus is formed by the convergence of the anterior rami of C5, C6, C7, C8, and T1. In the anterior triangle of the neck, behind the clavicle and into the axilla, nerve fibres interweave to form the trunks, the cords, and ultimately the radial median, and ulnar nerves. Major brachial plexus palsies are rare but when they do occur they are devastating to limb function. In civilian life most palsies are caused by motorcycle accidents, but they can be caused by penetrating wounds and traction to the limb during falls, or sport. Most clinicians classify injuries as either upper plexus injuries (Erb's) or lower plexus injuries (Klumpke's). There are three degrees of severity of plexus injury that affect the likelihood of recovery:

+ neuropraxia (traction of the nerve without loss of continuity)
+ rupture of the nerve or nerve root distal to the dorsal root ganglion (DRG)
+ Avulsion of the nerve root proximal to the DRG.

Neuropraxias can recover spontaneously but may take up to 2 years for functional recovery. Rupture distal to the DRG may recover after surgical repair or nerve grafting but recovery is never complete. Avulsed nerve roots never recover and the only chance of any functional recovery is with salvage surgery either involving stabilizing joint arthrodesis or tendon transfer. In permanent palsy there is severe weakness, numbness, and often unremitting pain. Pain is not helped by the usual analgesics but may be helped by carbamazepine, or transcutaneous electrical nerve stimulation (TENS).

The majority of individuals affected by these conditions are young men and if the dominant limb is involved this has a devastating effect on their ability to work. Such injuries are likely to be incompatible with occupations demanding safe lifting and handling. This requires appraisal of all aspects of the job and the workplace and will often require retraining and relearning of basic skills. Initial prolonged absence from work will need considerable patience from patient, colleagues, and employer, but with appropriate input and modification to the workplace many can return to full gainful employment.

The median nerve is damaged by lacerations around the wrist, either self-inflicted as part of a suicide attempt or accidental when the patient smashes a window. Less often the ulnar nerve is injured, usually around the elbow where it runs superficially. Because this site is remote from the hand, the functional outcome following ulnar nerve injuries is often poor. However, some improvement can be achieved if the repair is carried out by surgeons with particular experience of this condition. The ulnar nerve plays a major part in the innervation of the intrinsic muscles of the hand, and the motor problems that arise in the absence of recovery cause more handicap than the sensory loss. If surgery is indicated, the choice lies between simple release, medial epicondylectomy, or anterior transposition of the nerve.

For both the ulnar and median nerves two types of deficit result—motor and sensory. Resultant motor dysfunction is the more sensitive to the level of the laceration. Median and indeed ulnar nerve lacerations cause similar sensory dysfunctions as the major sensory target is distal to the division of the main nerve trunk. If the ulnar nerve is divided above the elbow there will be weakness in both flexion and extension of particularly the ulnar half of the hand. If, however, the injury is at wrist level normal flexion is likely to persist but the patient will be unable to straighten the fingers. Median nerve injuries at elbow level and above will result in poor flexion of the thumb and first and second fingers, but also an inability to oppose the thumb to the other fingers of the hand. If the injury is more distal the motor dysfunction will be the same but will pose, at this level, a more significant functional disability than an ulnar nerve lesion, preventing in many cases the patient from properly gripping a pen, hammer, etc.

Median nerve laceration around the wrist is extremely disabling, particularly if the dominant hand is injured, as the patient is initially left without any sensory innervation in the most important part of the fingers. The median nerve also innervates the muscles around the thumb, which enable the thumb to be brought into opposition and act as a post for the rest of the fingers. If this motor function is lost and not restored in any other way the functional deficit will be similar to the disability of an amputation. The lack of motor function in the thumb can, however, be compensated for if the more proximally innervated muscles of the forearm are intact as tendon transfer can be carried out especially if the ulnar nerve is intact. However, sensory deficit in the hand cannot be made up and the best option is to carry out meticulous repair of the median nerve to gain optimal sensory reinnervation.

Hand rehabilitation following nerve damage is to a great extent preventive. Nerve regeneration takes a long time and cannot be enhanced so permanent contractures can develop, which may prevent the patient from using the hand even after complete successful nerve regeneration has taken place. It is therefore important that during rehabilitation all joints in the affected extremity are treated regularly by a hand therapist. Between exercises a special splint may have to be worn ensuring the joints are placed in the most appropriate position to prevent contractures. After regeneration has taken place it may be necessary for the patient to be given a specific exercise programme in order to rebuild the strength of the affected muscles. As function has been impaired or is absent it generally takes twice as long for strength to return. Although partial sensation may have returned to the hand the input is not of the same quality as before the injury because the individual nerve cells do not grow back in exactly the same order as previously. If patients have had major sensory nerves repaired then sensory re-education may be necessary. The occupational physician should be very cautious in giving a long-term prognosis in these cases, which may take several years to achieve maximum recovery and which may be far from complete. There may be a permanent and significant functional deficit even in the best cases.

Congenital limb deformities

A clear distinction must be made between genetic abnormalities and congenital deformities. The former can produce the latter, but most congenital deformities do not have a genetic predisposition. Congenital limb deformities causing major functional disability are rare but minor deformities are relatively common. As a rule, the more proximal the deformity, the rarer and the more significant it is. Deformity may be classified as either the failure of formation of parts (transverse or longitudinal) or the failure of separation or differentiation of parts. Transverse failure of formations present as congenital amputation. Longitudinal failures (e.g. thalidomide) produce conditions such as radial club hand, cleft hand, or fibular hemimelia.

Commoner conditions such as duplications (e.g. polydactyly), hypoplasias, and hyperplasias are less serious. Surgery to improve function and not just appearance may include joint fusions, digit transplantation, limb shortening/lengthening, or even amputation. The commonest deformities presenting at birth to an orthopaedic surgeon are clubfoot (congenital talipes equinovarus, CTEV) and developmental dysplasia of the hip (DDH, previously called CDH). The majority of patients with CTEV and DDH are treated successfully in childhood and rarely have problems at work, but DDH may require hip surgery in later life.

Some genetic abnormalities produce orthopaedic conditions that may influence normal day to day activities. A number of autosomal dominantly inherited conditions are of interest including **osteogenesis imperfecta tarda** (the adult form of brittle bone disease), **classic dwarfism** (achondroplasia), and **neurofibromatosis.** Adults with achondroplasia can often cope well in the workplace provided they choose their jobs carefully and the workplace is ergonomically adapted. **Osteogenesis imperfecta** is an abnormality in the structure of collagen. This can either cause death *in utero*, severe deformity and growth retardation, or only minor bone fragility. A previous orthopaedic history will define an individual's suitability for particular employment so that avoidance of certain physical activities can be planned. Severe growth retardation can occur with this condition, and allowances in the workplace may be needed to accommodate those of marked short stature. However, the nature of the work must also be carefully considered. Any job requiring strong repetitive or forceful movements of the skeleton would be unsuitable. If aids can be reasonably provided to alleviate such situations then their procurement may be necessary to fulfil the requirements of the DDA.

Leg length inequality

Leg length inequality (LLI) may be due to an abnormally short or abnormally long limb. Any significant inequality in leg length is likely to interfere with a person's ability to cope with a physically demanding occupation. A short leg may be due to a congenitally short femur or tibia, congenital hemiatrophy, fracture malunion or growth plate injury. A long leg may be due to a congenital long limb in association with vascular anomalies or neurofibromatosis. Infection may destroy an epiphysis, causing shortening, or conversely, may cause overgrowth due to chronic osteomyelitis. LLI of less than 1.5 cm requires no corrective treatment. LLI of between 1.5 and 3 cm in an adult should be managed with a raised shoe. Discrepancies of more than 3 cm are not usually treated with a shoe raise, owing to its bulk and unacceptable appearance. LLI of more than 4 cm leads to marked asymmetry of spinal rotation. It is generally accepted that discrepancies over 2.5 cm can give rise to problems in the spine. Leg length discrepancies of this magnitude may be treated by lengthening the short limb or shortening the longer limb. In general, an average or tall individual with less than 5 cm discrepancy should undergo shortening of the opposite leg, as this involves less morbidity. The safe limit for lengthening is approximately 15% of the original bone length. Discrepancies greater than this are not correctable by one procedure and may require a combination of leg lengthening and contralateral leg shortening, or more than one lengthening procedure.

Amputations and prosthetics

Between 5000 and 6000 new amputees are seen in limb-fitting centres in England each year. The commonest reason for amputation is vascular insufficiency (54%) followed by diabetes (20%), trauma (11%), embolism (4%), and malignancy (4%).

Amputations and congenital limb deficiencies

The last national statistics for amputations were for 2002–3. A National Amputee Database has now been established. These statistics reflect only patients being referred to the Prosthetic Centres in England and therefore do not give the full incidence of new amputations. The figures, however, allow some points to be drawn. In 2002–3, 5565 patients were seen for the first time. Lower-limb amputations are more frequent than upper-limb amputations, the ratio being 18:1. The causes of lower- and upper-limb amputations are quite different and are shown for 2002–3 in Table 12.1. Limb deficiencies, or congenital growth anomalies, form a very small percentage of the whole. Functionally, the effect of an amputation is on mobility for lower-limb amputees and dexterity for upper-limb amputees. The extent of disturbance of function depends mainly on the level of amputation, the more proximal, the greater the disturbance.

However, it is worth noting that although one cannot walk without two legs, it is perfectly possible to do most activities with only one arm. As a rough guide, lower limb amputees will need 6 months before returning to work and upper limb amputees 3 months, although if the dominant arm was amputated rehabilitation may take longer.

Complications of amputation

Complications of amputations can be divided into immediate and late (see Table 12.2). Each of these complications can not only delay return to work but can limit working effectiveness or lead to further absence, with associated social and psychological problems.

In lower limb amputees there is an increased incidence of premature degenerative change in the joints of the contralateral limb, the knee more than the hip. In upper limb amputees there appears to be an increased incidence of shoulder and neck problems.

In addition to these medical complications there is the inconvenience of relying on a mechanical device, which itself requires maintenance and repair to provide reliable service. Individuals may require time off during working hours to attend for routine appointments.

Table 12.1 Amputation by principal cause (amputee statistical database for the UK 2002–3)

Upper limb	%	Lower limb	%
Trauma	57	Dysvascularity	70
Dysvascularity	10	Trauma	8
Neoplasia	9	Infection	6
Infection	2	Neoplasia	3
Other causes	22	Other causes	13
Total	100	Total	100

Table 12.2 Complications of amputation and their management

Complication	Treatment
Immediate	
1. Delayed healing	
Infection	Antibiotics
Ischaemia	Vasodilators Angioplasty Sympathectomy Higher amputation
2. Postoperative oedema	Stump elevation Exercises Elasticated stump sock Mobilization on an early walking aid
3. Phantom pain	Massage Analgesics Antidepressants Carbamazepine/other anticonvulsants Anticoagulants Behaviour modification
Late	
4. Late changes in stump volume	Adjust or refit socket
5. Stump abrasions	Adjust socket
6. Infected epidermoid cysts	Socket fit Stump hygiene Surgical excision
7. Neuromas	Adjust socket Neurectomy
8. Stress on other parts of the body	

Upper limb prosthesis

There are fewer than 100 upper-limb amputations per year in the UK. These amputations are carried out because of malignancy or severe trauma. A third group needing upper limb prostheses may be children with congenital loss of whole or part of the upper extremity. Children will generally have the best foundation for useful function of their upper limb prosthesis as they may, from an early age, develop the ability to use an advanced neurocutaneous electrically operated prosthesis.

The function that patients may be able to achieve with prostheses varies greatly: at one extreme is the patient who never accepts psychologically the loss of a limb and, as a result, rejects the whole concept of using a functional prosthesis and even sometimes a cosmetic prosthesis. Often, at the other extreme, are younger and otherwise fully fit individuals who are able to learn how a myoelectric prosthesis works and are able to operate it with such accuracy that even complex activities can be achieved, e.g. lifting a child using a normal hand and a myoelectric upper limb prosthesis.

Upper-limb amputations usually occur in younger patients as a result of trauma. Amputation in the upper limb can be devastating, usually more so than a loss of the corresponding part of the lower limb.

The most effective upper limb device is still the split hook, but technology is rapidly advancing. Artificial hands tend to be passive devices used for cosmetic purposes. Mechanical hands are bulky and heavy. 'Phantom limb' is present in all amputees to some degree but disappears more quickly in younger patients. Loss of a hand in an occupation requiring repetitive fine movements is likely to demand a change of occupation. Alternative jobs are possible but support of the employee may be critical, especially when the job involves contact with members of the public when the individual may feel awkward or embarrassed.

The amputee's job must be evaluated to make sure that the remaining limb is not placed at risk. Mechanization of the job is likely to be required to fulfil the requirement of the DDA to make reasonable adjustment and allow the individual to continue at work if at all possible. Voice-activated software would be beneficial for a worker using visual display equipment (VDE) to make sure that the remaining limb was not overworked. Dictating machines may be a substitute when the ability to write easily is lost because of a limb amputation and adaptations to telephones in the office may allow 'hands off' use.

Many occupations can be resumed following an **amputation of a lower limb**, but work in any of the emergency services, or jobs requiring climbing, ladder work, or scaffolding, are obviously excluded. An individual assessment of each case is essential. In below-knee amputations 75% of patients will walk with a prosthesis but with a 10–40% increase in energy expenditure. With an above-knee amputation only 20% are able to work because of the increased (65%) energy expenditure, although this is age related. Energy-storing feet and hydraulic joints allow efficient effective leg prostheses.

Careful examination of the workplace is essential to determine what part of a particular job can still be managed effectively. It is likely that most office-based and manufacturing jobs can still be done, providing adaptations in the workplace allow easy access and ergonomic adaptations are made to accommodate a wheelchair if necessary. Particularly in above-knee amputations in older people, the use of an electric wheelchair may facilitate movement about the workplace that would not be possible if long distances have to be walked. Employees who need to drive may have their vehicles adapted to hand controls.

The capabilities of those who have had amputations vary considerably and adaptation of the working conditions may well allow the individual to continue in their employment. In the foot, toe and ray amputations do not usually cause problems except in the case of the big toe and first ray. Through-ankle amputation provides better function than amputation through the hind foot, because it allows the use of a more effective prosthesis and better healing is obtained. Weight bearing is still possible through the stump even when the prosthesis is not worn.

The prosthetist is the person who tailors the fit of the artificial limb or prosthesis to the individual. This is a highly skilled job and requires knowledge of traditional materials, such as leather, metal, and wood as well as an increasing range of modern synthetics such as plastics, silicone, and carbon fibre. Prosthetic joints are becoming more sophisticated; for example energy-storing feet, which incorporate elastic materials that mimic normal gait more closely, and microprocessor-controlled knee units, which automatically control the rate of swing of the lower leg in relation to the speed of the gait.

Upper limb prostheses can be purely cosmetic, body-powered, or externally powered. Body-powered limbs can be adapted to a wide range of functions and very fine movements can be achieved. Servo-assisted mechanisms can augment weak muscles. Myoelectric prostheses, which are triggered by signals from muscle groups in the residual limb, are increasingly available. At present they still tend to be much heavier than body-powered limbs, are less reliable and offer relatively crude hand movement. In complex congenital deficiencies such as those with phocomelia (e.g. due to past use of thalidomide in pregnancy), individually designed prostheses may be required.

Rehabilitation of the amputee

Rehabilitation of the amputee requires multidisciplinary teamwork. Ideally, the team (surgeon, nurses, physiotherapist, occupational therapist, and rehabilitation physician) should assess the individual preoperatively. The technique of amputation is critical as satisfactory fitting of a prosthesis starts with the surgeon's fashioning of the stump, which must be viewed as an 'organ of locomotion'. Postoperatively the amputee will work on general muscle strength and specific stump exercises and be assisted in restoring independence in daily activities. Walking, using an early walking aid under the supervision of the physiotherapist, commences 5–7 days after the amputation. Rehabilitation continues following discharge from hospital, until the amputee has achieved maximum functional independence, and in the case of those of working age, has returned to suitable employment (see below).

Special work problems

A number of general and specific points should be borne in mind when advising both amputee and employer about working conditions. In general, employers should be made aware that a patient has an artificial limb. It is particularly important that adequate washing facilities can allow the amputee to attend to the limb and stump in reasonable privacy.

Individual assessment of the disability produced by a foot problem is necessary. Job adaptation may be necessary prior to, or during recovery from the operation. High stools allowing employees who normally stand to take the weight off their feet may be useful, and temporary reduction in walking duties may be necessary. An assessment of alternative footwear may be necessary to facilitate an early return to work. However, where safety boots are essential such adaptations may be unwise.

Lower limb amputees should avoid working at heights, climbing ladders, and habitually walking over uneven ground. Generally, the more proximal the amputation the more limited the mobility. Lower limb amputees may not be able to stand all day, but equally it is inadvisable to sit all day without periodically getting up and moving around. Bilateral lower limb amputees may need to use a wheelchair if they have stump or prosthetic problems. These employees, therefore, require wheelchair-accessible premises (see below). In the case of upper-limb amputation, there is little or no restriction on the clerical worker and manual workers can adapt remarkably well, with self-evident limitation. A full assessment by an occupational physician, including an employment evaluation, should always be performed before giving a definite opinion.

Use of walking aids and wheelchairs

Individuals who return to work using sticks or crutches experience particular difficulty with heavy spring-loaded doors (e.g. fire doors) and steps and stairs. The latter need to have at least one handrail to ensure safety. People using a walking frame generally find steps or stairs impossible to negotiate unless the depth of step accommodates the frame as well as the individual.

Individuals who require a wheelchair need suitable ramps over all steps and sills. Doorways and corridors need to be of suitable width to allow easy movement with adequate turning space. Particular attention must be given to toilet facilities. If the person has to work on more than one floor, then the use of lifts will be needed, with controls placed at an accessible height. Attention may also be required to desk heights, access to filing cabinets, and other working surfaces or furniture.

Bone and joint infection

Septic arthritis

Septic arthritis is a rare condition, which occurs by haematogenous spread, penetrating injury, or spread from neighbouring osteomyelitis. *Staphylococcus aureus* is the most frequent infecting organism; streptococci and coliforms account for most of the rest. In adults there is frequently an overlying wound or distal portal of entry, but this may be absent in the immunocompromised host. Previous arthritis is a predisposing factor. The classical signs are fever, erythema, effusion, and severely restricted range of movement. Treatment consists of joint drainage, antibiotics, and splintage. Prompt diagnosis and treatment are vital to avoid permanent damage to the cartilage. Tuberculous arthritis is occasionally seen in Europe, and this should not be forgotten when individuals travel widely during their working life. Septic arthritis is usually monoarticular. The order of frequency is hip, knee, ankle, sacro-iliac, wrist, and shoulder. A synovectomy can be considered in those with pronounced synovitis and an abscess may require drainage.

Acute infection of bone

Acute infection of bone occurs directly by contamination of an open wound (exogenous) or indirectly by haematogenous spread. It may occur as a complication of trophic ulcers in diabetics. The commonest causative organism is *Staphylococcus aureus* (80%). Osteomyelitis may become chronic as a result of inadequate treatment, a highly virulent organism, or impaired host resistance. Open fractures or penetrating injuries to bone may be complicated by osteomyelitis. Antibiotics are used immediately the diagnosis is suspected. Initial 'best guess' choice of antibiotic can be altered if blood cultures or pus allow specific organisms to be cultured. Open drainage is advised if there is swelling suggestive of an abscess or a sequestrum is identified. Splintage relieves pain and aids healing.

Hand infections

Infections of the hand usually follow an open injury and rarely occur by haematogenous spread from a distant focus. The commonest infecting organisms are *Staphylococcus aureus* (50–80%), streptococcal species, and coliform bacilli, but after an open wound any organism may be present. A human bite may be contaminated by *Eikenella corrodens* (and may be associated with an osteochondral fracture in up to 60% of cases if the bite has been incurred in a fight). *Bacteroides* and *Pasteurella multocida* are frequently isolated from animal bites. Infection of the nail fold (paronychia) often follows a minor penetrating injury. A chronic paronychia occurs in people whose occupation involves sustained immersion of the hand in water and is characterized by an inflamed eponychium with loss of the cuticle. Occupational infections include orf (sheep workers), erysipeloid (meat workers) pilonidal sinus (hairdressers), and infections with *Mycobacterium marinum* (swimming pool attendants). In cases of unusual tenosynovitis, consider the possibility of tuberculosis or *Mycobacterium kansaii*.

Infections of bone are likely to cause problems at work, mainly related to the time that is needed for a cure to be achieved. In rare cases persistence of a discharging sinus may make employment inappropriate in healthcare workers or where control of infection is vital.

Skeletal tuberculosis

Skeletal tuberculosis is caused by infection with *Mycobacterium tuberculosis* in the majority of cases, with *Mycobacterium bovis* and the rarer mycobacteria accounting for the rest. The incidence of skeletal tuberculosis is decreasing in the Western world, but not in Africa and Asia where there are 400 new cases per 100 000 population per year and one-tenth of all cases have skeletal tuberculosis. The spine is involved in 50% of those with disease of the musculoskeletal system. In tuberculous osteomyelitis any long bone may be affected. There are various regimens of chemotherapy using combinations of rifampicin, isoniazid, and pyrazinamide. Surgery is rarely required.

The length of time required for treatment to be effective especially in those with physically demanding jobs is likely to be a problem in most occupational situations. Whether any return to such posts is possible, or wise, depends on the site of infection and the stability of the bones and joints involved.

Trauma to the upper and lower limbs

In the industrialized world most severe injuries arise from road traffic accidents, which claim approximately 1 in 10 000 lives each year. Most deaths occur within the first hour following the injury, before the patient arrives at a hospital, and brain and thoracic injuries are the commonest causes. With improved emergency treatment at the roadside, more and more severely injured patients now reach hospital alive. Visceral injuries and cardiorespiratory complications must be treated first, with definitive treatment of musculoskeletal injuries delayed until after the patient's condition has been stabilized.

Tendons

The commonest tendon injuries arise from sharp injuries to the hands. The appropriate treatment depends on whether injury is to the extensor or to the flexor tendons. Extensor tendon injuries can be treated successfully with simple repair and immobilization for approximately 4 weeks, after which an equivalent rehabilitation period will lead to an acceptable functional outcome. Injuries to the flexor tendons of the fingers require skilled surgical repair and then postoperative rehabilitation by a dedicated hand therapist. A specially designed splint is used that passively flexes the fingers by means of a pulley but allows the patient to extend the fingers actively. Such a device will be necessary for 8–10 weeks before the patient is allowed to start active flexion exercises. Full rehabilitation may take up to 3 months after the initial repair. When flexor tendon repair has been delayed, a two-stage repair may be needed using spare tendons from other parts of the body after an initial operation has created a tunnel in which the grafted tendon can slide.

Ligaments

The commonest ligamentous injuries are about the ankle and knee. The commonest injuries to the knee are to the medial and lateral collateral ligaments. A more serious injury is to the ACL, which occurs with a torsional injury to the knee. Typical examples are the footballer who twists his knee or the skier who crashes. There may be a loud crack, immediate swelling, and severe pain. The injury causes instability of the knee, which may lead to secondary meniscal tears (see p. 270). No firm guidelines can be given regarding whether patients can work while on waiting lists for surgery to meniscal tears or cruciate ligament injuries. However, patients who for safety reasons require full use of their knees such as scaffolders, construction workers, and steeplejacks, or those who need to work on uneven ground, such as farmers, foresters, or emergency workers, should be directed towards less physically demanding work until surgery has been carried out. The same restrictions apply to carers who have to lift and support others. Office workers may return to work about 2 weeks after arthroscopic surgery for meniscal tears. Individuals who have physical jobs may not be able to return to work until normal muscle strength around the knee is re-established, particularly if they have been off work for a long time and developed significant muscle atrophy. Patients who have had surgery for reconstruction of ligaments may take up to a year to return to high physical activity and they will normally be required to wear a brace or plaster for 6–12 weeks after the operation.

A common site of ligamentous injury in the hand is the ulnar collateral ligament of the thumb (gamekeeper's or skier's thumb). This occurs when the ligament is stressed and subsequently ruptured due to radiovalgus trauma to the metacarpophalangeal joint. If it is completely unstable it is advisable to explore the injury and if necessary effect a repair. Postoperative rehabilitation requires 6 weeks in plaster followed by subsequent rehabilitation, which can normally be carried out by the patient himself. Depending on the dominant side, lighter work tasks can be carried out even in the immediate postoperative period and also during rehabilitation depending on the requisite grip strength in the affected hand.

Cartilage

There are three types of cartilage: hyaline, elastic, and fibrocartilage. Hyaline cartilage, which consists mainly of mucopolysaccharides, is the most common. Hyaline cartilage persists in adult life not only on the articular surfaces of joints, where it covers the opposing bone edges, but also in the supporting framework of the nose, larynx, trachea, and bronchi. Because of the mucopolysaccharides, hyaline cartilage has a very high concentration of water, which acts as a sponge, transforming the cartilage into a buffer, and acting as a barrier to mechanical trauma. However, if damaged, it is replaced not by new hyaline cartilage but by fibrocartilage, which does not have the same mucopolysaccharide content and is therefore not able to re-establish the same good mechanical shock-absorbing qualities. This is the reason why, after joint trauma, although no injuries may be discerned initially, the joint may develop osteoarthritic changes later when the original cartilage is replaced with a less mechanically favourable type.

Nerves (see also pp. 275 and 277)

Functional outcome

Several factors affect the functional outcome following a nerve injury. The best outcome is following a simple neuropraxia where the nerve fibre itself is not divided, or a crush injury that does not require surgical intervention. The least successful is any nerve injury that requires surgical intervention. The other important factor is the distance from the injured nerve to the target organ. Little if any function can be re-established following 2 years' lack of nerve supply. As the distance, in a mature adult, from the cervical spinal cord to the hand is in the region of 80 cm, with a regeneration growth of 1 mm per day the nerve-damaged hand is on the borderline as far as eventual function is concerned. Thus a significant delay in carrying out a surgical procedure may prevent a useful functional outcome even though the nerve eventually reaches the target organ. It is important therefore to establish as early as possible whether an injury has caused nerve damage requiring surgical intervention. If surgery is necessary, it should be carried out as soon as possible.

Age has been cited as an important factor for establishing good functional outcome following injury, but it is not clear whether this is a matter of age itself or size (and therefore a matter of growth distance). Experiments have not shown that young animals have superior regeneration to older ones under controlled conditions.

Hand injuries (See also p. 275–6)

Most nerve injuries are to the hand and therefore most often affect sensory nerves. When dealing with sensory nerves it is important to remember that the most significant disability following such injuries is not the loss of sensation but the neurogenic pain that such nerve lesions can cause. Two types of neurogenic disturbance can occur following such injuries.

1. The best known is **post-traumatic neuroma**, which normally occurs when the nerve has been completely transected and the proximal stump of the nerve has separated from the distal end. This prevents the growing axons from reaching the distal stump and they form a neuroma. Even small neuromas in the upper limb can cause significant pain and functional disability. It is important therefore that such nerve injuries are explored if possible and repair effected, as this significantly reduces post-traumatic neuroma formation. If a neuroma has formed, desensitization carried out by a specialist hand therapist can in some cases reduce discomfort. Utensils or tools with special handles that reduce direct compression of the neuroma can sometimes be useful. However, in most cases where a significant neuroma has formed, the best method of treatment is excision and grafting of the nerve if the distal end can be located. If that is not the case then transfer of the neuroma to a location that is less likely to be exposed to direct compression can help reduce the functional disability.

2. A less common problem is **post-traumatic Raynaud's syndrome**, which can occur after either crush or transection injuries. This often leads to cold intolerance, which, particularly for individuals who normally work in low temperatures or wet climates, may prove to be severely disabling. There is no proven treatment for this disorder but sympathetic blockade can be attempted using oral medication or a chemical sympathectomy by X-ray controlled injection. Guanethidine blockade, sympathetic stellate blockade, or transthoracic sympathectomy in well-selected patients can improve their work ability although some form of persistent disability always remains.

The hand is an extremely complex organ and critical organ and critical from almost any occupational point of view. It is also frequently injured in workplace accidents. Skilled repair of hand injuries, particularly to tendons is, therefore, essential and prolonged rehabilitation, under the care of a dedicated hand physiotherapist, may be required. The occupational physician has an important role to play in restoring the employee's confidence and preparing him for a return to employment by arranging, where possible, modified but rewarding employment at his normal place of work. This also requires sympathetic and supportive employers.

Limb reimplantation

Limb reimplantation is, for practical purposes only, carried out on upper extremities usually only around the wrist and more distally. Muscles in the extremities suffer permanent damage if they are deprived of their circulation for more than 6 hours. It is possible to reimplant a whole leg and achieve survival of structures such as bone and skin, but if the muscles do not function such reimplantations often cause more disability than amputation, which leaves a stump that may be fashioned for a useful prosthesis. As a result of these considerations, only whole-hand reimplantation is commonly attempted today. The intrinsic muscles of the hand may not work, but because of the function of the extrinsic long tendons and a hope of functional sensation in the hand, useful results can be achieved despite complete loss of the intrinsic muscles. Single-finger reimplantation is no longer advocated except when the thumb is involved. The reason for this is that reimplanted digits often lose their full range of movement and normal sensation. As, to all intents and purposes, a three-finger grip only is required, such patients will often avoid using such a disabled finger. Patients who have had reimplantation of a single finger have worse function than those who have had an immediate functional filling of the amputation stump. In addition rehabilitation following finger reimplantation can, due to prolonged healing problems and loss of sensation, be very long whereas revision of an amputation may enable a heavy labourer to return to work within a month with good permanent functional ability. Single finger amputation (either right or left) should not prevent an individual returning to work. However, many-finger amputations lead to problems of post-traumatic cold intolerance, which, apart from the milder degrees, does not seem to improve with time. This can also be the case even if the finger has been successfully reimplanted; quite often patients who have experienced significant limb injuries suffer as much from pain and cold intolerance as they do from actual loss of function as a result of reduced morbidity in the extremity. Obviously if an individual requires, for their particular occupation, to use all five fingers of both hands, or need normal mobility of all fingers, then such injuries can prove extremely limiting. With dominant hand injuries younger adults seem to be surprisingly able to compensate by increasingly using the non-dominant hand if only one hand is required. If both hands are required at normal strength and range of movement, such compensation cannot take place.

In assessing whether a patient with a partial amputation of the hand falls within the DDA, the functional disability must impair daily activities, not the patient's work. The loss of the little finger, for example, is unlikely to impair daily activities even though it may be incompatible with certain occupations, such as a professional pianist. In such a case the patient will not be disabled within the meaning of the Act. Each case must be carefully assessed by deciding whether there is a significant impairment of day to day activities.

Stress fractures

Fractures can arise from traumatic injury to healthy bone, repetitive strain to healthy bone, or during normal use of a pathologically weakened bone. Stress fractures occur in the absence of a specific precipitating event. They result from fatigue failure of normal bone after repeated normal loading.

Stress fractures are rare but can occur at sites repeatedly subjected to bending or twisting forces. One is the 'march fracture', so named because it occurs in soldiers, and affects the metatarsal neck. Stress fractures of the medial malleolus are seen most frequently in runners. These injuries present with a constant ache in the foot or ankle and the fractures are often not seen initially on plain radiographs. The diagnosis may be made with an isotope bone scan or MRI scan. Stress fractures of the patella and of the neck of the femur have been described in athletes participating in jumping or long distance running or walking. Stress fractures of the upper extremity are most frequently described in the hook of the hamate in individuals who use hammers presenting as a dull ache and an ulnar nerve neuritis.

Trauma of the upper limb

Shoulder

Shoulder injuries are common. Most are soft tissue problems with ligament and muscle strains predominant. **Anterior dislocation** of the shoulder is a common injury, usually caused by a fall or a wrenching external rotation force. Posterior dislocation is much less common. After dislocation, there is a risk in the long-term of a painful shoulder with limited movement or recurrent dislocation. Fitness for work following dislocation depends to a great extent on the method of treatment. Even a single dislocation treated with strict immobilization for at least 3 weeks can recur in up to 30% of cases in young men. Prognosis is good if there is no recurrence within 2 years. With recurrent dislocation treated with surgery there is a potential risk of further dislocation (5–10%), although the figure may be greater in physically demanding jobs. If a dislocation has recurred prior to application for a physically demanding job, a careful history and examination should be made to determine future risk, with specialist advice sought if the recurrence has been within 2 years or the 'apprehension test' (involuntary muscle spasm when the shoulder is put into a position that threatens dislocation, i.e. abduction and external rotation) is positive.

Injuries to the **acromioclavicular joint** often follow a fall directly on to the shoulder. This may cause instability or dislocation, which produces short-term pain but usually results in no disability or loss of function, but can take several months to settle. Jobs involving heavy lifting or the use of a shoulder harness can be affected and surgical stabilization may be required.

The majority of shoulder fractures are extra-articular and function is determined by the concomitant soft tissue injury. Articular fractures have a high incidence of avascular necrosis particularly when displaced. Avascular necrosis occurs in less than 10% of extra-articular fractures but in more than 60% of displaced articular fractures.[11]

Elbow

Fractures of the distal humerus in the working population are often high-energy injuries. However, 75% of patients have satisfactory results after internal fixation.[12] Significant post-traumatic OA occurs in approximately 12% of patients at 6-year follow-up. Fractures of the radial head and ulnar are extremely common and are usually caused by lower energy injuries. Ulnar olecranon injuries are invariably treated with internal fixation and early movement with the majority returning to full activities. Radial head fractures are common and caused by a fall on to the outstretched hand. These are often treated non-surgically but with displaced fractures surgery may be necessary especially if a dislocation is present.

Wrist

Fracture of the scaphoid is common and is caused by a forced dorsiflexion of the wrist usually from a fall on to an outstretched hand. An undisplaced fracture is treated in a forearm 'scaphoid' cast for 6 weeks. It is possible to work with such a cast if duties are light especially if the fracture is in the non-dominant wrist. Patients with a non-surgically treated scaphoid fracture, will be able to return to normal work. A displaced fracture or a non-union will require open reduction and fixation with a screw. In such a situation the patient will be able to resume light activities without plaster support 4–6 weeks after surgery, but heavy work should not be commenced until union has occurred. Avascular necrosis can occur and lead to OA in the wrist and permanent functional disability

Extra-articular fractures, e.g. Colles (dorsal displacement) or Smith's (volar displacement) make a good functional recovery, although 75% of patients experience subjective discomfort for up to a year following such injuries. Fractures that include an intra-articular extension, however, have a significantly worse outcome. Comminuted fractures have only a 50% satisfactory outcome. Factors associated with a poor outcome include a dorsal radial tilt of over 10° or radial deviation of greater than 10°. In younger adults with higher energy injuries arthritis is reported on X-ray in up to 65%, although only 30% of patients with radiological evidence are symptomatic.

Trauma of the lower limb

Hip fractures

Fractures of the hip either involve the acetabulum or the femoral head or rarely both. Significant fractures of the acetabulum are those that include the weight-bearing dome. Comminution is a significant prognostic sign and the presence of a joint articular step exceeding 2–3 mm is associated with a poor prognosis. A combined acetabular and femoral head fracture also has a poor prognosis. Patients over the age of 40 have worse results. Following acetabular fractures an accurate prognosis may not be given until approximately 1 year following injury. The functional recovery at 12 months reflects the final outcome. The majority of fractures of the proximal femur in the population of working age are extracapsular (and therefore extra-articular). Intracapsular fractures that are also mainly extra-articular are rare but are often caused by high-energy impact. Minimally displaced fractures are internally fixed *in situ* whereas displaced fractures need reduction and then internal fixation and have a high risk of avascular necrosis. Fractures of the femoral neck under 50 years of age are rare because of strong subcortical bone and if they occur are a sign of high-energy impact. Confirmation of bony union cannot be confirmed until 6 months postinjury and any subsequent arthritis should be evident within 1 year. Late segmental collapse of the femoral head can occur beyond 1 year.

Femoral fractures

Femoral shaft fractures are high impact injuries and occur mostly from road traffic accidents or a fall from a height. Surgical fixation with an intramedullary nail is usual and return to normal function should be expected. However, up to 6 months may be required before full recovery and other concomitant injuries often limit the rate of recovery. Intra-articular distal femoral fractures transgressing the knee inevitably produce a degree of loss of movement. Open reduction and rigid internal fixation produce the most satisfactory results. Anatomical realignment and early movement should obtain good function in more than 90% of individuals. The range of knee movement necessary for sitting is approximately 90°, for climbing stairs 100°, crouching 120° but for unrestricted movement for the majority of activities 125° is ideal. Recovery producing less than 90° of flexion or with a varus/valgus deformity greater than 15° results in significant disability.

Tibial fractures

Tibial shaft fractures are commonly caused by sports injuries but road traffic accidents often produce the more severe and often open, injuries. These are usually treated by surgical fixation using intramedullary nails but occasionally external fixation is required for more complex injuries. Owing to less soft tissue cover around the tibia healing is slower and complication rates are higher than in femoral fractures. **Tibial plateau** fractures are caused mainly as a result of a fall from a height involving a combination of axial loading and a valgus stress. Most of the remaining injuries are caused by lateral impact to the knee such as a strike by the bumper of a car. Medial plateau fractures are often of high-energy impact and have the worst results. These injuries require accurate open reduction and fixation and require specialist expertise. Long-term prognosis is significantly worse if there is coincidental ligament and meniscal injury. Tibial plafond (or pilon) fractures involve the ankle joint and are usually more severe than malleolar ankle fractures (see below). Recovery is slower and permanent articular surface damage more likely. Good function is achieved in 75% of patients following rigid internal fixation, although non-weight bearing is often required for 3 months postsurgery and return to active employment could be delayed by up to one year. Long-term sequelae of this injury may not be evident or full recovery achieved for 18 months–2 years.

The ankle

Ankle fracture accounts for approximately 10% of all fractures. It is the most commonly injured weight-bearing joint and fracture is frequent in the working age population. Ankle fractures are of two main types, malleolar fractures and tibial plafond fractures (see above). Malleolar fractures may involve the lateral malleolus, the medial malleolus and the posterior malleolus either individually or in combination. The mechanism and severity of the injuring force gives a direct indication of the likely outcome. Precise reduction of malleolar fractures is essential in obtaining a good result. After appropriate treatment of ankle injuries Lindsjo concluded that any significant post-traumatic arthritic symptoms should be evident by 18 months postinjury and depends on the congruity and stability of the joint.[13] Following accepted principles of internal fixation 90% of individuals return to the same occupation and 80% continue with sport at the pre-injury level. It is evident that an associated fracture to the posterior malleolus is a poor prognostic factor. Arthritis is evident in 30–40% of such patients in the long term.

The foot

The most debilitating fracture of the foot for manual workers is a calcaneal fracture. It is an occupational hazard for individuals who work at heights. Of all calcaneal fractures 75% are intra-articular. Displaced fractures are best treated by a specialist familiar with this particular injury and require internal fixation. Treated appropriately, 60% will have a good outcome. Others result in post-traumatic OA or shortening and widening of the heel, making boot fitting uncomfortable and walking on uneven surfaces hazardous. Residual symptoms of injury and recovery from the surgery can take 18–36 months to settle and final assessment for return to full active duties may take 2 years.

After open reduction and internal fixation (ORIF) of a fracture there is no absolute indication for removal of metalwork in an asymptomatic patient. If removal of percutaneous wires or stabilizing screws (such as diastasis screws in unstable ankle fractures or interlocking bolts in intramedullary nails) is an essential part of fracture management in the early stages, this will have occurred before fracture union. Issues about removing periarticular metalwork usually relate to soft tissue irritation or restriction of movement. There is an argument that screws inserted in subchondral positions to support articular surfaces in weight-bearing joints (such as tibial plateau or ankle pilon fracture) alter the biomechanics of cartilage wear and tear and should be removed before full activities are resumed. Following fracture union some prominent metalwork may need removing to allow full rehabilitation of joint mobility and muscle strength. Once metalwork is redundant after completion of bone healing there are no absolute indications to remove it. All indications are relative and should be discussed with the individual and the orthopaedic surgeon responsible for his/her care.

Non-union of fractures

Fracture non-union is rare. It is associated with either a high-energy injury, open fractures where infection is involved, inappropriate initial treatment, or in anatomical regions where bone blood supply may be compromised (scaphoid, talus, distal tibia). Surgery is usually necessary to internally fix the fracture fragments and bone graft and/or revascularize the fracture site. This clearly delays recovery but should enable return to full function. If non-union persists and an avascular necrosis develops within a joint, arthritis can occur. This may necessitate a joint replacement (i.e. subcapital hip non-union) or arthrodesis (i.e. scaphoid non-union).

Conclusions

Despite increasing efforts to improve safety on the road, and legislation on safety at work, traumatic injuries still continue to have a major impact on the working population. The majority of individuals, however, eventually return to work functionally intact.

Acknowledgements

The authors are grateful to the authors of the Trauma chapter in the previous edition, D. Snashall and B. Povlsen for allowing us to incorporate parts of it into this chapter.

References

1 Gabriel SE *et al*. Costs of osteoarthritis: estimates from a geographically defined population. *J Rheumatol* 1995; **22** (1 Suppl. 43): 23–5.

2 White PH. (1996) Future expectations: adolescents with rheumatic diseases and their transition into adulthood. *Br J Rheumatol* 1996; **35**: 80–3.

3 Klunder KB *et al*. Osteoarthritis of the hip and knee in retired football players. *Acta Orthop Scand* 1980; **51**: 925–7.

4 Reported on ALAMA (association of local authority medical advisors) website members forum Dec 2003 (www.alama.org.uk).

5 Seagroatt V. Elective total hip replacement: incidence, emergency readmission rate and post operative mortality. *BMJ* 1991; **303**: 1431–5.

6 Diduch DR *et al*. Total knee replacement in young active patients: long term follow up andfunctional outcome. *J Bone Joint Surg Am* 1996; **79A**: 575–82.

7 Insall JN. *Surgery of the knee*, pp. 587–695. New York: Churchill Livingston, 1996.

8 Daniel DM *et al*. Fate of the ACL injured patient; a prospective outcome study. *Am J Sports Med* 1995; **22**: 632–44.

9 Maletius W, Messner K. The effect of partial meniscectomy on the long-term prognosis of knees with localised, severe chondral damage. *Am J Sports Med* 1996; **24**(3): 258–62.

10 Saltzman C, Bonar S. Tendon problems of the foot and ankle. Orthopaedic knowledge update. *Foot Ankle*, 1st edn 1994; 269–82.

11 Sturzenegger M, Fornaro E, Jakob RP. Results of surgical treatment of multifragmented fractures of the humeral head. *Arch Orthop Trauma Surg* 1982; **100**(4): 249–59.

12 Wildburger R, Mohring M, Hofer HP. Supraintercondylar fractures of the distal humerus: results of internal fixation. *J Orthop Trauma* 1991; **5**(3): 301–7.

13 Lindsjo U. Operative treatment of ankle fracture-dislocations. *Clin Orthop Rel Res* 1985; **199**: 28–38.

Further reading

Apley AG, Solomon L. *Apley's system of orthopaedics and fractures*, (7th edn). Oxford: Butterworth-Heineman, 1993.

Barton MJ, Hooper G, Noble J, Steel MW. Occupational causes of disorders in the upper limb. *BMJ* 1993; **304**: 309–11.

Cranshaw AH (ed.) *Campbell's operative orthopaedics*, (8th cdn). St Louis, MO: Mosby Yearbook, 1991.

Doberman RH (ed.) *Operative nerve repair and reconstruction*. Philadelphia, PA: JP Lippincott, 1991.

Green DP (ed.) Operative hand surgery, 3rd edn. New York: Churchill Livingstone, 1993

Ham R, Cotton L. Limb amputation—from aetiology to rehabilitation. In: *Therapy in practice*, Vol. 23. London: Chapman & Hall, 1991.

Health and Safety Executive. *Work related upper limb disorders. A guide to prevention*. London HMSO, 1990.

Millender LH, Tromanhauser SG, Gaynor S. Occupational disorder management. *Orthop Clin North Am* 1996; **24**: 4.

Nugent IM, Ivory JP, Ross AC. *Key topics in orthopaedic surgery*. Oxford: Bios, 1995.

Review of artificial limb and appliance centre services. The report of an independent working party under the chairmanship of Professor Ian McColl. London: Crown Publishers, 1986.

Shepheard H, Bulgen D, Ward DJ. Rheumatoid arthritis—returning patients to work. *Rheum Rehab* 1981; **20**: 160–3.

Symmons D, Bankhead C. *Health care needs assessment for musculoskeletal diseases*. University of Manchester: Arthritis Research Council Epidemiology Research Unit, 1994.

Chapter 13

Rheumatological disorders

S. J. Ryder and H. A. Bird

Over 150 diseases can affect the musculoskeletal system. The vast majority are not caused by work, although work may become more difficult as a result of some.

In this chapter we consider mainly the commoner conditions:

- inflammatory polyarthritides, degenerative joint diseases, and some rarer conditions
- conditions affecting mainly muscles, tendons, connective, and soft tissue, including work-related upper limb disorders (WRULDs).

A patient may have more than one of these disorders, particularly in the upper limbs, and their interaction with the workplace may produce complex problems.

Some of the conditions considered in this chapter are also referred to in Chapter 12 (Orthopaedics) and spinal disorders are covered in Chapter 11.

Rheumatoid arthritis

Rheumatoid arthritis (RA) is the commonest of the three major inflammatory diseases; its current prevalence in the UK is about 1–2%. In a small number of subjects this disease will therefore complicate any musculoskeletal problems acquired at work. RA affects women two to three times as often as men and usually starts in the metacarpophalangeal joints of the hands with local involvement of the wrists. The disease is normally easily identifiable from circulating rheumatoid factors in the blood and the presence of a particular type of erosion on radiographs. Diagnostic confusion is unusual but may occur in the early stages before the specific blood and radiographic tests become positive. At this stage RA may also affect tendons, though it would still normally be distinguishable from tenosynovitis by its bilateral nature and by its systemic symptoms, including tiredness and malaise. Current theories on pathogenesis involve an as yet unidentified antigen, perhaps infective, superimposed on a genetic predisposition. RA is, therefore, not caused by work, though mechanical aspects are also important as potentially aggravating factors. If a unilateral stroke is superimposed on RA, the affected and less mobile side ultimately displays less joint damage. Whether this results from local neurological influences or is a direct mechanical effect is uncertain, but suggests a potentially damaging interaction between inflammatory arthritis and mechanical joint loading.

Juvenile RA and adult Still's disease are separate conditions characterized by sergonegativity and a different anatomical distribution of joint involvement. In particular the mandible is involved, to produce a receding chin.

RA can cause substantial joint deformity, with consequences for hand function, though it is now accepted that modern disease-modifying drugs can reduce bony damage, particularly if given in the early stages. Careful occupational therapy and ergonomic assessment is required for rheumatoid patients in the workplace so that their capabilities can be matched to suitable jobs. However, it is surprising how intricate movement can still be accomplished even with the most severely affected hands, particularly if thumb–finger grip is preserved. More widespread involvement, particularly of the lower limb, may necessitate substantial changes in working practices.

Prognosis should be guarded. At present there is controversy over whether RA shortens life expectancy (by perhaps about 10 years). In severe forms there is substantial morbidity with associated infections probably reflecting inadequate protection as a result of disordered autoimmunity. Recently, an increased incidence of cardiovascular disease, leading to myocardial infarction or embolic events, has been recognized as a co-morbidity independently of drugs that might predispose to this, perhaps reflecting inflammatory pathways common to both diseases. The work record may be at risk, although many patients are surprisingly resilient, retaining a will and motivation to work if at all possible.

A variety of prognostic markers have been suggested for use when the condition first presents. The most useful indicators of a poor prognosis are a strongly positive rheumatoid factor and the early presence of bone erosions. Multiple joint involvement and extra-articular features, older age at onset, and a lower level of formal education are all bad prognostic features.

Treatment is based on the principles that apply generally to arthritis, described later in this chapter. In addition, intra-articular and intramuscular steroid injections, and specific disease-modifying drugs for the control of RA all play a part, though management of the latter drugs normally requires hospital supervision. Conventional drugs such as sulphasalazine and methotrexate are nowadays often used in combination to provide greater efficacy. In addition, biological agents have recently obtained product licences, although these are expensive. At present the blockers of tumour necrosis factor α (TNF-α) (etanercept and infliximab) appear to offer more promise than blockers of interleukin-1 (anakinra). The next generation of these biological agents will soon become available. In addition to reducing joint deformity they seem to correct the fatigue that often accompanies RA. Many patients commencing on them enjoy a new lease of working life.

Replacement surgery is also available and is particularly successful for the hip, knees, and finger joints, although technically is not as easy as in osteoarthritis (OA) because of the bone friability associated with rheumatoid disease. As experience is gained with revision surgery, joint replacements are being performed at a younger age than previously, particularly if a single joint is preferentially involved or prevents the patient from working.

When considering the recruitment of an individual with known RA, a detailed history of the symptoms, the individual's physical limitations, and a careful functional assessment are essential. Although few employers may be willing to recruit an individual with aggressive disease, significant function limitations and an uncertain future, they must consider each case in the light of the requirements of the Disability Discrimination Act 1995 (DDA). Recommendations include the avoidance of work activity that would place the affected joints under significant mechanical strain, due either to force, repetitive movements or adverse postures. Indoor work requiring skill, rather than strength, is to be preferred.

If, as is more common, the symptoms first manifest themselves when an individual is in established employment, it may be necessary to consider ergonomic adjustments or the provision of handling aids if hand function is impaired. In extreme cases, relocation or retraining for less physically arduous tasks may help an individual to remain at work. Expert advice can be obtained from officers of the local Placing, Assessment and Counselling Team (PACT) or National Health Service occupational therapy department on writing aids, electrically operated devices or specialized hand-held tools.

Seronegative spondarthritis

This group of disorders comprises ankylosing spondylitis, psoriatic arthritis, colitic arthritis, Crohn's arthritis, and Reiter's disease and can be separated genetically, clinically, and serologically from RA. There is greater family clustering associated with the inheritance of the HLA-B27 antigen and rheumatoid factor is invariably negative (hence the term 'seronegative').

Initial involvement in the arm is most common at the interphalangeal joints of the fingers. In the lower limb the knee and ankle are affected and the sacroiliac joints in ankylosing spondylitis. These conditions are more likely to involve the enthesis (i.e. the site where the tendon is anchored to the bone) than in RA, often mimicking tennis elbow (lateral epicondylitis). They also sometimes improve with exercise, whereas RA is more likely to respond to rest.

In general the prognosis is better than RA, though vision can deteriorate significantly if there is substantial uveitis. Treatment is similar to that of RA, though the spinal involvement is more refractory to drug treatment, particularly requiring intensive physiotherapy to keep the spine mobile and to prevent ankylosis. Some disease-modifying drugs are effective but not as many as in RA, though TNF-α blockade seems particularly effective in this condition and is likely to be used more in the next few years, often allowing patients to return to work.

Ankylosing spondylitis

Work is beneficial for people with ankylosing spondylitis as activity reduces discomfort and the risk of spinal deformity. For many, the symptoms of the condition remain mild enabling them to work full-time and not causing absence. Although heavy physical work is not contra-indicated, those employed in less physically onerous or sedentary work are likely to require minimal work adjustments. Functional limitations are usually secondary to joint stiffness, particularly if free neck movements are essential for driving forklift trucks, passenger carrying vehicles, large goods vehicles, etc. Work requiring considerable spinal flexibility, such as work in confined spaces, may be contra-indicated. The maintenance of maximum spinal function is to be encouraged and regular physio-therapy classes are likely to help in preventing flexion deformities of the spine in the long-term.

Psoriatic arthritis

Frequent time off work rarely occurs in psoriatic arthritis, as the symptoms usually respond to appropriate treatment with non-steroidal anti-inflammatory drugs (NSAIDs) and treatment of the underlying skin condition. Where frequent severe exacerbations affect the joints of the feet, relocation to sedentary work may help but, for the majority, significant task and work modifications are unlikely to be required.

Connective tissue disorders

This third group of inflammatory conditions is less likely to involve the joints than the two described above, though arthritis may occur.

The cause of these various disorders is uncertain. Infective agents have been sought but not found. Prognosis depends mainly on whether there is renal involvement (and in the case of lupus, central nervous system involvement). If the kidneys are spared, prognosis is relatively good with a near normal life expectancy, though pregnancy may be complicated by other abnormalities, for example the antiphospholipid antibody syndrome, which is associated with arterial and venous thrombosis and recurrent spontaneous abortions and, when it occurs during pregnancy, with premature fetal death, especially in mid-pregnancy. This is in addition to the recent realization that atheromatus cardiovascular disease appears particularly common in this group of patients.

Systemic lupus erythematosus

The commonest disease among the inflammatory disorders of connective tissue that are not primarily diseases of the joints is systemic lupus erythematosus (SLE). Women are affected more frequently than men. Pain may occur in almost any joint, but often in the hands, and is associated with a photosensitive skin rash and Raynaud's phenomenon. At a later stage almost any other joint may become involved.

The prevalence of SLE, worldwide, averages 20–25 per 100 000 population (0.02%). The highest prevalence is in the West Indies and California, and women in their reproductive years account for 90% of patients.

Where the disease is mild, work modifications are unlikely to be required but in more severe cases, the systemic effects of the condition cause extreme fatigue and may require a change to less onerous, more sedentary work.

In extreme cases, with widespread organ involvement, long-term immunosuppressive treatment may be needed. Recently, B-cell suppression has been under investigation as a type of biological treatment, uniquely effective in this disease. Even so, employment exposing the individual to infection, e.g. hospital work or primary school teaching, especially if they are taking immunosuppressive medication, may be inappropriate, and the opportunity for relocation and retraining could enable the individual to remain in active employment.

Polymyalgia rheumatica

Polymyalgia rheumatica, a condition of the elderly and of uncertain aetiology, characterized by bilateral shoulder girdle stiffness and pelvic girdle stiffness, is closely associated with cranial arteritis that can cause visual symptoms leading to blindness. Because the disease normally occurs over the age of 60 years and is exceptionally rare below the age of 50 years, it is only occasionally encountered in the workplace, although this may change if people work until a later age. When treated with high doses of steroids it has a good prognosis.

Osteoarthritis

The heterogeneous group of conditions that share common pathological features of OA, in particular focal loss of the articular cartilage, is the subject of increasing interest as more predisposing causes are identified. This leads to a basic classification of primary (idiopathic or generalized) OA for which no obvious cause exists, and an expanding group of conditions that comprise secondary OA due to specific anatomical, inflammatory, or metabolic abnormalities.

- ◆ **Generalized (idiopathic) OA** affects many joints. Its frequency increases with age. Postmenopausal women are particularly vulnerable. The condition is invariably constitutional, an appropriate genetic background and perhaps hormonal factors all contributing to its causation. Sites commonly involved in the hand include the terminal interphalangeal joints where characteristic Heberden's nodes are found, and the base of the thumb. The presence of the disease at this latter site causes particular problems with workers who need regular fine apposition of the thumb as part of their job. Some argue that this condition is a natural consequence of ageing. Osteoarthritic hand involvement, for example, is found in 75% of women between the ages of 60 and 70 and in many of these it is relatively symptom-free.

- ◆ **Secondary OA** is usually localized to a single joint or group of joints unless it is secondary to a widespread metabolic abnormality in the body, either biochemical (such as ochronosis) or hormonal (such as acromegaly). A previous orthopaedic condition (such as Perthes' disease) may exist and this is more typical in the leg than the arm. Extreme hyperlaxity (suppleness) of the thumb base may accelerate damage at this joint. A fracture line into the joint cavity with resultant incongruity of the joint surfaces, the operation of meniscectomy, or injuries that damage ligaments causing joint instability, predispose to OA. Although the influence of major trauma of this sort is undisputed, the evidence that repetitive impulse loading (as in regular

jogging or in the use of vibratory power tools) predisposes to OA is much more contentious.
Many other factors impinge, among them being obesity.

Although diagnosis is ultimately made on radiographic change (or less certainly on clinical history if radiographic change has not yet occurred) support for the diagnosis may also come from negative blood tests. These include a normal erythrocyte sedimentation rate (ESR), normal plasma viscosity, normal C-reactive protein, a negative rheumatoid factor, and a negative antinuclear factor. Symptoms do not always correlate with X-ray changes.

Generalized OA presents in postmenopausal women or men over the age of 50. Secondary OA may present earlier, depending on the cause. Typical symptoms are pain, and sometimes swelling, around affected joints, particularly with exercise and sometimes after immobility.

The course of the condition varies according to the cause and classification. Prognosis varies but is normally much better than inflammatory polyarthritides, particularly with the advent of large joint replacement surgery, which is technically easier in OA than in RA because of the good bone stock found in the former condition.

Drug therapy centres on analgesics rather than anti-inflammatory agents though the latter may be required for inflammatory episodes. Many patients resort to over the counter folk cure, the evidence perhaps being strongest for the use of glucosamine in OA of the knee. Intra-articular steroid injection may assist a single affected joint and intra-articular hyaluronic acid has recently been advocated as an alternative strategy for patients failing to respond to steroids, providing joint lubrication, though the evidence for the efficacy of so-called 'disease-modifying' agents for OA is less convincing.

Management and the prevention of functional limitations require a strategy to maintain flexibility of affected joints and mobility, the strengthening of adjacent muscles, and the avoidance of secondary postural strains including those due to obesity. Work that facilitates movement and encourages flexibility of the affected joints, thus avoiding stiffness, is likely to be of benefit provided the tasks are not too physically onerous.

An ergonomic workplace assessment may be of benefit in assessing postural strains and giving appropriate preventative guidance. Where hand joints are affected, the provision of writing aids, the use of a Dictaphone, voice-activated control systems for computer work, or grasping aids may be of benefit. Where there are significant symptoms in the knee joints, mobility will be restricted and standing should be avoided, together with work activities requiring climbing, walking over rough ground, kneeling, or crouching.

Gout

Gout, an arthritis provoked by the release of uric acid crystals in the joint, must be distinguished from benign symptomless hyperuricaemia, which is found in a small proportion of the population. The big toe is the joint most frequently affected by gout; and after that the knee. Tophaceous deposits may be found, particularly on the ear.

Attacks tend to be acute and are nowadays treated effectively by high doses of NSAIDs. If attacks become more frequent, serum uric acid is particularly high or there is renal deposition of uric acid, long-term prophylactic treatment, normally with allopurinol, is indicated. Severe tophaceous gout affecting many joints is rarely seen nowadays. The condition therefore rarely interferes with employment.

Paget's disease

Paget's disease is an ill-understood metabolic condition of bone. Osteoclast-mediated bone resorption with subsequent compensatory overproduction of new bone causes the architecture to become distorted, and local pain occurs. Symptoms are often localized but the disease can affect any part of the body. Occasionally it is widespread, ultimately leading to bony deformity.

Pain is usually controlled by analgesics. If pain persists or if the alkaline phosphatase is unacceptably high, treatment with diphosphonates or calcitonin is recommended. Occasionally the disease mutates into an osteosarcoma.

The disease rarely proves troublesome in the workplace as it predominantly affects elderly people and adequate treatment is now available.

Algodystrophy

Algodystrophy, also known as Sudek's algodystrophy or reflex sympathetic dystrophy, may complicate WRULDs. Traditionally, an acute painful swollen extremity follows trauma, infection, or a burn. The complete florid form is virtually unmistakable. The difficulty arises with incomplete or atypical forms of the syndrome. All are characterized by loss of bone density, most accurately imaged with bone scintigraphy. This most commonly follows an acute event such as a Colles' fracture, myocardial ischaemia, or an acute hemiplegia. However, the trauma may be relatively mild, provoking claims for compensation. The rest that is often recommended to remedy reflex sympathetic dystrophy, particularly if enforced by immobilization of the affected limb in a plaster of Paris case, may also provoke similar symptoms. Pain tends to be localized to the bone and the bone is tender on palpation, sometimes to an exquisite degree. When the changes have been induced by work or trauma they are usually unilateral. Bilateral loss of bone density on radiography is more likely to suggest idiopathic osteoporosis, an affliction of elderly people.

Treatment requires adequate pain relief, wrist splintage to maintain good posture, and a graded exercise programme to maintain muscle tone and power and prevent further disability. Work adaptations may be needed following an ergonomic assessment, to facilitate the maintenance of neutral wrist and forearm postures; and the introduction of variety to the range of work tasks undertaken may prove of benefit. The provision of writing aids, power operated staplers and hole punchers, or modification of handheld tools requiring less application of force should be considered, when appropriate.

Some authorities draw attention to the similarity between mild algodystrophy and severe WRULD. It is conceivable that abnormality of the autonomic nervous system may be a more prominent feature of work-related conditions than has been appreciated in the past and it has been suggested that drugs active in algodystrophy may also be of some use in WRULD.

Hypermobility syndrome

The range of movement at a given joint varies from individual to individual. There are several reasons for this. The precise contour of the cartilaginous articulating surfaces varies between individuals, a shallow joint socket allowing a greater range of movement than a deep one. The chemical structure of the inherited collagen that gives stability to the joint capsule and surrounding tissues varies between individuals and may be further modified by stretching. Neuromuscular tone also varies, and can be influenced by training. As a result some people inherit very supple joints and others very stiff joints. Joints stiffen with age as collagen structure alters to render it more stable.

Because joints that are unduly supple require greater effort to control them, it can be postulated that patients with joint hypermobility may require greater muscular effort to perform a given task than their normal counterparts, with consequent earlier fatigue. We have an impression that some WRULDs may be more frequently encountered in hypermobile subjects standing at a conveyor belt performing repetitive actions than in the non-hypermobile subjects performing the same task alongside.

Joint hypermobility also predisposes to injury—the unstable joint may be uncoordinated and easily damaged. Minor injury probably predisposes to a traumatic synovitis that can mimic RA and even tenosynovitis. This has implications for differential diagnosis. Careful pre-placement assessment of patients with hypermobile joints will ensure that their employment will not lead to unnecessary injury. They may need physiotherapy to stabilize the joints used in the workplace as well as aids to assist writing if their hands are very supple.

Fibromyalgia

Until recently fibromyalgia was the non-specific rheumatological diagnosis by exclusion for which occupational predisposing factors could not be identified. Recently there have been attempts to formulate more precise diagnostic criteria based on the supposition that this widespread and diffuse musculoskeletal syndrome, with no evidence of synovitis or joint damage and no clear abnormalities on normal physical examination other than discrete tender areas in muscle on palpation, may be a pain-amplification syndrome. As 90% of patients have an age range of onset between 30 and 50 years, and the majority are female, hormonal factors may contribute. The pain and discomfort are widespread, with almost any joint in the body affected, and this has considerable consequences in the workplace. Associated features include fatigue, sleep disturbance, headaches, and irritable bowel syndrome. Investigations are invariably normal and the history of chronic fatigue syndrome, a diffuse condition in which tiredness predominates over pain, is regarded by some as being almost indistinguishable.

Pain may be relieved by analgesics though NSAIDs are less successful. A small nocturnal dose of an antidepressant in a dose lower than that conventionally used for the treatment of depression is often helpful. If amitriptyline causes too many side-effects, dothiepin is a proven substitute. The role of other antidepressants such as selective serotonin reuptake inhibitors, and indeed a wide variety of other compounds, is currently under investigation.

Compensation neurosis

In those seeking compensation, neurosis sometimes appears to dominate the clinical presentation. In other circumstances rates of musculoskeletal complaint vary considerably, even in those conducting similar work (being lower in the self-employed), and this suggests that psychosocial factors operate as well as mechanical ones.

Some patients may appear to overplay their symptoms, leading to suspicions of 'compensation neurosis'. Assessment of such cases is challenging, but some features that suggest the diagnosis are a histrionic presentation, widespread symptomatology, and an absence of a clear link between the ergonomic exposures and the site of the complaint.

Rarer arthritides

Many other arthritic conditions exist, sometimes inherited and others acquired, sometimes through infection. If a single joint only is involved, e.g. perhaps tuberculous arthritis of the wrist, an employee may be tempted, quite understandably, to attribute its occurrence to the workplace if by chance the condition occurs at the joint that is most frequently used. Clearly in this example the cause is independent, though work will certainly be rendered difficult until the condition is diagnosed and adequately treated.

Work-related upper limb disorders

There has been a considerable amount of confusion and controversy surrounding these conditions in recent years. The older term 'repetitive strain injury' (RSI) has justifiably fallen into misuse as the term 'injury', not always true, implies fault. Surveillance case definitions have been established by an expert group using the Delphi process[1] and, as this is considered to be an important step in establishing standard terms, they are used throughout this section to describe the various upper limb syndromes. More recently, an attempt to develop epidemiological criteria for soft tissue disorders of the arm has also been described.[2] To minimize confusion the expression WRULD is used here as an umbrella term covering both the specific anatomically defined syndromes not exclusively related to work, e.g. tenosynovitis, carpal tunnel syndrome, epicondylitis, etc. (discussed further below) and the non-specific, less well-defined, syndrome of non-specific diffuse forearm pain.

Although historical nomenclature can be confusing, it seems likely that workers have suffered upper limb symptoms in association with their work for centuries. Prior to the industrial revolution symptoms occurred in agricultural workers. These were perhaps most pronounced in the afflictions experienced by fish workers who, prior to the advent of refrigeration, had to work fast to fillet and prepare the catch once the trawlers had docked, before it decayed. Clerk's palsy, described 275 years ago, may have been a 'white collar' equivalent and epidemics of 'writer's cramp' described among male clerks in the British Civil Service in the 1830s were then attributed to the introduction of the steel nib, long before the advent of the computer. Interestingly, at a time when between only 4% and 10% of telegraphic staff in the USA were describing 'cramp symptoms', a simultaneous British epidemic caused up to 60% of a comparable workforce to describe symptoms within the period of 4 years.[3] By implication, local psychosocial factors are also important. The most recent reported epidemic has been in Australia with a peak incidence in the prevalence of WRULD in early 1985.[4] The growth of the Australian epidemic coincided with the introduction of a work compensation system that allowed lump sum payments for work-related disease. Once the emphasis had been removed from the term 'injury' and the criteria for qualification for compensation made more stringent, the epidemic quietly faded away.

The aetiology of WRULD is not clear. Studies from Australia[5] purporting to show histological abnormalities in affected muscles of patients complaining of pain due to chronic overuse are uncontrolled. Others have sought to explain the condition in terms of a pain amplification problem.[6] Factors that have been recently shown to be associated with these disorders are: task repetition,[7,8] magnitude of applied forces,[9] velocity of movement,[9] extreme positions of joints in terms of their range of movement,[9] psychosocial factors,[10] tendency to perfectionism,[11] stress,[10] and female gender.[12] There remain no definitive diagnostic criteria based on symptoms, clinical findings, or tests. There may be overlap with conditions presumed to be predominantly neurological such as focal dystonia and 'writer's cramp', the predominant condition for category A4 (cramp of the hand or forearm) of the work-related conditions that may qualify for industrial injury disablement benefit in the UK. Condition A8, more clearly defined as tenosynovitis, is also clear-cut as a separate entity. It remains to be established whether the symptoms may sometimes form the prodromal phase of a forearm tenosynovitis.

Certain features may occur in the history. There is a reasonable agreement on the importance of a change in technique or working practice in initiating symptoms or sometimes the total amount of a repetitive task can exceed a certain threshold, as when management requires a conveyor belt to be driven faster than it was before. There is agreement that symptoms are initially relieved by a short period of rest, perhaps just overnight, though as symptoms become more chronic not even the weekend or the 2–3 weeks of annual holiday will suffice. Symptoms are variously described as aching, soreness, or tingling. Frequently, symptoms are localized to a particular part of the musculoskeletal apparatus, normally that required for the particular ergonomic task in question. Sometimes they may be more widespread, which can cause confusion. The wrist, forearm, and elbow areas are most typically involved at the onset. There may be disturbance of sleep patterns and generalized fatigue is more common.

There are few consistent diagnostic clinical signs. Studies[13] have demonstrated that measurement of grip strength is helpful. Others have found an alteration in pain threshold when measured by an algometer, although this was not confirmed in a recent study.[14] There might be involuntary contraction of muscles and sometimes vasomotor changes, particularly prominent in workers in refrigerating plants.

In investigating the patient it is advisable, having taken a detailed history, to first arrange baseline investigations to exclude generalized conditions such as RA or fibromyalgia. Secondly, on clinical grounds, to exclude features that may also be present in the arm, which may contribute to symptoms. These include cervical spondylitis and Sudek's algodystrophy. Often a proportion of symptoms may be attributed to one of these causes. Thirdly, to attempt to identify specific anatomical sites as sources of symptoms. An assessment of the patient's psychosocial circumstances may also be helpful. Treatment should include a full explanation of the uncertainties of the diagnosis and reassurance as to a likely favourable outcome if aggravating movements and activities are avoided.

Most importantly, a workplace postural and ergonomic assessment should be undertaken and modifications introduced where appropriate. Recently risk filter and risk assessment worksheets have been developed,[15] which can be downloaded from the HSE website, as useful tools to assist with this process. Where several individuals have similar complaints, other possible factors also need to be considered including work rate, method of pay, excessive noise, heat or cold, or other factors that might increase levels of anxiety and muscular tension when at work. Individuals should be reviewed until resolution of their symptoms and, should this not occur, relocation might need to be discussed.

A judgment by Judge Prosser,[16] who found against the existence of this condition, may still have performed a good service, not only in discouraging people from seeking unreasonable damages in courts but in highlighting the dichotomy in a population from which prevalences varying from 5% to 60% can be alleged for the same condition. The view that WRULD has 'no place in the medical books' does not however accord with the two most recent major seminal textbooks of rheumatology, both of which have now devoted specific sections to this condition for the first time. Perhaps the more benign view of Judge Mellow, who recently awarded a record settlement to a typist who developed this condition while working for the Inland Revenue, is equally admissible. He commented that medical evidence on the subject 'would be worthy of medieval theology'. His apt statement 'while I do not rule out the existence of some wider diffuse condition, I do not find it proved to exist' acts both as a concise summary and indictment of current medical understanding (and dispute) on the condition.

Whatever the legal viewpoint, the Health and Safety Executive recognizes the existence of this condition by producing published guidelines[17] (recently revised) for its prevention that employers are now well advised to follow. Prevention concentrates on ensuring that all repetitive actions are performed in the position and style of maximum ergonomic advantage. Appropriate rest breaks should be provided to prevent the onset of symptoms. Job rotation may be a means of ensuring this. Workers should be encouraged to report symptoms and be referred early for occupational health assessment to establish the diagnosis, to receive advice on prevention and be referred for specialist treatment where necessary. Intervention in the early stages, when symptoms are reversible, gives the best chance of preventing chronic disease.

Disorders of the upper limb

Cervical spondylosis

Cervical spondylosis causes symptoms of local neck pain with restriction of movement, may be associated with distressing headaches and episodes of dizziness, and may cause referred pain in the upper limb or interscapular region. It is usually degenerative in aetiology, the frequency of cervical spondylosis increasing in all populations with age. In one study[18] the condition was identified on radiographic examination in 60% of women and 80% of men at the age of 49 years and in 95% of both sexes by the age of 90, but there was poor correlation between radiographic changes and symptoms. Degeneration is maximal in the discs and the apophyseal synovial joints of the middle lower cervical region. Dislocation of disc leads to instability with pressure on nerve roots causing neurological symptoms in the arms. Degeneration may progress at different rates in different people. Local mechanical factors predispose to symptoms, either exacerbation of pain (which may result from pressure of the disc on the ligaments of the spine) or neurological symptoms in the upper limb due to nerve root irritation or compression, including pain and paraesthesiae.

Symptoms may be induced by poor posture or by faulty movements of the neck. Conservative treatment focused on rest, intermittent use of a restrictive collar and adequate analgesic and NSAIDs normally suffices and surgery is only rarely required. Epidemiological studies[19] suggest that at any one time 9% of men and 12% of women over the age of 15 years will claim to have neck pain. The lowest prevalence of symptoms is found in sedentary office workers and the highest where work requires strenuous use of the arms. Workers on assembly lines seem to be particularly at risk. Many patients with proven radiological cervical spondylosis remain asymptomatic, so proof of an association with work can be contentious if the ergonomic history is not clear-cut. Only a small minority of subjects will demonstrate undoubted 'porter's neck'—so-called because bags of meal weighing 90 kg loaded on to the porter's head are unequivocally linked to radiological changes, including disc compression in the spine. Where a link is demonstrated between symptoms and the workplace, appropriate ergonomic and postural advice will prove to be essential in preventing a recurrence, but non-occupational causes of exacerbation of cervical spondylosis will also need to be excluded.

The frequency and severity of symptoms and degree of functional limitation vary considerably and the severity of changes on cervical spine radiographs are not a reliable guide to prognosis and fitness for work. Occupational factors may precipitate symptoms, particularly if work requires the head and neck to be held in a constant or constrained posture or there is strenuous physical effort of the shoulder girdle muscles as in heavy lifting, carrying or labouring tasks, including the use of vibratory tools. Working with the arms elevated above shoulder height or frequently extending the neck to look upwards should be avoided. For sedentary desk-orientated work, attention should be paid to seating, spinal posture, and the ergonomic layout on the desk, particularly if display screen equipment (DSE) is used. All commonly used articles should be within easy arm's reach, L-shaped workstations being provided where necessary to increase readily accessible work surface area. The availability of desk lecterns will help to avoid prolonged periods of neck flexion, and placing document holders adjacent to DSE will encourage an upright neck posture.

For the majority, the symptoms associated with acute exacerbations improve and permanent occupational restrictions are unlikely. Where permanent restriction of neck movement becomes established, driving motor vehicles or forklift trucks, or similar activities, may no longer be possible.

Often, degeneration at the cervical spine is associated with degeneration at the shoulder joint, either of the bony components of that joint or of the fibrous capsule. If the shoulder is unaffected, it is likely to be used with greater effect to compensate for the restricted range of movement at the neck. When the neck and shoulder are involved together, the disability is greater. Additionally, pain referred from the neck may appear to emanate from the shoulder joint even if that joint is relatively normal.

Disorders of the shoulder

The shoulder is a shallow ball and socket joint with a wide range of movement in many directions. To permit this degree of movement the capsule of the joint is loose and the various muscles attached to the proximal end of the humerus, the so-called 'rotator cuff', make a major contribution to the integrity of the joint. Most of the joints range of movement is achieved at the glenohumoral joint but symptoms arising from both the acromioclavicular ligament and the scapulothoracic joint also contribute to pain at the shoulder. The natural rhythm of elevation and abduction involves synchronized motor function at both the glenohumoral and scapulothoracic joints and the sternoclavicular joint is also stretched. The movements are facilitated by the bursae around the joints that ensure the smooth motion of contracting muscles and their ligaments over the bony prominences.

In patients over the age of 40 years the joint may have developed osteoarthritic change causing pain and restricted movements. This is most common in those engaged in heavy manual work but can occur in divers or compressed air workers who have developed aseptic bone necrosis. The dominant upper limb is more commonly affected. Otherwise local symptoms at the shoulder can be attributable to OA of the acromioclavicular joint, inflammation of the rotator cuff (tendinitis) or a tear in this structure, tendinitis of the long head of biceps tendon, and shoulder capsulitis (frozen shoulder). In occupational terms, shoulder tendinitis and capsulitis are the most important.

Shoulder tendinitis arises from symptomatic inflammation or degeneration of the tendons of the rotator cuff or biceps. Surveillance criteria[1] are: history of pain in the deltoid region and pain in one or more resisted movements of the shoulder joint, i.e. abduction—supraspinatus; external rotation—infraspinatus and teres minor; internal rotation—subscapularis and teres major. Biceps tendinitis gives rise to anterior shoulder pain and pain on resisted active flexion of the elbow (Speed's test) or supination of the forearm with the elbow flexed to 90° (Yergason's test).

Clinical features may include: a painful arc, which is more apparent on active than passive movement, pain that is worse at night, crepitus, subacromial tenderness, referred pain in the C5 distribution and pain and restriction of abduction of the shoulder beyond 80°. Tendon calcification may be seen on X-ray, and magnetic resonance imaging scanning may demonstrate appearances suggestive of inflammation. Tendon tears may be chronic or acute, partial or full thickness. The appropriate traumatic event should be sought in the history, which may or may not be work related.

The possible aetiology of tendinitis is more contentious. The symptoms may occur suddenly as a result of acute injury. For most, the onset is more gradual and is presumed to result from eccentric overload, possibly aggravated by instability that places the tendon at a greater mechanical disadvantage. The extent to which ergonomic factors in the workplace might contribute to this condition, which can also occur as a result of leisure pursuits and possibly spontaneously, requires careful consideration. Once present, most would agree that repetitive movements at the workplace can aggravate symptoms and healing may be correspondingly delayed if adequate rest is not possible. Treatment by injection of corticosteroids with lignocaine is usually quickly effective in tendinitis and bursitis. The condition can be prolonged, the mean duration of symptoms in a cross-sectional sample of industrial and service workers being in the order of 10 months.[20]

Shoulder capsulitis (frozen shoulder) is defined by Harrington et al.[1] as a condition characterized by current or past pain in the upper arm, with global restriction of glenohumeral movement in a capsular pattern. Surveillance criteria are: history of unilateral pain in the deltoid area and equal restriction of glenohumeral active and passive movement in a capsular pattern (external rotation > abduction > internal rotation). The condition is almost always unilateral but there is a 17% chance of developing it subsequently in the other shoulder over 5 years.

Underlying diseases such as diabetes mellitus, thyroid disease, infection, previous surgery, or cardiac disease may be associated. The prevalence in non-diabetics appears to be 2–3%. The prevalence in diabetics may be up to 20% and is associated with treatment with insulin. However, tests of immune function are usually normal. Careful ergonomic analysis and a full occupational history with exclusion of non-occupational contributory conditions would be required to prove beyond doubt that the frozen shoulder arose as a result of work. Recovery may be delayed if work requiring shoulder joint movement is continued, although local injection of corticosteroids and analgesics may reduce pain and the prognosis is favourable for a complete recovery. Full movements may not be regained for 12–24 months but surgical treatment may shorten this time.

Prevention

Shoulder pain is commonly experienced in the general population, 21% of respondents to a survey conducted in the Netherlands reported having shoulder pain at the time of questioning, similar figures have been reported from other countries.[21] Shoulder pain or specific disorders such as tendinitis, capsulitis, are especially frequent among workers in the following industries:[22] clothing, slaughtering and food processing, fish processing, repetitive assembly line work, and among supermarket cashiers. Relevant factors associated with symptoms are (1) biomechanical: repetitive tool use, vibrating tools and abduction of the arms >90°,[23] and (2) psychosocial: monotonous work[24] and poor job control. Prevention should be aimed at minimizing these factors. Work should be variable, without continuous repetitive work achieved by frequent breaks and job rotation. Vibration should be minimized and prolonged elevation of the arm above the shoulder avoided. Employees should be given opportunities to change working patterns and develop their jobs.

Epicondylitis of the elbow

Lateral epicondylitis (**tennis elbow**) and medial epicondylitis (**golfer's elbow**) are the commonest soft tissue lesions at the elbow. Both need to be distinguished from other causes of elbow pain such as OA, olecranon bursitis, or biceps tendinitis. A careful clinical examination is essential. Surveillance criteria[1] for diagnosis are: lateral epicondylar pain and epicondylar tenderness with pain on resisted extension of the wrist. Similar criteria apply to medial epicondylitis with pain on resisted flexion of the wrist. The measurement of pain-free grip strength is useful in assessing and monitoring the condition[25] and magnetic resonance imaging scanning may help with diagnosis in atypical cases.[26]

While the diagnosis is usually clear-cut, the aetiology is less certain. At some time 1–3% of the population may be affected by epicondylitis,[21,27] involvement of the lateral epicondyle being much more common than that of the medial. A sporting cause is relatively rare. It is most often found in non-athletes and not necessarily manual workers. Local trauma may play a part as in an acute wrenching injury, though this is more likely to aggravate established epicondylitis in the older patient. Ageing is associated with anatomical alteration at the enthesis, including changes in collagen content and increasing lipids that may predispose to injury. Repeated pronation and supination of the forearm, which may be an integral part of some jobs, will certainly aggravate the condition. Whether symptoms can arise *ab initio* from this action is more contentious. Even allowing for a clustering of the condition in families and a tendency for individuals affected to have widespread soft tissue lesions at other sites, not necessarily all simultaneously, the balance of probability is that this lesion can be induced at the workplace, particularly if the ergonomic insult corresponds with the use of the forearm muscles and, in turn, the enthesis affected.

Lateral epicondylitis is associated with the use of heavy tools, forceful and repetitive work, particular with the wrist in the non-neutral position.[28] For example, the use of power tools, such as saws, jack hammers, etc. may cause tennis elbow and although it is generally rare in athletes it does occur frequently in professional tennis players.

The condition is considered self-limiting, some patients improving with or without treatment within 1 year, but a majority still having symptoms after 1 year, particularly if they have persevered with the activity that caused it.[29] Recurrence does appear to be more common in manual workers and attributable to repeated grasping or lifting activity. Treatment, most commonly by intralesional steroid injection and advice to avoid aggravating activities, tends to be more ineffective in those who do not take a break from work or avoid its aggravating activities. Postural and ergonomic adjustments, task modification, or job rotation may need to be considered to prevent recurrence.

Medial epicondylitis has a high recovery rate (80% at 3 years), is associated with other WRULDs and appears to have no association with repetitive work.[30]

The mainstay of treatment is local steroid injection; however, recurrence rates are high. While in the short-term it is more effective than physiotherapy and no treatment, physiotherapy is significantly better than steroid injection in the longer-term (52 weeks). Physiotherapy is better than no treatment in the long-term but the difference is not statistically significant.[31] Other treatments may be effective. In a large systematic review,[32] there is some evidence of benefit from acupuncture, exercise therapy, manipulation and mobilization, ultrasound, diclofenac, and other physiotherapeutic techniques, i.e. phonophoresis and Rebox. Conversely, laser and electromagnetic therapy were shown to be ineffective. Surgery can be successful in cases resistant to conservative treatments but results in litigants can be disappointing.[33]

Carpal tunnel syndrome

Carpal tunnel syndrome (CTS) is regarded as the commonest peripheral nerve entrapment syndrome. It has an incidence of 99 per 10^5 in the general USA population.[34] It results from compression of the median nerve as it passes through the tunnel formed between the carpal bones and the flexor retinaculum, which it shares with the long flexor tendons and their synovial sheaths. Classic symptoms include numbness and tingling of the fingers (usually lateral 3½ digits), which is often experienced more diffusely in the hand. Pain is variable and can extend into the forearm and, occasionally, proximally. Symptoms are often worse at night and in the morning.

Examination commonly includes conducting Tinel's test (tapping over the carpal tunnel, which when positive causes tingling in the thumb and radial two and a half fingers) and Phalen's test (both hands are held tightly palmar-flexed opposite to a prayer position, creating at least a 90° angle between the forearm and the hand; a positive test is when numbness and tingling are produced when the hands are held in this position for approximately 30 seconds). The reported sensitivity of these tests is between 32%[35] and 93%[36] and their specificity ranges between 45%[37] and 100%.[38]

Investigations include nerve conduction studies, which have reported sensitivity of between 60% and 84% with a specificity of more than 95%. Harrington et al.[1] define surveillance criteria for the condition as: pain or paraesthesia, or sensory loss in the median nerve distribution, and one of: a positive Tinel's test, a positive Phalen's test, nocturnal exacerbation of symptoms, motor loss with wasting of abductor pollicis brevis, and abnormal nerve conduction time.

Associated factors are obesity, tobacco and alcohol use, RA and OA, diabetes, hypothyroidism, haemodialysis, pregnancy, and lactation. The condition may be bilateral, particularly if linked to a metabolic cause. CTS may also result from local space-occupying lesions, e.g. lipomas or a ganglion, etc.

A causal link with occupation remains unproven but with refined diagnostic techniques and more sensitive ergonomic analysis the balance of probability is now shifting to the acceptance that this can be a work-associated condition. NIOSH,[39] in a well regarded review, concluded that there is evidence of a positive association between exposure to highly repetitive work and forceful work. This evidence is stronger if the exposure is a combination of risk factors, e.g. force and repetition and force and posture. The condition is seen less frequently in patients who do not use their hands substantially, and occurs more often in the dominant hand. Workers using a keyboard seem to be particularly susceptible, though adequately controlled epidemiological studies to identify the precise causal factors are awaited. Musicians and meat cutters who may need to keep the wrist in a flexed position for long periods are particularly susceptible. A stamping or punching action involving the wrist also predisposes, presumably by regular direct compression. CTS is recognized as a prescribed industrial disease (A12) in association with work using hand-held vibrating tools.

By analogy with the cervical spine, an inappropriate occupation superimposed on an inherited or acquired propensity for the condition may together combine to cross a threshold allowing it to occur. At present, symptoms are undoubtedly intensified by occasions that involve persistent flexion and extension of the wrist, not necessarily confined to the workplace, and also simple activities such as grasping a steering wheel or holding a book.

Health surveillance of individuals whose work involves significant exposure to the risk factors described above will identify early evidence of disease and will enable the exposure to be eliminated or reduced to prevent its further development. Anecdotally, some employers in the USA are screening for delayed nerve conduction in workers entering repetitive jobs but the value of this as a predictive tool in asymptomatic individuals is unclear.

When the diagnosis has been established, the reduction or avoidance of possible work-associated factors: poor wrist and forearm posture, prolonged and extreme wrist flexion, forceful and repetitive wrist movement, direct pressure over the carpal tunnel, and the use of vibratory handheld tools may result in reduction or resolution of symptoms. The injection of steroids may relieve symptoms temporarily but is associated with relapse. The use of a wrist splint is often recommended but there is limited evidence of benefit and range of motion exercises appear to be associated with less pain and fewer lost days from work.[40] Where delayed nerve conduction is confirmed by electromyogram studies, surgical decompression of the carpal tunnel as a day-case procedure is often required to relieve symptoms. Resolution of symptoms is to be expected, enabling a return to unrestricted work activity.

Tenosynovitis of the wrist

This term **tenosynovitis** describes inflammation of the extensor or flexor tendon sheaths at the wrist. Surveillance criteria[1] for diagnosis are: pain on movement localized to the affected tendon sheaths in the wrist and reproduction of the pain by resisted active movement of the affected tendons with the forearm stabilized. Additional features that would give greater confidence in diagnosis are: history of crepitus and tenderness or swelling over affected tendon sheaths. It should be noted that the inflammation is of the tendon sheath rather than the tendon itself, which is painful on palpation. Crepitus is a fleeting sign and can be associated with triggering and occasionally with tethering, if the condition becomes chronic.

Treatment involves avoidance of the cause or aggravating movements, which are identified at a workplace ergonomic assessment; anti-inflammatory agents topically, orally or by intra-synovial injection of corticosteroids and local anaesthetic. Splintage is often recommended but prolonged use should be avoided to prevent muscle wastage and local osteoporosis. If surgery is required to relieve tethering, histopathological confirmation of the condition can be obtained. When the acute phase has resolved, return to work must be carefully planned if recurrence is to be avoided. Attention must be paid to good ergonomic principles to avoid excessive movement of the wrist, particularly at the extremes of its range of movement. Mechanization of the task, time restriction, job rotation, and job transfer need to be considered.

The distinctive nature of this condition has long been recognized in the UK as industrial disease A8. When it can be established that the inflammation was caused by manual labour, Industrial Injury Benefit can be claimed under the Social Security Contributions and Benefits Act 1992.

The term **de Quervain's tenosynovitis** is defined as painful swelling of the first extensor compartment containing the tendons of abductor pollicis longus and extensor pollicis brevis. Surveillance criteria[1] are: pain that is centred over the radial styloid and tender swelling of the first extensor compartment and either pain reproduced by resisted thumb extension or a positive Finkelstein's test (positive when ulnar deviation of the wrist with the fingers flexed over the thumb placed in the palm stretches the tendons and reproduces pain over the distal radius and radial side of the wrist). The condition should be distinguished from OA of the wrist or first carpometacarpal joint, wrist ligament strains and non-union of a scaphoid fracture.

As repetitive movement of the tendon in its sheath is a prime requirement in causation and the feature most distinctively lost when the condition is present, the ergonomic case for this being an occupational-related injury is extremely strong. It is more common in women than men, perhaps suggesting a hormonal influence (unless women are more likely to be ascribed repetitive tasks in the workplace), and the condition, like frozen shoulder, may be more frequently seen in association with certain diseases. Medical treatment as above is appropriate but surgical release may be required.

Trigger finger or **trigger thumb** (stenosing digital tenosynovitis) implies tenosynovitis of one of the flexor tendons to the finger or thumb. This characteristically occurs with repetitive gripping activities that increase pull and friction on the flexor tendons. Although it can be associated with other conditions (including RA, diabetes mellitus, sarcoidosis, and hyperthyroidism) a clear ergonomic history normally correlates with the anatomical abnormalities. In common with other forms of tenosynovitis, rest is beneficial and too early a return to the workplace delays the resolution of the condition. In the prevention of recurrence of symptoms, a postural and ergonomic assessment should be undertaken and, where required, alterations made to upper limb movements, work practices or workplace design. Modifications to handheld tools may also prove beneficial and, where groups of workers are similarly affected, automation of a process may be indicated.

Non-specific diffuse forearm pain

This is a diagnosis of exclusion. The merit of the use of this diagnostic term as an alternative to RSI or WRULD is that it contains no statement as to aetiology. It is defined by Harrington *et al.*[1] as: pain in the forearm in the absence of a specific diagnosis or pathology. Surveillance criteria are: pain in the forearm and failure to meet the diagnostic criteria for other specific diagnoses and diseases. Other features that may be present include loss of function, weakness, cramp, muscle tenderness, allodynia, and slowing of fine movements. It needs to be distinguished from the generalized pain syndromes such as fibromyalgia and referred pain.

Treatment consists of physiotherapy and avoidance of any precipitating factors. The guidance laid down in the section on WRULD with regard to workplace assessment should be followed and techniques to minimize exposure to precipitating factors such as breaks to allow recovery, job rotation, etc. should be followed. There is some evidence that a cognitive-behavioural therapeutic approach may be beneficial.[41,42]

Conclusions

Some common principles apply in the treatment and management of many of the conditions described above. This section includes aspects of self-management of these conditions for both employers and employees.

Many rheumatic conditions respond to rest. At the workplace this may comprise avoidance of the precipitating action or dilution of the action in the first instance. Changes in technique, posture, or equipment often alleviate symptoms. If not, attention should be directed to appropriate 'pacing' of the workload. For example, if 2.5 hours at a keyboard or on a production line cause symptoms, the maximum duration of working at any one time should be restricted to a lesser period (say 2 hours). The 8-hour day becomes correspondingly extended with half-hour breaks between each 2-hour working period.

If such attention to technique fails to remedy the situation, the total time spent at the workplace may have to be reduced. Ultimately a period of complete rest, perhaps of 1–2 weeks' duration, may be required with a cautious reintroduction to work. Splinting may help up to a point, particularly to stabilize movement of a joint at the workplace, but complete immobilization of part of a limb in a plaster of Paris case may cause disuse osteoporosis with worsening of symptoms and is generally to be avoided other than for brief periods of 10–14 days.

The patient can self-medicate by purchasing either paracetamol, which is a pure analgesic, or ibuprofen, which is an anti-inflammatory drug in oral or topical form. The general practitioner may prescribe from a much wider range of analgesics or NSAIDs. Practitioners are also empowered to prescribe these drugs in doses higher than those recommended on the packets purchased over the counter. Drugs of short half-life can be taken on an 'as required' basis a little before the circumstances that cause discomfort. If these circumstances persist throughout the day, a drug of longer half-life that is suitable for once daily dosing without any fall in blood concentration might be preferred.

An ergonomic assessment at the workplace is often valuable. Where direct access to professional advice from an occupational health department, an ergonomist, or occupational therapist is not available, the Disability Employment Advisor (DEA) at the local Job Centre should be contacted and will provide such a service through the Access to Work scheme.

If individuals are overweight, additional strain is placed on joints. When lower limb problems predominate, employees should be encouraged to diet to reach the optimum weight for their height.

A variety of physiotherapy techniques are available. These include short-wave diathermy, ultrasound, exercises, and hydrotherapy, among others. Relaxation techniques and acupuncture are gaining popularity. Physiotherapists may advise on the use of appliances that reduce pain such as a TENS machine.

Employees often resort to fringe medicine, consulting chiropractors, acupuncturists, reflexologists, and others. Chiropractice may be particularly helpful for degenerative conditions of the spine, providing there is no inflammatory component. Otherwise, controlled clinical trials for efficacy of these alternative treatments are often lacking, with the implication that improvement often depends on a brisk placebo response. Nevertheless, if the procedures allow patients to escape the side-effects of drugs, particularly NSAIDs, they should not be denigrated.

Selected references

1 Harrington JM, Carter TJ, Birrell L, Gompertz D. Surveillance case definitions for work related upper limb syndromes. *Occup Environ Med* 1998; **55**(4): 264–71.

2 Sluiter JK, Rest KM, Frings-Dresen M. Criteria for evaluation of the work-relatedness of upper extremity musculoskeletal disorders. *Scand J Work Environ Health* 2001; **27** (Suppl. 1).

3 Great Britain and Ireland Post Office Departmental Committee on Telegraphists Cramp Report. London: HMSO, 1911.

4 Hocking B. Epidemiological aspects of 'repetitive strain injury'. Telecom Australia. *Med J Aust* 1987; **147**: 218–22.

5 Dennett X, Fry HJH. Overuse syndrome: a muscle biopsy study. *Lancet* 1988; **339**: 905–8.

6 Kellgren JH. Observations on referred pain arising from muscle. *Clin Sci* 1938; **3**: 174–90.

7 Latko WA, Armstrong TJ, Franzblau A, Ulin SS, Werner RA, Albers JW. Cross-sectional study of the relationship between repetitive work and the prevalence of upper limb musculoskeletal disorders. *Am J Ind Med* 1999; **36(2):** 248–59.

8 Crumpton-Young LL, Killough MK, Parker PL, Brandon KM. Quantitative analysis of cumulative trauma risk factors and risk factor interactions. *J Occup Environ Med* 2000; **42**(10): 1013–20.

9 Arvidsson I, Akesson I, Gert-Ake H. Wrist movements among females in a repetitive, non-forceful work. *Appl Ergonomics* 2003; **34**(4): 309–16.

10 White PD, Henderson M, Pearson RM, Coldrick AR, White AG, Kidd BL. Illness behaviour and psychosocial factors in diffuse upper limb pain disorder: a case-control study. *J Rheumatol* 2003; **30**: 139–45.

11 Van Eijsden-Besseling MDF, Peeters FPML, Reijnen JAW, de Bie RA. Perfectionism and coping strategies for the development of non-specific work-related upper limb disorders. *Occup Med* 2004; **54**: 122–7.

12 Islam SS, Velilla AM, Doyle EJ, Ducatman AM. Gender differences in work-related injury/illness: analysis of workers compensation claims. *Am J Ind Med* 2001; **39**: 84–91.

13 Sande LP, Coury HJCG, Oishi J, Kumar S. Effect of musculoskeletal disorders on prehension strength. *Appl Ergonomics* 2001; **32**(6): 609–16.

14 Mitchell S, Reading I, Walker-Bone K, Palmer K, Cooper C, Coggon D. Pain tolerance in upper limb disorders: findings from a community survey. *Occup Environ Med* 2003; **60**(3): 217–21.

15 Graves RJ, Way K, Riley D, Lawton C, Morris L. Development of risk filter and risk assessment worksheets for HSE guidance—'Upper Limb Disorders in the Workplace' 2002. *Appl Ergonomics* 2004; **35**(5): 475–84.

16 Industrial Relations Law Report: IRL.R 571, 1993.

17 Health and Safety Executive (HSE). *Upper limb disorders in the workplace*. HSG60 (rev). Sudbury: HSE Books, 2002.

18 Schmorl G, Junghanns H. *The human spine in health and disease* (trans. EF Besemann). New York: Grune and Stratton, 1971.

19 Allender E. Prevalence, incidence and remission rates of some common rheumatic diseases or syndromes. *Scand J Rheumatol* 1974; **3**: 145–53.

20 Bonde JP, Mikkelsen S, Andersen JH, Fallentin N, Baelum J, Svendsen SW, Thomsen JF, Frost P, Thomsen G, Overgaard E, Kaergaard A. Prognosis of shoulder tendonitis in repetitive work: a follow-up study in a cohort of Danish industrial and service workers. *Occup Environ Med* 2003; **60**(9): E8.

21 Bongers PM. The cost of shoulder pain at work. *BMJ* 2001; **322**: 64–5.

22 Leclerc A, Chastang J-F, Niedhammer I, Landre M-F, Roquelaure Y. Incidence of shoulder pain in repetitive work. *Occup Environ Med* 2004; **61**: 39–44.

23 Svendsen SW, Bonde JP, Mathiassen SE, Stengaard-Pedersen K, Frich LH. Work related shoulder disorders: quantitative exposure-response relations with reference to arm posture. *Occup Environ Med* 2004; **61**(10): 844–53.

24 Harkness EF, MacFarlane GJ, Nahit ES, Silman AJ, McBeth J. Mechanical and psychosocial factors predict new onset shoulder pain: a prospective cohort study of newly employed workers. *Occup Environ Med* 2003; **60**: 850–7.

25 Smidt N, van der Winde DA, Assendelft WJ, Mourits AJ, Deville WL, DeWinter AF, Bouter LM. Intra-observer reproducibility of the assessment of severity of complaints, grip strength and pressure pain threshold in patients with lateral epicondylitis. *Arch Phys Med Rehab* 2002; **83**(8): 1145–50.

26 Mackay D, Rangan A, Hide G, Hughes T, Latimer J. The objective diagnosis of early tennis elbow by magnetic resonance imaging. *Occup Med* 2003; **53**: 309–12.

27 Kivi P. The aetiology and conservative treatment of humeral epicondylitis. *Scand J Rehab Med* 1982; **15**: 37–41.

28 Haahr JP, Andersen JH. Physical and psychosocial risk factors for lateral epicondylitis: A population based case-referent study. *Occup Environ Med* 2003; **60**: 322–9.

29 Binder AI, Hazelman B. Lateral humeral epicondylitis—a study of the natural history and the effect on conservative therapy. *Br J Rheumatol* 1983; **20**: 73–6.

30 Descatha A, Leclerc A, Chastang JH, Roquelaure Y. Media epicondylitis in occupational settings: prevalence, incidence and associated risk factors. *J Occup Environ Med* 2003; **45**(9): 993–101.

31 Smidt N, van der Winde DAW, Assendelft WJJ, Deville WLJM, Korthals-de Bos IBC, Bouter LM. Corticosteroid injections, physiotherapy, or wait-and-see policy for lateral epicondylitis: a randomised controlled trial. *Lancet* 2002; **359**: 657–62.

32 Trudel D, Duley J, Zastrow I, Kerr EW, Davidson RI, Macdermid JC. Rehabilitation for patients with lateral epicondylitis: a systematic review. *J Hand Ther* 2004; **17**(2): 243–66.

33 Kay NRM. Litigation epicondylitis. *J Hand Surgery* 2003; **28**(5): 460–4.

34 Von Shroeder HP, Botte MJ. Carpal tunnel syndrome. *Hand Clinics* 1996; **12**: 643–55.

35 Novak CB, Mackinnon SE, Brownlee R, Kelly L. Provocative sensory testing in carpal tunnel syndrome. *J Hand Surg Br* 1992; **17B**: 204–8.

36 Grunberg AB. Carpal tunnel decompression in spite of normal electromyography. *J Hand Surg Br* 1983; **8**: 348–9.

37 Seror P. Phalen's test in the diagnosis of carpal tunnel syndrome. *J Hand Surg Br* 1988; **13B**: 383–5.

38 Williams TM, Mackinnon SE, Novak CB, McCabe S, Kelly L. Verification of the pressure provocation test in carpal tunnel syndrome. *Ann Plast Surg* 1992; **29**: 8–11.

39 Bernard BP *et al.* (ed). *Musculoskeletal disorders and workplace factors: a critical review of epidemiological evidence for work-related musculoskeletal disorders of the neck, upper extremity and low back.* NIOSH, US Department of Health and Human Services, July 1997.

40 Feuerstein M, Burrell LM, Miller I, Lincoln A, Huang GD, Berger R. Clinical management of carpal tunnel syndrome: a 12-year review of outcomes. *Am J Ind Med* 1999; **35**(3): 232–45.

41 Spence SH. Cognitive-behaviour therapy in the management of upper extremity cumulative trauma disorder. *J Occup Rehab* 1998; **8**: 27–45.

42 Linton SJ. Early identification and intervention in the prevention of musculoskeletal pain. *Am J Ind Med* 2002; **41**(5): 433–42.

Chapter 14

Gastrointestinal and liver disorders

C. Astbury and J. L. Southgate

Many disorders affect the gastrointestinal tract and liver. A number of these have implications for employment and can significantly affect work capacity. They result in large numbers of consultations in primary and secondary care and hospital admissions in more severe cases.

Gastrointestinal disorders therefore have a high direct and indirect economic burden on society. A commonly attributed cause of short-term sickness absence of 1 or 2 days is gastrointestinal disease, usually described as 'stomach infection', 'tummy bug', or 'diarrhoea and vomiting'. How much of this significant sickness absence is genuine gastrointestinal disease is difficult to assess. However, recent studies in individuals with recognized gastrointestinal disorders have demonstrated increased sickness absence from work and significant impact on health-related quality of life. Advances in investigation, medical treatment, and surgery should improve symptom control and prognosis in many individuals enabling them to remain in employment.

The only absolute contraindication to employment is work that poses a significant risk of infection, such as food handling and some healthcare work. In assessing fitness for other areas of employment it is important to establish the level of symptoms, and degree of disability and prognosis, which may vary substantially in gastrointestinal or liver disorders. Therefore, individuals with the same diagnosis may function very differently in the workplace. Decisions about employment will need to take account of the previous history and course of the illness, previous work record, and the severity and frequency of symptoms as well as the likely progression of disease.

The Disability Discrimination Act (DDA) 1995 is likely to apply to disorders affecting the ability to control defecation. Therefore conditions that lead to regular minor faecal incontinence or to even infrequent loss of bowel control are likely to be defined as a disability under the Act. This will include many cases of ulcerative colitis and Crohn's disease. The occupational health practitioner has a key role in supporting employees with this disability who understandably may wish the details of their symptoms to remain medically confidential. Liaison with the employer about the nature of any support or adjustments required will be a key aspect of assessment of fitness to work.

Conditions likely to cause employment problems or risks to individuals and the public are:

+ gastro-oesophageal reflux and other oesophageal disorders

+ dyspepsia: peptic ulcer disease and non-ulcer dyspepsia

+ coeliac disease

+ chronic pancreatitis

+ inflammatory bowel disease

+ ileostomy and ileal pouch anal anastomosis

+ gastroenteritis and gut infections

+ functional gastrointestinal disorders

+ viral hepatitis

- chronic liver disease
- conditions requiring long-term enteral or parenteral nutrition
- obesity.

Investigations

Many gastroenterological investigations can be performed as day cases. Sedation is usual for colonoscopy and endoscopic retrograde cholangiopancreatograms; it is optional for a gastroscopy and usually unnecessary for flexible sigmoidoscopy. There is a tendency to use less sedation to reduce the associated risk of these procedures. However, due to the amnesic affect of the medication, it is advised that patients do not drive or operate machinery for 24 hours after sedation.

Increasingly, endoscopic surveillance is being performed to detect early colonic and, to a lesser extent, gastric cancers in patients with a strong family history.

Bowel preparation is necessary the preceding day for procedures such as a barium enema and computed tomography enema and colonoscopy, which will usually require brief periods of planned absence from work.

Oesophageal disorders

Gastro-oesophageal reflux

Gastro-oesophageal reflux is the reflux of stomach contents or acid into the lower oesophagus and, sometimes, the mouth causing a burning sensation. It is a very common complaint with 20–30% of Western patients experiencing intermittent heartburn or reflux. The majority have mild symptoms requiring little treatment; often patients self-medicate with over-the-counter preparations. Endoscopy is frequently normal in these individuals (endoscopy negative or non-erosive reflux disease) and treatment is aimed at symptom control. A proportion will have inflammation of the oesophagus, known as reflux or erosive oesophagitis.

Gastro-oesophageal reflux is probably caused by acid refluxing into the oesophagus, as a consequence of laxity of the lower oesophageal sphincter and delayed gastric emptying. Hiatus hernia occurs commonly and is not necessarily associated with reflux symptoms.

Atypical/extra-oesophageal symptoms, such as chest pain, globus, chronic cough, and hoarseness may occur in the absence of typical reflux symptoms. The most sensitive and specific investigation of gastro-oesophageal reflux is pH monitoring. This test is performed in conjunction with pressure measurements. A fine tube with either pressure sensors or a pH probe is passed through the nose to the lower oesophagus. Pressure recordings are made while the patient swallows. A separate pH probe measures the pH constantly and records this on a tape. The patient pushes a button whenever heartburn or chest pain is experienced, which marks the time on the tape. Positive symptom correlation is important to diagnose accurately symptomatic acid reflux.

Barrett's oesophagus is the precursor lesion to oesophageal adenocarcinoma and occurs as a consequence of chronic gastro-oesophageal reflux. It is a frequent finding in patients with reflux symptoms; however, a large number of patients remain undiagnosed.[1] Therapy is aimed not only at the relief of symptoms but also at prevention of malignant complications. New diagnostic procedures such as the topical application of stains during endoscopy—chromoendoscopy—may improve detection of premalignant change. Methylene blue staining of Barrett's oesophagus colours normal squamous epithelium only weakly, whereas Barrett's epithelium takes up more dye. Weakly stained areas within Barrett's epithelium represent centres of dysplasia. Chromoendoscopy may allow better detection of premalignant changes. Endoscopic treatments may offer

---

Box 14.1 NICE guidelines[3]

These recommend that patients who have gastro-oesophageal reflux disease should be offered a full dose of PPI for 1–2 months. If symptoms recur following initial treatment a PPI should be offered at the lowest dose possible to control symptoms, with a limited number of repeat prescriptions.

---

alternatives to oesophagectomy in selected patients with early cancer. At present the issue of regular endoscopic surveillance, usually every 1–3 years, is controversial.

Treatment

More recently studies have focused on pharmacological and surgical treatment of gastro-oesophageal reflux disease (see Box 14.1). There is no recent review on the non-pharmacological treatment. Although it is usual to discuss life-style changes and dietary modifications the evidence for the effectiveness of this advice is limited. There is a significant relationship between obesity and reflux, and patients with a high body mass index should be advised to lose weight. Smoking and alcohol decrease lower oesophageal sphincter pressure. Simple measures can be recommended, such as wearing loose clothes, avoiding caffeine, not eating late at night and raising the head of the bed.

The proton pump inhibitors (PPI) have revolutionalized the treatment of upper gastrointestinal disorders. Healing rates in erosive oesophagitis are more than 90% and as a result, complications of these conditions, which include oesophageal stricture, are less common. PPIs provide 50–65% symptom response in non-erosive reflux disease; they have also been used successfully in patients with atypical symptoms.[2]

Laparoscopic antireflux surgery, typically a Nissen fundoplication, may be offered to patients refractory to or requiring lifelong medical treatment. A partial fundoplication has fewer side-effects than a total fundoplication. Outcome studies claim 90% success rates at 5–8 years.[4] The surgical approach has the advantage of reducing both acid and bile reflux, which are thought to act synergistically in the aetiopathogenesis of Barrett's oesophagus.

Employment issues

The areas of work where gastro-oesophageal reflux disease may have an impact are those where the tasks involved are likely to increase intra-abdominal pressure and reflux symptoms. These include:

- frequent bending, stooping, crouching
- lifting or carrying of heavy loads
- regular work in confined spaces.

Although risks are potentially increased in such circumstances many patients are able to work without restriction. However, consideration may need to be given to reviewing manual handling risk assessments, to establish whether the tasks that aggravate symptoms can be eliminated or modified.

Oesophageal motility disorders

Achalasia is a disease characterized by failure of normal relaxation of the lower oesophageal sphincter on swallowing. Endoscopic balloon dilatation is effective at relieving obstruction. Surgical myotomy is reserved for refractory cases.

Chest pain

Some patients with chest pain of uncertain origin have a lower threshold of oesophageal pain. Anxiety exacerbates these symptoms. There is an abnormal visceral perception (see functional bowel syndrome), which is localized to the chest.

Dyspepsia

Dyspepsia is pain or discomfort in the chest or upper abdomen that is related to meals. It may be associated with a number of symptoms such as feeling bloated, burping, nausea or even vomiting.

NICE guidelines for the management of dyspepsia recommend urgent referral if certain 'alarm' symptoms are present (see Box 14.2). The guideline development group suggests patients should be seen within 2 weeks of referral.

Routine testing of patients (of any age) who present with dyspepsia and lack 'alarm' symptoms is not necessary. However, for patients over 55, endoscopy should be considered when symptoms persist despite *Helicobacter pylori* testing and acid suppression therapy and when patients have had one or more of the following: previous gastric ulcer or surgery, continued need for non-steroidal anti-inflammatory drug (NSAID) treatment, or increased risk of gastric cancer or anxiety about cancer.

In a recent prospective observational study the prevalence of gastric cancer was 4% in a cohort of patients referred urgently because of 'alarm' symptoms. Referral for (1) dysphagia, (2) significant weight loss, and (3) alarm symptoms in those aged over 55 years, would have detected 99.8% of the cancers in the cohort. These findings are supported by other retrospective studies. Retrospective studies have found that cancer is rarely detected in patients younger than 55 years without alarm symptoms but when found the cancer is usually inoperable.

In the UK, morbidity (non-trivial adverse events) and mortality rates for gastroscopy may be as high as 1 in 200 and 1 in 2000 respectively.

Peptic ulcer disease

Peptic ulcer disease is common; approximately 10% of the population of Western countries are likely to suffer a duodenal or gastric ulcer during their lifetime. However, peptic ulceration is the cause for dyspepsia in only 10% of patients. Hospital admission rates for duodenal ulcer have increased in patients over 75 years. This has coincided with an increase in the use of low-dose aspirin.

Infection by *Helicobacter pylori* is implicated in 90–95% of duodenal ulcers and 70% of gastric ulcers in patients not taking NSAIDs.

Box 14.2 Alarm symptoms that should prompt urgent referral for upper gastrointestinal endoscopy

- Chronic gastrointestinal bleeding
- Progressive unintentional weight loss
- Progressive difficulties with swallowing
- Iron-deficiency anaemia
- Epigastric mass
- Suspicious barium meal

Box 14.3 NICE guidelines on the management of peptic ulcer disease and non-ulcer dyspepsia

Intervention for peptic ulcer disease

- *H. pylori* eradication therapy for *H. pylori* positive patients
- Stop NSAID
- Full dose PPI for 2 months

Intervention for non-ulcer dyspepsia

- Treatment for *H. pylori* if present
- Symptomatic management
- Periodic monitoring
- Routine re-testing after eradication is not necessary if symptoms improve

Long-term management

Annual review of patients requiring long-term management of dyspepsia symptoms, encouraging them to try stepping down or stopping treatment, promoting on demand use of the lowest dose of PPI.

Incidence

In most of the UK the incidence of duodenal ulcer has been falling steadily since the 1960s, probably as a result of a decline in *H. pylori* infection as living conditions in childhood have improved. It remains high in areas such as Northern Ireland and Glasgow. *H. pylori* can be initially detected using a carbon-13 urea breath test or a stool antigen test or laboratory-based serology, where its performance has been locally validated. (Office-based serological tests for *H. pylori* are not recommended because of their inadequate performance.) Retesting after treatment is not possible with serology, which remains positive despite successful eradication.

Treatment

A 7-day twice daily triple therapy regimen, consisting of a full dose PPI with either metronidazole 400 mg and clarithromycin 250 mg or amoxycillin 1 g and clarithromycin 500 mg achieves rapid symptom relief and healing rates of approximately 90% of duodenal ulcers and 85% of gastric ulcers, with a relapse rate of approximately 5%.

NSAID toxicity in the upper gastrointestinal tract is the most common serious drug-induced toxicity reported to regulatory authorities. Prophylactic anti-ulcer treatment and eradication of *H. pylori* should be considered in patients at high risk, prior to commencing NSAIDs.

Selective Cox-2 inhibitors have a lower incidence of gastrointestinal side-effects. Long-term use of some Cox-2 inhibitors has recently been associated with an increased risk of cardiovascular disease. NICE guidelines recommend they be used in preference to standard NSAID in patients at high risk of serious gastrointestinal events. Their use should also be limited to patients without cardiovascular risk factors (see Box 14.4).

Box 14.4 NICE guidelines on the use of selective Cox-2 inhibitors

- Patients at high risk of gastrointestinal events on NSAIDs
- Age >65 years
- Long-term, high-dose NSAIDs
- Co-prescription of NSAID or aspirin with anticoagulants
- Serious co-morbidity (other than cardiovascular disease)

Patients with a previous history of upper gastrointestinal ulcers, bleeds, or perforations are considered especially high risk and as such, the use of even Cox-2 selective inhibitors should be considered carefully in this situation.

There is no clear association between peptic ulcer disease and other life-style factors. However, individual patients may be helped by life-style advice and there may be more general health benefits that make such advice important. Patients should be advised to avoid known precipitants they associate with their symptoms.

Employment issues

Generally, individuals with peptic ulcer disease are able to pursue any type of work. There may be increased periods of absence from work during the initial stages of investigation or diagnosis but once treated the prognosis is good.

Research into psychosocial factors as a cause of peptic ulcer disease has become less popular in recent years as more effective therapies have become available. The current view is of a multifactorial model of causation in which stress may increase vulnerability to other causative agents.

Some individuals experience exacerbation of symptoms of dyspepsia during periods of stress. This may impact upon attendance at work. If the underlying cause of stress is identified as coming from the workplace it should be addressed through management intervention in preference to controlling symptoms with long-term medication.

There is evidence that shift work is associated with peptic ulceration,[5] although the mechanism of this has not been established. The reasons suggested include increased alcohol intake and smoking in shift workers and irregular meals leading to changes in gastric acidity. There is evidence that smoking is more prevalent in shift workers and that shift workers have longer periods of low intra-gastric pH compared with controls. However, many individuals with peptic ulcer disease are able to work shifts without significant exacerbation of their condition. With recent advances in treatment there is not sufficient medical evidence to justify excluding individuals with peptic ulceration from shift work. Those experiencing problems should be advised to pursue modern medical treatment for their condition as this has a high success rate, which in most cases will enable them to continue with their normal employment.

Coeliac disease[6]

Coeliac disease is due to an allergy to gluten in wheat and results in inflammation and atrophy of the small intestine. Coeliac disease has a prevalence of 1:300 in England and Wales. Confirmation of the diagnosis depends on histological examination of the small bowel (duodenum or jejunum). There is considerable under-recognition of the condition that increased use of serological screening should correct. Coeliac disease presents at all ages and may present with clinical or

Table 14.1 Presenting features of coeliac disease

Fatigue	80–90%
Diarrhoea	75–80%
Asymptomatic iron/folate deficiency	85%
Vitamin D deficiency	15–30%
Vitamin K deficiency	10%

haematological features or is identified by serological screening of asymptomatic relatives. (Table 14.1 describes some common features.)

Serology can be performed for antibodies to tissue transglutamase (tTG), gliadin, or endomysium. IgG and IgA anti tTG antibodies can be measured easily and cheaply using enzyme-linked immunosorbent assay (ELISA) techniques. They are highly sensitive markers being present in 90% of patients with untreated disease and are relatively specific. Some high-risk groups for screening are listed in Box 14.5.

Symptoms improve rapidly on a gluten-free diet; however, histological improvement takes months. Food containing wheat, rye, and barley should be avoided. Oats should also be avoided as commercially available oat flour is contaminated with 10–15% wheat. Lifelong adherence to a gluten free diet usually results in complete restoration to normal health. Relapse of symptoms occurs if gluten is inadvertently or deliberately introduced into the diet.

Employment issues

The only restriction for employment of someone with coeliac disease is if they have to consume gluten-containing foods as part of their work. Travel is not usually a problem, although diet may be more restricted abroad.

Chronic pancreatitis

The number of hospital admissions for acute and chronic pancreatitis significantly increased in Britain over the last two decades. There was a 43% increase in admissions for acute pancreatitis and a 100% increase for chronic pancreatitis.[7]

The clinical presentation of acute pancreatitis is very variable. Physical findings vary from minimal to profound shock with an associated high case mortality rate. Excessive alcohol consumption, usually with binge drinking, is the cause in up to half the cases of acute pancreatitis. Other causes include gallstones, drugs (e.g. azothioprine), hyperlipidaemia, and following endoscopic retrograde cholangiopancreatogram.

Box 14.5 High-risk groups for coeliac disease

- Siblings of index cases and first-degree relatives
- Type I diabetes
- Patients with Down's syndrome
- Patients with IgA deficiency

Chronic pancreatitis is characterized by chronic severe epigastric pain, steatorrhoea due to exocrine insufficiency and diabetes as a consequence of endocrine dysfunction. The pain may be so severe as to require opiate analgesia or coeliac axis nerve blocks. Surgery may be effective in selected patients; however, it increases the incidence of diabetes and the need for enzyme supplements.

Employment issues

Uncomplicated recovery from acute pancreatitis will leave the patient symptom-free and without any increased risk of recurrence if alcohol is excluded and other predisposing factors are corrected. However, during exacerbations of chronic pancreatitis, pain, and the side-effects of medication are likely to prevent attendance at work. Reliability is likely to be a problem and may be related to alcohol misuse if this is the underlying cause. It is therefore important to obtain an accurate prognosis when advising on suitability for employment.

Inflammatory bowel disease

Crohn's disease is a chronic inflammatory process of the small and large intestines, which is associated with extra-intestinal features. It is characterized by areas of transmural inflammation interspersed by normal mucosa, so-called skip lesions, and may affect any part of the gastrointestinal tract from the mouth to the anus. (See Table 14.2.)

In contrast ulcerative colitis only affects the colon. The inflammation is superficial, but in continuum from the anus. There is characteristically a sharp demarcation between normal and inflamed mucosa, which may occur at any level in the colon. Inflammation may extend to the caecum (total or pancolitis), or affect only the rectum (proctitis). Distal disease may extend over time.

Clinical features

The incidence of colonic disease increases with age. The natural history of Crohn's disease is characterized by relapses between spontaneous or treatment induced remissions; however, about 15% of patients have non-remitting disease and 10% prolonged remission. Symptoms may be of insidious onset and initially non-specific so that diagnosis may be delayed for months or years. The symptoms and signs of Crohn's disease depend both on its site and the predominant pathological process, whether inflammatory, fibrosing, or fistulating:

- Active **ileocaecal Crohn's disease** usually presents with pain and/or a tender mass in the right iliac fossa. Diarrhoea is common. Patients with **extensive small bowel Crohn's disease** may have features of malabsorption with steatorrheoa, anaemia, and weight loss.
- **Active Crohn's colitis** is associated with diarrhoea and pain prior to defecation. Occult blood loss may cause iron deficiency anaemia. Active colitis may be associated with urgency.

Table 14.2 Anatomical pattern of involvement in adult Crohn's disease

Site	% of patients
Ileocolonic	45
Colon only	25
Terminal ileum	20
Extensive small bowel	5
Anorectal only	3
Other (gastroduodenal, oral only)	2

- In fistulating Crohn's disease sinus tracts may end blindly producing an intra-abdominal or psoas abscess. Alternatively fistulae may develop between adjacent bowel loops, bladder, vagina, and skin.
- Patients with **perianal Crohn's disease** may be relatively asymptomatic or experience mucoid or faeculant discharge or soiling, tenesmus, pruritis ani, or rectal bleeding.

In patients with ulcerative colitis, bloody diarrhoea is the commonest symptom and urgency of defecation the most troublesome. Symptoms are related to disease activity rather than extent.

In patients with chronic active inflammatory bowel disease there are frequently systemic symptoms including lethargy, weight loss, and low-grade fever.

Extra-intestinal manifestations

These occur more commonly with colonic disease.

Joint disease

Peripheral arthropathy affects 5–15% of patients (Table 14.3). Type I, pauci-articular, asymmetrical arthropathy is more often associated with disease activity than type II. Sacroiliitis is independent of disease activity and has been increasingly recognized since the advent of magnetic resonance imaging. It tends to be less severe than that seen in ankylosing spondylitis.

Eye disease

Episcleritis and scleritis occur more commonly in ulcerative colitis, and cause burning and itching. Anterior uveitis is a serious complication, more common in Crohn's disease. It is due to acute inflammation of the anterior chamber of the eye, causing severe ocular pain, blurred vision, and headaches. Prompt referral to an ophthalmologist is essential.

Skin disease

Erythema nodosum and pyoderma gangrenosum are associated with disease activity, and may precede the onset of bowel disease. Treatment of pyoderma should involve the dermatologists.

Treatment

Aminosalicylates are recommended as first-line treatment for mild to moderate Crohn's disease. In moderately high doses, aminosalicylates induce remission in 40–50% of patients with mildly active Crohn's disease.

Table 14.3 Frequency of extra-intestinal manifestations in inflammatory bowel disease

	Ulcerative colitis (UC)	Crohn's disease (CD)
Type I pauci-articular (<5 joints)	5–6%	10–15%
Type II polyarticular (>5 joints)	2–4%	5–10%
Sacroiliitis (MRI)	30–40%	40–50%
Episcleritis/scleritis	UC > CD	
Anterior uveitis	Uncommon	CD > UC
Erythema nodosum	1–3%	10%
Pyoderma gangrenosum	1%	8%
Aphthous ulceration		5–15%
Abnormal liver function test	5%	5%

In ulcerative colitis maintenance therapy with salicylates reduces the annual rate of relapse three to fourfold, however there is no evidence to support the use of maintenance therapy in Crohn's disease.

The standard treatment of active inflammatory bowel disease is corticosteroids. Approximately 65% of patients with active Crohn's disease given prednisolone achieve remission or improve symptomatically; however, at least half will relapse or become steroid-dependent 1 year after starting treatment. Steroids do not alter the natural history of the disease and their use should be restricted in dose and duration, so as to minimize side-effects.

Topical steroids can be used for mild distal colitis. More extensive disease or persistent symptoms require oral steroids. Seventy-five per cent of patients with mild to moderate ulcerative colitis will respond.

Immunomodulatory drugs, the thiopurines, azathioprine (the prodrug), and 6-mercaptopurine, given orally are effective steroid sparing agents in steroid-dependent and steroid-refractory Crohn's disease. Meta-analysis has shown a 56% response rate; however, it can take up to 4 months to work. These drugs are also effective in ulcerative colitis. Azathioprine should be used as maintenance treatment for several years and requires regular monitoring for side-effects, particularly bone marrow suppression. Current data suggest that the risk of relapse after 4 years of treatment is similar whether the drug is continued or stopped.

Intravenous cyclosporin has been shown to be effective in 60% of cases of severe ulcerative colitis failing to respond to intravenous steroids. Oral and intramuscular methotrexate is a useful adjunct to steroids in refractory Crohn's disease.

Anti-tumour necrosis factor antibodies are effective in refractory fistulating Crohn's disease. Repeated infusions may be necessary to maintain the response rate. There is an infrequent but increased incidence of lymphoma, serum sickness-like reaction, opportunistic infections, sepsis, and autoimmune disorders. Ultimately this disease-modifying therapy may prove the most cost-effective treatment to date.

Surgery for ulcerative colitis is necessary for patients who fail to respond to medical treatment and is likely in 1 in 50 patients within 5 years of the onset of proctitis, 1 in 20 with left-sided colitis and 1 in 3 with total colitis. In patients with ulcerative colitis a **panproctocolectomy** is curative.

Surgery for Crohn's disease is necessary more frequently; 70% of patients will have an operation within 15 years of diagnosis, and 36% will have required two or more operations. The symptoms recur in 30% within 5 years and in 50% by 10 years. Bowel should be preserved wherever possible to avoid short bowel syndrome; a defunctioning ileostomy allows time for the bowel to recover or limited segmental resections to be performed.

Ileostomy and ileal pouch anal anastomosis

An ileostomy may be fashioned temporarily or permanently. Stomal complications from a permanent ileostomy for ulcerative colitis occur in 75% of patients over 20 years. Intestinal obstruction occurs in 23% and stomal revision is necessary in 28%. Complications include electrolyte imbalance, dehydration, and intestinal obstruction. Stomas have a greater impact on the quality of life of females than males.

Ileal pouch anal anastomosis is increasingly being performed in patients with ulcerative colitis, with improved social, work capacity, and quality of life. Frequency of defecation up to six times per day may be a problem. There is a significant incidence of sexual dysfunction in males following the procedure. Seventy per cent of patients with a pouch will suffer a complication necessitating hospital admission, up to 30% develop pouchitis and excision of the pouch is necessary in about 10%.

Box 14.6 Factors associated with a worse prognosis in Crohn's disease

- Extremes of age
- Extensive small bowel disease
- Fistulating disease
- Stricturing
- Multiple operations
- Smoking

Prognosis

In Crohn's disease the prognosis appears to be affected by: the age at diagnosis, disease location, and disease behaviour (Box 14.6); these may be genetically determined, and are currently under investigation. Overall, there is a small increase in mortality.[8]

Despite an overall normal life expectancy for patients with ulcerative colitis, patients over 50 years of age and with extensive colitis at diagnosis have an increased mortality within the first 2 years after diagnosis, due to colitis-associated postoperative complications and co-morbidity.[9]

Employment issues

Most patients with Crohn's disease are able to lead a normal life and 90% of patients remain at work.[10] However, there is evidence that Crohn's disease adversely affects employment with long periods of absenteeism and early disability. Patients with Crohn's disease are twice as likely to have a sedentary occupation.[11]

The main problems for individuals with inflammatory bowel disease are recurrent or persistent abdominal pain and frequency and urgency of defecation. Frequent episodes may result in regular absence from work and employees may be referred for occupational health advice as a result of poor attendance linked to recurrent relapses. Allowances for absences related to the condition may be required as a reasonable adjustment under the DDA.

Mild relapses can be treated as an outpatient with little time away from work. Moderate or severe exacerbations will not be compatible with attending work and may require up to several months for recovery with medical treatment. Surgery will result in prolonged absence from work depending on the type of procedure. In many cases the longer-term prognosis after surgery will be favourable; therefore, employers may be prepared to be supportive in accommodating a prolonged period of recuperation. Extra-intestinal manifestations as described earlier in the chapter, may increase disability and impact upon work capacity particularly during relapses. Usually the associated joint disease is mild but pain and stiffness may prevent individuals from undertaking physically strenuous work, including manual handling. Restrictions and adjustments should be assessed on a case by case basis. Eye disease, although uncommon, will cause significant short-term disability until treated. Affected individuals will be unfit to work as a result of pain and visual disturbance.

Overall in inflammatory bowel disease symptom severity is twice as high for those unable to work, with inability to work being a marker of the global functional impact of the disease.[12]

In a small number of cases premature retirement on the grounds of ill health will be justified. The factors associated with a poorer prognosis have been discussed but a specialist prognosis should be obtained before final decisions are made about work capacity. The impact of symptoms will be greater in jobs where rapid and regular toilet access is not possible. This could include those working outside, peripatetic workers, those responsible for the supervision or safety of others and those undertaking paced work such as production line work where flexible breaks are not possible.

The National Association for Colitis and Crohn's Disease issues members with a 'Can't Wait' card although these words are not printed on it. The card has the following message on the back: 'Please help. Due to an illness which is not infectious our member needs toilet facilities urgently'. The card is recognized by a number of retailers and can be presented in shops and places displaying the NACC logo (see Appendix 8).

Employment issues for workers with intestinal stomas

Patients with stomas will have a disability under the DDA and therefore employers will need to consider what adjustments can be made to enable them to undertake their work. Although there is evidence that working life is disturbed for patients after surgery for stoma (reported by 63% of ileostomy patients 6 months or more after surgery), there are no absolute contraindications for any work.[13] The nature and siting of the stoma will have an influence on any restrictions so each case should be assessed individually. Potential problems are highlighted below but in problematic or potentially high-risk work situations advice can be obtained from the British Colostomy Association and the Ileostomy and Internal Pouch Support Group (see Appendix 8). Both of these provide support for patients and can offer practical advice and examples about how to overcome problems, which might arise in the workplace.

Physically strenuous work can cause difficulties for some patients with stomas. Development of a parastomal hernia can make manual handling difficult and uncomfortable. Other problems include increased risk of leakage and possible injury to the stoma itself. Work that involves high-risk manual handling, repetitive stooping and bending, and carrying heavy or awkward loads close to the body, may be problematic. However, not all patients will find this to be the case and there are cases of successful employment in safety critical work such as the emergency services.

Food handling is not contraindicated in patients with stomas, as there is no evidence of increased cross-infection risk. Providing there is not a problem with leakage and good hygiene is followed, people with stomas should not be excluded from this work.

Work in hot environments could potentially place employees with stomas at greater than average risk because of the increased potential for dehydration and electrolyte imbalance. This should be prevented by ensuring that adequate hydration is maintained. Patients visiting the Tropics should be instructed on the use of oral rehydration solutions.

Gastroenteritis and gut infections

Gastrointestinal infections can result in symptoms such as diarrhoea, which may affect ability to work. Fortunately many infections seen in this country are self-limiting. Travellers and the immunocompromised may develop more serious or prolonged infection. The elderly and young children are more susceptible, as are patients with hypochlorhydria or on antisecretory medication, such as PPIs. There is a strong case for instituting early empirical fluoroquinolone therapy in all high-risk patients with moderate to severe diarrhoea of infective type as most will prove to have salmonella, campylobacter, or shigella infections.

The most common and relevant infections are summarized in Table 14.4. Further information on infections in the immunocompromised can be found in Chapter 23.

Table 14.4 Enteropathogens responsible for infectious diarrhoea

	Blood in stool	Chronic diarrhoea
Viruses		
(Rotaviruses groups	–	–
Adenoviruses	–	–
Norovirus (Norwalk))	–	–
Bacteria		
Vibrio cholerae	–	–
Escherichia coli	+/–	–
Shigella spp.	+/–	+
Salmonella spp.	+/–	+
Campylobacter spp.	+/–	+
Yersinia enterocolitica	+/–	+
Clostridium difficile	+/–	+
Protozoa		
Giardia intestinalis	–	+
Cryptosporidium parvum	–	+
Entamoeba histolytica	+/–	+

+ = usually present; – = rarely present/absent; +/– = may or may not be present

Viral gastroenteritis

Viral infections are more common than bacterial infections in developed countries. Many viruses have avoided attention for many years due to the difficulty of detection and the inability to be cultured. Identification of the viruses responsible for outbreaks of gastroenteritis has improved in recent years with the use of the reverse transcriptase polymerase chain reaction.

Noroviruses[14–16] are the most common cause of epidemic gastroenteritis. Outbreaks affect families, schools, nursing homes, hospitals, and cruise ships. There have been reports of incidents at conferences, wedding receptions, and recreational camps. An outbreak has been reported following contamination of food by an asymptomatic food handler whose child had been unwell with watery diarrhoea.[17]

Noroviruses are highly infectious with a low infection dose and a large human reservoir; they affect all age groups and are able to be transmitted by various routes. Water contamination has been responsible for outbreaks at swimming pools and after paddling in communal untreated pools or drinking at decorative fountains such as those found in parks. Direct person-to-person and aerosol transmission is also important.

The patient should stay off work until asymptomatic and, in the case of food handlers and healthcare workers, for 48 hours after recovery to limit the extent of a potential outbreak.

Vibrio cholerae

Cholera is an acute dehydrating diarrhoeal disease. It is caused by infection of the small intestine by *Vibrio cholerae* 01 and 0139. Hypochlorhydria predisposes individuals to the disease. Death occurs in severe cases. It is transmitted primarily by ingestion of faecally contaminated water or food, for example seafood, rice, vegetables, or fruit. The two modern vaccines, the whole cell and the live attenuated vaccine have improved efficacy (50–85% sustained response). The main indication for vaccination is protection of a population at risk in an endemic area. Both vaccines may be recommended for travellers to high-risk regions. The live attenuated vaccine induces rapid protection at 1 week after a single dose. Oral rehydration therapy is the mainstay of treatment although quinolone antibiotics play a part.

Escherichia coli

Enteropathogenic *E. coli* (EPEC) commonly cause watery diarrhoea. Enterohaemorrhagic *E. coli* (EHEC) also known as Shiga toxigenic *E. coli* (STEC) cause bloody diarrhoea, haemolytic uraemic syndrome, and thrombocytopaenic purpura. Transmission of EHEC is foodborne, environmental (including direct contact with animals and their faeces and contaminated water supplies), or through person-to-person contact. The largest outbreaks tend to be foodborne and the serotype 0157:H7 is the best known EHEC. It has been cultured from asymptomatic carriers. Food handlers should not return to work until two negative stools have been obtained at 48-hour intervals.

Shigella spp.

Shigella dysentery is characterized by an invasive colitis. Of the four species (*S. dysenteriae*, *S. flexneri*, *S. boydii*, and *S. sonnei*) shiga toxin-producing *S. dysenteriae* is the most severe and *S. flexneri* the most common.

Systemic features, such as fever and headaches are common. Transmission is through the faecal–oral route. Recent reports of cases in sexually active men who have sex with men has highlighted the risk of transmission during oro-anal sexual practices. Asymptomatic and/or prolonged shedding of bacteria in the convalescent phase may contribute to this risk. Bacteria survive for several hours on hands or towels and only an extremely low dose of organisms is needed to cause disease. There is increasing antibiotic resistance but treatment with fluoroquinolones is effective.

Food handlers and healthcare workers should have three negative stool samples before recommencing work.

Salmonella infections

The prolonged bacteraemic illnesses of typhoid and paratyphoid fevers, caused by the exclusively human pathogens, *Salmonella typhi* and *paratyphi* A, B, and C are endemic only in countries where there is poor sanitation. Annually about 200 cases of typhoid fever are seen in the UK mostly in people after visiting relatives or friends in the Indian subcontinent.

In contrast the acute diarrhoeal illnesses caused by the animal adapted *Salmonella* spp. serotypes are an important public health problem, mainly in Western countries, where they are related to large-scale farming and processing of food. The dramatic rise can be partly attributed to the consumption of eggs infected by vertical transmission. A low infecting dose is necessary to cause human disease, and multiplication within eggs may occur during storage. Conventional cooking does not necessarily destroy the organism. Food may also be contaminated during preparation.

Watery diarrhoea occurs 12–72 hours after infection, accompanied by abdominal pain, vomiting, and fever. The illness lasts a few days and is usually self-limiting. Fatalities are rare but occur in the extremes of age. Adults excrete the organism for 4–8 weeks but all except food handlers and water workers can resume work after 48 hours symptom free.

The incidence of typhoid fever among those on short-term package holidays to endemic areas is extremely low. Attention to personal, water, and food hygiene reduces the risk to negligible levels and the need for vaccination should be based on the nature of the person's travel and not just on the destination. Visitors on a low budget back-packing holiday or those who will be living close to local people should have vaccine protection.

Immunization should be offered to laboratory staff who may handle *S. typhi*. There are three different vaccines: oral, 'whole cell' involving two injections, and a single injection Vi polysaccharide. The choice depends on the age of the patient, cost, adverse effect profile, and preferred route of administration.

Campylobacter enteritis[18]

Campylobacter jejuni has become the most commonly recognized cause of bacterial gastroenteritis in humans.[19] In Western countries the incidence of *C. jejuni* and *C. coli* infections peaks during infancy and again in young adults aged 15–44 years. Here most infections are acquired through the handling and consumption of poultry meat. In developing countries, where the disease is confined to young children, inadequately treated water and contact with farm animals are the most important risk factors. Many infections are acquired during travel.

The most common presentation is an acute self-limiting illness, characterized by diarrhoea, fever, and abdominal pain. Guillain–Barré syndrome is now well recognized as a postinfectious complication with an incidence of <1 in 1000 infections.[20]

Culture of the organism from stool using a selective media has made the diagnosis a simple procedure.

Fluoroquinolone resistance has been reported in *C. jejuni* since the late 1980s in Europe and Asia, and since 1995 in USA. The use of fluoroquinolones to treat animals used for food has accelerated this trend of resistance. In Australia where fluoroquinolones have not been licensed for use in food production animals, *C. jejuni* resistance is low.

Yersinia enterocolitica

Y. enterocolitica causes colitis, and is associated with systemic features and a non-purulent arthritis. Food products of porcine origin and contaminated water are the major source of human infection. Improvements have been made in food processing and in hygiene during slaughtering swine.

Clostridium difficile

Toxin-producing *C. difficile* is the commonest cause of nosocomial diarrhoea and represents a significant health service burden. It causes acute or persistent diarrhoea, associated with antibiotic treatment, particularly cephalosporins. The pathological hallmark is a pseudo-membranous colitis. Treatment is with oral metronidazole or oral vancomycin.

Giardiasis

The protozoan *Giardia lamblia* is prevalent throughout the world. In Western countries it is one of the most commonly isolated intestinal parasites, occurring primarily in waterborne outbreaks. Though it is a well-documented cause of illness among travellers from areas of low prevalence and during waterborne outbreaks in non-endemic areas, its role as a pathogen in highly endemic areas is controversial. Infection results from ingestion of mature cysts and the incubation period varies widely. The diagnosis of giardiasis is usually made by the identification of cysts in faeces or duodenal aspirates. A commercially available ELISA and a fluorescein-labelled monoclonal antibody test for identifying *G. lamblia* in faeces are more sensitive than routine microscopy. Treatment for giardiasis includes metronidazole and tinidazole.

Excretion of the cysts in the faeces is a potential source of infection especially in food handlers, although the risk for asymptomatic carriers is probably low.

Cryptosporidiosis

Cryptosporidium spp. belong to a group of intestinal coccidians, which infect the small intestinal mucosa. In recent years *Crypto parvum* has been recognized not only as a pathogen in healthy hosts but also among patients with AIDS. It has a prevalence of 1–4% in the UK and 15–16% in patients with HIV. There is a seroprevalence of 25–35% in the UK. Transmission is via water-borne spread, or person to person and occurs at any age. It is one of the most infectious pathogens known. It is also a recognized cause of travellers' diarrhoea.

The clinical presentation depends on the immune state of the host. In the immunocompetent the incubation period is 2 weeks and symptoms are very variable. The illness is usually self-limiting and resolves within 2–4 weeks. In the immunocompromised the illness rapidly progresses to copious watery diarrhoea and malabsorption. Biliary tract involvement with stricturing of the distal bile duct is also recognized. The diagnosis is made on identification of oocysts in the faeces using an acid-fast stain. The optimal treatment has yet to be defined. Microsporidia, *Isospora belli,* and *Cyclospora cayetanensis* are also found in immunocompromised patients.

Entamoeba histolytica

Amoebiasis has many clinical presentations. Most intestinal infections are asymptomatic resulting from non-pathogenic organisms. Some 90% of infections with pathogenic organisms are also asymptomatic. Clinically invasive amoebiasis only occurs in 10% and the most common presentation is acute colitis or acute right upper quadrant pain and fever. Amoebic liver abscesses can present acutely or subacutely without a history of diarrhoea. Microscopy of three separate stool samples has a 90% sensitivity rate. The false negative rate is high due to mistaken identity of leucocytes as amoeba. Serology in a non-endemic area is very useful in confirming the diagnosis. Table 14.5 summarizes the sources and clinical patterns of common food-borne diarrhoeal infections.

Employment issues

Gastrointestinal infections may temporarily impair work capacity, but the main issue for employment is the risk of the spread of infection. This risk is greatest with liquid stools; therefore all cases of gastroenteritis should be regarded as potentially infectious and individuals should refrain from work until free from diarrhoea and vomiting. This is particularly important for:

◆ food handlers
◆ staff of healthcare facilities in direct contact with susceptible patients or their food.

Each case must be assessed on an individual basis.

Transmission of infection by food handling

In spite of increased legislation, inspection, and education, there has been a steady increase in the incidence of food-borne illness with an increase in the availability of ready-to-eat foods.

British livestock waste spread on to agricultural land contains measurable levels of the zoonotic agents that cause most cases of bacterial gastroenteritis in the UK. Raw meat, poultry, eggs, and unpasteurized milk are commonly contaminated with these organisms.

The majority of food-borne infections occur due to a failure to follow good food preparation or manufacturing practices such as proper temperature control for cooking and storage of food, cross-contamination from raw to cooked foods and inadequate or inappropriate reheating of cooked foods.

Infected food handlers account for only a small proportion of food poisoning outbreaks. However, food handlers do play a significant part in *Staphylococcus aureus* food poisoning with transmission from infected skin lesions.

Definition of a food handler

A food handler is defined as a person employed in the production, preparation, storage, and transport of foodstuffs who is directly in contact with the product. This will include the manufacturing, catering, and retail industries. Those undertaking maintenance work or repairing

Table 14.5 Microbial pathogens responsible for food-borne diarrhoeal disease

	Source	Incubation period	Symptoms	Recovery
Bacteria that colonize the gut				
Salmonella spp.	Eggs, poultry	12–48 hours	Diarrhoea, blood, pain, vomiting, fever	2–14 days
Campylobacter jejuni	Milk, poultry	2–14 days	Diarrhoea, blood, pain, vomiting, fever	7–21 days
Enterohaemorrhagic *Escherichia coli*	Beef	1–14 days	Diarrhoea, blood, pain, vomiting, fever	7–21 days
Vibrio parahaemolyticus	Crabs, shellfish	12–18 hours	Diarrhoea, pain, vomiting, fever	2–30 days
Yersinia enterocolitica	Milk, pork	2 hours–12 days	Diarrhoea, pain, fever	1–3 days
Clostridium perfringens	Spores in food especially milk	8–22 hours	Diarrhoea, pain,	1–3 days
Listeria monocytogenes	Milk, sweet corn	8–36 hours	Diarrhoea, fever	
Preformed toxins				
Staphylococcus aureus	Contaminated food, usually by humans	2–6 hours	Nausea, vomiting, pain, diarrhoea	Rapid, few hours
Bacillus cereus	Reheated rice, bean sprouts	1–5 hours	Nausea, vomiting, pain, diarrhoea	Rapid
Clostridium botulinum	Spores geminate in anaerobic conditions, canned or bottled foods	18–36 hours	Transient diarrhoea, paralysis	Months

equipment in food handling areas, enforcement officers, and visitors to food handling areas who may touch surfaces that come into contact with unwrapped food should also meet the same health and hygiene standards as those involved directly in food handling.

People who handle only pre-wrapped, canned or bottled food or those involved in primary agriculture or harvesting processes are not considered as food handlers.

Food safety

The Department of Health guidance on food handlers' fitness to work was produced in 1995 to assist food businesses to meet their obligations under the regulations and to guide health professionals advising on a person's suitability to work as a food handler.[21] Occupational health specialists advising the food industry have developed additional guidance.[22]

Health screening of food handlers

On recruitment, prospective employees should be requested to complete a specific questionnaire to determine whether there are any medical conditions that would compromise food safety (see Table 14.6) as well as to determine fitness to undertake any special demands of the work such

Table 14.6 Fitness criteria for food handlers.[22] Reproduced with permission from Oxford University Press.

Site or condition	Pre-employment standard	Standard if in employment
Ear	Free of discharge and, if perforation of drum, no history of discharge in last year	Free of discharge
Throat		Unfit if purulent tonsillitis
Eyes		Unfit if infective conjunctivitis
Skin	Free of eczema or psoriasis on hands, forearms and face Free of purulent skin conditions affecting hands, forearms and face	Free of eczema or psoriasis on hands, forearms or face Free of purulent skin conditions affecting hands, forearms and face
Gastrointestinal		
Non- infective diarrhoea	Unfit if persistent watery stools (excluding individuals with colostomy or ileostomy)	Unfit if persistent watery stools (excluding individuals with colostomy or ileostomy)
Enteric fever, i.e. typhoid, paratyphoid (A, B &C)	Unfit if history of enteric fever unless stool testing has excluded the presence of persistent carrier status. 6 consecutive negative stool tests required at 2-week intervals	Unfit if suffering from acute enteric fever until persistent carrier status has been excluded. 6 consecutive negative stool tests required at 2-week intervals; starting 2 weeks after completion of antibiotic treatment. Household contacts of acute cases or people who have had contact with an acute outbreak should be excluded from food handling duties until three negative stool specimens have been collected at weekly intervals starting 3 weeks after last contact with the case or outbreak
E. coli O157 (Verotoxin producing strains)		Unfit until two negative stools obtained at 48-hour intervals
Salmonella, Shigella,* amoebic dysentery, cholera		Free of diarrhoea and vomiting for 48 hours*
Other infective causes of diarrhoea and vomiting		Free of diarrhoea and vomiting for 48 hours
Hepatitis A		Following acute illness, unfit until 7 days after onset of jaundice.

Shigella dysenteriae requires clearance by three negative stools.

as manual handling. Any positive responses should be followed up with medical enquiry and/or examination before employment commences. Stool examinations are not required routinely but should be undertaken if there is a history of illness that could be due to, or a history of contact with, enteric fever.

Prevention of microbiological contamination of food

Food handlers should be trained in the safe handling of food, have a good understanding of the principles of food hygiene and be aware of their obligation to report to management any infectious conditions that might arise during their employment. Local policies should state clearly the procedure that should be followed by food handlers if they develop infection or have been in contact with relevant conditions.

The most commonly reported conditions, which have implications for food handlers are diarrhoea and vomiting. It is important for employees to understand that diarrhoea implies a change in bowel habit, as some non-infectious bowel conditions (inflammatory bowel disease) may result in the passage of frequent loose stools.

Food handlers who develop symptoms of gastrointestinal infection should report immediately to management and leave the food handling area. Cases will need to be managed on an individual basis with medical investigation, stool sampling, treatment, and referral to the local consultant in communicable disease control depending on the nature, duration, and severity of symptoms and on the number of workers affected.

Gastrointestinal infections requiring special consideration include *Salmonella typhi* and *paratyphi*, *E. coli* and hepatitis A infections (see specific sections).

Functional gastrointestinal disorders

Definition

The term functional bowel disorder is used to define a complex of chronic or recurrent gastrointestinal symptoms that cannot be explained by structural or biochemical abnormalities.

These symptoms may coexist with organic disease so that, for example functional dyspepsia may be found in patients with *H. pylori* gastritis or biliary colic due to gallstones. Alternatively functional gastrointestinal disorders may persist after the resolution of an organic disease. Patients may present with irritable bowel symptoms in the absence of any inflammatory lesions after an episode of infective gastroenteritis (25% of cases) or during a phase of remission of ulcerative colitis.

Irritable bowel syndrome

Irritable bowel syndrome affects 9–12% of the population. Some 50% of patients attribute the onset of symptoms to a stressful event. Most patients do not seek medical care. Women are affected by irritable bowel symptoms twice as often as men, and are about three times more likely to seek healthcare.

Rome criteria have been developed to standardize diagnosis and aid the selection of patients for clinical trials. (See Box 14.7.)

Affected patients tend to have a higher incidence of psychiatric disease and psychosocial disturbance, are susceptible to stress and show a high degree of abnormal illness behaviour. There is an increased incidence of multiple somatic complaints. Patients with irritable bowel syndrome are over-represented in the gynaecology and surgical out patients and are more likely to undergo inappropriate surgery. Patients with functional gastrointestinal disorders exhibit visceral hypersensitivity.

> ## Box 14.7 Rome II criteria for the diagnosis of irritable bowel syndrome
>
> Twelve weeks or more in the last 12 months of abdominal discomfort or pain that has two of the following three features:
>
> ◆ relieved by defecation
> ◆ associated with a change in stool frequency
> ◆ associated with a change in stool consistency

Treatment and prognosis

Symptoms may last for many years with only 40% recovering over a 6-year follow-up. Coeliac disease, microscopic colitis, lactose intolerance, thyroid disease, early stage Crohn's disease, and bile salt malabsorption should be excluded, as should colon cancer in those over 45 years or in those with a positive family history. Treatment with loperamide, low-fibre diets, antispasmodics, and bile salt-binding therapy may help some patients.

Despite the benign nature of these disorders, many symptoms such as vomiting, bloating, faecal urgency, incontinence, diarrhoea, flatulence, and borborygmi can restrict social activities.

Employment issues

The majority of patients manage to remain in work despite their condition, although exacerbations may lead to up to twice the average absence from work. Symptoms may be made worse by occupational stress and the underlying work issues should be addressed in these cases. In severe cases the need for frequent defecation may substantially restrict travel or work and arrangements to facilitate ready access to a toilet at work may need to be put in place.

Viral hepatitis

Hepatitis A

Hepatitis A is transmitted by the faecal–oral route. It is uncommon with approximately 1000 infections notified per year in England and Wales. Most cases are sporadic but outbreaks can occur. With improvements in hygiene, infection has decreased in many parts of the world. This has rendered a large percentage of the younger population susceptible to the virus.

Clusters occur in families and in settings where potential for person-to-person faecal–oral spread is high, e.g. daycare centres, nurseries, primary schools. Cases have also been reported from eating virus-containing shellfish or cold food (particularly dairy products) contaminated by food handlers during the prodrome of the infection. Outbreaks have been recorded in male homosexuals and in injecting drug users.

Clinical features

Hepatitis A infection is anicteric in 50% of cases. The incubation period is 15–40 days and the patient is infectious while the virus is in the stools, from 2–3 weeks before to not more than 8 days after the jaundice is apparent. Patients feel unwell during the prodrome but often improve with the onset of jaundice. Lethargy may continue for 6 weeks or for as long as 3 months.

Box 14.8 Groups at high risk of hepatitis A

- Haemophilia
- Hepatitis B or C virus infection
- Liver cirrhosis
- Intravenous drug users with chronic liver disease
- Men who have sex with men

Diagnosis is based on the detection in the serum of IgM antibody to hepatitis A. The presence of IgG antihepatitis A antibody indicates either previous exposure or immunization.

Hepatitis A is usually a mild self-limiting illness but can occasionally result in severe or fatal disease. Individuals at particular risk of an adverse outcome include those more than 50 years old, those with liver cirrhosis of any cause, or with pre-existing hepatitis B or C virus infection.

Prevention of hepatitis A infection[23]

Hepatitis A vaccine should be offered to those at high risk from infection (see Box 14.8). It should also be used to prevent secondary cases and in outbreaks provided that the patients are informed that the latest date the vaccine is most likely to be effective is 7 days from the onset of illness in the primary case. Human normal immunoglobulin (HNIG) should be offered in addition or in preference to vaccine for contacts who are more than 7 days from onset of illness in the primary case, and for those at high risk of an adverse outcome.

Immunization is recommended for travellers to countries where hepatitis A infection is endemic. Current guidelines recommend a single dose of vaccine, which produces antibodies lasting at least 1 year.[24] A booster dose at 6–12 months will give immunity for up to 10 years and needs to be considered for groups at special risk.

Employment issues

Infected patients can resume or continue all forms of work (except food handling) as soon as they feel fit. Food handlers must refrain from work until jaundice has disappeared, or for 1 week after the onset of jaundice whichever is the longer. Those with anicteric hepatitis should remain off work for 1 week after serum transaminases have reached a peak.

Prevention of occupational exposure The only occupational group for whom routine immunizations are recommended are laboratory workers working directly with the virus. Serological evidence of previous infection (IgG HAV) should be checked before immunization. There is no evidence that most healthcare workers are at increased risk of hepatitis A and routine immunization of healthcare workers in residential institutions and with young children is not recommended. Immunization of workers who have direct exposure to untreated raw sewage should be considered as part of the control measures under the risk assessment required by the Control of Substances Hazardous to Health Regulations 1994. There is currently insufficient evidence to justify routinely immunizing all sanitation workers.

Hepatitis B

Intravenous drug use is the most frequently reported route of transmission in the UK and is identified as the risk factor in 50% of reported cases. Heterosexual sex is the risk factor in 18.5%, sex with an intravenous drug user in 3%, and men who have sex with men in 8%.[25] Other recognized modes of transmission include tattooing, needlestick injury, trauma, body piercing, and acupuncture. The number of cases attributed to heterosexual contact is stable, whereas the number of cases in men who have sex with men has decreased. For about a third of cases of acute hepatitis B infection no route of transmission is reported, but many of these may relate to intravenous drug use.[26]

Incidence

The infection is a global public health problem, with approximately 400 million people chronically infected. In England and Wales the estimated annual incidence of hepatitis B infection between 1995 and 2000 was 7.4 per 100 000.[26] Hepatitis B notification has increased 50% between 1990 and 2000. In England the highest prevalence is in the north-west. In Scotland it is in Glasgow; however, there has been a steady increase in many regions including the Grampian Region. This increase is probably due to intravenous drug use. Despite an effective vaccine most intravenous drug users are unvaccinated. More than 1 in 5 injectors is infected with hepatitis B. The incidence in South Asian immigrants is relatively high, and their main risk factors are medical treatment overseas and heterosexual contact. Vertical transmission from mother to child is particularly important in highly endemic areas.

Endemic transmission gives rise to only a small proportion of all new chronic infections in the UK, with the vast majority arising from immigration of established hepatitis B carriers.

Clinical features

Acute hepatitis B has an incubation period of 3–6 months, with a maximum infectivity immediately prior to the onset of jaundice. It is diagnosed by the presence of IgM antibody (HBcAb) to hepatitis core antigen, with or without hepatitis B surface antigen (HBsAg). A patient with resolving acute hepatitis is no longer infectious once hepatitis B surface antigen (HBsAg) is undetectable. Hepatitis B envelope antigen (HBeAg) correlates with a high degree of infectivity, while antibody to the envelope (HBeAb) demonstrates seroconversion with a low degree of infectivity.

A proportion of patients infected with hepatitis B virus progress to chronicity, defined as persistence of infection and presence of HBsAg for more than six months. The rate is 5–10% among adults. Inactive carriers of hepatitis B are healthy, have a low concentration of serum hepatitis B virus DNA (a measure of rate of viral replication, $<10^5$ copies/ml) or none, lack detectable HBeAg, have normal levels of alanine transferase and show little progression of liver disease.[27]

Patients with chronic hepatitis B have viral replication, high hepatitis B DNA concentrations, and biochemical evidence of hepatitis. Patients with chronic hepatitis B may test positive or negative for HBeAg. The HBeAg negative patients have a mutation (pre-core mutation) that permits viral replication but prevents production of HBeAg. These patients have a poorer prognosis.

Chronic hepatitis progresses to end-stage liver disease in 15–40% of patients.

Treatment

Antiviral agents may be used successfully to treat acute hepatitis B. However, there are no randomized controlled trials. The treatment for fulminant hepatitis B is transplantation. All patients with chronic hepatitis B should be offered treatment with antivirals.

Interferon-alfa is a host cytokine produced in response to any viral invasion. It has immunomodulatory, antiviral, and antifibrotic properties. It has been used in the treatment of chronic hepatitis B for more than 20 years and is associated with a higher HBV DNA inhibition rate and rate of HBeAg loss compared with controls, and it may have long-term beneficial effects in terms of HBV clearance, reduction of hepatocellular carcinoma, and prolongation of survival.

Pegylated (long acting) interferon-alfa is more effective than conventional interferon-alfa in the treatment of chronic hepatitis B as well as chronic hepatitis C, and is also associated with greater efficacy than conventional interferon in difficult-to-treat disease.

Lamivudine, a synthetic nucleoside (cytosine) inhibits viral reverse transcriptase. Treatment is associated with HBeAg seroconversion to HBeAb, and a reduction in HBV DNA levels. The response depends on a number of factors including the duration of treatment.

However, resistance occurs due to a mutation in the tyrosine–methionine–aspartate–aspartate (YMDD) motif in viral polymerase, which confers lamivudine resistance. Lamivudine has an excellent safety profile, even in patients with decompensated cirrhosis.

Adefovir dipivoxil, a nucleotide analogue of adenosine monophosphate, inhibits viral reverse transcriptase. Adefovir results in histological, virological, and biochemical improvement in both HBeAg-positive and HBeAg-negative chronic HBV. The rate of HBeAg seroconversion increases with prolonged treatment. Unfortunately resistance has now been observed. It may be useful as part of combination therapy, in HBV/HIV co-infection, hepatitis B-infected liver transplant recipients, and lamivudine resistance.

Prevention of hepatitis B infection

Hepatitis B immunization Worldwide the integration of hepatitis B vaccination into existing childhood immunization schedules has the greatest likelihood of long-term success; however, it is not currently policy in the UK. Active immunization against hepatitis B is safe and effective. The conventional schedule is a dose at 0, 1, and 6 months. This achieves a response rate exceeding 95%. Non-responders may benefit from additional doses of the vaccine. There is an accelerated schedule that allows the primary course to be administered within a period of 1 month. This schedule of day 0, 7, and 21, with a booster at 12 months, results in a seroprotection rate of 65% at day 28 and 99% at month 13. Seroconversion (anti-HBs antibody) should be checked 6–8 weeks after the final dose of each schedule. Antibody levels in excess of 10 mIU/ml are considered protective, although efforts are usually made to achieve levels above 100 mIU/ml for longer term protection. Some factors for poor response are listed in Box 14.9. Booster doses or a repeat course should be considered for those with a low response (10–100 mIU/ml) or no response (<10 mIU/ml) to the vaccine.

Vaccine protection lasts for 15 years, and because of strong immunological memory it continues after anti-HBs has become undetectable. There is no evidence to support the administration of routine boosters to those with a good initial response to the vaccine,[28] but these may have a role in immunosuppressed patients and those at a high risk of exposure. However the current

Box 14.9 Factors associated with a poorer response rate to hepatitis B immunization

- Age >40 years
- Obesity
- Chronic renal failure
- Haemodialysis
- Immunosuppression
- Organ transplants

Department of Health immunization guidelines still recommend a single booster dose 5 years after completion of the primary course in those who continue to be at risk of infection.[24]

Accidental exposure to hepatitis B virus

Passive immunity using hepatitis B hyperimmune serum globulin (HBIg) is effective if given within 48 hours of exposure. It is indicated for needlestick injury, other high-risk occupational exposure and sexual contacts of acute sufferers. Vaccination should be started simultaneously, with the first dose given in a site different from the HBIg. An accelerated four-dose immunization schedule (0, 1, 2, and 12 months) is preferred in this setting.

Employment issues

Approximately 50% of acute infections are mild and may be anicteric. Patients with more severe symptoms will be unable to work during the acute illness. Once recovery has taken place there should be no restrictions on employment (with the exception of some healthcare work—see below). Chronic carriers are usually in good health and are able to work normally. There is no evidence of risk of transmission of hepatitis B by casual contact in the workplace.

First aid Individuals who undertake first aid in the workplace should be advised that the risk of transmission of blood-borne viruses during normal first aid procedures can be minimized by standard cross-infection control procedures for all casualties. Training should be provided in how to prevent and deal with contamination and protective clothing such as disposable gloves should be provided to reduce the risk of exposure to blood-borne viruses.

Healthcare workers The specific problem of healthcare workers is addressed in Department of Health guidelines (Box 14.10).[29–31] These are regularly reviewed and updated. There are restrictions on the employment of healthcare workers who undertake **exposure-prone procedures.** These are procedures where there is a risk that injury to the healthcare worker could result in exposure of the patient's open tissues to the blood of the healthcare worker. Examples include surgery, obstetrics and gynaecology, and dentistry. Healthcare workers who are carriers of the hepatitis B virus and who are e-antigen positive must not perform exposure prone procedures. Healthcare workers who are e-antigen negative and who have a viral load (hepatitis B virus DNA) that exceeds 10^3 genome equivalents per millilitre should also be restricted from undertaking exposure prone procedures. It is possible that this may be relaxed for healthcare workers on antiviral treatment in the future.[32] The guidance recommends that advice on the work that e-antigen positive healthcare workers may perform should be sought from a specialist occupational physician.

Hepatitis C

The hepatitis C virus (HCV) is the most common chronic blood-borne pathogen. It is an emerging health concern across the world, with 170 million people chronically infected and at risk of liver cancer, cirrhosis, or liver failure. Modes of transmission include intravenous drug use, blood products, tattooing and, to a lesser extent, sexual intercourse. The six genotypes vary to a large extent, with as much as 34% nucleotide sequence disparity between two genotypes. The development of an effective vaccine may in part be hindered by this genetic heterogeneity.

Prevalence

HCV prevalence in Scottish childbearing women was found to be 0.3–0.4%. It was higher in deprived areas and among 25–29 year olds.[33] It is estimated that 0.4% or 200 000 people in England are chronically infected.

Box 14.10 Occupational indications for immunization against hepatitis B

- All healthcare workers including students and trainees who have direct contact with blood or bloodstained body fluids or patients' tissues including: doctors, surgeons, dentists, nurses, and midwives
- Laboratory staff in regular contact with blood or body fluids
- Mortuary staff
- Staff providing maintenance treatment with blood or blood products
- Blood transfusions service staff
- Any workers at significant risk of contaminated sharps injury, contamination of mucous membranes or skin lesions with blood or blood-stained body fluids
- Workers at significant risk of being bitten by patients or others
- Staff on secondment to areas of the world with a high prevalence of hepatitis B
- Others for whom immunization should be considered: ambulance and rescue services; staff at reception centres for people from high endemic areas; staff of custodial institutions; and some police personnel

Clinical aspects

Of those infected, 20–40% have been shown to clear infection naturally and have persistently negative HCV RNA on polymerase chain reaction (PCR). Hepatitis C infection progresses very slowly. Genotype 1, older age at first infection, co-infection with other viruses, particularly HIV and excess alcohol intake increase the progression rate.

Hepatitis C infection is characterized by a relatively long asymptomatic period of seronegative viraemia so that testing for HCV antibodies may miss patients with infection. HCV RNA testing is more accurate, but at present is not routine.

It is estimated that 5–20% of chronically infected people will progress to cirrhosis of the liver over a period of about 20 years. A small number (1–4% of those with cirrhosis) will progress to hepatocellular carcinoma each year.

Treatment

Case selection for antiviral therapy is crucial. Treatment is generally recommended for chronic hepatitis C patients, who are at increased risk of disease progression, such as those with elevated aminotransferase levels, hepatitis C viraemia, and portal fibrosis or moderate inflammation on liver biopsy. Certain groups of patients are not considered suitable for interferon therapy (see Box 14.11), as treatment is associated with significant side-effects (see Box 14.12). The most common side-effect is depression. However, mild to moderate depression can be treated with selective serotonin reuptake inhibitors.

The most effective therapy is pegylated interferon with ribavirin. Sustained viral response (absent viraemia 6 months after completing treatment) can be obtained in 54–56% of individuals infected with genotype 1 after 48 weeks of treatment.[34,35] Response rates are higher (75–85%) with genotypes 2 and 3 after only 6 months of treatment. Patients who have undetectable HCV RNA on PCR 6 months after treatment are extremely unlikely to relapse.

Box 14.11 Contraindications to interferon treatment

- Severe psychiatric disease
- Alcohol abuse
- Substance abuse
- Co-morbid conditions such as renal disease

Box 14.12 Side-effects of interferon treatment

- Depression: 30%
- Influenza-like symptoms: 25%
- Haematological abnormalities
- Autoantibodies
- Thyroid dysfunction
- Rare:
  - ocular toxicity
  - acute pancreatitis

Box 14.13 Factors associated with a sustained viral response[36]

Pretreatment

- Age <40 years
- Body weight <75 kg
- Mild disease on liver biopsy
- Genotype 2 or 3
- Hepatitis C RNA level <2 million copies/ml
- or <800 000 IU/ml

During treatment

- Early viral response (after 12 weeks of therapy)
- Compliance with treatment

Box 14.14 At-risk groups who should be tested for hepatitis C[37]

- Current injecting drug users
- Those who injected drugs at any point in the past
- Recipients of blood transfusions in the UK prior to September 1991 or blood products prior to 1986
- Recipients of organ and tissue transplants in the UK before 1992 or in countries where hepatitis C is common and donors may not have been screened
- Babies born to mothers known to be infected with HCV
- Children of mothers found to be infected with HCV
- Regular sexual partners of those infected with HCV
- Healthcare workers accidentally exposed to blood where there is a risk of HCV transmission
- Anyone who has received medical or dental treatment in countries where HCV is common and infection control may be poor (this will include recipients of blood transfusions and blood products where donations are not screened for HCV)
- People who have had tattoos, body piercing, and other forms of skin piercing in places with poor infection control procedures

Successful treatment enables regeneration of liver tissue and reduces the risk of liver failure and of hepatocellular carcinoma. The management of patients with HCV must also address quality of life issues by preventing or dealing with psychosocial factors and recommending life-style changes. Excess alcohol, central obesity, and insulin resistance increase the risk of disease progression and the development of type 2 diabetes mellitus, as well as reducing the efficacy of antiviral therapy.

Employment issues

Apart from the special problems of healthcare workers there are no specific contraindications for work and no risks of cross-infection in the workplace.

The risk of an individual surgeon acquiring the HCV has been estimated at 0.001–0.032% per annum.[38] Even in an area with an extremely high prevalence of HCV among its injecting drug using population, the risk of acquiring HCV through occupational exposure is low. Universal precautions should be observed however.

There is specific Department of Health Guidance about how hepatitis C infected healthcare workers should be managed in order to prevent the transmission of infection to patients.[39] Those who are HCV RNA positive should not undertake exposure prone procedures. The guidance contains current advice on which healthcare workers should be tested (see also ref. 31).

Chronic liver disease

Cirrhosis results from chronic liver injury. The most common causes are alcohol, hepatitis B, hepatitis C, and cryptogenic.

Alcoholic liver disease

Alcohol plays a part in 22 000 premature deaths per year in the UK. Deaths from alcoholic liver disease and admission rates to hospital have increased in the last decade.[40] The crude mortality from primary liver disease increased from 6.0 per 100 000 in 1993 to 12.7 per 100 000 in 2000. The increase is almost exclusively due to alcoholic liver disease.

Cryptogenic cirrhosis

Cryptogenic cirrhosis is likely to be the end result of non-alcoholic steatohepatitis. There is an increased prevalence of non-alcoholic fatty liver disease associated with an increase in obesity and insulin resistance.

Primary biliary cirrhosis

Increased use of diagnostic tests particularly autoantibody testing has meant that patients are often asymptomatic at the time of diagnosis. In a recent study 20% of initially asymptomatic patients had either died of liver disease or required liver transplant over long-term follow-up. The median survival was 9.6 years.[41] Patients with primary biliary cirrhosis may be troubled by extreme fatigue and intractable pruritis.

Treatment of complications of cirrhosis

Ascites and spontaneous bacterial peritonitis, hepatic encephalopathy, hepatocellular carcinoma, portal hypertension, and bleeding are major complications of cirrhosis. Oesophageal varices are treated endoscopically by band ligation and require fewer treatments than injection therapy. In alcoholic cirrhosis the prognosis is reasonable if the patient abstains from alcohol. In those with advanced liver disease continued drinking has a high mortality.

Diuretic treatment of ascites with spironolactone is often effective in mild cases. Diuretic refractory ascites may respond to vasopressin analogues, improving the systemic haemodynamics, the glomerular filtration rate and natriuresis. Paracentesis is effective but may increase the risk of bacterial peritonitis. Portosystemic shunts performed under radiological control or liver transplantation, where appropriate, are necessary in severe cases.

Encephalopathy is a potentially reversible neuropsychiatric disturbance in advanced liver disease. Subclinical encephalopathy can be diagnosed with an abnormal electroencephalogram and psychometric tests. Encephalopathy may be precipitated by a number of factors such as infection, gastrointestinal bleeding, constipation and drugs.

Hepatocellular carcinoma is seldom resectable, because it arises in cirrhotic livers and is often multifocal. Transplantation with restrictive selection criteria has improved the prognosis. Non-surgical methods such as chemo-embolization and percutaneous ethanol injection are used to prevent tumour progression either pre-transplant or as palliative therapy. Patients with one hepatocellular carcinoma nodule ≤5 cm in diameter, or two to three nodules ≤3 cm may be suitable for transplantation. However, because of a steadily increasing waiting time, a number of patients are excluded from orthotopic liver transplantation because of tumour progression.

Orthotopic liver transplantation

Approximately 3000 liver transplants are carried out each year in the UK.[42] The most common indications for transplantation are primary biliary cirrhosis, alcoholic cirrhosis and post-hepatitis C cirrhosis. Overall 1-year graft survival rate for first transplants is now 75%.

Employment issues

A specialist should optimize the care of patients with cirrhosis and decompensated liver disease before work is resumed. Although alcohol addiction and dependency are excluded from the definition of impairment under the DDA, the complications arising from alcoholism especially ascites and hepatic impairment will require individual assessment, to determine whether the patient is disabled within the meaning of the Act.

After successful liver transplantation 68% of individuals return to employment at 6 months. Physical fatigue is the main symptom limiting work activity in transplant recipients.

Patients with chronic or intermittent encephalopathy should not be employed in intellectually demanding work or jobs requiring a high degree of vigilance, including driving or operating machinery. Subclinical encephalopathy is less easy to detect, but may be as disabling in safety-critical work. Individual suitability for driving duties should be discussed with the medical branch of the Driver and Vehicle Licensing Authority (DVLA) (see Appendix 8—or refer to the website www.dvla.gov.uk). Patients who have been dependent on alcohol are barred from holding a vocational licence until they can demonstrate evidence of uninterrupted absence of dependency and misuse for 3 years. Confirmation of satisfactory liver enzyme tests and mean corpuscular volume as well as examination by a consultant with a special interest in alcohol abuse is required.

In patients with oesophageal varices there is no limitation on occupation once the varices have been treated. Patients with ascites may experience difficulty with lifting, bending, or stooping.

Guidelines for employees handling hepatotoxins

Hepatotoxins are metabolized at different rates, in an unpredictable nature. The reason for this is multifactorial, including genetic and environmental factors. In addition there is a complex interaction with other hepatotoxins, especially alcohol. In general patients with chronic liver disease with ongoing inflammation or liver damage should not work with hepatotoxins. All patients working with hepatotoxins should avoid alcohol misuse and enzyme inducing agents such as anticonvulsants, in particular phenobarbitone and phenytoin.

Obesity

Being overweight and obese are conditions in which weight gain (predominantly fat) has reached the point of endangering health. The prevalence has increased rapidly in the past two decades; since 1980 the prevalence of obesity has nearly trebled in the UK. Almost two-thirds of men and over half of women in the UK were either overweight or obese in 2001.[42] Obesity increases the risk of several serious chronic diseases and represents a significant economic burden. In 1998 over 18 million days of sickness were attributed to obesity with a total cost of £2.6 million in England.[43] Obesity is usually measured in terms of the Body Mass index (Box 14.15), with guidelines for clinically important ranges set out by the World Health Organization (Table 14.7).

Waist circumference can also be used as an indicator of central obesity. An increased waist circumference in men of >94 cm and women >80 cm is associated with insulin resistance, decreased

---

Box 14.15 Calculation of body mass index

$$BMI = \frac{(\text{weight in kg})}{(\text{height in metres})^2}$$

Table 14.7 The World Health Organization definition of obesity

Category	Body mass index
Normal	18.5–24.9
Overweight	25–29.9
Obese	
Class I	30.0–34.9
Class II	35.0–39.9
Class III	>40

high-density lipoprotein cholesterol, raised low-density lipoprotein cholesterol and triglycerides, hypertension, and decreased glucose tolerance known together as the metabolic syndrome.

Treatment

Several drug treatments are available with strict guidelines for use in obese patients. Orlistat inhibits lipase in the gastrointestinal tract and prevents absorption of 30% of dietary fat. Sibutramine is a selective serotonin and noradrenaline reuptake inhibitor. Both drugs cause sustained weight loss of 5–10% over 2 years.

The outcomes of bariatric surgery have improved steadily; the procedures work in one of two ways either by restricting the individual's ability to eat, e.g. gastric banding or interfering with the nutrient absorption, e.g. bypass surgery. Drawbacks to surgical therapy are lifelong rearrangement of the gastrointestinal tract, operative mortality (<0.5%) and morbidity (about 10%). None the less surgically induced weight loss is currently the most effective treatment for the severely obese patient.

Indications for drug or surgical treatment are:

◆ BMI >27.0 kg/m^2 and another significant disease (e.g. type 2 diabetes, high cholesterol)

◆ BMI >30.0 kg/m^2

Patients should also be offered advice, support, and counselling on diet, exercise, and behavioural changes.[45]

Employment issues

Obesity may affect the following factors relevant to the workplace:

◆ **Physical capability** in jobs requiring a high level of fitness, e.g. emergency services.

◆ **Mobility** in posts involving manual handling or entry to confined spaces

◆ The use of **personal protective equipment** and other equipment such as ladders.

◆ The risk of **heat stress** in individuals working at high temperatures.

◆ Concentration in safety critical work as a result of the increased risk of **sleep apnoea**.

BMI should be calculated for applicants where obesity could present an increased risk or specific work problems. Those with obesity may need to have further assessment including that of mobility. Functional assessments in the workplace may need to be undertaken to confirm fitness.

Prevention and treatment of obesity in the workplace

Occupational health units are likely to become increasingly involved in the prevention and treatment of obesity in the workplace. Two systematic reviews examined the use of workplace health promotion programmes and found evidence to support this as an effective intervention for overweight and obese adults.[45] As little as a 10 kg weight loss can have a significant benefit on blood pressure, serum lipids, glucose control in diabetics and mortality. Factors that appeared to be beneficial included dieting, supervision of exercise and personal counselling.

Nutrition

There has been a rapid growth in home enteral tube feeding, with over 20 000 adults and children on home enteral tube feeding and a growth of 16% per year. There is a peak in the 70–80-year age group. The commonest indication is cerebrovascular disease. Other indications include neurological disease, such as motor neurone disease, and cancers. Enteral nutrition is usually administered in the short term via a nasogastric tube, and longer term (more than 4 weeks) via a percutaneous gastrotomy tube. This may be placed endoscopically or radiologically. In the 16–64-year age group 25% of patients are capable of full normal activity, although the proportion of these in regular employment is not known. The feed often has to be given over a longer period and this and the underlying nature of the disease may have an impact on employment. The prognosis depends on the underlying disease but, almost inevitably, any patient on enteral tube feeding will be disabled within the definition of the DDA, therefore requiring reasonable adjustment in the workplace.

In 1998 there were 360 patients on home parenteral nutrition, increasing by <5% per year. Home parenteral nutrition peaks in the first decade and there is a second larger peak in the fourth decade mainly due to Crohn's disease. Other indications for parenteral nutrition are motility disorders, vascular disease and radiation enteritis. The mortality at 1 year is 4%, 11% return to oral feeding, and 82% remain on parenteral nutrition.[46] Some patients are able to live at home, maintain employment, and continue with most daily activities. The feed is usually administered overnight. Adjustments may need to be made during hot weather or to counteract excess fluid and electrolyte losses due to other causes. The complications (predominantly line sepsis) can result in frequent hospitalizations and may be life-threatening. Extensive training of the patient and caregivers and monitoring by a multidisciplinary team of professionals is essential.

Summary

Diseases of the gastrointestinal tract and liver rarely have safety implications in the workplace with the exception of blood-borne viruses in healthcare workers and gastrointestinal infections in food handlers. There is clear guidance about how these situations should be managed.

The main impact of gastrointestinal and liver disease on work relates to attendance as there is often a relapsing and remitting pattern. Despite this many individuals with these conditions achieve good control of symptoms and are able to work reliably. Inflammatory bowel conditions causing frequency and urgency of defecation may require adjustments under the DDA.

Advances in investigation and modern drug therapy have significantly improved the prognosis of some conditions such as peptic ulcer disease in recent years, so this condition is less likely to cause problems in the workplace.

The possible links with work-related stress in peptic ulcer disease, inflammatory bowel disease and functional intestinal disorders continue to be acknowledged although the mechanisms are poorly understood. Individuals with these problems should receive optimum therapy for their condition and the sources of work stress should be resolved through a risk assessment process.

Individuals with severe or chronic disease, resistant to current treatment, those experiencing significant constitutional upset and disabling side-effects from drug therapy will require a detailed occupational health assessment on a case by case basis to determine the prognosis and fitness to work.

Obesity is likely to be an increasing problem in the workforce particularly in occupations requiring high levels of physical fitness.

References

1 Jankowski J, Sharma P. Review article: approaches to Barrett's oesophagus treatment—the role of proton pump inhibitors and other interventions. *Aliment Pharmacol Ther* 2004; **19** (Suppl. 1): 54–9.

2 van Pinxteren B *et al*. Short-term treatment with proton pump inhibitors, H2-receptor antagonists and prokinetics for gastro-oesophageal reflux disease-like symptoms and endoscopy negative reflux disease. (Cochrane review). In *The Cochrane Library,* Issue 3(4)CD002095. Chichester: John Wiley & Sons, Ltd, 2004. Cochrane Database Syst. Rev.

3 NICE Guidelines. CG17 *Dyspepsia: managing dyspepsia in adults in primary care*, 2004.

4 Watson DI. Laparoscopic treatment of gastro-oesphageal reflux disease. *Best Pract Res Clin Gastroenterol* 2004; **18**: 19–35.

5 Nicholson PJ, D'Auria DAP (1999). Shift work, health, the working time regulations and health assessments. *Occup Med* 1999; **49**, (3) 127–137.

6 Ciclitira P. Guidelines for the management of patients with coeliac disease. *Clinical Practice Guidelines* BSG 2002 April, 2002.

7 Tinto A *et al*. Acute and chronic pancreatitis—diseases on the rise: a study of hospital admissions in England 1989/90–1999/2000. *Aliment Pharmacol Ther* 2002; **16**(12): 2097–2105.

8 Card T, Hubbard R, Logan RF. Mortality in inflammatory bowel disease: a population-based cohort study. *Gastroenterology* 2003; **125**(6): 1583–90.

9 Winther KV *et al*. Survival and cause specific mortality in ulcerative colitis: follow-up of a population based cohort in Copenhagen County. *Gastroenterology* 2003; **125**(6): 1576–82.

10 Bodger K. Cost of illness of Crohn's disease. *Pharmacoeconomics* 2002; **20**(10): 639–52.

11 Bernstein CN, Kraut A, Blanchard JF *et al*. The relationship between inflammatory bowel disease and socio-economic variables. *Am J Gastroenterol* 2001; **96**: 2117–25.

12 de Rooy EC, Toner BB, Maunder RG *et al*. Concerns of patients with inflammatory bowel disease: results from a clinical population. *Am J Gastroenterol* 2001; **96**: 1816–21.

13 Wyke RJ *et al*. Employment prospects for patients with intestinal stomas: the attitude of occupational physicians. *J Soc Occup Med* 1989; **39**: 19–24.

14 Khanna N *et al*. Gastroenteritis outbreak with norovirus in a Swiss university hospital with a newly identified virus strain. *J Hosp Infect* 2003; **55**(2): 131–6.

15 Widdowson MA *et al*. Outbreaks of acute gastroenteritis on cruise ships and on land: identification of a predominant circulating strain of norovirus—United States. *J Infect Dis* 2004; **190**: 27–36.

16 Lopman B *et al*. Increase in viral gastroenteritis outbreaks in Europe and epidemic spread of new norovirus variant. *Lancet* 2004; **363**: 682–8.

17 Daniels NA *et al*. A foodborne outbreak of gastroenteritis associated with Norwalk-like viruses: first molecular traceback to deli sandwiches contaminated during preparation. *J Infect Dis* 2000; **181**(4): 1467–70.

18 Butzler JP. Campylobacter, from obscurity to celebrity. *Clin Microbiol Infect* 2004; **10**(10): 868–76.

19 Allos BM. Campylobactyer jejuni infections: update on emerging issues and trends. *Clin Infect Dis* 2001; **32**(8): 1201–6.

20 Tam CC, Rodrigues LC, O'Brien SJ. Guillain-Barre syndrome associated with Campylobacter jejuni infection in England, 2000–2001. *Clin Infect Dis* 2003; **37**(2): 307–10.

21 Department of Health. *Food handlers' fitness to work. Guidance for food businesses, enforcement officers and health professionals*. London: Department of Health, 1995.

22 Smith T A *et al.* Code of practice for food handler activities. *Occup Med* 2005; **55**: 369–70.

23 Crowcroft NS *et al.* PHLS Advisory Committee on vaccination and Immunization. Guidelines for the control of hepatitis A virus infection. *Commun Dis Public Health* 2001; **4**(3): 213–27.

24 Department of Health. *Immunisation against infectious diseases.* London: Stationery Office, 1996. www.dh.gov.uk/green book/index.htm.

25 MacKenzie AR *et al.* Increasing incidence of acute hepatitis B virus infection referrals to the Aberdeen Infection Unit: a matter for concern. *Scott Med J* 2003; **48**(3): 73–5.

26 Hahne S *et al.* Incidence and routes of transmission of hepatitis B virus in England and Wales, 1995–2000: implications for immunisation policy. *J Clin Virol.* 2004; **29**(4): 211–20.

27 Aggarwal R, Ranjan P. Preventing and treating hepatitis B infection. *BMJ* 2004; **329**: 1080–86.

28 European Consensus Group on Hepatitis B Immunity (2000). Are booster immunizations needed for lifelong hepatitis B immunity? *Lancet* 2000; **355**: 561–5.

29 Health Service Guidelines HSG (93)40. *Protecting health care workers and patients from hepatitis B.* Department of Health 18 August 1993 and addendum EL (96) 77 (26 September 1996).

30 Health Service Circular HSC 2000/020. *Hepatitis B infected health care workers.* Department of Health (23 June 2000).

31 Department of Health. *Health clearance for serious communicable diseases: New health care workers.* Draft Guidance January 2003.

32 Department of Health. *Hepatitis B infected health care workers and oral antiviral therapy: consultation paper on implementing expert advice about a limited relaxation of restrictions on hepatitis B infected health care workers.* London: Stationery Office, 2004.

33 Hutchinson SJ *et al.* Hepatitis C virus among childbearing women in Scotland, prevalence, deprivation, and diagnosis. *Gut* 2004; **53**(4): 593–8.

34 Manns MP *et al.* Peginterferon alfa-2b plus ribavirin compared with interferon alfa-2b plus ribavirin for initial treatment of chronic hepatitis C: a randomized trial. *Lancet* 2001; **358**: 958–65.

35 Fried MW *et al.* Peginterferon alfa-2a plus ribavirin for chronic hepatitis C virus infection. *N Engl J Med* 2002; **347**: 975–82.

36 Pearlman BL. Hepatitis C treatment update. *Am J Med* 2004; **117**: 344–52.

37 Department of Health, Chief Medical Officer Update. *Hepatitis C testing quick reference summary* (August 2004).

38 Thorburn D *et al.* Risk of hepatitis C virus transmission from patients to surgeons: model based on an unlinked anonymous study of hepatitis C virus prevalence in hospital patients in Glasgow. *Gut* 2003; **52**(9): 1333–8.

39 Health Service Circular, HSC 2002/101. *Hepatitis C infected health care workers* (14 August 2002).

40 Fisher *et al.* Mortality from liver disease in the West Midlands, 1993–2000: observational study. *BMJ* 2002; **325**, 312–13.

41 Prince MI, Chetwynd A, Craig WL *et al.* Asymptomatic primary biliary cirrhosis: clinical features, prognosis, and symptom progression in a large population based cohort. *Gut* 2004; **53**(6): 865–70.

42 The Steering Group of the UK Liver Transplant Audit. The National Liver Transplantation Audit: an overview of patients presenting for liver transplantation from 1994 to 1998. *Br J Surg* 2001; **88**: 52–8.

43 Joint Health Service Unit on behalf of the Department of Health. *Health Survey for England 2001.* London: Stationery Office, 2002.

44 National Audit Office. *Tackling obesity in England.* Report by the Comptroller and Auditor General. London: Stationery Office, 2001.

45 Mulvihill C, Quigley R. *The management of obesity and overweight, an analysis of diet, physical activity and behavioural approaches.* London: Health Development Agency, 2003.

46 Elia M (ed.) *Trends in artificial nutrition support in the UK during 1996–2000*. A report by the British Artificial Nutrition Survey—a Committee of the British Association for Parenteral and Enteral Nutrition. Berkshire: BAPAN, 2001.

Further reading

Bloom S (ed.) *Practical gastroenterology*. London: Martin Dunitz, 2002.

Cook GC (ed.) *Gastroenterological problems from the tropics*. London: BMJ Publishing Group, 1995.

Greig E, Rampton D (ed.) *Management of Crohn's disease*. London: Martin Dunitz, 2003.

Tytgat GNJ (ed.) Functional gastrointestinal disorders. *Best Pract Res Clin Gastroenterol* 2004; **18**: 4.

Chapter 15

Diabetes mellitus and other endocrine disorders

E. R. Waclawski and G. V. Gill

Diabetes

Classification

There are two major subgroups of diabetes:

1. **Type 1 diabetes** (formerly insulin-dependent diabetes or IDDM). This is due to absolute insulin deficiency following autoimmune destruction of pancreatic beta cells. Though it can occur at any age, the vast majority of cases are under 30 years of age at diagnosis, and most are in their teens or twenties. Insulin is required from diagnosis for life.

2. **Type 2 diabetes** (formerly non-insulin-dependent diabetes or NIDDM). Peripheral resistance to the action of insulin is common in this syndrome, though there may be partial insulin deficiency also. The majority of patients are obese and over 30 years of age, though Type 2 diabetes is being seen now at younger ages. Type 2 diabetes makes up about 80% of the total diabetic population, and is particularly common in certain groups such as the elderly and Asian immigrants. Though there is a genetic component, Type 2 diabetes is very much a 'lifestyle disease'.

As mentioned above, all Type 1 diabetes is treated with insulin. Type 2 diabetes is treated with diet and exercise initially, usually followed by oral agents. Many patients, however, progress to needing insulin treatment. As the use of insulin can be associated with hypoglycaemia, from the viewpoint of driving and potentially hazardous occupations, a useful subdivision of diabetic patients is into those who are 'insulin-treated' (i.e. all Type 1 and some Type 2 patients), and those who are 'non-insulin treated' (all Type 2 patients).

Recent advances in diabetes

The last 5 years has seen significant changes in the practice of clinical diabetology, and the available drugs and insulin preparations in common use. These changes have affected both Type 1 and Type 2 diabetic patients. The major new treatments and innovations are described below.

Thiazolidinediones

Traditional drug treatment of Type 2 diabetes is with sulphonylureas and metformin. However, in the last 5 years a new class of oral hypoglycaemic agents has become available. These are the thiazolidinediones, or as they are more commonly known, the 'glitazones' (the two currently available are pioglitazone and rosiglitazone). These operate by increasing the sensitivity of the insulin receptor, which is of course an ideal mode of action as insulin resistance is the hallmark of Type 2 diabetes.[1] They can be used alone, or in combination with metformin or sulphonylureas. At the time of writing, in the UK they are not licensed for 'triple therapy' (with both sulphonylureas and metformin), though this seems safe and effective, or with insulin. The glitazone drugs have a potency similar to mid-range doses of sulphonylureas or metformin, and are generally well tolerated. They can sometimes cause fluid retention or mild anaemia, and should not be used when there is liver dysfunction.

Insulin secretagogues

These are also known as meglitinides, and in the UK the available preparations are repaglinide and nateglinide.[2] They act similarly, but not identically, to traditional sulphonylureas. Insulin secretion from the pancreatic beta cell is stimulated by closing potassium channels. This leads to a more physiological pattern of insulin release, in particular preserving 'first-phase' or early insulin release. They can be used alone or in combination with other oral agents. Like traditional sulphonylureas, they can occasionally cause hypoglycaemia as a side-effect, and they also have to be taken in multiple daily doses with meals. As there is no convincing evidence of long-term superiority over traditional sulphonylureas, they are not as yet widely used.

Insulin analogues

Insulin analogues—sometimes known as 'designer insulins'—belong to no species; their amino acid chains have been subtly altered from the human insulin molecule, leading to significant changes in absorption characteristics.[3] Two short-acting insulin analogues are available—Lispro and Aspart. These have absorption characteristics closer to physiological insulin secretion, and their use may be associated with lower postprandial peaks of blood glucose, and a reduced risk of pre-meal hypoglycaemia. There are also two long-acting analogues—Glargine and Detemir.[4] These are once daily insulins with a relatively smooth 24-hour absorption profile, which reduce hypoglycaemic risks, particularly nocturnally. Long-term experience with analogue insulins is lacking, and improvements in overall glycaemic control (as measured by HbA1c) rarely occur. Reductions in hypoglycaemia however are a definite benefit from these insulins, and so they clearly have relevance to safety at work for insulin-treated diabetic subjects.

Insulin delivery

Continuous subcutaneous insulin infusion (CSCII) is a technique that dates back to the late 1970s, but has undergone a resurgence of interest in the last few years. Though modern devices are small, they are unacceptable to some patients, and costs are high. However, CSCII—when used in enthusiastic and motivated patients, can improve HbA1c levels, often with reduced hypoglycaemic events.[5] Good patient selection is vital. A completely new method of insulin delivery will shortly become available—inhaled insulin.[6] This is obviously attractive as it avoids injections, although for most Type 1 diabetic patients using modern syringes or pens this is not a major issue. The delivery device is also rather cumbersome. It may be that inhaled insulin will have a more useful place in Type 2 diabetes that is inadequately controlled despite maximum doses of oral agents. Such patients are generally more reluctant to start insulin injection treatment, and may find inhaled insulin a more attractive option.

Pancreas transplantation

Segmental pancreas transplantation for Type 1 diabetes is a well-established technique. However, it is technically more difficult than many other transplant procedures. In the past it was performed typically at the same time as a renal transplant.[7] 'Solo' pancreas transplants are, however, increasingly being performed in selected patients. The simpler and more attractive procedure of islet cell transplantation is gradually increasing.[8] Immunosuppression is still needed, however, and the number of islets transplanted to achieve a successful graft is large—often in excess of the equivalent of two donor pancreas glands. Nevertheless, these exciting advances are leading to some patients with effectively 'cured' diabetes.

Diabetes and employment

Individuals with diabetes can still encounter largely unjustifiable difficulties in finding and keeping work because of their condition. However there is now evidence that having diabetes does not decrease the chance of entry into the labour market and does not result in higher unemployment in young people with Type 1 diabetes.[9,10]

The previously identified under-representation of diabetes in the workforce[11] may indicate prejudice against their employment, or a failure always to declare their diabetes to their employer or occupational health service. The risk of hypoglycaemia and visual impairment may legitimately debar those with poorly controlled Type 1 diabetes from jobs where safety is an important factor, but people with diabetes are not invalids and most can work normally and should not be discriminated against in job selection. Severe late complications can lead to lower employment rates, even in young people with diabetes, and lead to reduced income.[12,13] Diabetes UK provides useful information on the employment implications of diabetes in a wide range of occupations.[14,15] Such information helps employers to familiarize themselves with the condition and to recognize that the work record of those with diabetes is good and that they make perfectly satisfactory employees.

Diabetes is normally treated by dietary advice and insulin for Type 1 diabetes and dietary advice with or without the addition of oral hypoglycaemic agents or insulin for Type 2 diabetes. The Disability Discrimination Act provides that where an impairment is being treated or corrected the impairment is to be treated as having the effect it would have without the measures in question. This applies even if treatment results in the effects of disease being completely controlled and masked. In addition the Act provides for a person with a progressive condition to be regarded as having an impairment which has a substantial adverse effect on their ability to carry out normal day-to-day activities before it actually does so. Where a person has a progressive condition, they will be treated as having an impairment that has a *substantial* adverse effect from the moment any impairment resulting from that condition first has some effect on ability to carry out normal day-to-day activities. The effect need not be continuous and need not be substantial.

Within the meaning of the Disability Discrimination Act Type 1 diabetes must be regarded as a disability. Type 2 may be different, as people with this type of diabetes may be asymptomatic and have no complications. Where complications such as retinopathy exist, and such complications can be found at initial presentation in some cases, they will be covered by the Act as they indicate evidence of a progressive condition. (See also Chapter 3.)

Prevalence, morbidity, and mortality

Epidemiology of diabetes

Type 1 diabetes has a current UK incidence rate of about 20 per 100 000 head of population per year.[16] Rates vary greatly geographically (being higher in northern countries, e.g. Finland, Scotland), and the incidence appears to be increasing, particularly in young children.[17] Type 2 diabetes makes up about 80% of the total diabetic population. Its prevalence is rapidly increasing worldwide, due to factors such as obesity and migration with the adoption of Western habits. In the UK, current prevalence rates are in the order of 3% or more, with higher rates in areas with large ethnic communities or elderly populations.[18]

Morbidity and mortality of diabetes

Diabetes is said to be the commonest cause of blindness in the working age-group. Coronary heart disease is increased by a factor of two to three. Diabetes is the second leading cause of fatal kidney disease and a diabetic patient is many times more likely to need an amputation.[19] It should be emphasized, however, that only a minority of people with diabetes develop disabling complications.

Recent studies of sickness absence and diabetes indicate that rates are higher than in the non-diabetic population.[20–25] Prolonged absence however, is mainly associated with a minority of diabetic employees who have complications of the disease. Life expectancy is reduced in all age groups, mainly as a result of renal failure and vascular disease. There is great variation, however, and many diabetic people live for 40 years or more after the onset of the disease without developing serious complications. Though there is evidence that the outlook has improved, those people with complications of diabetes experience a loss of earnings.[13,26,27] Therefore prevention of complications and their early detection and management by regular screening is important clinically and economically for people with diabetes. Traditional mortality figures are often based on actuarial studies, which are now very dated.

The prevalence of diabetes and its complications as a cause of ill-health retiral is still greater than would be expected, indicating that the increased morbidity is still present in the working population. Improved methods of control of diabetes and more effective treatment for end-stage renal failure have improved the prognosis.

Clinical aspects affecting work capacity

Management of Type 1 diabetes

There are a large number of insulin regimens. Once daily systems should no longer be prescribed. Twice daily regimens are common (usually with 30%:70% mixtures of short and intermediate-acting insulins). These can be given by conventional syringe or by injector pen. For those with a variable life-style, multiple injection treatment (MIT)—as above—with a pen injector is often acceptable and effective. Flexible regimens with MIT and pen injectors are now used quite commonly, and allow for greater variation in times of meals, and a better quality of life. Such systems can also facilitate shift work, particularly if the person is educated to vary insulin doses and diet according to the varying work patterns.[28] Continuous subcutaneous insulin infusion (CSII) and pancreatic transplants are less common.

The major guideline for insulin treatment is that any method that works should be continued; there is no merit in making changes for their own sake. The objectives are always that the patient should feel well, hypoglycaemia should be uncommon, mild and preceded by warning, and blood glucose control should be acceptable—in that order.

Insulin was originally extracted from animal pancreas, at first cattle, later pigs. In the last 10–20 years it has been made by genetic engineering and most insulin made this way is now identical to the human insulin molecule, and is termed 'human insulin'. There are minor chemical differences between the different species of insulin. Their actions, however, are essentially the same. Bovine insulin (now little used) is slightly less potent than porcine and human insulin and the latter are of similar potency. Claims that human insulin may be particularly associated with hypoglycaemia and/or hypoglycaemia unawareness have not been substantiated. Nevertheless, most diabetologists believe that if patients prefer a particular insulin species, then they should be allowed to exercise a choice.

New recombinant human insulin analogues: The short-acting insulins Lispro and Aspart have more rapid 'physiological' absorption than standard short-acting insulins. Their use is not usually associated with improved HbA1c levels, but can improve postprandial glucose control and reduce hypoglycaemia. They can also be given with meals, rather than the traditional 20–30 minutes before (but the value of this practice is doubtful).[29] The long-acting analogues Glargine and Detemir have a relatively smooth 24-hour absorption profile (unlike existing traditional insulins) and can be given at any time of day (provided that the timing is regular). These are promising insulins, as standard intermediate-acting insulins have enormously variable absorption profiles. The use of long-acting insulin analogues sometimes—but by no mean always–reduces HbA1c levels, and they can reduce hypoglycaemia, particularly at night.[30] The association of analogue insulin use with reduced hypoglycaemic risks has obvious implications for increased safety at work.

It is hardly ever possible to achieve consistently normal blood glucose levels in Type 1 diabetes throughout the 24-hour period, and intensive attempts to do so may lead to frequent hypoglycaemia.[31] People with diabetes should maintain a blood-glucose concentration of between 4 and 10 mmol/litre for most of the time. There is nearly always variation in glycaemia due to differences in food intake and exercise levels, and the inherent imperfections of current insulin treatment and delivery systems. Self-treating of blood glucose is an important advance, but it can have the drawback of undermining confidence and producing worry unless it is seen in context, and is combined with an appropriate education programme.

Management of Type 2 diabetes

Type 2 diabetes is managed with diet alone, diet and oral hypoglycaemic agents (OHAs), or diet and insulin. Patients are frequently obese and the main objective of dietary control is to reduce body weight, principally by controlling fat intake. Excessive intake of refined carbohydrates is not advisable. High fibre intake seems to be beneficial for all types of diabetes, as fibre delays carbohydrate absorption and reduces blood glucose excursions.

Oral hypoglycaemic drugs are of five types:

1. **Biguanides** (e.g. metformin). Biguanides act by reducing glucose release from the liver, and enhancing glucose uptake by the tissues. Metformin is the only member of this class of drugs available in most countries (including the UK). Metformin is of moderate potency, does not cause hypoglycaemia, but is prone to be associated with gastrointestinal upsets (notably diarrhoea). The well-known side-effect of lactic acidosis is in fact very rare, especially if the drug is not given to patients with renal dysfunction. Metformin also tends to cause slight weight loss and is indicated mainly for obese Type 2 diabetes.

2. **Sulphonylureas** (e.g. glibenclamide, gliclazide, chlorpropamide, tolbutamide, and glipizide). The sulphonylureas act mainly by stimulating pancreatic insulin release. They can cause hypoglycaemia, especially after unaccustomed exercise, high alcohol consumption, and/or inadequate food intake. This is less common with shorter-acting sulphonylureas, such as tolbutamide, or gliclazide; but is more common with glibenclamide and chlorpropamide.[32] Sulphonylureas may also be associated with weight gain. This class of drugs is predominantly indicated for normal weight Type 2 diabetic patients.

3. **Glucosidase inhibitors**. The only drug currently available in this group is acarbose. This drug partially inhibits the enzymes that control carbohydrate absorption from the gut. Acarbose is not associated with hypoglycaemia or weight gain, but diarrhoea and flatulence (due to undigested carbohydrate) are common side-effects that limit the drug's usefulness.

4. **Insulin secretagogues ('Meglitinides')**. These drugs have a rapid onset of action and short duration of activity, and should be administered shortly before each main meal. Repaglinide can be used as monotherapy for those who are not overweight or for those in whom metformin is contraindicated or not tolerated. Netaglinide is licensed in the UK only

for use with metformin. These drugs act similarly to sulphonylureas, and similarly can cause hypoglycaemia.

5. **Thiazolidinediones ('Glitazones').** These drugs reduce peripheral insulin resistance, leading to a reduction in blood glucose concentration. Pioglitazone and rosiglitazone are licensed for use in the UK. Glitazones can be used as monotherapy or in combination with either metformin or a sulphonylurea drug. The UK National Institute for Clinical Excellence (NICE) recommends that metformin and/or sulphonylureas should remain first-line therapy, with glitazones substituting for either drug if intolerance occurs (usually with metformin). 'Triple therapy' remains unlicensed in the UK, but not in many other countries. It is a safe and effective treatment strategy. Glitazones can cause fluid retention and weight gain. Liver function testing is required during the first year of treatment.

Modern concepts of control

The landmark DCCT and UKPDS trials showed that 'tight' control of diabetes can reduce the risk of long-term complications in both Type 1 and Type 2 diabetes, respectively.[33,34] Increasing emphasis is therefore placed on achieving not only clinical well-being but also optimal blood glucose levels. Ideally this should be indicated by glycosylated haemoglobin levels of <7% (which reflects control over the previous 4–6 weeks) though clinically this is hard to achieve in most cases. Self-monitoring of blood glucose is useful especially in younger insulin-treated patients. Self-monitoring gives information on low blood glucose levels, as well as high, and can thus give warning of impending hypoglycaemia. Blood glucose strips are now included in the drug tariff in the UK and are readily available. Careful regulation of insulin dosage together with blood glucose monitoring, reduces the risk of hypoglycaemia and enables individuals to cope more easily with variations in daily work patterns. Blood glucose testing is a vital part of management for insulin-treated patients who might otherwise experience difficulty in coping with certain types of employment (for example those involving shift work).

Cardiovascular risk reduction

It has been recognized for many years that cardiovascular disease (notably coronary heart disease) is the leading cause of death in diabetes, and that reduction of standard risk factors (such as smoking, hyperlipidaemia, and hypertension) is an important component of care for the diabetic patient. However, clear evidence-based targets have been lacking until the recent completion of several major adequately powered randomized controlled trials. Current advice can be summarized as follows.

Hypertension   The UK Prospective Diabetes Study (UKPDS)[35] hypertension wing compared strict and routine hypertensive control. Enormous benefits in morbidity and mortality were obtained by tight control–roughly equivalent to a blood pressure of less than 140/80 mmHg. No specific drug showed benefit, and this finding has been supported by other studies. An exception arises when renal complications are present (microalbuminuria or nephropathy), when angiotensin-converting enzyme (ACE) inhibitors or angiotensin II receptor blockers (ARBs) have definite benefit (whether or not hypertension is present). Even tighter blood pressure control should be aimed for—below 130/80 mmHg is a widely accepted figure. The UKPDS was entirely a Type 2 study, and clear targets for blood pressure control in Type 1 diabetes are lacking, but it seems reasonable to apply similar targets.

Lipids   The Joint Society Tables[36] have been widely used in the UK and are available as a computer package and also as colour risk charts. They are, however, based on outdated subgroup analysis from the Framingham Study. They undoubtedly underestimate the risk in diabetes, and in particular do not take into account the considerable independent added risk from microalbu-minuria. Two recent studies suggest that a 'statins for all' policy may be advisable. The HPS (Heart Protection Study)[37] and CARDS[38] (Collaborative Atorvastatin Diabetes Study) trials used simvastatin 40 mg daily and atorvastatin 10 mg daily respectively, in large randomized placebo-controlled trials. Major cardiovascular outcome benefits were observed, independent of the initial lipid levels. These studies involved predominantly Type 2 patients, but there was a Type 1 cohort in the HPS trial. Questions remain as to how best to manage raised triglycerides and/or low high-density lipoprotein in diabetic patients, but ongoing studies will help clarify these issues in the near future.

Other risk factors Smoking is a major coronary risk factor, with significantly additive effects in diabetic subjects. Unfortunately attempts at smoking cessation often fail. Support groups and nicotine replacement therapy are helpful, but relapses are common. Glycaemic control, though of undoubted benefit in preventing or retarding microvascular complications, remains of unproven benefit in improving macroangiopathy-related outcome. Tight glycaemic control (HbA_{1c} <7.0%) did, however, almost reach statistical significance in reducing large vessel disease outcome in the UKPDS, and it would seem reasonable to include optimized glycaemic control in the risk factor package (though without diverting attention from the huge proven benefits of blood pressure and lipid control).

Special work problems caused by diabetes

The work record of people with diabetes

In recent years there is more general awareness of employment issues in diabetes, in part associated with the requirements of the Disability Discrimination Act. The result has been wholly beneficial. Employers seem much less likely to operate overall bans for diabetic persons, while diabetic employees are better able to manage and less inclined to conceal their condition.

Occupations closed to those with insulin-treated diabetes are usually those in which hypoglycaemia could be highly dangerous, e.g. airline pilots and large goods vehicle drivers. The risk here comes not from the diabetes itself but from its treatment. It has traditionally been considered unwise for those taking insulin to work in potentially hazardous environments, e.g. with moving machinery, in foundries, on scaffolding, and fighting fires. But even here there is room for latitude. Much depends on the exact nature of the work, the adequacy of diabetic control (in particular the frequency and warnings of hypoglycaemia), and the good sense of the patient.

The situation with UK fire fighting is of particular interest. In common with other emergency and armed services, applicants with existing Type 1 diabetes are not accepted for employment. Those who develop diabetes that requires insulin while in service, however, are assessed on an individual basis. Criteria such as those mentioned above are used, and considered jointly by an occupational physician and a diabetologist. This situation seems sensible as it takes into account the great variability of control, education, and motivation among those with insulin-treated diabetes, as well as the potential for employment-related risk assessment. This approach may be applicable to other potentially dangerous occupations, and has led Diabetes UK to publish guidelines for such employment (see p 355).[39]

Restrictions on the employment of those with diabetes treated without insulin are much less stringent. Although hypoglycaemic episodes can occur with sulphonylurea tablets (and may be serious and prolonged[32]), they are less common. If the physician is satisfied with treatment over a period of time, and especially if the patient monitors his or her own blood glucose levels, the risk of hypoglycaemia is remote and will rarely be a bar to employment. There are exceptions, for example in air crew and train drivers. Treatment with metformin, acarbose, or glitazones does not carry hypoglycaemic risk (unless combined with insulin, sulphonylureas, or insulin secreta-gogues when they may potentiate the hypoglycaemic actions of these agents).

The suitability of a diabetic person for employment also depends on their general health. In the case of diabetes this means freedom from sight-threatening retinopathy, severe peripheral or autonomic neuropathy, advanced ischaemic heart disease, serious renal failure, or disabling cerebrovascular or peripheral vascular disease.

With the improved general knowledge of diabetes, and more positive attitudes to the disease (as well as its improved management in recent years), the work performance of most diabetic persons is very good and their rate of unemployment is no worse than for other people.[9,10] They are, however, likely to have about 1.5–2 times as much time off work, but in well-controlled cases the excess is small or nil.[20–25] This is especially true of those on diet and/or oral hypoglycaemic agents. Good medical treatment and good liaison between physician and occupational health staff are important in controlling diabetes and minimizing its effects. Treatment has improved greatly in recent times, and with better self-monitoring of blood glucose and newer types of insulin and treatment regimens, the trend is likely to continue.

Working patterns and diabetic treatment

There is, in general, no reason why a diabetic person on insulin should not undertake shift work, though diabetic workers do experience more problems with shift work than non-diabetic work-ers.[21] Most sensible and well-motivated diabetic shift workers can rapidly learn how to adjust their treatment, especially if they are measuring their own blood glucose levels and using multi-ple insulin injection techniques, particularly with long-acting insulin analogues such as Glargine or Detemir. Thus, shiftwork should not be an automatic bar. One recent development in shift patterns may complicate matters. This is the introduction of shorter shift cycles in which day, evening, and night shifts may follow each other at 2-day intervals. This may test the ingenuity of the most intelligent insulin-treated diabetic worker. Such problems can occur in different types and grades of employment, for example supervisors and managers may also be required to undertake such shiftwork or work irregular hours. The use of long-acting analogues can help, with short-acting insulin given with meals, whatever time that may be. People with Type 2 dia-betes can normally undertake shift work though it is generally less well tolerated in the older workforce where most of the cases of Type 2 diabetes will occur.

Complications of diabetes

There are two acute diabetic complications that can cause coma or clouded consciousness.

Diabetic ketoacidosis may occur if there is serious loss of control of diabetes, resulting in hyperglycaemia, dehydration, and acidosis due to the accumulation of ketones. Ketoacidosis occurs mostly in Type 1 diabetes. As onset is gradual ketoacidosis does not cause sudden collapse at work. It only rarely leads to significant sickness absence.

Hypoglycaemia can occur in either type of diabetes when treatment is with insulin, or more rarely, with sulphonylurea tablets. It may cause confusion and clouded or lost consciousness, and so is a much more serious problem from the work standpoint. The majority of insulin-treated diabetic persons receive ample warning of impending hypoglycaemia (e.g. sweating, nausea, palpitations, etc.), take preventive steps (i.e. take glucose) and experience neither loss of control nor unconsciousness. In some, however, hypoglycaemia can develop suddenly and without warning. This is why many employers have reservations about diabetic workers on insulin work-ing in potentially hazardous situations. The majority, however, rarely experience serious hypogly-caemia, and the risks have been exaggerated. None the less, safety is a factor that has to be considered by employers and occupational physicians when deciding on the placement of those with insulin-treated diabetes at work. It may be important for some to have regular breaks when they can carry out blood tests, consume snacks, or take insulin. A study of the impact of hypoglycaemia at work found that severe hypoglycaemia was uncommon. Serious morbidity, including accidents or injuries associated with hypoglycaemia at work, was very uncommon.[40] Improvements in treatment regimens and education may have reduced hypoglycaemic problems at work. Evidence suggests that when hypoglycaemia occurs, it is usually outside working hours.

Insulin regimens in Type 2 diabetes are important in relation to hypoglycaemia risk and work performance. Thus, a common initial regimen for Type 2 patients poorly controlled on maximal oral agents is to continue these tablets, and add night-time isophane insulin. This lowers the fasting blood glucose level, allowing oral agents to act more effectively. As isophane insulins generally act for only 10–12 hours, there is little if any effect on daytime hypoglycaemia risk. There is also evidence that hypoglycaemia in insulin-treated Type 2 patients is less frequent than in Type 1 diabetes,[41] though with regard to severe episodes there is conflicting evidence.[42]

As mentioned, sulphonylureas are much less likely to cause serious hypoglycaemia than insulin, and there are relatively few jobs barred to those on these drugs. The guiding principle must always be to assess the risk of hypoglycaemia, and whether or not its development might put the diabetic employee or others at risk. Unfortunately, many occupational guidelines do not recognize the different modes of action of oral hypoglycaemic agents, and 'tablets' are considered as having identical risk profiles. This is not the case, as metformin, acarbose, and glitazones do not have hypoglycaemic potential.

A relatively small proportion of people with diabetes develop significant long-term complications in employment, usually after many years of diabetes. From the work viewpoint the most important are retinopathy, which can lead to visual impairment and blindness; neuropathy, either sensory or autonomic (which may cause postural hypotension); nephropathy, which can lead to renal failure, and foot ulceration, which occasionally necessitates amputation. Furthermore, there is an increased risk of coronary artery disease, stroke, and peripheral vascular disease. Treatment of complications may occasionally give rise to fresh problems: for example, 'pan-retinal photocoagulation', sometimes used in the treatment of retinopathy, may cause significant diminution in peripheral visual fields. However, it must be emphasized that few working age persons with diabetes develop such severe and disabling complications. Those individuals who hold driving licences and develop significant complications should be advised to notify the licensing authorities; often they will still be able to continue driving.

Transplantation of the kidney can improve quality of life and, in combination with pancreatic transplantation, has been shown recently to increase the likelihood of being employed compared with kidney transplantation alone.[43]

Diabetes, pregnancy, and employment

Pregnancy and diabetes co-exist in three different contexts:

◆ pregnancy occurring in a woman with pre-existing Type 1 diabetes

◆ pregnancy occurring in a woman with pre-existing Type 2 diabetes

◆ gestational diabetes, i.e. diabetes occurring *de novo* in pregnancy.

With a markedly declining age of onset in many people with Type 2 diabetes, pregnancy in women with already diagnosed Type 2 disease is increasingly seen. Regardless of prior treatment, such patients will almost always be moved on to insulin during the pregnancy. Gestational diabetes is also frequently treated with insulin. 'Tight' glycaemic control is well known to improve the outcome of pregnancy in diabetes, whether diabetes is pre-existing or new in onset, and intensified four times daily regimens are often used (short-acting insulin with meals, and intermediate-acting insulin at night).[44]

Pregnant diabetic patients are generally young, with little or no complications and co-morbidity, and are intensively cared for by combined obstetric/diabetes teams. As such, patients generally remain well throughout pregnancy, and those who wish are usually able to carry on their employment. There are two provisos, however—hypoglycaemic risk and entitlement to drive. Intensive insulin therapy is often associated with an increase in hypoglycaemic episodes, and this may have employment implications, depending on the occupation. Such 'hypos', however, are usually mild (i.e. self-correctable). In a study of diabetic patients treated with either two or four daily insulin injections, there was no significant difference between those on two or four insulin injections daily and the occurrence of severe hypoglycaemia (needing third party assistance for correction).[44] The risk of significant hypoglycaemia is greatest in those with pre-existing Type 1 diabetes.

The second issue concerns driving. Those with pre-existing Type 2 diabetes, or gestational diabetes, are likely to begin insulin treatment during pregnancy, and may be able to discontinue it after delivery. Nevertheless, they must observe the driving regulations for insulin treatment in general. In the UK, they must inform the DVLA (Driver Vehicle Licensing Agency), and there will be checks of control (in particular hypoglycaemia occurrence), and restrictions on the type of vehicle that can be driven. This may occasionally affect employment involving driving as part of the work schedule.

Pension schemes

In the past difficulty in arranging associated life insurance has sometimes been given as a reason for not employing those with diabetes. The attitude of different insurance companies to diabetes has varied considerably.[45] Diabetes UK can give useful advice on insurance matters. Section 10 of the Code of Practice on Employment and Occupation indicates that an employer must not discriminate against a disabled person in the opportunities it affords him for receiving pension or insurance-related benefits, or by refusing him, or deliberately not affording him, any such opportunity. Pension scheme trustees and insurance providers also have responsibilities under the Disability Discrimination Act. These recent changes to the Disability Discrimination Act and accompanying code are important for those with diabetes and other disabilities.

Diabetes in employer-sponsored health insurance

Health care expenditure has been shown to be higher for those with diabetes than in all health care consumers. However, when compared with individuals with other chronic diseases (heart disease, HIV/AIDS, cancer, and asthma) people with diabetes were not more expensive for employers' insurance plans.[46]

Advisory services

The diabetic specialist, family practitioner, and occupational health services should be able to give advice in cases of employment difficulty. The diabetes specialist and/or family practitioner can provide detailed medical information, while the occupational physician is best placed to assess the suitability for a particular occupation. For especially difficult decisions, the combined opinions of specialists in diabetes and occupational medicine are particularly useful.

Disability Employment Advisers based at Department for Work and Pensions Job Centres can advise and help anyone with diabetes and disabilities affecting their work to find or keep suitable employment. Careers officers and teachers should also be able to advise diabetic school leavers. Diabetes UK is a comprehensive source of information.

Guidelines for employment

Diabetes UK and the American Diabetes Association publish guidance for employers and occupational health services[47] and the current situation can be summarized as follows:

1. **Diabetic persons treated with diet alone** should be able to undertake virtually any occupation, provided that they do not have significant disabling complications of the disease.

2. **Diabetic persons treated with diet and oral hypoglycaemic agents** can undertake most occupations, subject to being free from disabling complications. However, currently they are not recruited to the armed forces or emergency services (fire brigade, police force, and ambulance service). They are also not usually permitted to work in air traffic control, pilot transport aeroplanes, or work on off-shore oil platforms. The criteria relating to main line train driving have recently been relaxed. This occupation is now open to applicants and employees with diabetes receiving oral hypoglycaemic agents provided they are well controlled, under regular specialist supervision, monitor their blood glucose levels, do not suffer from any significant complications and do not experience hypoglycaemia. Vocational drivers with uncomplicated diabetes, which is well-controlled by diet alone or with oral agents are usually allowed to continue driving large goods and passenger carrying vehicles, subject to not suffering from any significant complications. Merchant Seafarers (see Appendix 2) and deep sea fishermen are allowed to remain at sea subject to regular medical reviews. As mentioned, almost all employment regulations for those with diabetes on oral agents do not differentiate between the type of drug used and therefore fail to differentiate between the risk of sulphonylurea-induced hypoglycaemia as compared with the safety of metformin and acarbose.

3. **Diabetic persons treated with insulin** should not work in situations where sudden attacks of hypoglycaemia are a significant risk, and a likely source of danger to themselves or others. For this reason they are usually not permitted to drive LGVs or PCVs, enter the armed and emergency services, fly aeroplanes, drive trains, or continue as seafarers or divers. It may be undesirable for them to work in some other severely hazardous surroundings. They may also be barred from certain occupations such as railway signal operators because of the possible risks to the safety of others.

Regulations do not differentiate between insulin treated Type 2 and Type 1 diabetes (hypogylcaemic risk is generally lower in the former). Also isophane insulin taken at night in Type 2 diabetes will not increase the risk of daytime hypoglycaemia.

Guidelines on recruiting insulin-treated diabetic applicants to occupations are usually fairly clear; but the situation is often unclear when someone already in employment develops insulin-requiring diabetes. The case with fire fighters has already been mentioned and the approach of individual assessment is increasingly being applied elsewhere (e.g. police, armed forces, etc.). However, though employment may be continued the nature of the job may alter; for example in the police force new diabetic personnel on insulin treatment may not necessarily lose their jobs but there will be restrictions (e.g. driving at high speed and membership of armed response units will not be allowed).

Finally, the Diabetes UK Working Party on Driving and Employment has produced guidelines for the employment of insulin-treated diabetic persons in potentially hazardous occupations. These suggest the factors to be considered when a policy of individual consideration is adopted, and they provide a sensible framework for the safe employment of insulin-treated diabetic persons.

Box 15.1 Diabetes and potentially hazardous occupations (after reference 39)

1. People should be physically and mentally fit in accordance with non-diabetic standards.
2. Diabetes should be under regular (at least annual) specialist review.
3. Diabetes should be under stable control.
4. People should self-monitor their blood glucose, and be well educated and motivated in diabetes self-care.
5. There should be no disabling hypoglycaemia and normal awareness of individual hypoglycaemic symptoms.
6. There should be no advanced retinopathy or nephropathy, nor severe symptomatic peripheral or autonomic nerve damage.
7. There should be no significant coronary heart disease, peripheral vascular disease, or cerebrovascular disease.
8. Suitability for employment should be re-assessed annually by both an occupational physician and a diabetes specialist; and should be based on the criteria outlined above.

Conclusions and recommendations

A few studies of employment and diabetes in the UK[21,23,24] indicate some increase in sickness absence. Recent research on the impact of hypoglycaemia at work indicated that severe hypoglycaemia was uncommon. Serious morbidity including accidents or injuries associated with hypoglycaemia at work was very uncommon. Information is still needed on the impact of particular work activities on diabetic control, especially shift work and vocational driving. Because of the paucity of definitive information, the advice given to diabetic workers is often arbitrary and employment decisions are taken with little supporting evidence. Physicians should take care to inform employers and potential employers factually about diabetes and to dispel any prejudice that might exist.

The introduction of **self-testing** and modern systems of treatment have enabled those with diabetes to cope more easily with irregular work patterns. Careers officers and teachers need to know more about diabetes, so that they can give school-leavers accurate advice and enable them to make sensible career plans. A sustained effort is required to educate employers and persuade them to take a more objective view of diabetic workers.

Significant changes have occurred in relation to pensions and group insurance services in the latest Employment and Occupation Code of Practice that are of benefit to those with diabetes and other disabilities.

It is essential that each individual case be assessed on its own merits with full consultation between all medical advisers. Diabetes *per se* should not limit employment prospects, for the majority with diabetes have few, if any, problems arising from the condition and make perfectly satisfactory employees in a wide variety of occupations.

Considerable improvements in the treatment of people with Type 1 and Type 2 diabetes have occurred in the past few years. These improvements are associated with better quality of life and reductions in the incidence of long-term complications. Over time these will lead to longer, healthier working lives for people with diabetes. There is also evidence that those with severe renal complications can benefit from advances in transplant surgery and have improved quality of life and ability to work. Finally, rapidly progressing transplant technology (notably islet cell transplants) may begin to deliver a true 'cure' for diabetes (at least Type 1) in the not too distant future.

Endocrine disorders

Thyroid disease

Thyroid over- or underactivity is fully treatable and should have little or no long-term employment effects.

Hypothyroidism

In adult life hypothyroidism (primary, or secondary to hypopituitarism) is usually insidious and can easily be missed. Increasingly with frequent 'routine' thyroid function testing, hypothyroidism is diagnosed early.

In untreated hypothyroidism, performance at work (and elsewhere) is likely to be affected. Poor memory and concentration and slowing of mental and physical activity are likely to lead to decline of efficiency both physically and mentally. Treatment with thyroxine is simple and effective and needs to be continued indefinitely. A patient with well-controlled hypothyroidism can lead a normal life in all respects.

Hyperthyroidism

Thyroid overactivity ('thyrotoxicosis') presents classically with agitation, tremor, sensitivity to heat, tachycardia, and loss of weight. The diagnosis is not usually difficult though it must be differentiated from acute and chronic anxiety states. In some cases, however, especially in older patients, thyrotoxicosis may present asymptomatically ('apathetic toxicosis'), non-specifically, or as sinus tachycardia or atrial fibrillation. If the diagnosis is still not made the patient may develop severe heart failure.

Treatment is effective with drugs, thyroidectomy, or radioiodine. There should be no long-term employment problems.

Pituitary disease

Growth hormone deficiency in childhood can be effectively treated with replacement therapy, which is now produced using recombinant DNA techniques (Somatropin). The academic achievements of individuals are no different from siblings or the general population.[48–51] However, their later employment prospects appear to be less favourable with some studies suggesting that fewer are in employment, have a lower professional scale than siblings and are also on lower income.[48,52] The reasons for this are unclear but it does not appear to be related to treatment. Adults with growth hormone deficiency have decreased psychological well-being and the numbers receiving a disablement pension tend to be higher than expected.[46] Pituitary hormonal disorders can result from pituitary adenomas. If very large and extending supratentorially, they can affect the visual fields (classically a bitemporal hemianopia), which may affect ability to drive or work near moving machinery for example. Formal perimetry can help to define the extent of the problem and whether it will result in a restriction from specific duties.

The long-term sequelae of treatment for paediatric craniopharyngioma has been shown to impact on employment. Conservative surgery and radiotherapy together resulted in a more consistent level of employment and tertiary education than other groups (conservative surgery, radical surgery, shunting).[53]

Hypoadrenalism

Underactivity of the adrenal glands (Addison's disease) may be due to primary adrenal disorders (usually autoimmune destruction), or to pituitary underfunction, leading to reduced adrenocorticotrophic hormone secretion. The result is reduced adrenal cortisol secretion leading to symptoms and clinical features such as postural dizziness, increased pigmentation, and even hypoglycaemia. Once diagnosed, however, treatment with hydrocortisone replacement is straightforward and there are no long-term health or employment implications.

Insulinoma

Finally, this rare but important endocrine syndrome should be mentioned. An insulinoma is a tumour of the pancreatic beta cells leading to autonomous insulin overproduction and consequent unpredictable hypoglycaemia. This has serious implications for employment as the patient is unable to prevent hypoglycaemic attacks. The condition is cured by removal of the tumour. However, in some cases tumour localization is difficult or the patient may be too frail for surgery. In these cases a combination of dietary advice and the drug diazoxide is used.

References

1 Yki-Jarvinen H. Thiazolidinediones. *N Engl J Med* 2004; **351**: 1106–18.

2 Dornhorst A. Insulinotropic meglitinide analogues. *Lancet* 2001; **358**: 1709–16.

3 Barnett AH, Owen DR. Insulin analogues. *Lancet* 1997; **349**: 47–51.

4 Younis N, Soran H, Bowen-Jones D. Insulin glargine: a new basal insulin analogue. *Q J Med* 2002; **95**: 757–61.

5 Pickup JC, Mattock M, Kerry S. Glycaemic control with continuous subcutaneous insulin infusion compared with intensive insulin injections in patients with type 1 diabetes: meta-analysis of randomised controlled trials. *BMJ* 2002; **324**: 705–8.

6 Amiel SA, Alberti KGMM. Inhaled insulin. *BMJ* 2004; **328**: 1215–16.

7 White SA, Nicholson ML, London NJM. Vascularised pancreas allotransplantation–clinical indications and outcome. *Diabetic Med* 1999; **16**: 533–43.

8 Robertson RP. Islet transplantation as a treatment for diabetes–a work in progress. *N Engl J Med* 2004; **350**: 694–705.

9 Ardran M, MacFarlane I, Robinson C. Educational achievements, employment and social class of insulin-dependent diabetics: a survey of a Young Adult Clinic in Liverpool. *Diabetic Med* 1987; **4**: 546–8.

10 Bergers J, Nijhuis F, Janssen M, van der Horst. Employment careers of young Type 1 diabetic patients in the Netherlands. *J Occup Environ Med* 1999; **41**(11): 1005–10.

11 Waclawski ER. Employment and diabetes: a survey of the prevalence of diabetic workers known by occupational physicians, and the restrictions placed on diabetic workers in employment. *Diabetic Med* 1989; **6**: 16–19.

12 Ingberg CM, Palmer M, Aman J, Larsson S. Social consequences of insulin-dependent diabetes mellitus are limited: a population-based comparison of young adult patients vs healthy controls. *Diabetic Med* 1996; **13**(8): 729–33.

13 Kraut A, Walld R, Tate R, Mustard C. Impact of diabetes on employment and income in Manitoba, Canada. *Diabetes Care* 2001; **24**: 640–8.

14 *Diabetes employment handbook*. London: Diabetes UK, 1997.

15 *Diabetes and employment*. London: Diabetes UK, 1997.

16 Karvonen M, Tuomilehto J, Libman I, LaPorte R. A review of the recent epidemiological data on the worldwide incidence of Type 1 (insulin-dependent) diabetes mellitus. *Diabetologia* 1993; **36**: 883–92.

17 Metcalfe MA, Baum JD. Incidence of insulin-dependent diabetes in children under 15 years of age in the British Isles during 1988. *BMJ* 1991; **302**: 443–7.

18 Zimmet P, McCarthy D. The NIDDM epidemic: global estimates and projections—a look into the crystal ball. *IDF Bull* 1995; **40**: 8–16.

19 Morrish NJ, Stevens LK, Fuller JH, Keen H, Jarrett RJ. Incidence of macrovascular disease in diabetes mellitus: the London cohort of the WHO Multinational Study of Vascular Disease in Diabetics. *Diabetologia* 1991; **34**: 584–9.

20 Waclawski ER. Diabetes and Employment. MFOM Thesis, Faculty of Occupational Medicine, Royal College of Physicians, 1989.

21 Robinson N, Yateman NA, Protopapa LE, Bush L. Employment problems and diabetes. *Diabetic Med* 1990; **7**: 16–22.

22 Griffiths RD, Moses RG. Diabetes in the workplace. Employment experience of young people with diabetes mellitus. *Med J Aust* 1993; **158**: 169–71.

23 Poole CJ, Gibbons D, Calvert IA. Sickness absence in diabetic employees at a large engineering factory. *Occup Environ Med* 1994; **51**: 299–301.

24 Waclawski ER. Sickness absence among insulin-treated diabetic employees. *Diabetic Med* 1990; **7**: 41–4.

25 Skerjanc A. Sickness absence in diabetic employees. *Occup Environ Med* 2001; **58**(7): 432–6.

26 Sarter G, Nystrom L, Dahlquist G. The Swedish Childhood Diabetes Study: a seven-fold decrease in short-term mortality? *Diabetic Med* 1991; **8**: 18–21.

27 Holmes J, Gear E, Bottomley J, Gillan S, Murphy M, Williams R. Do people with type 2 diabetes and their carers lose income? (T2ARDIS-4). *Health Policy* 2003; **64**(3): 291–6.

28 Robinson N, Stevens LK, Protopapa LE. Education and employment for young people with diabetes. *Diabetic Med* 1993; **10**: 983–9.

29 Ahmed ABE, Badgandi M, Howe PD. Interval between insulin injection and meal in relation to glycated haemoglobin. *Pract Diab Int* 2001; **18**: 51–6.

30 Anonymous. Update on insulin analogues. *Drug Ther Bull* 2004; **42**: 77–80.

31 Egger M, Davey-Smith G, Stettler C, Diem P. Risk of adverse effects of intensified treatment of insulin-dependent diabetes mellitus: a meta-analysis. *Diabetic Med* 1997; **14**: 919–28.

32 Stahl M, Berger W. Higher incidence of severe hypoglycaemia leading to hospital admission in type 2 diabetic patients treated with long-acting versus short-acting sulphonylureas. *Diabetic Med* 1999; **16**: 586–90.

33 Diabetes Control and Complications Trial Research Group. The effect of intensive treatment of diabetes on the development and progression of long-term complications in insulin-dependent diabetes mellitus. *N Engl J Med* 1993; **329**: 977–86.

34 Stratton IM on behalf of the United Kingdom Prospective Diabetes Study Group. Association of glycaemia and macrovascular and microvascular complications of Type 2 diabetes—Prospective observational study. *BMJ* 1998; **321**: 405–12.

35 UK Prospective Diabetes Study Group (UKPDS). Tight blood pressure control and risk of macrovascular and microvascular complications in type 2 diabetes: UKPDS 38. *BMJ* 1998; **317**: 703–13.

36 Wood D, Durrington P, Poulter N, McInnes G, Rees A, Wray R. Joint British Recommendations on prevention of coronary heart disease in clinical practice. *Heart* 1998; **80** (Suppl.2): S1–29.

37 Collins R, Armitage J, Parish S, Sleigh P, Peto R for the Heart Protection Study Collaborative Group. MRC/BHF Heart Protection Study of cholesterol-lowering with simvastatin in 5963 people with diabetes: a randomised placebo-controlled trial. *Lancet* 2003; **361**: 2005–16.

38 Colhoun HM, Betteridge DJ, Durrington PN *et al* on behalf of the CARDS investigators. Primary prevention of cardiovascular disease with atorvastatin in type 2 diabetes in the Collaborative Atorvastatin Diabetes Study (CARDS): multicentre randomised placebo-controlled trial. *Lancet* 2004; **364**: 685–96.

39 *Diabetes and potentially hazardous occupations.* London: Diabetes UK, 1996.

40 Leckie AM, Graham MK, Grant JB, Ritchie PJ, Cowie HA, Frier BM. Frequency, severity, and morbidity of hypoglycaemia occurring at work in people with insulin-treated diabetes. *Diabetologia* 2001; **44**(Suppl. 1): A66.

41 Henderson JN, Allen KV, Deary IJ, Frier BM. Hypoglycaemia in insulin-treated type 2 diabetes: frequency, symptoms and impaired awareness. *Diabetic Med* 2003; **20**: 1016–21.

42 Leese GP, Morrison W, Wang J *et al.* Frequency of severe hypoglycaemia requiring emergency treatment in type 1 and type 2 diabetes. *Diabetes Care* 2003; **26**: 1176–80.

43 Knight RJ, Daly L. The impact of pancreas transplantation on patient employment opportunities. *Clin Transplant* 2004; **18**: 49–52.

44 Nachum Z, Ben-Shlomo I, Weiner E, Shalev E. Twice daily versus four times daily insulin dose regimens for diabetes in pregnancy: randomised controlled trial. *BMJ* 1999; **319**: 1223–7.

45 Jones KE, Gill GV. Insurance company attitudes to diabetes. *Pract Diabetes* 1989; **6**: 230–1.

46 Peele PB, Lave JR, Songer TJ. Diabetes in employer-sponsored health insurance. *Diabetes Care* 2002; **25**(11): 1964–8.

47 American Diabetes Association. Hypoglycaemia and employment/licensure. *Diabetes Care* 2004; **27** (Suppl. 1): S134.

48 Dean HJ, McTaggart TL, Fish DG, Friesen HG. The educational, vocational and marital status of growth hormone deficient adults treated with growth hormone during childhood. *Am J Dis Child* 1985; **139**: 1105–10.

49 Mitchell CM, Joyce S, Johanson AJ, Libber S, Plotnick L, Migeon CJ, Blizzard RM. A retrospective evaluation of psychological impact of long-term growth hormone therapy. *Clin Pediatr* 1986; **25**: 17–23.

50 Dutch Growth Hormone Working Group. Rikken B, van Busschbach J, le Cessie S, Manten W, Sperman TR, Grobbee R, Wit JM. Impaired social status of growth hormone deficient adults as compared to controls with short or normal stature. *Clin Endocrinol* 1995; **43**: 205–11.

51 Rosen T, Wiren L, Wihelmsen L, Wiklund I, Bengtsson BA. Decreased psychological well-being in adult patients with growth hormone deficiency. *Clin Endocrinol* 1994; **40**: 111–16.

52 Hakkart-van Roijen L, Beckers A, Stevenaert A, Rutten FF. The burden of illness of hypopituitary adults with growth hormone deficiency. *Pharmacoeconomics* 1998; **14**(4): 395–403.

53 Graham PH, Gattamaneni HR, Birch JM. Paediatric craniopharyngiomas: a regional review. *British Journal of Neurosurgery* 1992; **6**(3): 187–93.

Chapter 16

Haematological disorders

J. C. Smedley and R. S. Kaczmarski

Introduction

Few haematological disorders are caused or exacerbated by work. However, the most common haematological disorders may affect capacity to work. Mild haematological derangements (e.g. iron deficiency anaemia, anticoagulant treatment) are common, but have only minor implications for employment. Conversely, genetic and malignant haematological diseases, although comparatively uncommon, are complex and affect young people of working age. Malignant disease has a profound impact on work ability during the treatment and early recovery phases. However, with important recent advances in clinical management there is now much greater potential for return to work during treatment, and a growing population of survivors in whom it is important to address employment issues.

Evidence base

An exploration of the evidence for this chapter revealed little research upon which to base advice about fitness for work related to haematological disease. It is difficult to find prevalence rates for specific disorders in the working population, so the likelihood of an occupational physician encountering haematological disease in fitness for work assessments is based on occurrence in the general population. Searching of the Clinical Evidence and Cochrane databases using key words for haematological diseases identified randomized controlled trials for treatment regimens (mainly for leukaemia and lymphoma), but little information about functional rehabilitation. Therefore, this chapter relies primarily on traditional textbook teaching, and recent reviews of advances in clinical management.

Chapter structure

The major determinants of functional capacity are similar for many haematological conditions, their treatment and associated complications. In order to avoid repetition the common treatments, complications and symptoms are covered under 'Generic Issues' below. Where appropriate, the reader is referred to other chapters in this book.

Disease-specific summaries

This section provides a brief summary of the more common haematological disorders that an occupational physician might encounter when advising about fitness for work. It is not intended to be a comprehensive clinicopathological guide to each condition and further information can be found in the haematology reference texts cited at the end of the chapter.

Haemoglobinopathies

Sickle cell disease (SCD)

Epidemiology and clinical features SCD is a collection of inherited disorders that are characterized by the presence of abnormal haemoglobin (HbS). Homozygous sickle cell anaemia (HbSS) is the most common, but the doubly heterozygote conditions with haemoglobin C and beta thalassaemia respectively (HbSC and HbSβthal) also cause sickling disease. The disorders are common in West Africa, the Middle East, and parts of the Indian subcontinent, and have become established through migration in northern Europe and North America. It has been estimated that 12 000 people in the UK have SCD. Occupational physicians working in London, the West Midlands, and Yorkshire might expect to see a few cases annually. However, outside these areas the condition will be encountered less frequently. The main clinical features in SCD arise from the sickle-shaped deformation of red blood cells, due to crystallization of HbS at low oxygen concentrations. This leads to chronic anaemia through reduced red cell survival (typical haemoglobin levels 7–9 g/dl), and to episodes of vascular and microvascular obstruction. Patients develop both acute 'crises' (vaso-occlusive/painful, aplastic or haemolytic), which at their most severe can be life-threatening, and insidious multisystem damage from repeated infarction. Box 16.1 shows the wide range of end-organ effects.

Recent advances Modern management of SCD in developed countries has dramatically increased the life expectancy for patients (from 14 years in the early 1970s to 50 years in 2003). Consequently more SCD patients are likely to be working than in previous decades. Newer treatments include hydroxyurea, which increases the production of fetal haemoglobin (an inhibitor of the HbS polymerization). Patients are monitored regularly to detect end organ damage and facilitate early intervention. Transfusion therapy may be indicated where continuing organ damage is detected. Laser therapy reduces the complications of proliferative retinopathy. Joint replacement may be indicated for patients with severe joint disease. Allogeneic stem cell transplantation (SCT) is undertaken for the most severely affected individuals, although this is indicated mainly in children. SCT offers a definitive cure, but has long-term consequences as discussed below.

Functional limitations in sickle cell disease Fitness for work can vary markedly, and adjustments must be based on an individual functional assessment. The most severely affected patients are unlikely to be fit for work, but moderately and mildly affected individuals should have reasonable work capacity. The main functional issues are listed in Box 16.2. Anaemia is usually well tolerated by sickle cell patients and symptoms are less prominent at low haemoglobin levels

---

Box 16.1 Organs and systems affected by sickle cell disease

- Spleen (splenic infarcts leading to auto-splenectomy)
- Bones and joints (bone infarcts, avascular necrosis particularly of the hip and shoulders, osteomyelitis, and arthritis)
- Kidney (renal acidosis and glomerular sclerosis leading to renal failure)
- Brain and spinal cord (stroke and cognitive impairment)
- Eye (retinal infarcts and haemorrhages, retinal detachment, and central retinal artery occlusion)
- Lungs (acute lung syndrome, interstitial fibrosis, and pulmonary hypertension)
- Skin (leg ulcers)
- Gall bladder (pigment gall stones)
- Blood (anaemia)

Box 16.2 Potential functional and occupational restrictions in sickle cell disease

- Impaired exercise tolerance (anaemia, pulmonary hypertension)
- Reduced mobility (bone/joint disease, stroke)
- Impaired visual acuity (retinopathy)
- Decreased performance (cognitive impairment due to cerebrovascular events, depression, chronic pain)
- Susceptibility to infection (impaired white cell function, hyposplenism, post bone marrow transplant)
- Infectious carriage of blood-borne viruses
- Frequent absence from work (painful crises, complications of chronic organ failure)

(down to 7 g/dl) compared with other causes of anaemia. Poor performance at work might be due to a number of factors, including untreated depression or cerebral infarctions. Therefore, it is particularly important to make a careful assessment, liaising with the treating clinician to arrange cognitive screening, magnetic resonance imaging, and a therapeutic review where appropriate. The effects of chronic transfusion therapy are considered under Generic issues. Depression is common among patients with moderate to severe disease. Despite the need for opiate analgesia in severe painful crises, the incidence of drug dependence is very low.

Adjustments to work It is important to ensure a working environment without extremes of temperature, and employees must have access to drinking water to manage their hydration. If mobility or exercise tolerance is seriously impaired, care might be needed over improved access to work (ramps or lifts) and reducing physically demanding work. Adjustments for visually impaired employees are covered in Chapter 9. Particular care should be taken in jobs that expose the individual to risk of infection, to ensure that prophylactic antibiotics and pneumococcal vaccine are given. Travel requirements should be carefully considered, including access to medical care and safe blood for transfusion in the event of a sickle crisis abroad. Commercial air passenger travel is safe, but special care should be taken to ensure adequate hydration on long haul flights. Additional care is also necessary during pregnancy in employees with SCD. This group have a higher incidence of gestational hypertension, pre-term birth and small for gestational age infants. A lower threshold for recommending abstention from work during pregnancy should be adopted, but close liaison with the responsible clinicians is strongly recommended. Some occupations are contraindicated for individuals with HbSS. Jobs that are physically demanding, or which have a risk of exposure to severe extremes of heat, cold, dehydration or hypoxia (e.g. foundry work, diving, compressed air work, armed forces) are unsuitable. Joint Aviation Authority standards on fitness for work exclude individuals with SCD from certification as flight crew on civil aircraft.

Pre-employment assessment Pre-employment assessment raises important questions about the disclosure of a tendency for high rates of absence. The possibility of frequent absence should be based on clinical history and previous absence record. Managers should be informed if frequent absence is likely *and* will be critical to the organization. However, an individual with homozygous SCD is likely to fulfil the definition of disability under the Disability Discrimination Act 1995, and the prospective employer has a duty to make reasonable adjustments. In this situation adjustments might be considered to include the allowance of a higher level of absence compared with 'able' peers.

Sickle cell trait Heterozygotes for sickle haemoglobin (HbAS) have no clinical anaemia. There are no employment consequences other than restriction of activities that are associated with a risk of severe hypoxia (diving, compressed air work or work at altitude above 12 000 feet). Certification for civil air-crew would be considered on an individual basis.

Thalassaemia

Epidemiology and clinical features The thalassaemias are a heterogeneous group of genetic disorders of haemoglobin synthesis. The disorders are most common in the Mediterranean countries, the Middle East, India, and South-east Asia, although they occur sporadically in all populations. Thalassaemia is rare in the UK (800 cases). The common clinical features are anaemia and splenomegaly, and the most severely affected are individuals with homozygous beta thalassaemia (thalassaemia major). These patients have severe transfusion-dependent anaemia, and can develop complications of iron overload (cardiomyopathy, liver failure, and endocrine failure including diabetes mellitus) by teenage years. Even with careful management of iron overload with chelation therapy, life expectancy in thalassaemia major is 20–30 years. However, milder forms of the disease (thalassaemia intermedia) require transfusion less frequently. In heterozygous beta thalassaemia (β thalassaemia trait) anaemia is asymptomatic (with haemoglobin levels usually >9 g/dl).

Recent advances Genetic screening has reduced the overall incidence of thalassaemia in the UK, so fewer cases of this condition are encountered in the workplace. SCT offers a cure, but introduces other implications for work.

Functional limitations in thalassaemia With good medical management patients with thalassaemia major are able to function normally in education and employment with allowance for hospital attendance. However, when complications arise, even with advances in disease management, there are likely to be severe limitations on adults with thalassaemia major in the workplace. Other variant forms of thalassaemia and interactions with structural haemoglobin abnormalities (e.g. haemoglobin E/β thalassaemia) cause a range of clinical manifestations. Therefore functional assessment should be undertaken according to the individual clinical features. Functional impairment is related to the degree of anaemia (see below) and haemoglobin levels are usually kept at about 9–10 g/dl in transfusion dependent patients. A checklist of the limitations on fitness for work is shown in Box 16.3.

Adjustments to work in thalassaemia The main aim is to match the physical job requirements to fatigue and impaired exercise tolerance. Increased susceptibility to infection is also important, and care should be taken in jobs that might expose individuals to infection. Infection with blood-borne viruses secondary to treatment is important only where infection might be passed to others because of the nature of the work, for example healthcare workers undertaking exposure prone procedures. Adjustments for those on chelation therapy are covered below (p. 376). Thalassaemia major would disqualify patients from work as commercial air-crew. However, air-crew certification for those with thalassaemia minor would be considered on an individual basis, provided full functional capacity is demonstrated.

Coagulation disorders

Therapeutic anticoagulation

Treatment with coumarin anticoagulants and antiplatelet drugs is common. Based on data from the 1990s, it has been estimated that 500 000 people in the UK take warfarin. Overall functional

> ### Box 16.3 Potential functional and occupational limitations in thalassaemia
>
> ◆ Reduced capacity for physical work (impaired exercise tolerance due to anaemia, cardiac failure; small stature due to endocrine complications, hypothyroidism, osteoporosis bone pain and fractures due to hypoparathyroidism)
>
> ◆ Increased susceptibility to infection (splenectomy, diabetes mellitus, bone marrow transplantation)
>
> ◆ Infectious carriage of blood-borne viruses (secondary to transfusion)
>
> ◆ Requirement for iron chelation

impairment is more likely to relate to the underlying disorder than anticoagulant therapy. Increased bleeding tendency varies between individuals, but is proportional to the anticoagulant effect, measured by the international normalized ratio (INR). For most indications (venous thromboembolism, atrial fibrillation, cardiac mural thrombosis, cardiomyopathy, and prior to cardioversion) the target INR is 2.5, but for mechanical heart valve prostheses, antiphospholipid syndrome and recurrent venous thromboembolism while on warfarin, the target INR is 3.5. Advances in treatment include self-management of anticoagulant therapy using near patient devices (portable coagulometers). For the future, newer drugs (e.g. new direct thrombin inhibitors, which are given at fixed doses) will eliminate the need for anticoagulant monitoring. The risk of bleeding while on oral anticoagulants increases significantly with INR >4.5, and the risk is low in well-controlled patients. Therefore employees on therapeutic anticoagulation can work normally and adjustments are not necessary unless anticoagulant control is erratic. *Extremely* heavy physical work or work where there is an *extremely* high risk of cuts or trauma should be avoided.

Antiplatelet therapy with aspirin has no important implications for fitness for work.

Inherited clotting disorders: haemophilia and Von Willebrand's disease

Epidemiology and clinical features Haemophilia A is the most common of the hereditary clotting factor deficiencies, with a prevalence in the general population of 30–100 per million. This sex-linked disorder results in deficiency of Factor VIII (FVIII) of the clotting cascade. FVIII levels below 1% (0.01 U/ml) give rise to a severe bleeding tendency. Conversely, above 5% FVIII the clinical syndrome is mild. The primary symptom of the haemophilias is haemarthrosis, usually in the large weight-bearing joints (knees, ankles, and hips). Other features include muscle haematomas, less commonly haematuria, and rarely intracranial bleeds. Parenteral administration of FVIII is indicated for prophylaxis and management of bleeding episodes. A FVIII level of 30% of normal activity is required for haemostasis, but spontaneous bleeding is usually prevented at levels over 20%. Long-term sequelae include the development of FVIII antibodies (inhibitors) in 10–15% of patients, and degenerative joint disease resulting from repeated haemarthrosis.

Haemophilia B (hereditary Factor IX deficiency) is clinically similar to haemophilia A, but is treated with FIX replacement. Von Willebrand's disease is another of the inherited clotting disorders. It differs from classical haemophilia in its autosomal inheritance, and bleeding tends to be mucocutaneous (epistaxis, gastrointestinal, cutaneous bruising) rather than into joints and muscle. Treatment of Von Willebrand's disease is with desmopressin (DDAVP) or concentrates of von Willebrand factor and FVIII.

Box 16.4 Potential functional limitations in haemophilia

- ◆ Impaired tolerance of extremely heavy physical work (risk of bleeding into muscles or weight-bearing joints)
- ◆ Impaired mobility (degenerative joint disease)
- ◆ Infectious carriage of blood-borne viruses

Recent advances A serious problem with transfusion-related infections arose in the 1980s. The use of pooled plasma products gave rise to high exposure to blood-borne viruses in these patients compared with recipients of individual blood components. Over 50% of haemophiliacs treated in the USA and Europe died of HIV before the advent of effective treatments. Many patients were also infected with Hepatitis C before screening of blood products was introduced, and morbidity due to chronic hepatitis is still seen among older haemophiliacs. The uncertainty of new variant Creutzfeld–Jakob disease (nvCJD) with plasma products remains a concern. Improvements in the safety of blood products, in particular the production of recombinant clotting factors, represent a major advance (see multiple transfusion below, page 376). Consequently, young haemophiliacs currently entering higher education and employment are rarely infected with blood-borne viruses. Ultimately, it is hoped that gene therapy will cure these conditions in the future.

Functional limitations in haemophilia Limitations (Box 16.4) relate mainly to the risk of acute joint bleeds, and longer-term degenerative joint disease. The former affects ability to undertake physically strenuous work, although the risk of bleeding can usually be controlled in all but the most severe cases by regular factor replacement.

Adjustments to work in haemophilia Adjustments (Box 16.5) will depend entirely on the severity of the bleeding disorder. Patients with mild haemophilia can work normally in any job. Even with severe FVIII deficiency (below 1%) some patients have very infrequent problems with bleeding, and few if any adjustments to work will be required. Very heavy physical work or work that is associated with a high risk of injury would be contraindicated in an individual who has frequent large joint bleeds. Examples include mining, heavy construction, armed forces, fire fighting, and the police service. Healthcare workers who undertake exposure prone procedures should be screened for blood-borne viruses. Special care is needed if an individual is required to travel for work, or to work in isolation. Arrangements for the safe storage of factor replacement, and access to sterile distilled water (diluent), sterile needles, syringes, and other equipment for administration are needed. Some freeze-dried concentrates of Factors VIII and IX can be stored at room temperature (up to 25°C or 77°F) for up to 6 months, but general advice is to keep all

Box 16.5 Adjustments to work in haemophilia

- ◆ Provide facilities for self-treatment
- ◆ Avoidance of extremely heavy physical work or work associated with a high risk of injury
- ◆ Improved access to work and sedentary work if mobility restricted
- ◆ Extreme care with foreign travel. Avoid remote areas with poor medical facilities

products in a refrigerator at 2–8°C (36–46° F). Clearly in hot climates adequate refrigeration is essential. Documentation may be required by customs to carry medical equipment, and it is essential that appropriate insurance covers haemophilia-related complications. Work in very remote areas with poor hygiene arrangements or medical facilities, is contraindicated in haemophilia, except for very mild cases that are unlikely to require replacement therapy. Significantly affected haemophiliacs would be excluded from certification as commercial air crew, but very mildly affected cases might be considered for certification on an individual basis provided there was no history of significant bleeding episodes.

Thrombophilia

The annual incidence of venous thromboembolic disease (VTE) is between 1 and 3 per 1000 per year. Deep vein thrombosis and pulmonary embolism (PE) are most common, but other sites (upper limbs, liver, cerebral sinus, retina and mesenteric veins) are affected infrequently. VTE causes significant mortality and morbidity: 1–2% of patients will die of PE and up to 20% of patients go on to suffer significant debility due to the post-thrombotic syndrome (chronic leg oedema, varicose veins, and venous ulceration). Risk factors for VTE include inherited and acquired medical conditions, and external factors play a significant part (Table 16.1).

The pathogenesis and risk factors for VTE and arterial thrombosis are distinctly different. In VTE age is the single greatest risk factor, and stasis, immobilization, and prothrombotic abnormalities are common. Atheroma, smoking, hypertension, or hypercholesterolaemia do not increase the risk of VTE.

The majority of cases of VTE are managed initially with low molecular weight heparin (LMWH) followed by warfarin. The advantage of LMWH is that it can be administered out of hospital without the need for blood monitoring. Warfarin dosing needs to be monitored and titrated regularly to achieve an appropriate anticoagulant level. The duration of anticoagulation will depend on the circumstances, severity of the VTE event, and predisposing factors, varying from 3 months to lifelong treatment. As a result of the investigation of patients with VTE for genetic predisposition, an increasing number of asymptomatic family members are found to carry genetic mutations that confer an increased thrombotic risk. These patients require counselling about risk factors including enforced immobility, and advice on appropriate

Table 16.1 Risk factors for venous thromboembolic disease

Inherited	Acquired	External
• Antithrombin deficiency (ATIII)	• Age	• Immobilization
• Protein C (PC) deficiency	• Previous venous	• Surgery and trauma
• Protein S (PS) deficiency	thrombembolism	• Oral contraceptives
• Factor V Leiden (FVL)	• Malignancy	• Hormone replacement therapy
• Prothrombin 20210A	• Polycythaemia	
• Dysfibrinogenaemia	• Essential thrombocytosis	
• Elevated FVIII, IX, XI	• Paroxysmal nocturnal	
	Haemoglobinuria (PNH)	
	• Pregnancy	
	• Antiphospholipid syndrome	

preventive measures. There is an increasing body of evidence to associate VTE with long-haul (>3000 miles) air travel. This risk is likely to be significantly increased in patients with a thrombophilic tendency. It is good practice for all long-haul passengers to exercise during flight, walk around if possible, maintain a good fluid intake and limit alcohol consumption. Graduated compression stockings may also be worn. For 'high-risk' patients, immediately before the flight, a single dose of LMWH at a prophylactic dose may be given.

There are significant issues for employment in thrombophilic patients. Patients who have suffered deep vein thrombosis or PE may have residual problems of reduced exercise capacity, mobility and pain. Long-term problems related to post-phlebitic limb and cardiac problems due to pulmonary hypertension, may develop many years following the original event. Patients, and known carriers of risk factors, in sedentary jobs should be encouraged to mobilize frequently. Appropriate precautions need to be taken during long-haul travel. Thrombophilias associated with a significant history of clotting episodes would exclude from certification as civil air crew. Because of the low incidence of disorders that cause a genetic predisposition to VTE, screening of frequent long-haul occupational travellers is not indicated.

Malignant haematological disorders

Epidemiology Haematological malignancies, although individually rare, comprise 8–10% of all cancers in the UK (Table 16.2).

This heterogeneous group of conditions ranges from acute leukaemias, which may be rapidly fatal, to chronic conditions for which no intervention is required. They are characterized by impairment of bone marrow (BM) function and immunity. Although many are aggressive in nature, some of the treatable conditions have the highest cure rates among all malignant disorders.

Clinical features and recent advances:

Acute leukaemias Acute lymphoblastic leukaemia (ALL) is the commonest malignancy in children, and contemporary cure rates above 80% represent one of the success stories in modern cancer therapy. Over the last 15 years research has aimed at maintaining high cure rates, while reducing long-term side-effects. Thus craniospinal radiotherapy is given only to poor-risk

Table 16.2 Epidemiology of haematological malignancies

Disease	Number of cases/yr (UK)	Median age at onset
Childhood acute lymphoblastic leukaemia	450	3–7
Adult acute lymphoblastic leukaemia	200	55
Childhood acute myeloblastic leukaemia	50	2
Adult acute myeloblastic leukaemia	1950	65
Non-Hodgkin lymphoma	8450	65
Hodgkin disease	1400	30
Chronic lymphocytic leukaemia	2750	66
Chronic myeloid leukaemia	750	50
Myelodysplastic syndrome	3250	70
Myeloma	3300	65

patients rather than routinely, and boys are now treated for 3 years to prevent testicular relapse. BM transplantation (BMT) would only be considered for children with poor risk or relapsed disease. Long-term follow-up studies have shown that children treated with standard chemotherapy regimens, who did not receive radiotherapy, can be considered cured after 10 years. Thus the majority of long-term survivors of childhood ALL entering working life will not require continuing medical care. For those who received radiation, follow up would continue in view of late side-effects. For ALL presenting in adulthood, the prognosis is markedly worse, with 5-year survival figures of only 30–35%. Transplantation is therefore a first-line option for many patients. Because craniospinal radiotherapy is integral to the regimen, adult survivors of ALL are more likely to have co-morbidities and will require long-term follow-up.

Acute myeloid leukaemia (AML) is predominantly a disease of adults. Studies have shown a steady improvement in survival in patients up to age 60 with intensification of treatment over the last 25 years. Current therapies for AML involve a risk-based approach to treatment. Patients are stratified into good, intermediate, and poor risk groups and transplantation is reserved for intermediate/poor risk patients (see below). Overall 5-year survival is 40% (range 17–73%) in adults and 67% in children. Standard treatment protocols involve four to five courses of intensive multidrug chemotherapy with prolonged hospitalization, during which time patients can develop a wide range of medical problems. Patients are unable to work during this period, which usually lasts 6–8 months. Thereafter, full recovery from the effects of treatment can take up to 1 year. When the disease is in remission patients are able to return to work and lead normal lives. Some patients have residual treatment-related problems, including incomplete recovery of blood counts with consequent anaemia, infection or bleeding risk, and respiratory, cardiac, or renal dysfunction. All patients should continue on long-term hospital follow-up.

Chronic leukaemias The incidence of **chronic lymphocytic leukaemia (CLL)** appears to be increasing, with involvement of younger patients. However, the increased availability of blood counts (e.g. through health screening) has promoted earlier diagnosis among asymptomatic patients, who may previously have remained undiagnosed for years. The disease often runs a benign course, and no survival advantage is gained from earlier intervention. Indications for treatment include symptoms of sweating, fever, or weight loss, evidence of anaemia or thrombocytopenia or rapidly rising lymphocyte count. Patients with CLL require long-term follow-up. All patients are immunocompromised, are particularly susceptible to respiratory infections, and should receive influenza and pneumococcal vaccines. Some patients, particularly those with underlying chronic pulmonary disease, may benefit from immunoglobulin therapy. CLL remains incurable with conventional treatment. Treatments range from simple oral alkylating agents, fludarabine, combination chemotherapy, the monoclonal antibody Alemtuzumab (MabCampath), through to transplantation (see pp 371–4). Although newer drugs achieve higher rates of complete remission it is not clear whether this translates to improved survival over established treatments. Purine analogues and Alemtuzumab produce profound immunosuppression through loss of T-cell-mediated immunity. Patients are susceptible to opportunistic infection including reactivation of cytomegalovirus and pneumocystis carinii pneumonia (PCP), and current guidelines recommend prophylaxis against pneumocystis carinii for a year post treatment.

Chronic myeloid leukaemia (CML) occurs at all ages. Patients present with elevated white blood cell counts and splenomegaly. The disease follows a chronic phase of variable duration (a few months to 10 years). However, patients will eventually transform to acute leukaemia. The only current cure for CML is allogeneic transplantation. Recently Imatinib, the first of a new generation of drugs, has revolutionized treatment. It targets the known molecular cause of the disease. Imatinib is administered orally, and is generally well tolerated. It is now the treatment of choice in patients with chronic phase CML but, because of uncertainty about the long-term prognosis, allogeneic transplantation is still undertaken in young patients with a sibling donor. Patients require outpatient monitoring, but during treatment usually remain well and lead a normal life. In an attempt to improve outcome, there are ongoing trials of using higher doses of Imatinib and combination with interferon. Side-effects of interferon are common and include flu-like symptoms, myalgia, headache, and nausea in up to 50% patients. These may affect a patient's stamina and ability to attend and perform at work.

The **myelodysplastic syndromes (MDS)** predominantly affect the elderly, but do occur in adults of working age, particularly where there has been exposure to prior chemo/radiotherapy. They are characterized by peripheral blood (PB) cytopenias and a risk of transformation to acute leukaemia. The only curative treatment is SCT (see p 371). However, supportive care, involving blood transfusion and antibiotics for intercurrent infections, remains the treatment of choice for the majority. Transformation to acute leukaemia may be treated with intensive chemotherapy, but has a poor prognosis. The prognosis for MDS is very variable and depends on the number of cytopenias, BM blast percentage and chromosomal abnormalities present. Median survival varies from 67 (low risk) to 4 months (high risk). Low-risk patients may remain well, continue in work and require only occasional follow-up. However, those who are transfusion dependent require more frequent and prolonged hospital attendance and are unlikely to tolerate work. In older patients co-morbidity, particularly chronic cardiac or respiratory disorders, may compound functional incapacity.

Lymphomas—Hodgkin's disease is predominantly a condition of young adults, and modern treatment achieves cure rates of 90%. Multidrug chemotherapy, radiotherapy, or combination protocols result in significant impairment of ability to work. Treatment lasts 6–8 months and transplantation is indicated for non-response or relapse. On recovery (6–12 months post-treatment) the majority of patients would be expected to return to a full and active life.

Non-Hodgkin's lymphomas (NHL) comprise the largest group of haematological malignancies and their incidence is increasing in Western societies. There are over 40 histological subtypes, but they can be classified clinically as aggressive (high-grade) or indolent (low-grade) disease. High-grade NHL comprises 30–40% of all NHL diagnosis. Standard treatment comprises combination chemotherapy given for 6–8 courses over a period of 4–6 months. Response rates vary according to a prognostic index that includes disease stage at presentation and performance status. Overall 40–60% achieve complete remission, with a 5-year survival of 30–40%. The addition of the monoclonal antibody Rituximab to chemotherapy has improved complete remission rates to 75%. Improved supportive care, intensive dose scheduling and newer treatments are also improving prognosis. Thus increased numbers of long-term survivors of high grade NHL, now return to employment. Unlike high grade NHL, where long-term survival is dependent on disease cure, low grade NHL is incurable with standard treatment regimens. It often runs an indolent course, and treatment is only required if the patient becomes symptomatic. Median survival exceeds 10 years. Increasingly patients are diagnosed on routine health screening and blood tests. Others present with lymphadenopathy, fevers, sweats, weight loss, BM failure due to marrow infiltration, or disease involvement of other organs (gut, lungs, central nervous system). Many patients can be managed conservatively and will be able to continue with their daily lives, unaffected by treatment. Progressive and symptomatic disease requires treatment with single or multiple drug regimens. Transplantation may be considered in selected patients (see below). Many cases can be well controlled with oral chemotherapy, which produces few side-effects and allows patients to continue with normal daily activities and employment. Patients require regular hospital follow-up to assess disease response and drug toxicity. As the underlying conditions are incurable, fitness to work depends on individual functional assessment.

Multiple myeloma Although myeloma is predominantly a disease of the elderly, many people of working age are affected. Haematological and immunological effects of myeloma include anaemia and immuneparesis. Biochemical effects include chronic renal failure, hypercalcaemia, hyperviscosity (due to high paraprotein levels), and gout. Lytic bone lesions can cause bone pain, pathological fractures, and vertebral involvement with cord compression and paralysis. Myeloma is incurable for the majority of patients, but considerable advances have resulted in the development of novel drugs. The principles of treatment are tumour reduction with multi-agent chemotherapy, followed (in younger patients only) by high dose chemotherapy and autologous SCT (see below). Current clinical trials are evaluating the role of immunomodulatory drugs (IMiDs), including thalidomide, in treatment regimens and as postchemotherapy maintenance. Skeletal disease is treated with radiotherapy, and bisphosphanates are effective in treating hypercalcaemia, bone pain and preventing fractures. Median survival is 54 months in transplanted patients (42 months in patients receiving conventional treatment).

The ability to continue to work during or after treatment for myeloma may be severely affected. Anaemia and fatigue are common. Thalidomide treatment may contribute to somnolence, and is associated with a significant risk of venous thromboembolism and neuropathy. Heavy manual or lifting work may exacerbate skeletal symptoms and risk of fractures.

Adjustments to work in malignant haematological diseases

Patients are usually absent from work during the acute phase of treatment, which can last up to a year depending on the condition. Once disease is controlled or in remission, short-term adjustments may be needed for rehabilitation of patients who have impaired marrow function. Long-term alterations are needed in some jobs to manage the life long susceptibility to infection. Possible adjustments for generic issues are summarized in the sections below.

Joint Aviation Authority (JAA) standards on fitness for aircrew recommend exclusion for acute leukaemia and for initial applicants with chronic leukaemia. The Aeromedical Section of the Joint Aviation Authority would consider certification for individuals with treated lymphoma or acute leukaemia that was in full remission. Re-certification for an established aircrew member would be considered for CLL stages O, I (and possibly II) without anaemia and minimal treatment, or 'hairy cell' leukaemia provided haemoglobin and platelet levels are normal; although regular follow would be required by the JAA. If anthracycline has been included in chemotherapy regimens cardiological review would be required for certification.

Generic issues

Stem cell transplantation (SCT)

SCT is a highly advanced medical procedure that carries significant risks of major morbidity and mortality. The principles behind SCT differ between autologous and allogeneic procedures (See Glossary p 380). Autologous SCT allows intensification of chemo/radiotherapy to myeloablative doses to treat the underlying condition. Thus the SCT functions as a 'rescue' allowing reconstitution of marrow function. Standard allogeneic transplantation, while also allowing the use of myeloablative chemo/radiotherapy, transplants the donor's immune system. The donor (graft) immune response to the recipient (host) accounts for the graft versus host disease (GvHD), which is the major complication of allogeneic transplantation. However, the same immune response is also directed at the underlying disease (leukaemia) creating a graft versus leukaemia (GvL) effect. It is clear that the GvL effect plays a major role in the long-term cure achieved by allogeneic SCT.

Table 16.3 Numbers and reasons for bone marrow transplantation in the UK, 2003

	Transplants performed	
Conditions	**Allograft**	**Autograft**
Acute myeloblastic leukaemia	230	41
Acute lymphoblastic leukaemia	110	23
Chronic myeloid leukaemia	111	3
Chronic lymphocytic leukaemia	14	17
Myelodysplastic syndrome	88	2
Myeloma	26	605
Hodgkin's disease	14	160
Non-Hodgkin lymphoma	81	460
Haemoglobinopathy/anaemias	45	0
Severe combined immune deficiency (SCID)	18	0
Inborn errors of metabolism	8	0
Autoimmune disorders	4	4
Solid tumours	2	107
Others	34	3
Total	785	1425

British Society of Blood and Marrow Transplantation data.

Indications for stem cell transplantation and survival

The indications for SCT (in both adults and children) and number of procedures performed in the UK are shown in Table 16.3.

Many factors influence the outcome of SCT, including type of transplant, age, underlying disease, and stage at time of transplant. As age is one of the principal determinants of outcome, it is generally accepted that autologous transplants should be limited to patients under 65 years, sibling allografts to 60 years and alternative donor allografts to 45 years. However, improvements in supportive care and transplant techniques, are pushing the age boundaries for allografting ever upwards. Based on European Group for Blood and Marrow Transplantation (EBMT) registry data of 60 000 autologous and allogeneic SCTs performed between 1969 and 1998, the overall projected probability of survival at 20 years is 38%. However, this may reach 90% for children undergoing sibling SCT for certain conditions. During the transplant procedure itself and in the early post-transplant period the patient would be unable to perform work. Recovery from treatment may take months or years and will depend on success of the procedure in curing the underlying condition and any long-term side-effects (see p 373).

Fitness for work in stem cell donors

Haemopoietic stem cells can be derived from bone marrow (BM) or peripheral blood (PB). Donors can be the patient himself (autologous) or a family or volunteer donor (allogeneic). Collecting stem cells involves either a BM harvest or PB stem cell (PBSC) collection. Marrow (1000–1200 ml) is harvested under general anaesthesia from the posterior iliac crests. Marrow donors usually recover fully from the procedure within 1–2 weeks, during which time they are advised to refrain from work. Occasionally, a BM harvest can cause or exacerbate back problems. The principle of PBSC collection depends on giving a course of the haemopoietic growth factor, granulocyte colony stimulating factor (G-CSF). Transient side-effects include flu-like symptoms and bone pain due to the G-CSF injections, and hypocalcaemia during the apharesis process.

Late effects of chemo/radiotherapy and stem cell transplantation for haematological disease

For many patients with haematological malignancies cure or control of the underlying disease is not accompanied by restoration of normal health. Late complications contribute to both chronic physical and psychological illness. These include toxicity from treatment regimens, immune deficiency, autoimmune syndromes, infectious complications, endocrine dysfunction, growth impairment in children, cognitive dysfunction and learning difficulties, secondary malignancies, chronic GvHD, and psychological and psychiatric disturbance.

Cardiovascular complications

Chemotherapeutic drugs and radiation may lead to impairment of cardiac function including cardiomyopathy, arrythmias, pericarditis, pericardial thickening, coronary artery disease, decreased ventricular mass, and impaired contractility. Cardiac dysfunction may also occur secondarily to pulmonary complications. Regimens that avoid or limit radiation, and trials of radioprotection therapies serve to limit this complication in the future.

Respiratory complications

Radiation and certain drugs may produce a pneumonitis, leading to pulmonary fibrosis. Lung shielding and fractionating radiation doses aim to reduce the incidence and severity of these problems. Respiratory infections are a major cause of morbidity and mortality in all patients undergoing treatment for haematological diseases. The risk of late infection is related to the degree of immunosuppression, pre-existing lung damage from infections during treatment, and late drug/radiation damage. Patients are at risk of opportunistic infections with, *Pneumocystis carinii* (PCP), fungi, cytomegalovirus (CMV), tuberculosis (including reactivation of disease) as well as respiratory bacterial and viral infections. Antimicrobial prophylaxis is often required for prolonged periods, particularly in SCT patients. Patients should receive vaccinations according to recommended schedules (Table 16.4).

Immunodeficiency

The underlying pathology, chemo/radio/immunotherapy and associated chronic complications, will all contribute to the immunodeficiency of patients who have undergone treatment for haematological malignancies or SCT. The major manifestation is infection, but secondary malignancies and autoimmune syndromes also occur. There are no adequate measures of immune function, and decisions regarding antimicrobial prophylaxis and vaccination schedules are largely based on clinical and time post-treatment criteria. Antibiotic prophylaxis is given for PCP, hyposplenic patients (see below), antivirals for CMV, varicella zoster (VZV)/herpes simplex and antifungal prophylaxis, particularly for patients on steroids. Antibody responses to vaccinations are poor in patients with absolute CD4 counts $<100 \times 10^6/l$ (T-helper lymphocytes carrying the CD4 antigen). Thus vaccinations are likely to be ineffective in severely immune compromised patients. Furthermore, live vaccines may pose a risk to patients. Vaccinations are therefore deferred to allow sufficient degree of immune reconstitution, to be effective without posing a risk. Table 16.4 shows the European Group for Blood and Marrow Transplantation recommendations for immunizations post-SCT.

Table 16.4 Recommended vaccinations in patients with stem cell transplantation

Vaccine	Allo SCT	Auto SCT	Timing post-SCT
Tetanus toxoid	All	All	6–12 months
Diphtheria	All	All	6–12 months
Inactivated poliovirus	All	All	6–12 months
Pneumococcus	All	All	6–12 months
H. Influenzae B	All	All	6–12 months
Influenza virus	All	All	Season-dependent
Measles	Individual recommendation based on risk/benefit assessment		>24 months postallogeneic stem cell transplant

Vaccination schedules are important for those who are likely to be exposed to infection at work, in particular healthcare workers. If response to vaccines is inadequate they may need to be restricted from work that carries a high risk of exposure, e.g. work with infectious tuberculosis patients.

Endocrine, neurological, and ophthalmological dysfunction

Hypothyroidism occurs in patients who receive total body irradiation or mediastinal radiotherapy. Learning difficulties occur in children receiving intensive craniospinal irradiation; hence this treatment is now only given to patients with a poor prognosis. Radiation and neurotoxic chemotherapy are known to cause leucoencephalopathy, cerebral atrophy, and demyelination. Cyclosporin, used for post-transplant immune suppression, may cause cerebellar dysfunction and seizures. Vinca alkaloids and thalidomide commonly cause peripheral neuropathy. This may be irreversible and cause significant problems with pain and functional impairment. Cataracts are common in patients who received steroid drugs and particularly radiation treatment. Keratoconjunctivitis sicca occurs in 25% of allogeneic SCT recipients and is related to chronic GvHD

Secondary malignancies

The development of second malignancies is recognized as a potential late complication of chemotherapy or radiation. The overall relative cancer risk compared with the general population is 6.4. Patients should not smoke, and environmental and occupational exposure to carcinogens (e.g. sun exposure, etc.) must be minimized.

Chronic GvHD

This is one of the common and significant problems affecting survivors of allogeneic SCT. Up to 60% of patients surviving more than 4 months after allogeneic SCT develop chronic GvHD. It is characterized by profound immune suppression with concomitant infection risk (see above), and involvement of skin (scleroderma-type picture also affecting mouth, eyes, muscles, and joints), the gastrointestinal system (affecting nutrition, bowel and liver function) respiratory system, and marrow (variable cytopenias). Principles of management include prophylaxis and early treatment of infections, continued immune suppression and symptomatic management of complications. The commonest drugs used are corticosteroids and cyclosporin A, but a wide range of treatments are available or under evaluation. However, these treatments compound the risk of infection and secondary malignancy.

Table 16.5 Indications for splenectomy and causes of splenic insufficiency

Indications for splenectomy	Causes of hyposplenism
• Trauma	• Congenital aplasia
• Malignancy	• Haematological disorders
• Autoimmune conditions (immune thrombocytopenic purpura, auto-immune haemolytic anaemia)	• Sickle cell disease
	• Myelofibrosis
• Diagnostic	• Lymphomas
• Hereditary haemolytic anaemias (e.g. hereditary spherocytosis pyruvate kinase deficiency)	• Autoimmune disorders
	• Coeliac disease
	• Inflammatory bowel disease
• Hypersplenism	• Splenic infiltration
	• Splenic irradiation
	• Splenic embolization

Splenectomy and hyposplenism

The spleen is the largest single accumulation of lymphoid tissue in the body and contains 25% of the T-lymphocyte and 10–15% of the B-lymphocyte pool. It also performs a major role in phagocytosis of blood-borne bacteria and senescent and damaged red cells. Thus, the spleen fulfils a major role in protecting against bacterial, viral, and parasitic infections.

The causes of splenic insufficiency are summarized in Table 16.5. These patients are at risk of overwhelming bacterial infections particularly involving encapsulated organisms, *Streptococcus pneumoniae* (pneumococcus), *Haemophilus influenzae*, and *Neisseria meningitidis*.

Guidelines recommend immunization for patients undergoing splenectomy or with hyposplenism (Table 16.6). In patients undergoing elective splenectomy, vaccinations should be given at least 2 weeks prior to surgery. In addition, lifelong antibiotic prophylaxis with penicillin (erythromycin if allergic to penicillin) is advised to all patients. Despite these measures severe infections still occur, and patients should carry a 'Splenectomy Card' and a 'MedicAlert 'bracelet. Infection should be treated with a broad-spectrum penicillin and it may be advisable for patients to carry an emergency supply of this when away from home. During travel to affected areas,

Table 16.6 Recommended vaccination schedule for splenectomy patients

Vaccine	Schedule
Pneumococcus	Re-immunization recommended every 5 years or based on antibody levels
Haemophilus influenza B (HiB)	Included as part of routine childhood vaccinations since 1993
Meningococcal C	Now part of routine childhood vaccinations
Conjugate vaccine	Older and non-immune patients should receive single dose
Influenza vaccine	Annual vaccination recommended

> ## Box 16.6 Adjustments to work for hyposplenic/splenectomized employees
>
> - Ensure immunizations up to date, and on prophylactic antibiotics
> - Avoid exposure to bacterial pathogens
> - Care with travel, carry antibiotics, and fastidious compliance with antimalarial prophylaxis
> - Avoid working in remote areas with poor medical facilities

patients should be advised of the increased risk of severe malaria infections and must adhere scrupulously to antimalarial prophylaxis.

There are no guidelines or data on which to base recommendations for employment, and the adjustments suggested in Box 16.6 are based on traditional textbook teaching about increased risk of infection. Hyposplenic or splenectomized employees should be able to undertake almost any kind of work, and restrictions to employment are very few. The exception is work that carries a risk of exposure to encapsulated pathogens and potentially infective biological material, and foreign travel. Individual susceptibility must be considered in addition to generic risk assessment in this situation.

Repeated transfusion

Repeated transfusion with whole blood or blood products is used in the management of haemoglobinopathies, bleeding disorders, and haematological malignancies. Long-term transfusion can give rise to a number of clinical problems (Box 16.7), including iron overload. Clinical sequelae include cardiac, endocrine and liver damage. The treatment of choice is with parenteral chelation. Desferrioxamine is usually administered by subcutaneous infusion (rarely by indwelling intravenous catheter) over 12 hours three to five times a week. Travel must be planned to ensure adequate treatment facilities, including documentation for medical equipment carriage for

> ## Box 16.7 Complications of multiple treatment with blood products
>
> - Iron overload
>   - cardiomyopathy
>   - liver failure
>   - endocrine failure
> - Infection with blood-borne viruses
>   - chronic hepatitis
>   - HIV infection
>   - infectious carriage of blood borne viruses (relevant for healthcare employees)

foreign travel. Local healthcare provision should be adequate for handling complications including infection.

Transmission of infection is much less of a problem since the introduction of rigorous measures to reduce the incidence of infection in blood products. UK blood donors are routinely screened for syphilis, hepatitis B and C, HIV1, HIV2, HTLV I, and HTLVII In addition, selective screening includes CMV (where patients are deemed to be susceptible) and malaria and *Treponema cruzi* (where donors are judged to have a risk of exposure). Since the mid-1980s pooled plasma products such as clotting factor concentrates have undergone viral inactivation processes (heat, solvent-detergent, monoclonal antibodies). Moreover, some products are now produced using recombinant technology, removing the risk of infection completely. Table 16.7 shows the risk of transfusion related infection in 2000. Three possible cases of transfusion-related transmission of nvCJD have been recorded. Since 1999 all UK blood cellular products had had 99.9% of the white cells removed in order to reduce the risk of vCJD, and since 2004 plasma for children born after 1996 (the year in which UK meat was deemed to be safe) has come from non-vCJD endemic areas (North America).

Fitness for work resulting from infection with blood-borne viruses is covered in Chapters 14 and 23. Infectivity is only an issue where others in the workplace might be exposed to blood or body fluids from the infected employee (mainly in healthcare or dentistry). However, the risk of acquiring a transfusion-related infection is extremely low, and regular screening for infection for employment purposes is usually inappropriate.

Anaemia

The main symptoms associated with chronic anaemia that are relevant for fitness for work are fatigue, breathlessness, and impaired exercise tolerance. These symptoms are variable and depend, among other things, on the patient's age, level of fitness, and co-morbidity (including cardiovascular and respiratory disease and cancer). In general chronic anaemia is better tolerated than acute anaemia because of adaptive mechanisms for improved oxygen delivery to the tissues. Measurable physiological changes do not occur until the haemoglobin falls below 7 g/dl. However, when functional assessment scales have been used in patients with anaemia haemoglobin concentrations above 12 g/dl were associated with less fatigue and a better quality of life. Advances in the treatment of chronic anaemia include the use of recombinant erythropoietin. Individuals who have anaemia with haematocrit <32% would be disqualified as aircrew.

Fatigue

Fatigue is commonly experienced by patients with haematological disorders and is well recognized as the most prevalent and functionally debilitating symptom of cancer and its treatment. It is related to a number of factors including disease activity, treatment, anaemia, and sleep disturbance, but the specific aetiology of this symptom is not well understood. The reduction in energy

Table 16.7 Estimated risks of transfusion-related viral infection in the UK in 2000

Viral pathogen	Estimated risk per unit of blood screened in UK
Hepatitis B	1/50 000–1/170 000
Hepatitis C	1/200 000
Human immunodeficiency virus	1/2 000 000

levels with cancer-related fatigue is often disproportionate to physical effort required to perform tasks. Moreover, fatigue has dimensions other than purely physical, including emotional, behavioural, and cognitive elements. Fatigue that is sufficiently severe to threaten employment has serious psychosocial consequences for the individual, and it is important to ensure that employers are aware of the effect of fatigue on workability. The main difficulties with assessing the impact of fatigue on fitness for work are the subjective nature of the symptom and the variability between individuals. Several instruments have been developed to measure fatigue in clinical settings, either through self-report scales or fatigue diaries. In theory these self-report scales (e.g. Piper Fatigue Scale, Functional Assessment of Cancer Therapy Scale) might be useful for repeated measurements, including the recording of symptoms prior to return to work and regular monitoring during a work rehabilitation programme. However, most of the available literature focuses on fatigue as a measure of treatment outcome rather than functional assessment for work, and these instruments have not been validated in the workplace setting.

During the treatment phases most patients with haematological malignancy will not be well enough to work. However, fatigue can last for months (or even more than a year) after treatment. It is important to identify chronic fatigue symptoms, as adjustments to work may enable a productive return. Strategies for managing cancer-related fatigue include promotion of acceptance, positive thinking, and education about treatment and prognosis. Energy conservation strategies have been found to be helpful in the setting of cancer treatment, including increasing sleep time, pacing and restriction of activities, restoring attention and concentration (by pleasant diversionary activities), and physical exercise. The literature in this field comes from the treatment and early post-treatment phase of malignant diseases. However, these findings suggest that practical adjustments to allow pacing of work activities with rest and graded exercise will be beneficial for the individual and allow earlier return to work. On literature searching, no studies that specifically and directly assessed interventions for the workplace management of fatigue were found. Therefore the evidence for recommendations in Box 16.8 for rehabilitation back to work is indirect, based on intervention studies in cancer patients.

Bleeding

Many haematological disorders and their treatments will affect bleeding tendency through the failure of thrombopoiesis. In patients with thrombocytopenia bleeding tendency is typically

---

Box 16.8 Suggested adjustments to work in employees with chronic anaemia- or cancer-related fatigue

- Flexible working arrangements
- Part-time work
- Late starts and early finishes
- Minimize night work or shift work
- Encourage frequent breaks and job variety to help maintain attention
- Support from manager and peers to encourage positive attitude and progression towards normality
- Reducing very heavy physical work
- Arrangements to allow working from home

Box 16.9 Markers of significantly high risk of bleeding in haematological conditions (threshold for advising restriction from heavy physical work or work associated with risk of injury)

- Haemophilia: Factor VIII activity below 5%
- Therapeutic anticoagulation: INR>4.5
- Marrow suppression due to chemotherapy, radiotherapy; marrow failure due to leukaemia, myelodysplasia, aplastic anaemia——platelet count—<20 × 10^9/l

---

manifested as spontaneous skin purpura, mucosal haemorrhage, and prolonged bleeding after trauma. Prophylactic platelet transfusion is indicated at counts below 10×10^9/l, and counts are maintained above 50×10^9/l in patients who are undergoing invasive procedures including liver biopsy. Bleeding in haemophilia is discussed above. Therapeutic anticoagulation, if managed carefully, is unlikely to cause bleeding that is relevant for work. Adjustments to work in bleeding disorders are indicated by the risk of haemorrhage due to physical activities. There are no specific evidence-based guidelines, but clinical markers for increased risk of bleeding are listed in Box 16.9. These are based on indirect evidence of thresholds for platelet transfusion from standard haematological texts.

Psychosocial aspects

Haematological disease may have a considerable impact on psychosocial function. Many of the specific diseases described in this chapter are life-threatening and chronic in nature. There is a high incidence of associated psychological morbidity that must be taken into account in planning rehabilitation in the workplace. Depression is more prevalent among patients with haematological disease including haematological cancers, haemoglobinopathies and haemophilia. Surveys in cancer survivors have shown that 35% had symptoms of psychological distress. Even patients in long-standing remission have a high rate of psychiatric disorders (37%) including depression in 13%. It is important to be aware of psychosocial morbidity when returning to work, as treatment can usefully be facilitated. Support at home and at work improves the outcome of psychological problems.

Conclusions

In recent years there have been major advances in the management of many haematological conditions. As a result there have been real improvements in long-term survival and workability, particularly among patients with haematological malignancies. More of these patients will return to the employment market than previously and, with the exception of a few jobs that are contra-indicated, adjustments to work will enable them to work efficiently and safely.

Further reading

CancerBACUP. *Coping with fatigue; cancer related fatigue: what it is and how to handle it.* CancerBACUP Booklet, 2004. http://www.cancerbacup.org.uk

Hoffbrand AV, Pettit JE (eds) *Essential haematology*, (3rd edn). Oxford: Blackwell Scientific Publications, 1993.

Hoffbrand AV, Lewis SM, Tuddenham EGD (eds) *Postgraduate haematology*, (4th edn). London: Arnold, 2001.

Joint Aviation Authority Manual of Civil Aviation Medicine. Haematology, Chapter 6. http://www.jaa.nl/licensing/manual/06%20%Haematology.pdf

Jones P. *Living with haemophilia* (5th edn). Oxford: Oxford University Press, 2002.

Serjeant GR, Serjeant BE (eds) *Sickle cell disease*, (3rd edn). Oxford: Oxford University Press, 2001.

Glossary

Allogenic BMT — Bone marrow transplant using stem cells from the bone marrow of a matched donor

Allo-graft — See Allogenic BMT

Autologous BMT — Bone marrow transplant using stem cells from the patient's own bone marrow

Chapter 17

Cardiovascular disorders

A. E. Price and M. C. Petch

Introduction

Cardiovascular disorders affect fitness to work in two ways. First, an individual may suffer from symptoms on effort that limit his or her working capacity. Such disability is quantifiable and can often be alleviated by effective treatment, such as heart surgery. The second and much more difficult problem is the risk of sudden incapacity, especially in individuals who appear perfectly well. This may take the form of a simple faint, or loss of vision through systemic embolism, or a ruptured aortic aneurysm, or Stokes Adams attack, or even sudden cardiac death as a result of ventricular fibrillation. Assessment of this risk and the consequent effect on the individual and his/her colleagues at work is possible in populations who may be identified as being at high or low risk of incapacity. One example would be an individual who has extensive ventricular damage following a heart attack thereby placing him in a high-risk category. Yet he may feel very well, and may defy the poor prognosis, for a while. Explaining this concept to a lorry driver who has lost his job is not easy. While the instantaneous risk of sudden incapacity is very small, the consequences can be unacceptable, as when the London bus driver lost consciousness at the wheel while approaching a bus stop, with the result that several people in the bus queue were killed.

Limitation of working capacity and the risk of sudden incapacity can both be well judged in populations by specialist opinion. Nowadays this must be backed by objective data, usually derived from the results of 'non-invasive' tests such as echocardiography and exercise testing. Unfortunately disease progression can be unpredictable and individuals judged to be at low risk from further cardiovascular events can nevertheless suffer incapacity, just as those high-risk individuals may escape that fate. For this reason some employers unfairly reject employees who have a heart 'problem', even those whose risk of incapacity is demonstrably no greater than their peers. Occupational medical advisers can help to achieve the difficult balance between restricting the liberty of the individual, and protecting that individual and others from the effects of sudden incapacity.

Sometimes cardiovascular symptoms are out of all proportion to the objective evidence of disease. This may be due to the profound psychological disturbance that can follow the development of cardiovascular disease (CVD). The victim is typically an overweight manual worker in his forties, a smoker, who has always enjoyed robust good health. A heart attack proves devastating and he never returns to work despite prompt treatment, a full cardiac recovery, and the demonstration of only modest coronary disease. Atypical chest pains and tightness, shortness of breath, dizzy spells, loss of fitness, fatigue, and depression persist despite attempts at rehabilitation, reassurance, and treatment often including myocardial revascularization. Such individuals deserve sympathy and support. Their management is, however, extraordinarily difficult and retirement on grounds of psychological ill health may be the only option.

Clinical aspects affecting work capacity

Coronary heart disease

Epidemiology

Heart disease is common both in the population at large and in those of working age. CVD, including stroke and high blood pressure (BP), is responsible for more costs than any other disease or injury. Heart disease can claim the ultimate cost as the most common cause of death.

CVD is the main cause of death in the UK, accounting for over 240 000 deaths per year. The main forms of CVD are coronary heart disease (CHD) and stroke. Death before retirement age is commonly attributed to CVD, accounting for 36% of premature deaths in men and 27% of premature deaths in women. CHD is responsible for 120 000 deaths a year in the UK and is responsible for 23% of deaths before the age of 65 years in men and 13% in women. Significant advances in acute medical care have, however, brought reductions in mortality from CHD over the last 10 years. Morbidity rates have not seen that same fall; in fact, rates have risen especially in older individuals over the last 20 years. Two million people in the UK suffer from angina, 680 000 people have heart failure, and 270 000 will suffer a heart attack each year—highlighting the significance of CVD as a cause of morbidity.[1]

A recent study of self-reported work-related illness shows that record numbers of workers feel that they have an illness that was caused by or made worse by their work, equating to 2.3 million people and 33 million working days lost. These figures show a prevalence estimate for CVD caused or made worse by work of 80 000 individuals during the study year, with each person reporting work-related illness taking an average of 23 days off through sickness in the year.[2] This equates to 1.84 million days lost to work-related CVD, with associated costs to industry of approximately £120 million. In essence, the issue of heart disease and work is significant in terms of individuals affected, industry, health service resources, and national resources.

Death from CHD may be sudden, from ventricular fibrillation. In the WHO Tower Hamlets study[3] 40% of heart attacks (defined as myocardial infarction (MI) or sudden death from CHD) were fatal and 60% of deaths occurred within 1 hour of the onset of any symptoms. This early high mortality has been amply reinforced by more recent studies, and persists despite advances in treatment. Heart attacks tend to occur more frequently in the morning, or towards the beginning of shift-work, as compared with other times of the day.[4] Their onset may be associated with unaccustomed vigorous effort and acute psychosocial stress.[5]

Clinical features

CHD usually presents as chest pain, either MI or angina; it may also present with symptoms resulting from arrhythmia (including sudden death), or heart failure, or be detected incidentally by electrocardiography. Anyone with chest pain who is suspected of suffering from MI or an acute coronary syndrome should be taken urgently to the nearest coronary care unit where prompt treatment can save lives. After recovery the risk of further cardiac events (i.e. sudden death, recurrent MI or need for myocardial revascularization) is assessed by the combination of clinical features and simple investigations (see below).

Assessment

The risk of sudden disability and death through ventricular fibrillation is the major factor affecting work capacity among victims of CHD. The risk is greatest in the early days following an acute coronary event. Those with severe myocardial damage and/or continuing myocardial ischaemia form a high-risk group. The extent of ventricular damage may be judged by the presence of heart failure, gallop rhythm, and estimation of left ventricular function using simple imaging techniques such as **echocardiography**. The presence of residual areas of myocardial ischaemia may be judged by a recurrence of cardiac pain or the development of angina pectoris that may be confirmed by **exercise testing**. An exercise test may also reveal cardiovascular incapacity in other ways, namely exhaustion, inappropriate heart rate and BP responses, arrhythmia, and electrocardiographic change, especially ST segment shift. In practice, the exercise test in combination with the opinion of an accredited specialist is generally sufficient to assess fitness for work. This is reflected in the guidance material relating to vocational drivers (see Chapter 28). Individuals who are free of symptoms and signs of cardiac dysfunction and who can achieve a good workload with no adverse features, have a very low risk of further cardiac events. This applies particularly to younger individuals whose employers need have little hesitation in taking them back to work.

An ability to reach stage 4 of the Bruce protocol on a treadmill is judged to place an individual at such low risk of further cardiac events that vocational driving may be permitted. The DVLA guidelines are the result of careful deliberation by the Honorary Medical Advisory Panel and are now being applied more widely to other groups of workers whose occupation may involve an element of risk to themselves or others should that individual suffer cardiovascular collapse. Most employees, however, are not required to demonstrate such high levels of cardiovascular fitness and lower levels would be acceptable for those in more sedentary and low-risk occupations.

Those whose early investigations are inconclusive will require further tests, often including **radionuclide imaging** to assess both ventricular function and myocardial perfusion. This noninvasive technique is, however, not readily available in District Hospitals. Those who have continuing symptoms, or whose non-invasive investigations are unsatisfactory will be recommended to undergo **coronary angiography** with a view to myocardial revascularization. This is mildly unpleasant and hazardous with a risk of groin complications around 1 in 300, and catastrophes including stroke and death, about 1 in 1000. Facilities for angiography are now widely available. Most angiograms are undertaken as day case procedures.

Management strategies: medical

Life-style management and drug therapy have transformed the management of all manifestations of CHD. Employers have a duty to support and reinforce community measures by discouraging smoking, encouraging healthy activities during rest and recreational hours, and by providing a healthy diet at work. The public health White Paper[6] has decreed that smoking in enclosed workplaces must be banned by 2007, along with a ban on smoking in all public places by June 2007. Employees in the hospitality industry will only be partially protected—discussions continue. This is to be encouraged because evidence exists to show that smoking bans in the workplace impact beneficially on worker health. For example, a study in Helena Montana[7] revealed a drop of almost 40% in hospital admission of MI during the 6-month period following a ban on smoking in workplaces.

The prognosis of patients following MI is improved by thrombolysis and subsequent treatment with aspirin. Nitrates, beta-adrenergic antagonists, and calcium antagonists alleviate the symptoms of myocardial ischaemia. Diuretics and angiotensin converting enzyme inhibitors improve the symptoms and survival of patients with heart failure. Statins improve prognosis and reduce the risk of subsequent events in all groups of patients with CHD. These and other cardiovascular drugs are generally well tolerated and seem remarkably free from long-term side-effects. Many owe their efficacy to their vasodilating action; hence hypotension and faintness are possible complications.

Following an acute coronary event or MI, assessment of prognosis along the lines outlined above is recommended: those with no complications and good exercise tolerance may return to work in 4–6 weeks. A few will take longer. Patients with persistent angina or an abnormal exercise test should be assessed with a view to myocardial revascularization. All patients will require life-long medication, with aspirin and a statin as a minimum.

Coronary angioplasty and stenting (percutaneous coronary intervention)

Balloon angioplasty was introduced by Andreas Gruntzig in 1977 and for years was bedevilled by a high recurrence rate. The development of the coronary stent led to a substantial reduction in the restenosis rate. A stent is a tubular metal mesh that is delivered on the balloon in a collapsed state, down the artery and subsequently deployed at very high pressure (e.g. 16 atmospheres) into the arterial wall. The angiographic results are truly remarkable and relief of symptoms can be equally dramatic. Complex, distal, and multiple stenoses can be safely treated. The introduction of drug eluting stents for selected cases—currently smaller arteries and long lesions—has reduced the restenosis risk to almost zero. About half of all procedures are now urgent or emergency cases; for these, but not for elective cases, consent is usually obtained in order to proceed directly to stenting, following diagnostic angiography.

Success rates are of the order of 97%. Disasters, often necessitating surgery, occur in about 1 in 500 procedures. Groin haematomas are an unusual but well recognized complication. Return to work within 1 week is commonplace. Angioplasty has not yet been shown to improve the long-term survival of patients with CHD in a randomized controlled study, unlike surgery. But most cardiologists believe that opening up a major coronary artery should improve prognosis.

Coronary artery bypass grafting (CABG)

This is more complex but is also remarkably safe with most centres reporting mortality rates of about 1% for elective operations. Recovery is rapid and most patients resume work within 2–3 months of surgery and most are relieved of their angina. Patients who were working before surgery generally do so afterwards, and restrictions that may have been appropriate previously should no longer be relevant. Unfortunately, surgery constitutes a dramatic event that may prompt overprotective attitudes among family members, friends, employers, and even medical advisers. Many individuals who could and should return to work fail to do so for this reason rather than because of continuing incapacity. Waiting times, both for coronary angiography and bypass surgery, have been such that many patients do not return to work because they have lost their jobs. One study showed that of those who had lost more than six months work before operation, fewer (35%) returned to work than those who had lost less than 6 months.[8] This situation is changing because more resources are being devoted to myocardial revascularization, and many people who would have had CABG, are being rapidly and successfully treated by coronary stenting.

No special restrictions are usually necessary after return to work. Coronary graft stenosis and occlusion, however, leads to a recurrence of angina at a rate of about 4% per annum. This is generally less severe than previously but will affect long-term occupational planning. CABG for left main stem or three-vessel disease improves prognosis.

Rehabilitation programmes are now well established in many hospitals. These enable many patients to make a full physical and psychological recovery following a cardiac event such as MI or CABG.

Return to work after the development of coronary heart disease

Studies on the likelihood of returning to work after the onset of heart disease have shown that several different issues are involved.

The nature of the original cardiovascular event that led to the individual stopping work. CHD can range from acute MI to angina treated with coronary artery bypass, angioplasty or drugs alone. Whichever form it takes, the important issues for return to work are the persistence of chest pain during exercise, the risk of arrhythmia and the level of left ventricular function especially if this affects exercise capacity. In addition the possibility of silent ischaemia needs consideration for high-risk individuals. Interestingly, while angioplasty ensures a more speedy return to work than CABG, long-term employment prospects are the same in both treatment groups.[9]

Associated hypertension with symptoms such as headache, dizziness, or general malaise may make return to work difficult. The physical and psychological impact of work may induce worsening hypertension and compound the problem. Where possible, treatment regimens should be effective and stabilized prior to return to work.

The residual loss of function following the cardiac event. Functional capacity of the individual should be assessed prior to return to work. For cardiac disease an exercise stress test will give the information required. Assessment of individuals with cardiac failure may need additional investigation. Whereas cardiac failure once meant that a return to work was unlikely, improvements in treatment regimens now mean that more people with heart failure can return to work. Whatever condition gave rise to the cardiac failure needs treatment and the more effective this is, the more likely is the individual to return to work.

The prognosis of the causative CVD. Prognostic indicators are well documented for most cardiovascular problems. Where the prognosis is poor and the risk of recurrence high, return to work may be inappropriate and create unrealistic expectations for the patient and his family.

The nature of the individual. Psychological factors may play a much bigger part in whether an individual returns to work than medical/clinical factors. Research has shown some useful pointers regarding the likelihood of an individual returning to work after a cardiac event.

- Independent of the prognosis of the CVD, the longer an individual is off sick, the harder it is to return them to work.
- If the cardiac event happened at work, return can be more difficult.
- The older the patient, especially if a pension is available, the more unlikely it is he will return to work.
- Where the job is seen as unrewarding/unfulfilling, a patient is less motivated to return to work. In addition, if the job is seen as dangerous or damaging to health, return will be more difficult.
- When redeployment/retraining is difficult to achieve due to certain individual factors such as education, adaptability, or even personality, the likelihood of returning that individual to work is reduced.
- Attitude of employer:
  - fear of further illness at work and subsequent litigation can act as a barrier to return to work. Many employers take a defensive stance in this situation.
  - reluctance to consider rehabilitation/redeployment will make return to work more difficult.
  - a 'cardionoxious' work environment in the organization which can be physical or related to the culture of the organization will hinder a return to work.
- Attitude of the individual:
  - fear of future illness
  - lack of motivation/understanding of the illness
  - benefits of the 'sick role'.

  ◆ Attitude of the State
    • sickness benefit may be generous and with low paid jobs better than being at work
    • safety-related medical standards and acceptability of 'risk' are covered by legislation and regulatory authorities, which if overcautious, can prevent some people returning to work

In all cases, return to work should be phased whenever possible, both in terms of time and intensity.

Return to work

In all cases, when work is resumed, the levels and duration of activity should be increased progressively; returning to work implies a level of sustained activity well above that achieved by most who are recovering at home or who are undertaking hospital rehabilitation programmes.

Psychological difficulties may be experienced even by those with no signs of cardiac damage. Anxieties of both the patient and spouse or partner have been shown to affect the ability of men surviving MI to return to work; half may have some anxiety or depression and, of those, half may have severe symptoms persisting, if untreated, a year later.[10]

In general, physical activity is good for the heart. The degree of physical activity must take into account patients' previous fitness and the results of exercise testing, etc. Patients with stable angina pectoris can safely work within their limitations of fitness but should not be put in situations where their angina may be readily provoked. Although it may be possible to be dogmatic in giving advice about physical work, guidance about the psychological stresses associated with managerial duties must be individually tailored.[11] Personality has a small influence on survival following MI.

The existence of patterns of coronary-prone behaviour is well embedded in Western business culture. The results of epidemiological and clinical studies have been conflicting; the idea that psychological stress has a role in the aetiology of CHD is nevertheless a persistent one and owes much to the work of Friedman and his colleagues who suggested that modification of hectic work patterns marked by long hours, competitiveness, time urgency, and aggression (so-called type A behaviour) as part of other stress reduction measures may be beneficial.[12]

Not everyone will be able to go back to their own work after a coronary event. In light engineering it has been observed that after 1 year about half those returning were fully fit, requiring no job change. The remainder had some limitation of fitness; half required a job change.[8] About one-tenth of all those returning to work had severe limitations of fitness requiring a change of work. Work responding to emergency calls may place unacceptable demands on the cardiovascular system and such duties should be avoided. Heavy physical work, the need to climb up and down stairs, rapid and tight pacing of repetitive operations, such as component assembly, technical skill, and the stress of responsibility will all be relevant. In most situations a full working day must be managed from the day of restarting despite professional advice to the contrary. Tiredness, which will often be more burdensome initially, usually resolves over the subsequent days or weeks. It may be helpful to arrange temporary shorter hours, perhaps curtailing both ends of the day, so as to avoid rush-hour travelling. This recommendation can usually be accomplished by a defined time through which the hours can be extended towards the full working day. By defining this time period, the perceived stress on colleagues and the employer would be reduced rather than leaving the period of phased return open-ended.

The stress of managing or supervising may be underappreciated and consideration will need to be given to the time necessary to catch up with events that the employee will have missed while being away, and to allow a gradual resumption of responsibilities. The requirements of overtime work, meetings that occur early or late in the day, and the managerial responsibility that may be exercised all demand understanding For some, shortening the hours of work temporarily signals to the organization that the employee is not yet fully recovered, and perhaps encourages those who have been managing in the employee's absence to continue to do so for a further period of time.

Psychological stress may arise from a variety of circumstances peculiar to the patient, his relatives, friends (and others), or his particular working circumstances. These factors are usually the source of discouragement and may delay recovery. In the present climate of employment many individuals will take the opportunity to cease work and hope to obtain favourable financial terms; many will be disappointed.

Formerly, vocational drivers, i.e. those holding large goods vehicle (LGV) and passenger carrying vehicle (PCV) licences, rarely regained their licences following the development of heart disease and then only after extensive testing including angiography. This situation has now changed, partly because of our better understanding of the natural history of CHD, our ability to identify high-risk populations, and because of the availability of more effective treatments. Those at low risk of cardiovascular collapse can be identified by a combination of clinical factors and 'non-invasive' testing.

Screening for coronary disease

Those populations at high risk of sudden incapacity can be identified once their disease has declared itself. But silent coronary disease is extremely common. For example coronary angiography in patients being investigated before heart valve replacement, has revealed disease in approximately one-third.[13] Sudden death may be the first manifestation of coronary disease.

Many cardiac events will therefore occur in those who appear to be fit—approximately one-quarter in studies of road traffic accidents for example. These may well be sudden and cannot be predicted. One solution to this problem is to attempt to screen employees for 'silent' myocardial ischaemia. This may be justifiable in certain groups of individuals and has been adopted by the US Air Force for example. The usual screening measures are a clinical examination and an exercise test. Exercise-induced electrocardiographic ST segment change in an asymptomatic individual has a variety of causes; using the criterion of 1 mm ST segment depression about one-third will turn out to have coronary disease on angiography.[14] Screening for asymptomatic CHD in this way cannot therefore be recommended *routinely* because of the high incidence of false positive results. Simple clinical features such as age, male sex, history of chest pain, smoking habit, or a strong family history of premature CHD, and physical examination are better methods of assessing apparently asymptomatic individuals. If there is a strong clinical suspicion of CHD and a certain diagnosis is essential, then coronary angiography should be undertaken. This policy, however, would only be justifiable in those with very high-risk occupations. In the future other imaging techniques will become available and may well change this view; at present electron beam computerized tomography (EBCT) appears to be the most promising non-invasive technique.

Congenital and valvular heart disease

Individuals with congenital heart disease and also young people with acquired heart disease may ask for specific career advice. Generally this is likely to relate to careers that have defined medical standards at pre-employment such as the armed forces and other 'safety critical' jobs. Early discussions can help to develop appropriate expectations and informed career choices for these individuals.

Individuals suffering from congenital heart disease will generally be detected in childhood and should seek *specialist* advice before entering employment. Employers should not be deterred from taking on young people who have undergone cardiac surgery for the correction of congenital defects in childhood, as many lead a normal life and are capable of full-time employment. Acquired valve disease, usually degenerative aortic stenosis or mitral regurgitation, is most commonly seen nowadays in those beyond working age but the condition of mitral valve prolapse deserves emphasis because it affects some 2% of the population and carries an excellent prognosis; it often presents as an auscultatory finding at a pre-employment medical examination, may be associated with electrocardiographic change, and may sometimes lead to a false diagnosis of significant heart disease.

The satisfactory results of valve surgery have led to the practice of early operation, before left ventricular function declines. Many mitral valves can be repaired nowadays, leading to full functional recovery and no need for medication. The use of catheter techniques is expanding; percutaneous balloon valvotomy is now the treatment of choice for pulmonary stenosis in children and rheumatic mitral stenosis, as are *occlusion* devices for closing the smaller atrial septal defects.

Following replacement of the aortic or mitral valves by mechanical or biological prostheses patients generally recover rapidly and resume work fully 2–3 months after the operation. Those with mechanical valves need to take anticoagulants indefinitely and are thus at slightly increased risk from bleeding, serious bleeding occurring at a rate of some 2% per annum. Sudden failure of mechanical valves is extremely uncommon. Biological valves undergo slow deterioration and do fail suddenly, some years after implantation. They are therefore used rarely in people of working age.

Cardiac arrhythmias

Transient cardiac arrhythmias (e.g. extrasystoles) are extremely common and do not usually indicate heart disease. They may be provoked by a variety of substances, e.g. alcohol, coffee. Assessment by a specialist is recommended for those with persisting symptoms. A few individuals will suffer recurrent arrhythmias. The commonest is atrial fibrillation, which affects 2% of the population at some time in their lives and tends to be paroxysmal in individuals of working age. Drug treatment is sometimes required and for some an opportunity to withdraw from work and rest for a short period may be necessary. For others with supraventricular tachycardia curative treatment is now available in the form of catheter ablation of the accessory electrical pathway that subserves the re-entrant tachycardia.

The prognosis for individuals with more serious arrhythmias occurring in the context of heart muscle disease is determined by the underlying cardiac pathology, which is often myocardial scarring as a result of CHD. Continued employment for these individuals may be inadvisable. Complete heart block generally requires permanent pacing (see below) but first- and second-degree block may be incidental findings in otherwise healthy people that requires no further action.

Syncope

Syncope, other than a simple faint, requires specialist evaluation including a neurological review if appropriate. Following unexplained syncope, provocation testing and investigation for arrhythmia must be implemented. If the results are satisfactory return to work is recommended including (re-)licensing for vocational drivers after 3 months. Careful follow-up is mandatory.

Pacemakers and implantable devices

Pacemakers

The presence of an implanted cardiac pacemaker to maintain regular heart action is entirely compatible with normal life including strenuous work. The underlying heart condition for which the pacemaker was implanted may, however, impose its own restrictions.

The indications for cardiac pacing are widening as the efficacy of this form of treatment improves; modern pacemaker technology allows pacing of atria and ventricles, variation in the output of the generator, facilities for telemetry, etc.

Virtually all pacemakers have the capacity to sense and be inhibited by the patient's own heart rhythm. Somatic muscle action potentials and electromagnetic fields can in theory interfere with the pacemaker, causing temporary cessation of pacing. Usually the interference will be brief and the pacemaker will revert to a fixed-rate mode so that symptoms will be minimal.

Implantable cardioverter defibrillators

The implantable cardioverter defibrillator (ICD) is now the preferred treatment for individuals with ventricular tachycardia and/or fibrillation whose arrhythmia is refractory to drugs or myocardial revascularization. Generally, the individual will have experienced at least one cardiac arrest. The device is implanted by a cardiologist under local anaesthetic but is tested under general anaesthetic. Both ventricular tachycardia and fibrillation can be detected and treated, for the former by antitachycardia pacing and the latter by a DC shock. In either event transient impairment of consciousness is possible and hence certain jobs, e.g. vocational driving, are not permitted.

Hypertension

Hypertension carries the risk of sudden disability from stroke; discovery of this condition may require cessation of employment where a serious accident risk exists. When considering the need to continue in employment, well-controlled hypertension may be risk-free. Powerful drug regimens may carry the risk of hypotension with resultant giddiness and fatigue. Central nervous system side-effects may affect judgement and the performance of skilled tasks. But modern antihypertensive therapy with beta-adrenergic and calcium antagonists, diuretics, and angiotensin-converting enzyme inhibitors is generally free from side-effects.

Patients with controlled hypertension can expect to manage most varieties of working activity. Frequent postural changes occasionally prove troublesome due to altered central and peripheral vascular responses. Very heavy physical work and exposure to very hot conditions with high humidity may result in postural hypotension. Provided BP readings can be maintained under satisfactory control and are checked regularly, heavy goods and public service vehicle driving is allowed.

Other circulatory disorders

Peripheral vascular disease may cause intermittent claudication that limits the victim's mobility. Medical treatment is relatively unsatisfactory; surgical/interventional treatment can be very successful. The prognosis depends upon any associated coronary disease. The presence of an aortic aneurysm also indicates arterial disease and a liability to vascular catastrophe. Cerebrovascular disease is commonly accompanied by CHD, to the extent that most stroke victims die a cardiac death. All these groups of patients should be carefully assessed, both clinically and by non-invasive investigations, with particular attention being paid to the likelihood of cardiac involvement.

Raynaud's phenomenon, on the other hand, is a benign, albeit distressing, complaint. Underlying causes should be excluded; vibrational trauma from work with chain saws or pneumatic hammer devices must be avoided. Sufferers should work in a warm environment and be allowed to wear gloves and heated socks if indicated.

Special work issues

Physical activity

As a general rule activities that cause no undue symptoms can be undertaken safely. Careful history taking will identify what activities are possible, initially by eliciting activities of daily living (ADL) then correlating these with equivalent work activities. A useful model to quantify what individual workers are capable of in terms of physical activity is that of metabolic equivalents or METS. This can also be compared with the results of exercise testing in that: Stage 1 of the Bruce Protocol is 4.6; Stage 2 is 7.0; Stage 3 is 10.1; Stage 4 is 12.9 METS.

Table 17.1 describes the different levels of physical activity using ADL along with occupational activities.

Jobs that may require extreme physical effort, for example those in the emergency services, may be unsuitable for anyone with CHD. Each case must be judged on its individual merit and specialist advice taken as required.

Lifting weights

Only the very fit and confident might reasonably attempt heavy work, such as lifting 40–100 lb (23–45 kg). Many employees may quite comfortably manage medium work, such as lifting 25–50 lb (11–23 kg) perhaps at the rate of once a minute, providing they do not have any other physical limitations. The presence of support for the weights and keeping them at waist height eases the strain considerably, and if the task only requires the weights to be slid along benches or roller tracks, then the effective strain will be reduced by some 50%. Those with moderate to severe restriction may need to be confined to a maximum of 10 lb (4.5 kg) or an equivalent degree of force on levers, turning wheels, and similar machine controls. In any work organization there may be a few jobs requiring lightweight detailed work or simple checking, which are suitable for those who are quite severely disabled. Some patients have sufficient skills to learn inspection tasks that may be physically much less stressful. Other opportunities may be found in material and production control, progress chasing, recording, indexing, etc., which may allow continued work in fairly heavy industries.

Physical effort requirement well above normal, such as work in foundries and forges, may well be reasons for barring such employment in patients with heart disease, especially those with symptoms of shortness of breath or angina.

Rapid and tightly controlled pacing of work, such as on assembly lines, has not been shown to be a precipitating factor for MI and should not inhibit a normal return to work after a heart attack. If employees were managing satisfactorily before their infarction they may well manage afterwards if they are not severely disabled by shortness of breath or angina. Returning to their own work, where social support is provided by former rather than new colleagues, may be less of a problem than trying a new task.

Psychosocial hazards

As early as 1958 evidence began to emerge that exposure to 'occupational stress and strain' was much higher in young male coronary patients than in equivalent healthy controls.[15] At the same

Table 17.1 Some metabolic equivalents (METS)

1–2 METS
Doing seated ADLs (eating, performing facial hygiene, resting)
Doing seated recreation (sewing, playing cards, painting)
Doing seated occupational activities (writing, typing, doing clerical work)
2–3 METS
Standing ADLs (dressing, showering, shaving, doing light housework)
Standing occupation (mechanic, bartender, autorepair)
Standing recreation (fishing, playing billiards, shuffleboard)
Walking (2.5 mph)
4–5 METS
Doing heavy housework (scrubbing floor, hanging out washing)
Canoeing, golfing, playing softball, tennis (doubles)
Social dancing, cross country hiking
Swimming (20 yards/min)
Walking 4 mph (level), 3 mph (5% gradient)
Bike ride 10 mph
6–7 METS
Heavy gardening (digging dirt, manual lawn mowing, hoeing)
Skating, water skiing, playing tennis (singles)
Stair climbing (<27 ft/min)
Swimming (25 yards/min)
Walking 5 mph (level), 3.5 mph (5% gradient)
8–9 METS
Active occupation (sawing wood, digging ditches, shovelling snow)
Active recreation (downhill skiing, playing ice hockey, paddleball)
Bike riding (12–14 mph)
Stair climbing (more than 27 ft/min)
Swimming 35 yards/min
Walking 10 mph (level), 3 mph (15% gradient)

ADL = activity of daily living

time, Friedman *et al.* published their findings showing a significant relationship with serum cholesterol levels and blood clotting times and a cyclical variation of worker-related stress in a group of accountants.[16] While these early reports were viewed with scepticism, the relationship always seemed plausible and now enjoys support from many more studies that have continued to demonstrate a relationship between work-related stress and the development of CVD.

A major contributor to this field is Karasek who introduced the concept of the 'Job Strain Model'.[17] Karasek postulated that strain occurs where there is excessive psychological workplace demands coupled with low job decision latitude. Social isolation has been added to this combination more recently as an additional deleterious factor. Karasek also postulated that work, where high demands were coupled with high decision latitude, led to increased learning with the likelihood of improved coping mechanisms and improved health outcome measures, i.e. high demands were not deleterious of themselves, it was the coupling with lack of control. A detailed analysis of studies of job strain and ischaemic heart disease in men[17] showed that when taken together, a significant positive relation existed between exposure to low control and/or job strain and the subsequent development of CVD. Cohort studies also demonstrate the temporal nature of the association.

One mechanism by which job strain could predispose to CHD is by increasing BP levels. Where casual BP readings are used, this correlation is very limited. For ambulatory BP measurements, the associated rise with job strain exposure extends beyond work periods into leisure time and evidence exists that reduction in the levels of 'exposure', i.e. job strain, reduces the likelihood of morbidity in this group—said by Heinberg to be 'the most conclusive evidence of causality'.[18] Obesity is another factor that has been shown in some studies to be significantly associated with job strain and a study of American chemical operators in 1990 showed that even after controlling for socio-demographic factors, those workers exposed to higher levels of job strain smoked more than comparable workers in lower job strain roles.[19] There is, therefore, some evidence building that job strain impacts on the likelihood of development of CVD via changes in BP and other cardiac risk factors.

Another measure of the psychological impact of work is the effort–reward model, which looks at effort/reward imbalance in the workplace. The Whitehall Study[20] showed that exposure to high effort and low reward at work was associated with double the risk of newly reported CHD over 5.3 years. Work that requires employees to maintain a high level of vigilance to prevent major incidents/accidents presents a greater psychological burden than many jobs. Such work includes professional drivers, air traffic controllers, sea pilots, etc. Epidemiological studies have shown some association between this type of work and CVD outcomes.[17]

Shift work is recognized as an occupational risk factor for CVD. There is, unfortunately, no agreed definition of shift work but it usually applies to fixed work at night, roster work, and specific shift patterns—of which there are many. The number of people working shifts appears to be increasing. Many people have second jobs. In Europe about 18% of the workforce works at night 25% of the time and even more work outside normal hours.[21] This means that shift work is one of the most common work environment risk factors for CVD. However, shift work is unlikely to be eradicated since society requires that some work outside of normal hours continues so that attempts to modify the impact of shift work on cardiovascular health will need to be by manipulating and reducing the links that shift work has with the development of CVD.

It has been postulated that the link between shift work and CVD is via three pathways—mismatch of circadian rhythms, social disruption, and behavioural changes. The mismatched circadian rhythm relates in part to eating patterns—eating more calories at night than during the day has been associated with higher cholesterol levels.[22] MI rates and angina are higher in the early morning and this parallels markers of neurohumoral activation. It has therefore been suggested that mismatch of oxygen supply to cardiac muscle may precipitate this increased rate of angina. Workers requiring extra-cardiac effort at this time may be at greater risk. Shift work impacts on the availability of social support and lack of social support is well recognized as a risk factor for CVD. Finally, shift work often leads to behavioural changes, which are risk factors for CVD. These include higher smoking rates, altered eating habits—snacks or missed meals—and one study showed that shift workers, though not significantly heavier than non-shift workers, had more centrally deposited adipose tissue—another risk factor for CVD.[23] Exercise levels and alcohol consumption were no worse in shift workers than non-shift workers.

The INTERHEART case–control study[24] has reinforced the link between psychosocial risk factors and the risk of acute MI. Multiple elements of stress—work, home, and financial, along with the incidence of major life events in the preceding year showed a significant correlation with the risk of MI. Additional questions relate to locus of control and the presence of depression. The study examined 11,119 cases from 52 different countries and hence is valid in multiple populations and ethnic groups. A third more cases experienced several periods of work stress than controls (odds ratio 1.38; 99% confidence interval 1.19–1.61) and permanent work stress was experienced by twice as many cases than controls (odds ratio 2.14; 1.73–2.64). Population attributable risks (PARs) i.e. the proportion of all cases attributable to the relevant risk factor if causality were proven was calculated. The PAR for stress at work and depression were both 9%, when the PAR for financial stress was 11%. The PAR for low locus of control was 16%. Combining all risk factors gave a PAR of 33%, If this effect is truly causal then psychosocial factors are much more important than commonly recognized.

The conclusion that psychosocial factors are important in the development of CHD is now inescapable, such that efforts should be made in the workplace to reduce these factors. The relative contribution as compared with traditional risk factors, and how best to ameliorate their impact are questions that merit urgent clarification.

Toxic substances

Work involving exposure to certain hazardous substances may aggravate pre-existing CHD and careful consideration should be given to patients who are returning to jobs involving exposure to chemical vapours and fumes. Methylene chloride, a main ingredient of many commonly used paint removers, is rapidly metabolized to carbon monoxide in the body and in poorly ventilated work areas, blood levels of carboxyhaemoglobin can become elevated enough to precipitate angina or even MI. A blood carboxyhaemoglobin level of 2–4% has been shown to be associated with impairment of cardiovascular function in patients with angina pectoris.

Smokers, especially pipe smokers, will have an elevated blood carboxyhaemoglobin due to their smoking, which will obviously be additive to any carbon monoxide in the workplace potentially increasing their risk of adverse cardiac events.

The World Health Organization[25] recommends a maximum carboxyhaemoglobin level of 5% for healthy industrial workers and a maximum of 2.5% for susceptible persons in the general population exposed to ambient air pollution; this level may also be applied to workers whose jobs entail specific exposure to carbon monoxide, e.g. carpark attendants, furnace workers, etc. There is a good correlation between carbon monoxide levels in the air with blood carboxyhaemoglobin, in accordance with the Coburn equation*, and the WHO guideline level of 2.5% implies an 8-hour occupational exposure average, well below the current occupational exposure standard of 50 p.p.m. In fact, to ensure that the 2.5% carboxyhaemoglobin level is not exceeded, the ambient carbon monoxide concentration should not be higher than 10 p.p.m. over an 8-hour working day: equivalent to exposure to the current occupational exposure standard (50 p.p.m.) for no more than 30 minutes. Occupational exposure to carbon disulphide in the viscose rayon manufacturing industry is a recognized causal factor of CHD but the mechanism remains unclear.

Reports of sudden death from angina are well recognized in dynamite workers, particularly after a period of 36–72 hours away from work and following re-exposure, an effect almost certainly related to direct action of nitroglycerine on the blood vessels of the heart or peripheral circulation. Persons with clinical evidence of CHD should avoid occupational exposure to these substances.

---

*See *J Clin Invest* 1965; **44**:1899–1910.

Solvents, such as trichloroethylene or 1,1,1-trichloroethane, may sensitize the myocardium to the action of endogenous catecholamines resulting in ventricular fibrillation and sudden death in workers receiving heavy exposure in poorly ventilated workplaces.[26] Chlorofluorocarbons (CFCs) are still widely used as propellants in aerosol cans and as refrigerants—CFC-113 has been implicated in sudden cardiac deaths and CFC-22 has been reported to cause arrhythmias in laboratory workers using an aerosol preparation. Certain industrial workers will need proper assessment of their workplace by an occupational physician with an occupational hygienist, so that they can be advised on their suitability for work handling chlorinated hydrocarbon solvents or involving exposure to gases.

There are no formal medical requirements for workers who have to enter confined spaces where there may be hazards of oxygen deficiency or a build up of toxic gases. Persons with heart disease or severe hypertension may need to be excluded. Certain occupations may require the use of special breathing apparatus either routinely (e.g. asbestos removal workers), or in emergencies (e.g. water workers handling chlorine cylinders). The additional cardiorespiratory effort required while wearing a respirator, combined with the general physical exertion that may be required, usually means that persons with a previous history of CHD are excluded from such work.

Hot conditions

Working in hot conditions may prove difficult for some patients with heart disease. High ambient temperatures or significant heat radiation from hot surfaces or liquid metal, added to the physical strain of heavy work, will produce quite profound vasodilatation of muscle and skin vessels. Compensatory vascular and cardiac reactions to maintain central BP may be inadequate and lead to reduced cerebral or coronary artery blood flow. The resulting weakness or giddiness could prove dangerous. As many cardioactive drugs have vasodilating and negative inotropic actions, some reduction in dosage may be necessary.

Cold conditions

Cold is a notorious trigger of myocardial ischaemia and caution must therefore be exercised for individuals who suffer from CHD. Impaired circulation to the limbs will result in an increased risk of claudication, risk of damage to skin (frostbite), and poor recovery from accidental injury to skin and deeper structures.

Travel

Following a cardiac event such as MI, individuals should convalesce at home and not travel. They should then be assessed by a specialist at 4–6 weeks. Those with no evidence of continuing myocardial ischaemia or cardiac pump failure can then travel freely within the UK for pleasure. Business and overseas travel is more problematical because the physical and psychological demands are greater. Additional difficulties for the overseas traveller include the uncertain provision of coronary care facilities in some countries and the justifiable reluctance of insurance companies to provide health cover. Such travel is best deferred until 3 months have elapsed and any necessary further investigations and treatment have been carried out to ensure cardiovascular fitness.

Overseas travel for those with continuing cardiovascular unfitness need not be ruled out. Utilizing the airport services for disabled travellers can ease a passenger through customs, passport control, etc., at major airports like Heathrow. Modern aircraft can be very comfortable. The cabins are kept at a pressure equivalent to 6000 feet (2000 metres) so that those with angina are not likely to experience an attack; most developed countries have an excellent coronary care service.

Businessmen with continuing cardiac disorders may therefore fly to Europe and North America with very little risk. Flights in unpressurized aircraft, work in undeveloped countries or in remote areas of the world, and work in a hostile environment (both climatic and political) is best avoided. Aircrew are subject to CAA guidelines whose advice should always be sought (See also Appendix 5).

Cardiac deaths are uncommon in trekkers or workers at high altitude (8000–15 000 ft/ 2440–4570 m). The increase in cardiac output at altitude will exacerbate symptoms in those who already experience symptoms at sea level, but asymptomatic individuals with CHD are unlikely to be at special risk.

Ordinary driving may be resumed 1 month after a cardiac event provided that the driver does not suffer from angina that may be provoked at the wheel. Vocational driving may be permitted at 6 weeks, subject to a satisfactory outcome from non-invasive testing (see Chapter 28). Ordinary driving licence holders do not need to notify the DVLA, Swansea if they have made a good recovery and have no continuing disability, but vocational drivers must notify the DVLA. Insurance companies vary in their requirements but most policies are temporarily invalidated by illness. (See also Chapter 28 for details.)

Electromagnetic fields

Industrial electrical sources such as arc welding, faulty domestic equipment, engines, antitheft devices, airport weapon detectors, radar and citizen-band radio, all generate electromagnetic fields that can, in theory, affect pacemakers and ICDs; but the patient has to be very close to the power source before any interference can be demonstrated. Any pacemaker abnormality is usually confined to one or two missed beats or reversion to the fixed mode. The number of documented cases of interference in the UK is less than three a year.[27,28] ICD discharges are equally rare.

If pacemaker patients are expected to work in the vicinity of high-energy electric or magnetic fields capable of producing signals at a rate and pattern similar to a QRS complex (e.g. on some electrical generating and transmission equipment and welding) then formal testing is recommended. The cardiac centre responsible for implanting the pacemaker will usually provide a technical service for this purpose, thus enabling the risk of interference to be defined precisely. Magnetic resonance imaging machines are found in certain chemical laboratories and many hospital radiological departments. Patients with pacemakers and ICDs should not be subjected to magnetic resonance imaging. Persons with implanted devices are generally advised to avoid work that may bring them into close contact with strong magnetic fields. If a patient should experience untoward symptoms or collapse while near electrical apparatus then he should move/be moved away, but the likely cause of the symptoms will be unrelated to the device. Patients with implanted devices carry cards that identify the type of pacemaker, the supervising cardiac centre, etc. Further advice is readily available from the British Pacing and Electrophysiology Group (see Appendix 8 for the address).

Patients with ICDs may have severe underlying heart disease and may well not be able to work. But if they can work then this should be in a safe electromagnetic environment. There has been one report of a patient who collapsed in the vicinity of an electronic antitheft surveillance system in a bookstore and who was shown to have ICD malfunction.[29] The advice for patients with these devices is to explain to the attendant that they have an ICD or pacemaker and not to loiter in the vicinity of shop doors or airport detector gates.

There has been considerable interest in the possibility that mobile telephones might interfere with pacemakers and ICDs. Studies have shown that this is a theoretical possibility and that re-programming of a pacemaker can be achieved under exceptional circumstances if the telephone is held close (less than 20 cm) to the pacemaker. In practice no clinically significant interference has yet been reported, but individuals are advised to use the hand and ear furthest from the pacemaker and not to 'dial' with the telephone near to the pacemaker.

Physical hazards

Raynaud's phenomenon can be caused by the use of vibrating tools and work processes that transmit vibration to the fingers (vibration-induced white finger). Common situations are the use of power-saws, pneumatic chisels, and rough grinding of metal objects. Further advice on fitness in users of vibrating tools can be found in Appendix 6.

Cuts and bruises from accidental contact with furniture, machinery, etc., or from dropped objects, may not heal at all well in the presence of circulatory restriction, and there could be a risk of the onset of gangrene and the subsequent need for disabling operations. Limbs at risk need adequate protection continuously while at work.

Varicose veins of the legs present similar problems; accidental injury may lead to severe blood loss and protection is essential. Work routines involving standing still are difficult to cope with but some walking is helpful. Sitting for long uninterrupted periods may aggravate ankle swelling and, if the hip and knee are awkwardly flexed, there could be some risk of vascular thrombosis. (See also Chapter 16.)

Where an occupation has a trauma risk that cannot be eradicated, individuals with vascular disease merit very careful consideration.

The future of work

Current trends in working life for most people are not improving. Many workers spend longer hours at work, often with deteriorating work conditions and work environments. A study in Europe in 1996 showed that 23% of employees worked more than 45 hours a week. Similarly, in America working hours have increased by 3.5 hours up to 47 hours a week between 1977 and 1996.

Changes have also occurred in relation to the nature of work in industrialized nations over the past four decades. The main changes relate to increased workload demands and increasing pace of work. Some increase in job decision latitude or control over work tasks has occurred but at an insufficient rate to compensate for the increased demands. Men and women are working harder now than 25 years ago. New systems of work organization have been introduced by employers to bring about increased productivity, better quality of goods/services and of course increased profitability. These systems go under various euphemisms—lean production, total quality management, or modular manufacturing. Very often such changes are introduced without consultation with workers—80% of US workers want to have a better say in decisions about their job.[30]

The features of lean production such as downsizing, outsourcing, 24-hour working, increased overtime and increased worker flexibility have all been made easier by the loss or reduction of union influence. Downsizing and excessive overtime can have negative effects on workers' health; in addition such changes often act as serious barriers in returning an individual back into work after a period of illness. These same issues need to be taken into account when assessing individuals at pre-employment to ensure work suitability and also impact on decisions relating to ill-health retirement as it may be very difficult to introduce reasonable adjustments or redeploy in such organizations. It is important to remember that many of these organizational changes result in negative effects on health and indeed contribute to increased CVD risk particularly in the lower socio-economic groups.[31]

Two other groups at work need consideration—that is women and the elderly worker. Most women now work. Women tend to work in service industries—office work, sales, healthcare, and teaching. This type of work is often associated with a higher prevalence of job strain and with a lower level of job control than in most men's jobs. The additional impact of family responsibilities for many women adds to these stressful exposures. In spite of the increasing involvement of women in paid work, women still spend more hours in child caring and housework than men. In western Europe women spent an average of 35 hours a week in childcare and housework before 1975 and 31 hours after 1975. Men spent 8 and 11 hours, respectively, during the same period.[31] In the Framingham Study,[32] employed women with three or more children had a higher incidence of CVD than employed women with no children, or housewives with three or more children. Women who work shifts or long hours appear to have an increased rate of hospitalization for MI, whereas for men, moderate overtime may be protective. This gender difference may be explained by the difficulties women find in combining family responsibilities with irregular or long working hours.

By 2020 the UK population will include 19 million people over 60 years of age. This is the population bulge that followed World War II, which is having major implications for the population at large. In 1975, 95% of 55–65-year-old men worked; by 1999 the figure had fallen to 60%. Since then the UK government has undertaken various initiatives to get older people to continue working longer. If these initiatives are successful, individuals will continue to work beyond the retirement age of 65. Since much CVD is more common in an ageing population, it is likely that these demographic changes will impact on *all* aspects of heart disease and work. (See also Chapter 26.)

Legal aspects

It is clear from the preceding that work can be 'cardionoxious' for many reasons—chemical, physical, and psychosocial. In the UK the level of cardiotoxicity is subject to a variety of regulations that are designed to ensure that all work is assessed in terms of its impact on health. The Management of Health and Safety at Work Regulations (1999) imposes this duty on employers and is backed up by more specific legislation, which, for example, considers chemical hazards (Control of Substances Hazardous to Health (COSHH) Regulations 2002).

The Working Time Directive aims to limit excessive working hours but will not necessarily alter shift patterns, which may, over time, impact adversely on cardiovascular health.

The Disability Discrimination Act 1995 is designed to minimize discriminatory practice at work. Disability is defined by the Disability Discrimination Act as 'a physical or mental impairment, which has a substantial and long-term adverse effect on a person's ability to carry out day to day activities'. In certain cardiovascular conditions this will be obvious but in others it may not be. Importantly, assessment of whether an individual is legally disabled is done after discounting the beneficial effect of any medication/treatment they are receiving or have received (e.g. angioplasty or surgery).

References

1 *Coronary heart disease statistics*. British Heart Foundation Strategic Database, 2003.

2 Jones JR, Huxtable S, Hodgson JT, Price MJ. Self Reported Work-Related Illness in Great Britain 2001–2002. Results from a household survey. London: National Statistics HSE.

3 Tunstall-Pedoe H, Clayton D, Morris JN, Brigden W, MacDonald I. Coronary heart attack in East London. *Lancet* 1975; **ii:** 833–8.

4 Muller JE *et al*. Circadian variation in the frequency of onset of myocardial infarction. *N Engl J Med* 1985; **313**: 1315–22.

5 Mittleman MA, Maclure M, Tofler GH, Sherwood JB, Goldberg RJ, Muller JE. Triggering of acute myocardial infarction by heavy physical exertion. *N Engl J Med* 1993; **329**: 1677–83.

6 *Choosing health: making healthier choices easier*. Public Health White Paper CM6374. Department of Health, 2004.

7 Sargent R *et al*. Reduced incidence of admissions for myocardial infarction associated with public smoking ban before and after study. *BMJ* 2004; **10**: 1136.

8 Nagle R, Gangola R, Picton-Robinson I. Factors influencing return to work after myocardial infarction. *Lancet* 1971; **2**: 454–6.

9 Hlatky MA, Boothroyd D, Harine S, *et al*. Employment after coronary angioplasty or coronary bypass surgery in patients employed at the time of revascularisation. *Ann Intern Med* 1998; **129**: 543–7.

10 Clark DB, Edward FC, Williams WG. *Cardiac surgery and return to work in the West Midlands. Cardiac rehabilitation*, pp. 61–70. Proceedings of the Society of Occupational Medicine Research Panel Symposium, London, 1983.

11 Cay EL. *The influence of psychological problems in returning to work after a myocardial infarction. Cardiac rehabiliation*, pp. 42–60. Proceedings of the Society of Occupational Medicine Research Panel Symposium, London, 1983.

12 Friedman M, Thorensen CE, Gill JJ. Alteration of type A behaviour and its effect on cardiac recurrence in post myocardial infarction patients. Summary results of the recurrent coronary prevention project. *Am Heart J* 1986; **112**: 653–5.

13 Enriques-Sarano M, Klodus F, Garratt KN, Bailey KR, Tajik AJ, *et al*. Secular trends in coronary atherosclerosis—analysis in patients with valvular regurgitation. *N. Engl J Med* 1996; **335**: 316–22.

14 Froelicher VF *et al*. Angiographic findings in asymptomatic aircrew with electrocardiographic abnormalities. *Am J Cardiol* 1977; **39**: 31–8.

15 Russek HI, Zohman BL. Relative significance of heredity, diet and occupational stress in coronary heart disease in young adults. *Am J Med Sci* 1958; **235**: 266–75.

16 Friedman M, Rosenman RH, Carroll V. Changes in the serum cholesterol and blood clotting time in men subjected to cyclical variations in occupational stress. *Circulation* 1958; **17**: 852–61.

17 Steenland K *et al*. Research findings linking workplace factors to cardiovascular disease outcomes. *Occup Med* 2000; **15**: 7–68.

18 Heinberg S. Evaluation of epidemiologic studies in assessing the long term effects of occupational noxious agents. *Scand J Work Environ Health* 1980; **6**: 163–9.

19 Green KL, Johnson JV. The effects of psychosocial work organisation on patterns of cigarette smoking among male chemical plant employees. *Am J Public Health* 1990; **80**: 1368–71.

20 Bosma H, Marmot MG, Hemingway, Nicholson AC, Brunner E, Stansfield SA. Low job control and risk of coronary heart disease. In: Whitehall II (Prospective Cohort Study). *BMJ* 1997; **314**: 558–65.

21 Wedderburn A. *Statistics and News: BEST 6*. Luxembourg: European Foundation for the improvement of Living and Working Conditions, 1993.

22 Lennermas M, Akerstedt T, Hambraeus L. Nocturnal eating and serum cholesterol of three-shift workers. *Scand J Work Environ Health* 1994; **20**: 401–6.

23 Nakamura K, *et al*. Shift work and risk factors for coronary heart disease in Japanese blue collar workers. Serum lipids and anthropometric characteristics. *Occup Med* 1997; **47**: 407–15.

24 Rosengren A, Hawker S, Ounpuu S *et al*. Assocation of psychosocial risk factors with risk of acute myocardial infarction in 11,119 cases and 13,648 controls from 52 countries (the INTERHEART Study): case-control study. *Lancet* 2004; **364**: 953–62.

25 WHO (World Health Organization). Carbon monoxide. *Environmental health criteria*, No. 13. Geneva: WHO, 1979.

26 Boon NA (editorial) Solvent abuse of the heart. *Br Med J* 1987; **294**: 722.

27 Gold RG. Interference to cardiac pacemakers—how often is it a problem? *Prescribers J* 1984; **24:** 115–23.

28 Sowton, E. Environmental hazards and pacemaker patients. *J R Coll Phys* 1982; **16:** 159–64.

29 Santucci PA, Haw J, Trohman RG, Pinski S.L. Interference with an Implantable Defibrillator by an electronic anti-theft surveillance device. *N Engl J Med* 1998; **339:** 1371–4.

30 US Departments of Labor and Commerce: Fact finding report. *Commission on the Future of Worker Management Relations.* Washington DC, US: Departments of Labor and Commerce, 1994.

31 Belkic K *et al.* The workplace and cardiovascular health: conclusions and thoughts for a future agenda. *Occup Med* 2000; **15:** 307–21.

32 Haynes SG, Fernlieb M. Women, work and coronary heart disease: prospective findings of the Framingham heart study. *Am J Public Health* 1980; **70:** 133–41.

Chapter 18

Respiratory disorders

K. T. Palmer and S. B. Pearson

Introduction

Respiratory illnesses commonly cause sickness absence, unemployment, medical attendance, illness, and handicap. Collectively these disorders cause the loss of 14% of available working days (approximately 38 million days per year) in men and 11% of work days in women (5 million days per year). In the 16–64-year-old population, they account for about 18% of general practitioner consultations, 10% of all hospital admissions, and 3–9% of all deaths. Ten per cent of working-aged men and 5% of working-aged women receive invalidity benefit because they are too disabled to work.

Respiratory disease may be caused, and pre-existing disease may be exacerbated by the occupational environment. More commonly, respiratory disease limits work capacity and the ability to undertake a particular job. Finally, respiratory fitness in 'safety critical' jobs can have implications for work colleagues and the public as well as for the affected individual. Within this broad picture, different clinical illnesses pose different problems. For example, acute respiratory illness commonly causes short-term sickness absence, whereas chronic respiratory disease has greater significance in long-term sickness absence and work limitation; and the fitness implications of respiratory sensitization at work are very different from non-specific asthma aggravated by workplace irritants.

Occupational causes of respiratory disease represent a small proportion of the total burden, except in some specialized work settings where particular exposures predominate and give rise to particular disease excesses. The corollary is that the common fitness decisions on placement, return to work and rehabilitation more often involve non-occupational illnesses than occupational ones. By contrast, statutory programmes of health surveillance revolve around specific occupational risks (such as spray painting with isocyanates) and specific occupational health outcomes (such as occupational asthma).

In assessing the individual it is important to remember that respiratory problems are often aggravated by other illnesses, particularly disorders of the cardiovascular and musculoskeletal systems.

Methods of assessing respiratory disability

General considerations

Respiratory fitness needs to be assessed in the context of the intended employment and its particular elements and demands. However, a number of general questions will influence the decision-making:

1. Does the combination of work and respiratory fitness result in an immediate foreseeable risk to the individual's health and safety, or that of others?

2. May present or anticipated future standards of health and safety be compromised?

3. If so, how great are the risks likely to be?

4. Is the work in the 'safety critical' category, in which the worker has substantial responsibility for the safety of colleagues or members of the public?

5. Can the work be discharged effectively, and can reasonable levels of attendance be anticipated?

6. Are there special considerations in placement, health review, or workplace adaptation?

7. Are particular policies required in selection, control, and monitoring?

8. Are there legal standards or other codes of good practice that need to be observed?

These questions are not particular to respiratory fitness assessments, but quite commonly occur in people with respiratory illness (e.g. the importance of aerobic capacity in the emergency rescue worker or the manual labourer; the risk posed to members of the public by tuberculosis in a healthcare worker, or pneumothorax in an airline pilot; the potential for life-threatening asthma following occupational sensitization).

Physicians in the UK have responsibilities under the Health and Safety at Work etc. Act 1974 (to place people in safe employment) and the Disability Discrimination Act 1995 (to ensure that disabled workers are not discriminated against unfairly on health grounds). The dual requirements of these two Acts challenge physicians to weigh matters carefully. They need, for example, to consider the likely duration of illness and its prognosis in the individual; the weight of evidence for incapacity on the one hand and risk on the other; and the scope for reasonable accommodation by the employer. These points are touched on elsewhere, but here we emphasize the complexities in making blanket judgements in respiratory fitness assessment:

♦ many aspects of lung function can be objectively measured, but, except at extreme departures, a poor correlation exists between measurements and handicapping symptoms (motivation may perhaps be more important);

♦ assessment of workplace demands and risks may be limited in scope or in their relevance to individual circumstances; and

♦ many conditions improve given sufficient time, appropriate treatment, proper environmental control, or work modification.

Fitness assessment should be made in this light. An employer's failure to control potentially modifiable respiratory hazards (dusts, fumes, etc.) may be construed not only as a failure of control (under Regulation 6 of the Control of Substances Hazardous to Health Regulations 1994), but a failure to make a reasonable accommodation under the Disability Discrimination Act.

Some organizations and public services apply pre-defined fitness standards; many others conduct routine measures of respiratory function, and apply pre-determined protocols and decision algorithms. These initiatives aid fitness assessment, but it should be noted that the status of these procedures under the Disability Discrimination Act, and their inter-relation to health and safety legislation, has not yet been adequately tested in the law courts.

Measurements of lung function

Respiratory disease produces impairment in lung function, and this, if severe enough, will interfere with the ability to perform some work tasks. Whether a given level of lung function impairment causes work difficulty depends on the nature of the job and the presence or absence of coexisting disease. The duration, intensity and pattern of work, the environmental conditions (such as temperature, humidity, dust, and fume content), and the attitude and personality of the individual all play a part. Pulmonary function testing is, therefore, only one component in the process of assessing fitness for work.

In an occupational setting lung function tests are used routinely in one of two ways. First, as a single set of measurements performed at a point in time (typically the pre-employment assessment, or during or following illness), to assess lung function in relation to accepted norms; and second, as serial measurements over time, to monitor disease control or progression, or detect adverse occupational effects at an early stage. Used in the second way, the diagnostic value of the testing is probably higher.

Standard lung function tests are conveniently classified into measurements of airways function, measurements of static lung volume and measurements of gas exchange. Measurements of airways function (for example, spirometry and PEF) should be routinely available in occupational healthcare, and can be augmented, under medical supervision, by tests of response to bronchodilator medication; the other tests, as well as measurements of bronchial responsiveness to inhaled histamine or methacholine, require specialist facilities, and are generally employed in secondary care investigation and research settings.

Spirometry is performed by taking a maximal inspiration and then blowing as hard as possible into the machine, and continuing to blow until the lungs are empty. The volume of gas expired is plotted against time to produce a spirogram (see Figure 18.1). The trace should be a smooth curve, and there should be good reproducibility between successive measurements, with super-imposition of traces. The volume of gas expired in the first second (FEV_1) is a measure of the speed of airflow. The total volume expired is the forced vital capacity (FVC). The absolute values obtained depend upon age, height, sex and racial origin, and values need to be compared with appropriate 'predicted normal values'.[1] Measurement of relaxed vital capacity can be used to assess the extent of any gas trapping in obstructive pulmonary disease where relaxed VC is usually greater than FVC, but the measurement is technically more difficult and less reproducible than FVC.

A number of basic points of technique need to be observed to minimize measurement errors.[2] Spirometry equipment needs to be calibrated at regular intervals, and checked for leaks, wear and tear, and blockages. Spuriously low results can occur if inspiration is incomplete, if partial leakage occurs (around the mouthpiece or in the tubing), or if expiratory effort is submaximal. The FVC is commonly underestimated because the blow is finished early, and this is apparent in

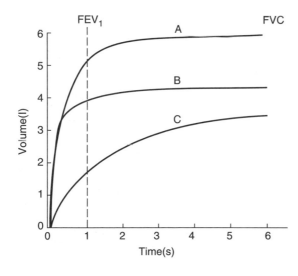

Fig. 18.1 Spirograms illustrating obstructive and restrictive patterns of abnormal ventilation: A, normal spirogram; B, restrictive deficit; C, obstructive deficit.

tracings that fail to attain a plateau. Variable effort is indicated by wobbly curves and poor reproducibility. Subjects should be encouraged to repeat the procedure until three acceptable curves are achieved (the best two FVCs should be within 5% or 1/10 of a litre of one another). The documented values should be the highest values from *any* of the three chosen curves. Benchmark standards and a more detailed account of these techniques have been provided by the British Thoracic Society and Association of Respiratory Technicians and Physiologists[3] and by the American Thoracic Society.[4] Other factors that need to be considered include variation between observers and between machines and recent infections, irritant exposures, and exercise.

Sometimes, despite encouragement and multiple attempts, subjects are unable to produce acceptable tracings. This commonly results from an inability to master the technique, but there is evidence in some of these cases that so-called 'test failure' is a marker of incipient health problems.[5]

Two main patterns of ventilatory abnormality can generally be defined, namely obstructive and restrictive. Obstruction arises in asthma and in chronic obstructive pulmonary disease (COPD), and tends to produce a diminution in FEV_1 greater than that in FVC. The ratio of FEV_1 to FVC should normally be greater than 0.7 (70%), but in airflow obstruction lower values arise. Restrictive lung changes are caused by diffuse inflammatory and fibrotic diseases of the lung parenchyma, such as fibrosing alveolitis and asbestosis, by pleural disease and by respiratory muscle weakness; and in this case FEV_1 is reduced, but so too is FVC, so that the ratio of FEV_1 to FVC is preserved (and often increased).

When interpreting lung function tests, however, it needs to be remembered that the range of normal values is generally large, two standard deviations being approximately 20% of the average value. This means on the one hand that a healthy individual can appear to have deficient lung function simply because he lies in the lower tail of the normal Gaussian distribution; and on the other hand that an individual with impaired lung function can still remain within the normal range of values. In the latter case, if he has moved from the top of the predicted normal range for a particular parameter to the bottom, the fall will represent 40% of the population mean. Hence, serial patterns are more informative than a single snapshot. Furthermore, the pattern of a number of different measurements should be considered, rather than one single index of lung function. For example, in chronic airflow limitation the FEV_1 will be reduced but this will also be associated with a reduction in $FEV_1/FVC\%$ and an increase in residual volume (RV) and functional residual capacity (FRC). This pattern of results would indicate significant airflow limitation for that individual, even if FEV_1 remained within the normal range for the population.

Measurements of airflow such as FEV_1 and peak expiratory flow (PEF) are influenced most by disease in the larger airways, where most of the resistance to flow lies. The cross-sectional area of the bronchial tree increases approximately exponentially with distance from the trachea as the bronchi divide, and resistance to flow falls concomitantly. Narrowing in the peripheral airways of less than 2 mm in diameter has little effect on FEV_1 and PEF unless the damage is extensive. This means that early disease in small airways, such as that caused by smoking and toxic fume damage, is poorly reflected in these measurements.

Most modern spirometers will also present the information in the form of an expiratory flow-volume curve, plotting flow against volume expired between maximal inspiration (total lung capacity or TLC) and maximal expiration (RV). From these curves additional information such as flow at 25% or 75% FVC may be obtained. Flows towards the expiratory end of the flow-volume curve represent flow in smaller airways, but accuracy of measurement, reproducibility, and reference ranges are all less precise for these low flows than they are for FEV_1, so these tests are not generally helpful in assessing fitness for work.

PEF measures the highest flow recorded during a forced expiratory manoeuvre and is measured with a peak flow meter. The subject is asked to perform a short, sharp, hard blow into the meter. It is usual to take the best of three attempts, providing the readings are reproducible. As with simple spirometry, a number of errors are possible, particularly variable subject effort, errors in reading PEFs and transcribing them to a diary, and incomplete returns. A great deal of instruction and encouragement are required to obtain adequate data. Self-treatment with bronchodilators and corticosteroids may affect the record, but the influence of the first of these factors can be minimized by recording PEFs before drug delivery. Upper respiratory tract infections can cause large (20%) falls in PEF for a week or more, making interpretation difficult. The effect is most marked in the late stages of infection.

PEF measurements are usually made serially over time, and used in one of two ways: to assess the degree of control achieved in patients with established asthma; and to look for work-related changes in situations where occupational asthma is suspected (The later section on asthma describes this last application more fully).

The Wright peak flow meter scale is non-linear and over-represents flows in the mid-range and under-represents flows in the high and low ranges.[6] Recent changes require that peak flow meters used in the UK must have a scale that conforms to the EU standard EN13829. Adjustments have also been made to the tables of predicted normal values.

Measurements of **static lung volumes**, such as TLC and RV, involve advanced techniques, including helium (or other inert gas) dilution and body plethysmography; they require a specialized pulmonary function laboratory and skilled technicians, but may be useful in clarifying diagnoses. Thus, in airflow obstruction, all static lung volumes are increased, but the increase in RV is proportionately greater than in TLC because of gas trapping; while in restrictive lung disease, such as pulmonary fibrosis, all lung volumes are reduced.

Measurements of **gas exchange** such as oxygen consumption ($\dot{V}O_2$) during incremental exercise, CO_2 production ($\dot{V}CO_2$), and arterial blood gases, are useful in assessing disability, especially in those with interstitial lung disease or emphysema. However, the findings reflect total cardiorespiratory function as well as peripheral muscle deconditioning, require a sophisticated laboratory, and are time-consuming to perform. Simpler tests of exercise capacity such as shuttle walk tests and 6 or 12-minute walks are more suitable for use in the field, but still require skilled technical help and time.[7,8] Carbon monoxide diffusion, expressed as transfer factor (TLCO), or gas transfer coefficient (KCO), measures the uptake of carbon monoxide from the lung to the blood. Carbon monoxide is of similar molecular weight to oxygen, and is bound to haemoglobin, so its uptake provides a measure of oxygen diffusion. It is reduced in interstitial lung disease and in emphysema, but it is also affected by other factors such as smoking habits, haemoglobin levels, and resting cardiac output. Again its measurement requires a dedicated lung function laboratory and skilled technicians. In the clinical setting the portable pulse oximeter provides a simple inexpensive guide to diffusion, and can be used to detect desaturation of haemoglobin at rest and during exercise in patients with pulmonary fibrosis or COPD.

Several other tests are used as adjuncts to diagnosis. Asthma in an occupational setting is sometimes investigated by **serology**, **skin prick tests**, or by **bronchial provocation challenge**. Immunological responsiveness (sensitization) to workplace agents may be detected by the identification of specific IgE antibodies using radioallergosorbent tests (RAST) or enzyme-linked immunosorbent assays (ELISA); or in response to a specific challenge to the skin or airways. The usefulness of these investigations varies from one agent to another. They also depend on identification of the suspected agent, and in the case of skin prick and provocation tests, may depend on obtaining a correct formulation of the material, or achieving a representative challenge. The subject is more fully discussed later (see p 409).

Screening questionnaires

In occupational health practice, screening questionnaires are widely used to assess respiratory fitness. This is particularly true prior to certain job placements, and periodically in certain jobs that may affect respiratory health.

The best known respiratory questionnaire is the MRC standardized questionnaire on respiratory symptoms.[9] This was devised for the epidemiological investigation of chronic bronchitis, but has since been adapted in a variety of ways to assess respiratory symptoms and risk factors in working groups. The original questions on sputum production had a high sensitivity and specificity in relation to measured sputum production, but these questions are of limited interest today. Several other versions have been tried, including the European Community for Coal and Steel (ECSC) questionnaire, the American Thoracic Society and the Division of Lung Disease (ATS-DLD-78) questionnaire, and the International Union Against Tuberculosis and Lung Disease (IUATLD) questionnaire. (For sample questions, and an assessment of their validity, see Toren *et al.*[10]) Venables *et al.*[11] have proposed a simple nine-item panel of questions for use in asthma epidemiology that correlate well with tests of bronchial hyper-responsiveness, and a simple extension to cover work-related symptoms (Table 18.1).

Work limitation arises most commonly from the sensation of breathlessness, and for monitoring and documentary purposes this can be graded on a clinical scale, such as the one proposed by the Medical Research Council (Table 18.2).

Chest radiography

Chest radiography plays an important part in monitoring patients exposed to fibrogenic dusts such as asbestos, silica, and coal dust.[12] It is a requirement, upon entering employment for the first time, and at regular intervals, in certain professions such as airline pilot and commercial diver. It is also valuable in the assessment of workers exposed to tuberculosis who develop

Table 18.1 Screening questions used in the epidemiological investigation of asthma (adapted from Venables *et al.*[11] with permission)*

Current health (during the last 4 weeks)	
If you run, or climb stairs fast do you ever:	
cough?	Yes/No
wheeze?	Yes/No
get tight in the chest?	Yes/No
Is you sleep ever broken by:	
wheeze?	Yes/No
difficulty with breathing?	Yes/No
Do you ever wake up in the morning (or from your sleep if a shift worker) with:	
wheeze?	Yes/No
difficulty with breathing?	Yes/No
Do you ever wheeze:	
if you are in a smoky room?	Yes/No
if you are in a very dusty place?	Yes/No

*Answers of 'yes' to three of the nine questions correspond to a sensitivity of 91% and a specificity of 96% for current bronchial hyper-responsiveness.

Table 18.2 The MRC breathlessness scale

1. Troublesome shortness of breath when hurrying on level ground or walking up a slight hill
2. Short of breath when walking with other people of own age on level ground
3. Have to stop for breath when walking at own pace on level ground

persistent respiratory symptoms. (Some of these aspects of surveillance and fitness assessment are more fully described in later sections.)

However, the routine application of chest radiography in many other traditional situations has fallen into disfavour. For example, it is no longer considered helpful in routine surveillance of asymptomatic healthcare workers with potential tuberculosis exposure; likewise, the yield in asymptomatic workers who work with lung carcinogens is considered too low to justify the cost or radiation risk. Indeed, for the common round of health problems (upper respiratory tract infections, asthma, and COPD), decisions on fitness for work seldom rest upon the outcome of radiography.

In the detection of pleural and interstitial lung disease more information is obtained by computed tomography scanning than radiography, but the procedure is expensive and its routine application for screening cannot presently be justified. It is also quite difficult presently to interpret the findings of a sensitive technique that frequently reveal changes in asymptomatic individuals.

Clinical conditions and capacity for work

Asthma

Asthma has a prevalence in the adult population of about 5%. It is a condition of variable airflow limitation associated with bronchial hyper-responsiveness and symptoms of cough, breathlessness, and tightness of the chest. The predominant physical sign is wheeze. Onset in childhood or early adult life is frequently associated with the syndrome of atopy, characterized by elevated IgE antibody levels, positive skin prick tests to common inhaled antigens, and an increased incidence of eczema and allergic rhinitis. Childhood symptoms often remit in early adult life, but frequently recur in middle age. Onset in middle life is not usually associated with manifestations of atopy, and the condition tends to be more persistent and more likely to progress in severity with time.

There are some difficulties in defining asthma. Wheeze is a highly prevalent symptom in the community, and many people with occasional wheeze do not have asthma. Conversely, subjects with bronchoconstriction do not recognize the symptom as often as might be supposed.[13] A further difficulty arises in distinguishing between chronic asthma and COPD, as there may be overlap between the classical features of asthma (such as wheeze and reversibility) and those of COPD (sputum, dyspnoea, and irreversible airflow obstruction). It is important, therefore, for doctors making a fitness assessment to decide whether the diagnosis is truly asthma, and whether some response to treatment is likely. A more detailed history, including smoking habits, periodicity, and remission of symptoms and precipitating factors is essential. Ideally this should be supported by diurnal measurements of PEF and evidence of responsiveness to bronchodilators. This assessment should recognize that hyper-responsiveness can be exaggerated during and following recent infection. However, simple screening questions and a single measurement of lung function and bronchodilator responsiveness may prove misleading. The most usual pattern on spirometry is to observe an obstructive deficit (low FEV_1 with an abnormal FEV_1/FVC % ratio), but these measurements, though highly specific, have a relatively low sensitivity[14] in a disorder characterized by variable airflow limitation. Another common mistake is to confuse asthma with recurrent chest infection, especially in those who smoke. One unfortunate consequence of this mislabelling is to undertreat asthma, and to limit employment opportunities thereby.

In the worker with established asthma, fitness and placement judgements may hinge on a number of important questions.

How severe is the condition?

Hyper-responsive airways represent a biological continuum. Asthma varies from mild disease with intermittent symptoms, through mild-to-moderate persistent disease requiring regular prophylactic treatment, to severe disease requiring regular high-dose inhaled steroids, or more rarely, continuous oral steroids. It is difficult to estimate how often disease falls into the different categories of severity, but it is widely considered that most asthma is relatively mild and amenable to treatment. In employment terms asthma accounts for 2% of all lost working days in men, and these typically fall in the winter months when viral respiratory infections are more prevalent.

In the common situation where asthma is mild, infrequent, or amenable to simple treatment, job placement decisions are straight forward. Adequate control may require only occasional use of a bronchodilator at times of unusual exertion or intercurrent infection. The anticipatory use of an inhaler (before exertion, and in the early stages of respiratory infection) will further ameliorate any problem, though short-term work modification may be helpful, and brief spells of sickness absence can arise (on average about 1–2 weeks a year[15]). Under these circumstances the label 'asthmatic' may be unhelpful, leading simply to misinformed and prejudicial decisions on work fitness. Disease at the moderate to severe end of the spectrum poses more concern. At the extreme end, brittle asthma may be severe and life-threatening. A particular worry arises if the workplace is far removed from medical care facilities, and emergency transfer is expensive, disruptive, or technically difficult. **Two thousand people in the UK still die of asthma every year.**

A broad indication of disease activity can be gained from the frequency of bronchodilator use and the degree of sleep disturbance. In more severe disease it is essential to know whether, or how often a patient has been admitted to hospital with asthma; whether or not he has ever required ventilation because of asthma; or received emergency intravenous therapy; or takes regularly prescribed oral steroid medication. A number of guidelines on assessing disease severity have been produced by specialist societies, such as those recently published by the British Thoracic Society and Scottish Intercollegiate Guidelines Network.[16] The American Thoracic Society has proposed some guidelines for assessing residual disability in *controlled* asthma. These relate to the degree of reversibility of airways obstruction or hyper-responsiveness, and the minimum drug dose required to maintain asthma control.[17]

An alternative approach, particularly in physically demanding jobs, is to measure changes in lung function during representative work tasks. Exercise tests are not specific enough to be used routinely in pre-placement screening, but in subjects with active troublesome disease a fall in FEV_1 >15% may be a useful indicator of current work handicap.

Are there any work factors that are liable to aggravate constitutional asthma?

Asthmatic airways are hyper-responsive to a wide range of non-specific irritants that are commonly encountered at work, as well as many highly prevalent environmental allergens. Extremes of temperature and humidity, irritant dusts and fumes, pollens and house dust mites may all provoke or aggravate constitutional asthma, as may work stress and heavy physical exertion. This can pose temporary or enduring employment problems to asthmatics in a wide range of occupations, from cold store workers in refrigeration plants through to outdoor workers in construction and farming. In practice, however, it is not easy to predict the sensitivity of a sufferer to irritant conditions. The degree of susceptibility to different irritant stimuli varies considerably between individuals: for example, airways that bronchoconstrict in response to cold air may be less sensitive to dusts, and vice versa. In general, individuals with severe disease tend to be most vulnerable to irritant conditions, but not to the point where generalized judgements can be applied. (Thus, severe asthmatics with a significant component of fixed airways obstruction may be less susceptible to non-specific irritants than those with severe labile asthma.)

Can the principal aggravating factors be removed or limited?

For example, can irritant fumes or dusts be better controlled by exhaust ventilation or different work practices? Can less irritating materials be used? Can the process be enclosed? Can respiratory protection be used to limit exposure? If physical exertion is a limiting factor, can the effort of the work be reduced (e.g. by providing a lifting aid)? These are areas in which occupational health practitioners need to be particularly influential.

Has optimum treatment been offered, or could disease control be improved?

There is a growing appreciation that asthma tends to be undertreated, and that insufficient use is made of long-term prophylactic treatment, especially inhaled corticosteroids. Regular use has been shown to have a beneficial effect on attack frequency, sleep disturbance, hospital admission rates, and absenteeism, and recently consensus guidelines have emerged on the optimum management of adult asthma.[16] The well-educated patient should be able to self-monitor, self-medicate and self-refer. Deteriorating serial peak flow and worsening nocturnal symptoms should trigger an increase in medication and early medical attendance; while in brittle asthma, a home supply of oral steroids has enabled earlier treatment in those most in need, and has transformed employment prospects in some individuals. The latest British Guidelines[16] provide a detailed stepwise approach to the treatment of asthma. It is important, before reaching irrevocable placement decisions, to determine whether better control is possible.

Might the patient have occupational (sensitization) asthma?

This is an important question to consider when asthma begins or recurs in adulthood, and a vital question to consider in industries from which case reports often arise (Table 18.3).[17] The possibility is suggested if symptoms are worse at work, or on work days, better when away from work (at weekends and on holiday), and deteriorate upon return to work. A similar picture can arise from a non-specific response to irritant conditions, as described above, and the distinction between these possibilities is important. The reason is that occupational asthma may result in severe bronchospasm, and sensitized workers may react to amounts of material so tiny that workplace controls cannot be guaranteed to afford reliable protection. By contrast, it is more realistic

Table 18.3 Agents most frequently reported to cause occupational asthma and occupations that often give rise to such reports[17]

Agents	Occupations
Isocyanates, flour & grain dust, colophony and fluxes, latex, animal products, aldehydes, wood dust	Paint sprayers, bakers & pastry makers, nurses, chemical workers, animal handlers, welders, food processors, timber workers

to achieve the control measures that ease the problems of aggravated asthma due to irritants, so the prospects for continued healthy employment are correspondingly brighter.

In practice it may be difficult to distinguish between the two diagnoses: irritant industrial exposures often coexist with the presence of a workplace sensitizer, and workers with pre-existing asthma are not immune to occupational sensitization. A separate diagnostic problem arises in sensitized workers who manifest late asthmatic reactions, rather than immediate ones. Symptoms often arise at night-time, and thereby mimic the pattern of constitutional asthma.

FEV_1 is an insensitive indicator of occupational asthma, and alternative investigations are required to secure a diagnosis. Agents that cause occupational asthma can be classified broadly into those that sensitize by the induction of specific IgE antibodies (e.g. laboratory animal proteins, platinum salts, and halogenated anhydrides), and those like isocyanates, western red cedar and colophony that sensitize by other poorly understood means, and have mute or inconsistent antibody responses. Hence, for some causes of occupational asthma the detection of specific IgE antibodies may serve as an indicator of sensitization, as may a positive skin prick test. Examples include latex sensitivity in healthcare workers, flour and enzyme sensitivity in bakery workers, sensitivity to acid anhydrides, and sensitivity to animal products in exposed workers. These tests can be specific and relatively sensitive for some agents,[19,20] and can be used in case investigation. (The predictive value of a test depends not only on its sensitivity and specificity, but also the prevalence of the disorder in the population tested, so they tend to be less helpful in screening.) But the distinction between sensitization and frank occupational asthma is an important one to draw. Skin prick and serological tests do not in themselves indicate work-limiting disease. Corroborative evidence is required before making placement decisions.

If the patient is still exposed, and fit for further exposure, the standard investigative tool is serial measurement of PEF.[21] A pattern is sought of exaggerated PEF variability and a fall in mean PEF level around times of exposure. Normally, several readings a day (at work and away from it) will be required over a 3–4-week period—at least four per day to ensure adequate sensitivity and specificity.[17] Care is needed in the execution and interpretation of the test, and the variability of occupational asthma needs to be differentiated from normal diurnal changes in PEF and other determinants of airways responsiveness (exercise, treatment, infection, etc.). The record must cover a period in which the potential for exposure exists, and this may require some planning if exposures are intermittent or infrequent. It is important to keep to the same pattern of measurement at work and on rest days. The minimum standards to be met with serial peak flow measurements in an occupational setting are described in the British Asthma Guidelines.[16]

Different PEF patterns can arise in affected workers, dependent on their response and recovery times. An immediate response and a short recovery interval will generate obvious PEF dips related in time to work, but late responses will produce dips at home, and those that occur at night can readily be confused with constitutional asthma. Slower recovery times may result in a day on day decline in the working week, with recovery at weekends. If recovery is protracted, ordinary work breaks may be insufficient for recovery, and a week on week decline ensues, leading to a nadir of persistently low values. Recovery may take weeks or months away from exposure, a pattern readily misdiagnosed as COPD, especially in smokers. Diagnosis has traditionally been based on the relatively subjective approach of pattern recognition by an experienced physician, but rule-based quantitative approaches have been suggested, and computerized diagnostic algorithms have been developed with some success.[22,23] PEF, if conducted according to validated standards, is dependable with good agreement on interpretation between experts and few false positive results, but it may miss about 20% of cases.[17] Questionnaires and history-taking by experts display the obverse pattern to some extent, of relatively poor specificity but good sensitivity.

The 'gold standard' for diagnosis is bronchial provocation challenge test (BPT) or inhalation challenge test with the suspected sensitizer: a simulated industrial exposure conducted under controlled conditions, with FEV_1 and responsiveness to histamine or methacholine measured serially. A late response, in particular, is taken as evidence of an allergic response; bronchial hyper-reactivity can also be demonstrated for 2–3 days after the challenge. The procedure entails some risk of severe bronchospasm, and needs to be undertaken in a specialist hospital unit. The patient has to be admitted prior to the procedure, to ensure an adequate (exposure-free) baseline, and kept in for a day or so afterwards to measure late responsiveness. Because of its risk and cost, BPT is usually reserved for special circumstances, which include the investigation of mixed exposures and novel agents, and situations of significant diagnostic uncertainty. Although it is often assumed that BPT is always correct, false negatives can arise if testing is conducted with the wrong material or too low an exposure and standardized procedures have not been defined for many agents of interest.

Occupational asthma is important and comparatively common (over 400 causal agents have been identified and about 1000 new cases are diagnosed annually by UK specialists). It may account for about 9–15% of adult onset asthma.[16,17] It can result in acute severe bronchospasm in the workplace and chronic ill-health during employment. For some sensitizing agents, such as isocyanates, non-specific bronchial hyper-responsiveness is known to persistent for several years after leaving employment.

There is good research evidence now that early re-deployment can mitigate against the risk of continuing symptoms, and thus improve the long-term prognosis.[24] Several studies have shown that prognosis is worse for those who remain exposed for more than 1 year after symptoms develop compared with those removed earlier.[25,26] A comprehensive highly recommended systematic review, undertaken by Nicholson et al. on behalf of the British Occupational Health Research Foundation and the Faculty of Occupational Medicine, draws attention to the benefits of early withdrawal from exposure (Table 18.4).[17]

In the UK, the Control of Substances Hazardous to Health (COSHH) Regulations 1994 require health surveillance programmes to be conducted where there is a reasonable risk of disease

Table 18.4 Evidence-based guidelines on the need to withdraw from causal exposures in subjects with occupational asthma

Statement	Strength of evidence*
The likelihood of improvement or resolution of symptoms or of preventing deterioration is greater in workers who have: no further exposure to the causative agent	2+
relatively normal lung function at the time of diagnosis	2+
shorter duration of symptoms prior to diagnosis	2+
shorter duration of symptoms prior to avoidance of exposure	2+
Redeployment to a low exposure area may lead to improvement or resolution of symptoms or prevent deterioration in some workers, but is not always effective	3
Air-fed helmet respirators may improve or prevent symptoms but not for all workers who continue to be exposed to the causative agent	3

2+ means evidence from well-conducted case-control or cohort studies with a low risk of confounding or bias and a moderate chance of causality; 3 means evidence only from non-analytic studies (e.g. case reports). Adapted from Nicholson et al.[17]

occurrence. Guidance on the contents of suitable programmes has been provided by the Health and Safety Executive. Periodic symptom enquiries, measurements of lung function and review of sickness absence reports are advised, the exact schedule being based on an assessment of risk.[27] The effectiveness of health surveillance in detecting early reversible disease has not been rigorously established so far, and the directions that have the most impact are not well defined.[17] None the less, screening, early detection of symptoms and prompt action are seen as vital ingredients in fitness assessment of workers from high-risk industries.

The strong presumption is that those with occupational asthma should be redeployed and removed from further exposure to the sensitizing agent that caused their asthma. The American Thoracic Society suggests that such subjects should be regarded as fully and permanently debarred for jobs that give rise to further exposure to the causal agent,[18] and the review by Nicholson et al.[17] offers persuasive evidence on the wisdom of this policy.

Some doctors perceive a difficulty in employees who develop mild occupational asthma with normal pulmonary function when exposures are low or occasional. The pressure to continue in work (and preserve earning power) has to be balanced against the longer-term risks of deterioration, chronicity of symptoms, and fixed airflow limitation. There is a commonly held view that differences exist between sensitizers in their potency to sensitize, and in the severity and persistence of the symptoms they provoke. Isocyanate asthma, for example, may be induced by minute concentrations and may result in severe asthmatic attacks at work. It is also known to persist after exposure ceases, albeit with some improvement. More than half of those affected by small molecule asthma remain symptomatic after 2 years away from work, and in this group the disorder is usually permanent. Asthma resulting from sensitization to large molecules, such as flour dust, by contrast, is considered often to be milder with a better prognosis.

With respiratory protection, modification of their job to reduce exposure and effective treatment, many bakery workers have continued to work successfully. Other sensitized workers have also continued in employment, wearing higher level respiratory protection. Under these circumstances close medical supervision is essential and the ever-present risk of control failures should be borne in mind. Every effort should be made to explore work and process modifications that minimize the risk. Ideally patients should withdraw permanently from all further exposures; but if not, they should be aware that progression of symptoms can and sometimes does occur despite great care and redeployment to work areas of lower exposure.[17]

Some authorities have recommended *pre-employment* policies that restrict the employment of workers perceived to be at greater risk of occupational asthma. Atopic individuals appear to be at increased risk from some agents that induce specific IgE such as animal proteins, while smokers are at a greater risk of asthma from platinum salts, phthalic anhydride, green coffee bean, snow crab, and ispaghula. But for other agents, such as isocyanates and red cedar, *lower* risks have been described in atopics and smokers,[28] and in general these risk factors are so common as to form a poor basis for health-based pre-placement selection. However, prudence would dictate that symptomatic asthmatics should not be newly employed in environments known to contain respiratory sensitizers, as supervening occupational asthma will be more difficult to detect than in normal people, and may be more troublesome.

Chronic obstructive pulmonary disease

COPD is common, affecting 9–11 % of the population in the UK. In England and Wales it is estimated that about 1.5 million people have COPD.[29] Smoking leads to a syndrome of chronic mucus production with goblet cell hyperplasia (simple chronic bronchitis), and also to a condition of chronic airflow limitation with airways narrowing and emphysema. It appears that exposure to industrial dust and fumes may contribute to both syndromes, although smoking tobacco is a more important cause.

The principal symptoms in COPD are cough, sputum, and breathlessness on effort. Frequently, however, the symptoms and signs are non-specific and detection of latent airflow limitation is delayed until disease is more advanced. Some authorities have therefore advocated annual spirometry to aid earlier detection in smokers, and people with recurrent respiratory symptoms or a family history of premature lung disease.[29,30] There have been several guidelines published for the diagnosis and management of COPD over the years, of which the most recent and most comprehensive is that published by the National Collaborating Centre for Chronic Conditions commissioned by the National Institute for Clinical Excellence (NICE).[29] Currently, a further set of guidelines is being prepared by the American Thoracic Society and the European Respiratory Society (see www.ersnet.org).

In assessing the fitness for work of a person with COPD for employment, a number of matters need to be considered, and these broadly parallel those described earlier for asthma.

Is the problem primarily one of mucus hypersecretion or of airflow limitation?

Mucus hypersecretion by itself does not limit capacity to work, and in the absence of airflow limitation simple chronic bronchitis is compatible with a wide range of normal employment. Infective exacerbations and sickness absence may be more frequent, although a programme of winter influenza vaccinations may ameliorate the problem. In these circumstances a medical label may be unhelpful and prejudicial to employment prospects. Frequently, however, mucus hypersecretion coexists with airflow limitation, which can be a real cause of disability.

If airflow limitation is present, how severe is it and what is its functional effect?

Emphysema is defined in pathological terms, but in life its presence can be presumed when there is an obstructive pattern on spirometry with evidence of increased static lung volumes (TLC), gas trapping (disproportionate increase in RV with reduced RV/TLC ratio) and impaired gas transfer (TLCO). Although FEV_1 may be normal despite significant small airways disease, there is a broad correlation in COPD between FEV_1 and breathlessness, and it provides a better guide to disability than PEF. In general terms, people with FEV_1 values of less than 60% but greater than 40% predicted tend to show moderate disability, while those below 40% predicted tend to display severe disability. Spirometry predicts prognosis in COPD. Ventilatory failure (hypercapnia) is unusual if the FEV_1 is more than 1.5 litres.

Measurements of lung function and maximum oxygen uptake ($\dot{V}O_{2max}$) should, in principle, provide a fair guide to work capability in patients with airflow limitation, and two broad approaches have been adopted towards the objective assessment of impairment:

1. banding spirometric findings according to their likely impact on function (Table 18.5 summarizes various international guidelines on the relation between FEV_1 and severity of disease).

2. comparing the measured $\dot{V}O_{2max}$ with the approximate energy demands of a range of common occupations and occupational activities (using a scheme such as that in Table 18.6, or the US Department of Labor's job by job analysis of work demands[31]).

Unfortunately, the energy demands of work vary through time as the component activities of a task vary; individuals also vary in their oxygen requirements for a given task because of personal and job-related factors (e.g. differences in their metabolic efficiency and different working methods); and finally, resting lung function tests explain only a small part of the variance in $\dot{V}O_{2max}$.[32] The subjective appreciation of breathlessness usually proves to be the limiting factor.

Table 18.5 Grading the severity of airflow obstruction using FEV_1: Some international guidelines

	Mild	Moderate	Severe
ATS	>50	35–49	<35
ERS	>70	50–69	<50
BTS	60–79	40–59	<40
GOLD	>80	40–59	<40
NICE	50–80	30–49	<30

All values represent percentage of predicted normal FEV_1. ATS, American Thoracic Society; ERS, European Respiratory Society; BTS, British Thoracic Society; GOLD, Global Initiative for Chronic Obstructive Lung Disease; NICE, National Institute for Clinical Excellence UK.

Hence, 'objective' measurements of disability provide no more than a rough guide to work capacity.[33,34] Crudely speaking, those with 'slight' impairment (Table 18.5) can manage most ordinary work, whereas those with 'moderate' impairment fail to meet the physical demands of many jobs, and those with 'severe' impairment do not cope in most jobs. However, given wide individual variation and scope for job modification, fitness decisions still depend on subjective medical judgements.

Has optimum treatment been offered, or could disease control be improved?

In individuals with airflow limitation due to COPD there is scope for therapeutic improvement, but the scope is much less than for asthma. Detailed guidance on the steps for treating COPD of different levels of severity is to be found in recent consensus documents, for example, the recent NICE guidelines.[29] Inhaled β-agonists are less effective than in asthma, and need to be used in

Table 18.6 The energy cost of some occupational and reference activities

Activity	Cal/ml	MET*	Activity	Cal/ml	MET*
Rest	1.0	1.0	Plastering	4.1	3.5
Sitting	1.2	1.0	Ploughing (tractor)	4.2	3.5
Standing	1.4	1.0	Wheeling barrow	5.0	4.0
Watch repair	1.6	1.5	(115 lbs, 2.5 mph)		
Sweeping floor	1.6	1.5	Carpentry	6.8	5.5
Machine sewing	1.8	1.8	Tree felling	8.0	6.5
Armature winding	2.2	2.0	Shovelling	8.5	7.0
Playing piano	2.5	2.0	Ascending stairs	9.0	7.5
Radio assembly	2.7	2.5	(27 ft/min, 17lb load)		
Driving car	2.8	2.5	Planing	9.1	7.5
Making beds	3.9	3.0	Ascending stairs	16.2	13.5
Bricklaying	4.0	3.5	(54 ft/min, 22 lb load)		

Adapted from Rusk HA (ed): *Rehabilitation medicine*. St Louis: CV Mosby, 1977 (with permission). *MET = Metabolic equivalent. One MET = 3.5 ml/kg per min of oxygen consumed (or the amount of basal oxygen consumption at rest).

doses that often provoke tremors. Anticholinergic agents, such as ipratropium bromide or the longer-acting tiotropium may be more effective,[35,36] and in disease of moderate severity either or both may be employed on a regular basis or long-acting β-agonists substituted for shorter-acting ones. Bronchodilators may improve breathlessness and exercise tolerance, even in the absence of measurable bronchodilation.

The inflammation of COPD tends to be less responsive to steroids than in asthma, but there is evidence in patients with more severe COPD (FEV_1 <50% predicted) that regular use of inhaled corticosteroids will reduce the number of exacerbations and slow the rate of decline in health status despite little improvement in lung function. In COPD, tests of reversibility using oral steroids do not predict response to inhaled steroids.[29]

Theophyllines have only a modest bronchodilatory effect, but may modify small airways function and gas trapping and can be used usefully in combination with other bronchdilators. Beneficial effects on exercise tolerance have been reported, but not consistently. In users, plasma theophylline levels should be monitored, in view of the narrow therapeutic range of these drugs and their propensity to cause side-effects and drug interactions. Mucolytic drugs have no effect on lung function, but reduce the number of exacerbations and the number of days of COPD illness.

Graded exercise programmes increase exercise tolerance in symptomatic patients with moderately severe COPD and symptomatic breathlessness (MRC grade 3 or greater). Programmes of rehabilitation should be tailored to individual patient needs. Ingredients include disease education, including smoking cessation, and a review of medication and an assessment of psychological and nutritional needs. Patients should be encouraged to commit to an ongoing exercise programme.

It is very important to encourage COPD sufferers to stop smoking. In people with smoking-induced COPD the rate of decline in FEV_1 is increased from an average value of 20–30 ml per year seen in non-smokers to a value of about 60–80 ml per year. In smokers with moderate impairment of lung function the rate of loss of function returns to normal upon smoking cessation, but the benefit in severe COPD and in industrial disease is less certain. Thus, an important preventive role for the occupational health service is to educate and to provide support for attempts to stop smoking, especially in employees with COPD. Useful guidelines for smoking cessation have been provided by the British Thoracic Society.[37]

Finally, intercurrent infections require prompt treatment to prevent acute deteriorations and chronic airways damage.

Are there any work factors that are liable to aggravate COPD?

In workers who develop troublesome progressive airflow limitation, continuing employment may still be possible in more sedentary work, or under a modified work schedule. Exercise physiology experiments on leg effort and degree of dyspnoea have shown that a doubling of work intensity causes a fourfold increase in effort and dyspnoea, whereas a doubling in the duration of work causes only a 30% increase.[38] Thus, one possible strategy may be to conduct less arduous work spread over a longer time period. Better process control (dust and fume control at source, assisted mechanical lifting, etc.) may also extend the range of employment possibilities, and these measures should all be considered before declaring the worker unfit.

Are there special work problems for COPD sufferers?

The wearing of respiratory protective equipment (RPE) may increase the effort of work. Some RPE, like self-contained breathing apparatus (SCBA) can be bulky, heavy or awkward; while some RPE systems, such as canister respirators and half-face masks increase the work of breathing, requiring the wearer to inspire air against the resistance of a filter. It may be possible, instead, to provide a filter-free 'active' system (air-fed respirators blow a stream of fresh air across the face behind a visor, the positive pressure generated preventing the ingress of hazardous fumes), but even these require extra weight to be carried around while physically active; and the choice of system may be limited by the circumstances (for example, the need to attain very high degrees of protection may necessitate SCBA, and work in oxygen deficient atmospheres may necessitate the carriage of gas cylinders). Fitness decisions need to be made in the light of residual lung capacity, the work in question and the options for process control over and above RPE use.

The presence of emphysema, particularly bullous disease, increases the risk of spontaneous pneumothorax and is thus a bar to employment in certain occupations that involve changes in barometric pressure (such as diving and air flight—see p 423).

Interstitial lung disease

The important diseases in this group include interstitial fibrosis, chronic pulmonary sarcoidosis, and extrinsic allergic alveolitis. All these conditions can produce pulmonary fibrosis. In functional terms they reduce pulmonary compliance, make the lungs stiffen, reduce static lung volumes and impair gas transfer. $FEV_1/FVC\%$ is usually preserved, but airflow limitation may be present in addition to fibrosis. These conditions are all associated with radiological abnormalities, but high resolution computed tomography scanning is more sensitive than plain radiography in assessing the extent of disease.

Pulmonary fibrosis may be cryptogenic, secondary to other clinical disorders (such as rheumatoid arthritis, systemic sclerosis, inflammatory bowel disease, sarcoidosis, and chronic allergic alveolitis), or due to occupational contact with fibrogenic dusts. A number of professional groups, including miners and quarrymen, stone dressers, foundry fettlers and construction workers, are at special risk, although this fact may go unrecognized.[12]

Established fibrosis from whatever cause frequently progresses, although the rate of progression can be very variable. In the case of fibrogenic dust disease, progression may occur despite removal from the industry,[39,40] although early identification and withdrawal from exposure may result in a better long-term outcome. It seems prudent therefore to identify this disorder at an early stage and to recommend avoidance of further exposure. Unfortunately, there are no unique symptoms or signs, and disease onset is insidious (over a decade or longer). Gradually progressive dyspnoea may be erroneously attributed to simple ageing, particularly when the potential for exposure is overlooked. A programme of regular surveillance in high-risk professions obviates this problem. In Britain there is a legal requirement to conduct health surveillance in asbestos workers under certain conditions,[41] and the programme and the physician need to be approved by the Health and Safety Executive (HSE).

Tests of pulmonary function are not diagnostically specific, so plain radiography provides the mainstay of screening programmes. (Radiography is considered to be about 80% sensitive in asbestosis and silicosis, and other diagnostic methods such as high resolution computed tomography may one day be used in preference.)

Table 18.7 details two model surveillance programmes advocated by the World Health Organization.[42] These include radiography, symptom enquiry, and spirometry. In the UK, guidance has been provided by HSE, though this is somewhat different in its content. In the case of crystalline silica exposure, the HSE advocates surveillance in employees who are regularly exposed to levels exceeding 0.1 mg/m^3 8-hour TWA[43] (generally in quarrying, certain heavy clay activities, and the refactory and foundry industries). A 2-yearly programme of chest radiography and respiratory questioning is suggested, but spirometry is not advocated on a serial basis. According to the Executive, the number of respiratory episodes should be determined, by

Table 18.7 WHO recommendations for health screening of workers exposed to asbestos or silica

Agent	Surveillance procedure	Interval/frequency*
Silica (crystalline quartz) dust exposure	Chest radiograph	At baseline, after 2–3 years of exposure, then every 2–5 years
	Spirometry + symptom questionnaire	At baseline, then annually, or at the same frequency as chest X-ray
Asbestos exposure	Chest radiograph	At baseline, then: —every 3–5 years if less than 10 years since first exposed —every 1–2 years if longer than 10 years but less than 20 years —annually if longer than 20 years since first exposure
	Spirometry + symptom questionnaire + physical examination	Annually, or at the same frequency as the chest X-ray

*In both cases, surveillance should be life-long. Adapted with permission from: Wagner GR. Asbestosis and silicosis. *Lancet* 1997; **349**: 1311–15. © The Lancet Ltd.

questioning and perusal of sickness absence records, and evidence sought of any serial trends that may suggest disease onset. Pre-employment assessment should identify those more vulnerable to respiratory infection (those with COPD and asthma, for example), and should include enquiry about current symptoms, a chest X-ray and baseline spirometry. Old tuberculosis may become reactivated in silica-exposed workers, so a history of earlier respiratory tuberculosis should also be sought. For health surveillance in asbestos workers, HSE provides guidance for its Appointed Doctors.

X-rays may be scored against a standard set of ILO films, based on the presence, profusion, size and shape of opacities.[44] In coal worker's pneumoconiosis, category 1 changes can occur without evidence of impaired lung function. Such workers can continue to work under surveillance. Category 2 change and above is associated with increasing impairment of lung function, and warrants removal from contact with fibrogenic dust, as does simple silicosis and asbestosis.

Established fibrotic lung disease is irreversible, and presently untreatable. Oral corticosteroids and other forms of immunosuppression such as cyclophosphamide or azathioprine, have been tried, but the results are disappointing. The drugs are, however, effective in early extrinsic allergic alveolitis and sarcoidosis in preventing fibrosis and have some effect in some forms of interstitial pulmonary fibrosis.

The principal disability is breathlessness on effort, which is often accompanied by significant falls in arterial oxygen levels. Spirometry and measurements of $\dot{V}O_{2max}$ and arterial pO_2 in representative exercise (i.e. appropriate to the conditions of work) provide a basis for fitness assessment; the general considerations are the same as those for COPD with airflow limitation. Affected workers may remain gainfully employed in less manual work, but disability tends to progress with time, and a periodic medical review is appropriate. All forms of pulmonary fibrosis are probably associated with an increased risk of bronchogenic carcinoma.

Extrinsic allergic alveolitis (EAA) is a hypersensitivity pneumonitis, provoked principally by occupational allergens, such as mouldy hay and bird excreta. In its acute form it produces a mild systemic flu-like illness, with fever, aches and pains, malaise, and dry cough. Symptoms develop within a few hours of exposure. Mild attacks resolve spontaneously, but severe attacks may require corticosteroid therapy. The condition is self-limiting if contact with the offending protein ceases or if adequate respiratory protection is provided. However, chronic exposure can cause pulmonary fibrosis and permanent respiratory disability. Established fibrosis is unresponsive to treatment, so regular surveillance (radiography and lung function testing) is appropriate for those with continuing potential for exposure.

Respiratory infections

Acute upper respiratory tract infections

These are very common. Occupational environments that are enclosed with little natural ventilation favour the spread of prevalent respiratory infections, particularly viral ones. These contribute importantly to short-term sickness absence, but are self-limiting and pose no special difficulties in fitness assessment.

More serious are a range of viral upper respiratory tract infections that may be complicated by chest problems or protracted debility. *Influenza* is a highly infectious condition that involves a longer period of sickness, and a greater risk of complicating illness (tracheobronchitis, pneumonia, exacerbated COPD). Some occupational groups such as healthcare workers and teachers, are a particular risk and may benefit from prophylaxis with influenza vaccine. Vaccination in these worker groups is also important in limiting risk to clients. It can be recommended in those with pre-existing lung diseases such as asthma and COPD, irrespective of occupation.

Glandular fever and the other infectious mononucleoses are relatively common in young adults, and cause a protracted period of illness and work difficulty. A severe tonsillitis occurs, often associated with palatal petechiae, cervical lymphadenopathy and a palpable spleen. The diagnosis is confirmed by the finding of atypical mononuclear cells on the blood film. In glandular fever the Paul-Bunnell test is positive in about 60% of patients during the first week of illness, and abnormal liver function tests arise half the time.

Although these diseases are self-limiting, it is not uncommon to feel tired and fatigued for 3–6 months after the acute stage of illness. Sufferers who lack their normal stamina are often signed off as unfit to attend work, although a modified work programme with phased rehabilitation is a more constructive approach. Ideally this would encourage the sufferer to work his normal duties, but only for a part of the week to begin with, the hours gradually increasing as his stamina assumes more normal levels.

Chronic fatigue syndrome, which typically arises as an upper respiratory tract infection with incomplete recovery, requires a similar approach. A comprehensive review by the Royal Colleges of Physicians, Psychiatrists and General Practitioners has recommended planned and mutually agreed incremental increases in physical activity as the cornerstone of treatment.[45]

Some respiratory infections may be occupationally acquired—for example, Q fever in slaughterhouse workers and veterinary surgeons and legionella pneumonia in industries using humidification and water cooling plants, but these are uncommon occurrences. Occasionally respiratory infection may be transmitted from workers to members of the public, and vice versa, as well, the most important example being tuberculosis in healthcare workers.

Tuberculosis

Tuberculosis is a respiratory infection spread by infected droplets from person to person. In England and Wales, since 1950 the number of cases fell 10-fold from about 50 000 per year to 5085 per year in 1987, but there is now good evidence that this decline has ceased and the number of cases is increasing again. Around nine million new cases occur each year world-wide, 95% of which arise in low income countries. Migrants from these countries bring with them an increased risk of tuberculosis. In England and Wales the 1993 Medical Research Council survey showed a incidence of 4.3/100 000/year for white people, but the rate was 27 times higher in people from India and more than 30 times greater in people from Africa. In 1998, 56% of cases reported in the UK were in people not born in that country. In countries with a high prevalence of tuberculosis, the advent of HIV disease is promoting the disease in working-aged people. The same effect is apparent in the HIV-positive population of New York. In the UK, where the reservoir of tuberculous infection is mainly in elderly people, HIV has been less of a factor but this is now changing with increasing numbers of HIV positive cases of TB being diagnosed in patients arriving from high-risk countries. Worldwide about 1.8 million people die from tuberculosis each year of whom 1 in 7 have HIV infection.

Cross-infectivity in tuberculosis arises principally in the close domestic contacts of patients with smear positive sputum. The British Thoracic and Tuberculosis Association survey[46] found that about 9–13% of close contacts of smear positive index cases developed disease. In casual contacts the risk was 0.3%, and in close contacts of smear negative index cases only 0.5% of non-Asian and 2.8% of Asian subjects developed tuberculosis. (The risk of cross-infection with non-respiratory tuberculosis is very low.) The principal risk, therefore, lies with close contacts of smear positive cases. In an occupational setting each case needs to be assessed individually in the light of the clinical details of the index case and the working environment. In the UK, cases of tuberculosis must be notified by law to the Health Protection Agency, who will institute screening of people at risk, usually via an advisory local chest service.

Figure 18.2 summarizes the guidelines of National Institute of Clinical Excellence (NICE) on pre-employment screening for healthcare workers.[47] Doctors, nurses, physiotherapists, post-mortem technicians, laboratory workers, and others at risk of contact should be assessed and protected as necessary. Students, locums, agency staff, and contract ancillary workers may easily be overlooked, and should be included in assessment procedures, as should laboratory technicians in commercial and private research facilities.

At the pre-employment stage, details should be sought of any symptoms suggestive of tuberculosis, and of previous BCG vaccination or the presence of a BCG scar. A tuberculin test (preferably the Mantoux test) or interferon-gamma test is only necessary in new employees who do not have either a definite BCG scar or documentary evidence of previous BCG. If the tuberculin test proves negative (or Heaf grade 1), a BCG vaccination should be offered. It is not necessary to inspect the site after the vaccination (unless as a means of quality control of the technique of administering BCG). In British studies vaccination has been shown to reduce the risk of active tuberculosis by 70–80%. Quite often, a strongly positive tuberculin test arises. Formerly, this was taken to be suggestive of current infection and further investigation (chest radiography) ensued; but recent evidence suggests this is unnecessary in the absence of symptoms. An exception may be made for individuals with strongly positive reactions who come from tuberculosis endemic areas.

BCG vaccination is contraindicated in HIV-positive individuals. Potential employees in groups, or from countries, with a high prevalence of HIV infection, should be considered for HIV testing before BCG vaccination in tuberculin-negative individuals. HIV-positive healthcare workers should not be employed in areas where there is a risk of contacting active tuberculosis.

During employment, routine periodic chest radiography is neither necessary nor effective in screening. Awareness and early reporting of suspicious symptoms is the mainstay of detection.

If a worker contracts tuberculosis, treatment will initially comprise at least three first-line drugs (isoniazid, rifampicin, and pyrazinamide), with the addition of a fourth drug (usually ethambutol) if the possibility of drug resistance is considered significant. Treatment should be supervised by a physician (usually a chest physician) experienced in the management of tuberculosis.

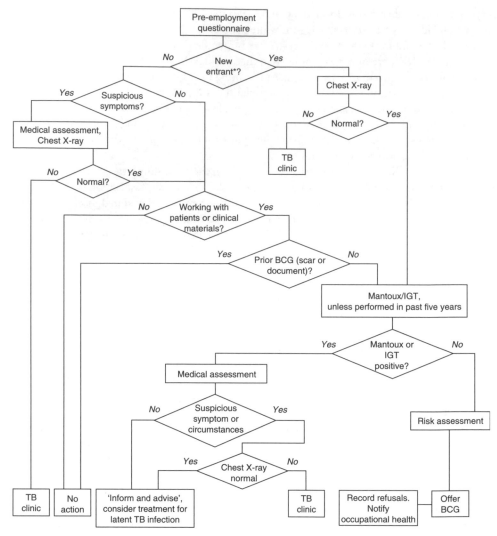

*New entrants = people arriving in or returning to the UK from a high-incidence country
(as defined by HPA website **www.hpa.org.uk**).

Fig. 18.2 Guidance on the protection of health care workers[47] © 2006, Royal College of Physicians.
Reproduced with permission.

Providing sensitivity results are available, continuation therapy can be reduced to isoniazid and
rifampicin after 2 months of treatment, and then needs to be maintained for a further
4 months. In fully sensitive infections (the majority in the UK), the patient is non-infectious after
2 weeks of treatment, and it is not usually necessary to restrict work after 2–3 weeks of treatment.
Caution may be appropriate, however, where there is reason to suspect drug resistance, and in
healthcare workers who deal with vulnerable patient groups (such as the immunosuppressed and
young children). An infectious risk should be assumed until drug sensitivities are known or the

sputum is known to be negative on culture. Drug resistance should be suspected in patients who have relapsed from earlier treatment and those who come from areas where drug resistance is common (e.g. Africa, the Indian subcontinent, and certain parts of the USA such as New York). HIV infection is a risk factor for drug-resistant tuberculosis. Problems may also arise in patients who are poorly compliant with treatment.

Neoplastic disease

Lung cancer

The most important aetiological risk factor for lung cancer is smoking. A number of occupational risk factors are also well-recognized, asbestos exposure being numerically the most important. In workers who both smoke and have asbestos exposure, the risk from lung cancer is substantially higher (roughly speaking, the risk from asbestos multiplied by the risk from smoking). Occupationally related lung cancers may also arise in the extraction of chromium from its ore, the manufacture of chromates, nickel refining, and exposure to polycyclic aromatic hydrocarbons, cadmium compounds, arsenic (in mining, smelting, and pesticide production) and bis-chloromethyl and chloromethyl methyl ethers.

The different histological types of lung cancer vary in their growth rate. In the absence of treatment, a patient with adenocarcinoma is likely to survive for about 2 years from the time of diagnosis, a patient with a squamous cell tumour for about 1 year, and a patient with a small cell tumour for about 4 months. Small cell tumours metastasize early, and are rarely amenable to surgical cure; but 85% respond to combination chemotherapy. The median survival is thus extended to about 8 months in patients with extensive disease, and to about 14 months in patients with limited disease; but a minority survive longer (10% for 2 years, 4% for 5 years). During this period, patients often enjoy a good quality of life, and can sometimes continue in light work.

For non-small cell lung cancer (adenocarcinoma, squamous carcinoma, and undifferentiated tumours), chemotherapy is much less successful, and the preferred treatment is surgical resection. Radiotherapy is usually used as an adjunct to surgery, or for the palliation of specific problems, such as haemoptysis and localized bone pain. Unfortunately, most tumours present when advanced, and other smoking-related lung disease often limits resectability. About 25% of patients are suitable for surgery. Of these, about a third survive for 5 years (65–85% in the absence of lymph node, chest wall, and metastatic involvement; but about 25–35% when there is ipsilateral mediastinal lymph node involvement). The 30-day operative mortality is about 6% for pneumonectomy and 3% for lobectomy. Patients below retirement age who undergo successful resection may well be able to return to work, though the choice of employment will depend on the physical demands of the job and the residual lung function after resection.

Mesothelioma

Mesothelioma is a rare tumour in the absence of asbestos exposure. It is a malignant condition affecting the pleura, or less often the peritoneum. The tumour arises after a long latent period— rarely less than 20 years from first exposure, and typically 35–40 years. This means that cases tend to arise after retirement.

The incidence of the tumour is rising in the UK, reflecting a greater use of asbestos during, and after the Second World War. In 1984 there were 534 cases in men and 84 cases in women, but by 1991 the annual total had risen to 1009. It is estimated that by 2020 there will be 3000 cases per year. A gradient of risk exists for different fibre types, greatest for crocidolite (blue asbestos) and least for chrysotile, with amosite occupying an intermediate position.

Mesothelioma often presents with chest wall pain, breathlessness, and pleural effusion. It progresses mainly by local invasion, although distant metastases can sometimes occur. Involvement of the chest wall, diaphragm, mediastinum, and neck root is common, and results in local pain, restricted chest movement, dysphagia, obstruction of the great veins, and pericardial involvement. The condition is incurable and most patients die within 2 years of presentation. It is rare for a patient with mesothelioma to be able to continue for long in active employment. A recent consensus statement by the British Thoracic Society Standards of Care Committee[48] offers a good summary of the condition and its management.

Other diseases of the pleura

One of the commonest manifestations of pleural disease is pleural effusion. Effusions that result from inflammatory processes are exudates, with a high protein content (>30 g/litre). Underlying causes include infection, collagen vascular disease, malignancy, and pulmonary infarction. Pleural malignancy, pulmonary infarction, and asbestotic pleurisy can also produce blood-stained effusions. Effusions of low protein content (transudates, protein <25 g/litre) may arise in cardiac failure and low protein states such as nephrotic syndrome and cirrhosis of the liver.

Fitness decisions require accurate information on the cause of the effusion and its prognosis. Investigation by aspiration, examination and culture of the fluid, and closed pleural biopsy normally enable the various possibilities to be distinguished, but otherwise thoracoscopy with biopsy, or open pleural biopsy are necessary.

When inflammatory effusions resolve, they frequently leave behind an area of pleural thickening, and adhesions that obliterate the pleural space. If extensive, this thickening can restrict lung movement, and produce chest discomfort and breathlessness on exertion.

At work, asbestos exposure frequently causes pleural plaques, which are circumscribed areas of thickening on the parietal pleura that may gradually calcify. They are composed of areas of hyaline fibrosis, a few millimetres up to 1 centimetre in thickness. Plaques are discovered radiographically (and seldom become evident within 15 years of first exposure), but they do not obliterate the pleural space, and produce no impairment of lung function or other disability. Their presence does not correlate well with that of pulmonary fibrosis (asbestosis), nor do they predicate the occurrence of mesothelioma (which is related to levels of exposure, but no more common in those who develop plaques than in those who do not). They tend to be discovered accidentally, and do not require work restriction or redeployment.

Asbestos exposure sometimes leads to pleurisy and haemorrhagic exudative pleural effusion. Effusion may also be discovered as an incidental radiographic finding. The majority occur 10–15 years after first exposure. They may persist for several months, recur after drainage, or affected both sides in sequence over a year or 2. Biopsy simply shows non-specific pleural inflammation. These pleural effusions may lead on to adhesions and diffuse pleural thickening. This latter condition, if extensive enough, produces restriction of lung expansion, dyspnoea, and work limitation. (Bilateral pleural thickening is therefore a prescribed disease.) There is no evidence that simple pleural plaques progress to diffuse pleural thickening, which is a different entity.

Smoking

Smoking is a major cause of respiratory disability, being the principal cause of both COPD and lung cancer. These two diseases together account for the majority of deaths from respiratory disease. The heavier the smoking the greater the risk. It is clearly good preventive practice to offer help and support to those who want to stop smoking and to make the workforce generally aware of the risks. The benefits of smoking cessation in COPD have already been discussed.

Smoking at work has major health implications for the smoker, but also some consequences for their colleagues. Patients with lung disease, especially asthma, are vulnerable to the irritant effects of a smoke-filled environment, and there is growing evidence that passive smoking is harmful: the children of smoking parents are more vulnerable to respiratory infections than those of non-smoking parents; the non-smoking wives of male smokers have somewhat higher risks of lung cancer than the wives of non-smokers; and the US Environmental Protection Agency has concluded that environmental tobacco smoke (ETS) is a carcinogen that accounts for some 2000 deaths per year in non-smokers in the USA. Although the health effects of ETS are small compared with active smoking, the large number of people exposed make ETS an important public health problem. The evidence has been summarized by the Royal College of Physicians of London.[49] A political mandate exists currently to extend the number of public places in which smoking is banned, to protect the health of third parties. Responsible employers should therefore give serious thought to establishing non-smoking policies in the workplace.

Special work problems and restrictions

Sometimes work is conducted in adverse environments, or in safety critical roles characterized by a requirement for high standards of respiratory fitness. Such is the case in airline pilots and cabin crew, commercial and military divers, caisson workers, and members of the armed forces, police, and rescue services. A number of these work activities involve changes in gas pressure and composition, and the use of breathing apparatus to extend the range of hostile environments in which work can be conducted; and all require a general level of fitness that transcends simple respiratory health.

The fitness standards required of pilots and commercial divers, and the physiological demands of their work are more fully described in Appendices 2 and 5 and elsewhere,[50,51] but reference is made here to some of the respiratory aspects of the work.

Flying and diving result in ambient gas pressure changes that pose major respiratory problems. The lung walls rupture at transmural pressures of about one-tenth of an atmosphere (10 kPa); the muscles of the chest tire within minutes if transmural pressures exceed 5 kPa; and the airways become easily irritated by changes in pressure and humidity. The fall in ambient pressure encountered in aeroplane ascent may thus result in pneumothorax, if gas trapping occurs in the chest (as might arise in bullous disease, asthma, or recent chest trauma). Similarly, ascent from a commercial or military dive may result in trapped gas at higher than ambient pressure seeking a means of escape, and causing pulmonary barotrauma or decompression sickness. Pneumothorax, peribronchial rupture, mediastinal emphysema, and air emboli are all well-recognized outcomes.

Related problems arise from altered oxygen tensions. The lowered partial pressure of oxygen (PaO_2) at elevated altitudes may aggravate hypoxia in air crew with existing airways disease; and, in fighter pilots, the problem may be exacerbated by physiological shunting in the dependent parts of the lung during high-G turns.

High standards of respiratory fitness are required in these categories of work, from the viewpoint of personal safety and well-being, and (especially in the case of aircrew) because of their responsibility for expensive equipment and other lives. In new entrants, a history of spontaneous pneumothorax, asthma, or obstructive respiratory disease is normally a bar to employment, as are most radiographic abnormalities.

In established workers who develop chest disease the criteria are slightly less stringent: it may, for example, be possible for well-controlled asthmatics, or patients with a pleurectomy or pleurodesis, to continue as members of an aircrew. The standards are set down respectively by the Civil Aviation Authority and Armed Services for flight fitness, and the HSE in the UK for fitness to dive.[52] In each of these cases, regular assessment is required by approved medical assessors, followed by certification of continuing fitness. Assessments include a number of subsidiary investigations, such as an annual chest X-ray in divers, as well as a detailed appraisal of other health issues, as described in Appendices 1–3.

Intercurrent respiratory illness is a temporary bar to diving and flying. Failure to equilibrate pressures across the Eustachian tube in catarrhal illness, and air trapping in the sinuses can cause decompression trauma, so diving and flying are best avoided until natural recovery has occurred. Professional divers who have recently surfaced (decompressed) sometimes wish then to fly: this may represent a further extreme of decompression, and they should be advised to refrain from flying until a minimum of 12 hours has elapsed.

Recommended minimum fitness standards for workers in the UK **Armed Services** are laid down in a Joint Services System of Medical Classification (JSP 346). New applicants with active tuberculosis, chronic bronchitis, or bronchiectasis are normally rejected, but if disease appears for the first time in service, the worker is individually assessed. Current asthma, or recurrent wheeze requiring recent treatment (within the past 4 years), is treated similarly; while those with a more distant history are tested for exercise-induced decrements of FEV_1. The occurrence of pneumothorax requires individual assessment, and depends on the nature of the work and the success or otherwise of surgical treatment.

The Armed Services use the 'PULHHEEMS' system to rank fitness for a number of physical and mental attributes against an eight-point scale of descriptors. Respiratory fitness is not separately identified in the rubric, although the P scale (physical fitness) encompasses cardiorespiratory fitness. Between Services and between jobs there may be some differences. For example, the fitness standards in RAF air-flight crew are more stringent than for ground personnel, such as engineers and technicians. However, for many jobs the minimum standard (fit with training for heavy manual work, including lifting and climbing, but not to endure severe or prolonged strain) precludes sufferers of significant chest disease.

UK regulations require **fire service workers** to have their FEV_1 and FVC measured by a doctor, and to have their aerobic capacity ($\dot{V}O_{2max}$) measured in a step test prior to employment. The regulations stipulate that a duly qualified medical practitioner must be satisfied that these measurements are compatible with the fitness requirements of firefighting, but refers to these only in general terms. Guidance by the Home Office, however, recommends a $\dot{V}O_{2max}$ standard of 45 ml/kg per min for recruit firefighters, and various age-related values for serving firefighters. The guidance further recommends regular fitness ($\dot{V}O_{2max}$) assessments and a 3-yearly health surveillance programme that involves measurement of height, weight, pulse, blood pressure, and visual acuity, as well as FEV1 and FVC, but the performance standard for spirometry is not specified. To assist Fire Service Medical Advisers with the interpretation and application of these rules, the Association of Local Authority Medical Advisers (ALAMA) has produced guidance on respiratory fitness for firefighters,[53] and this provides the basis of the further details that follow.

Firefighters are required to operate in very adverse environments, to wear breathing apparatus, and to perform physically arduous tasks. Intercurrent illnesses provide no more than a temporary bar to active duties, but conditions of airflow limitation may jeopardize employment prospects. Rescue workers may encounter irritant or sensitizing fumes and many products of combustion; some of these will exacerbate asthma, and some, including products of PVC combustion, may incite new asthma (reactive airways dysfunction syndrome or RADS). Active asthma on application often leads to rejection. If there is a prior history, or disease develops during employment, the circumstances should be individually assessed, but recurrent, severe, or refactory symptoms may precipitate medical retirement, as may poor performance on spirometry (≤ 2 SD of predicted). Established COPD of more than slight severity (as defined by the

British Thoracic Society. FEV_1 <60%), and chronic restrictive lung disease are generally considered incompatible with active fire fighting duties at the recruitment stage, and their development during employment generally leads to early retirement. The occurrence of pneumothorax should trigger individual review, but a successful pleurodesis may enable active duties to continue. Finally, the development of lung cancer would generally lead to rejection or retirement, but a successfully resected benign tumour is not a definite bar.

References

1 Standardised Lung Function Testing. Official Statement of the European Respiratory Society. *Eur Respir J* 1993; **6** (Suppl 16).

2 Cotes JE, Chinn DJ, Reed JW. Lung function testing: methods and reference values for forced expiratory volume and transfer factor. *Occup Environ Med* 1997; **54**: 457–65.

3 British Thoracic Society and the Association of Respiratory Technicians and Physiologists. Guidelines for the measurement of respiratory function. *Respir Med* 1994; **88**: 165–94.

4 American Thoracic Society. Standardization of spirometry: 1994 update. *Am J Respir Crit Care Med* 1995; **152**: 1107–36.

5 Eisen EA, Dockery DW, Speizer FE, Fay MA, Ferris BG, Jr. The association between health status and the performance of excessively variable spirometry tests in a population-based study in six US cities. *Am Rev Respir Dis* 1987; **136**: 1371–6.

6 Miller MR. Peak expiratory flow meter scale changes: implications for patients and health professionals. *Airways J* 2004; **2**(2): 80–2.

7 Singh SJ, Morgan MDL, Walters SS *et al*. The development of the shuttle walk test of disability in patients with chronic airways obstruction. *Thorax* 1992; **47**: 1019–24.

8 McGavin CR, Gupta SP, McHardy GJR. 12 minute walking test for assessing disability in chronic bronchitis. *BMJ* 1976; **1**: 822–3.

9 Medical Research Council on the Aetiology of Chronic Bronchitis. Standardized questionnaires on respiratory symptoms. *BMJ* 1960; **ii**: 665.

10 Toren K, Brisman J, Jarvholm B. Asthma and asthma-like symptoms in adults assessed by questionnaires: A literature review. *Chest* 1993; **104**: 600–8.

11 Venables KM, Farrer N, Sharp L, Graneek BJ, Newman Taylor AJ. Respiratory symptoms questionnaire for asthma epidemiology: validity and reproducibility. *Thorax* 1993; **48**: 214–19.

12 Wagner GR. Asbestosis and silicosis. *Lancet* 1997; **349**: 1311–15.

13 Stenton SC, Beach JR, Avery AJ, Hendrick DJ. Asthmatic symptoms, airway responsiveness and recognition of bronchoconstriction. *Respir Med* 1995; **89**: 181–5.

14 Stenton SC, Beach JR, Avery AJ, Hendrick DJ. The value of questionnaires and spirometry in asthma surveillance programmes in the workplace. *Occup Med* 1993; **43**: 203–6.

15 Jones PW. Assessment of the impact of mild asthma in adults. *Eur Respir Rev* 1996; **6**: 57–60.

16 British Thoracic Society and Scottish Intercollegiate Guidelines Network. British Guideline on the Management of Asthma. *Thorax* 2003; **58** (Suppl. 1): 1–94.

17 Nicholson PJ, Cullinan P, Newman-Taylor AJ, Burge PS, Boyle C. Evidence-based guidelines for the prevention, identification and management of occupational asthma. *Occup Environ Med* 2005; **62**: 290–9.

18 American Thoracic Society. Guidelines for the evaluation of impairment/disability in patients with asthma. *Am Rev Respir Dis* 1993; **147**: 1056–61.

19 Slovak AJM, Hill RN. Laboratory animal allergy: a clinical survey of an exposed population. *Br J Ind Med* 1981; **38**: 38–41.

20 Tee RD, Gordon DJ, Hansham ER. Occupational allergy to locusts: an investigation of the sources of the allergen. *J Allergy Clin Immunol* 1988; **81**: 517–25.

21 Burge PS. Single and serial measurements of lung function in the diagnosis of occupational asthma. *Eur J Respir Dis* 1982; **63**: 47–59.

22 Bright P, Burge PS. The diagnosis of occupational asthma from serial measurements of lung function at and away from work. *Thorax* 1996; **51**: 857–63.

23 Burge PS, Pantin CF, Newton DT *et al.* Development of an expert system for the interpretation of serial peak expiratory flow measurements in the diagnosis of occupational asthma. Midlands Thoracic Society Research Group. *Occup Environ Med* 1999; **56**: 758–64.

24 Chan-Yeung M, MacLean L, Paggiaro RL. Follow-up study of 232 patients with occupational ashma caused by Western Red Cedar. *J Allergy Clin Immunol* 1987; **79**: 792–6.

25 Malo JL, Cartier A, Ghezzo H *et al.* Patterns of improvement in spirometry, bronchial hyperresponsiveness and specific IgE antibody levels after cessation of exposure in occupational asthma caused by snow-crab processing. *Am Rev Respir Dis* 1998; **138**: 807–12.

26 Gannon PF, Weir DC, Robertson AS, *et al.* Health, employment and financial outcomes in workers with occupational asthma. *Br J Ind Med* 1993; **50**: 491–6.

27 Health and Safety Executive. *Medical Aspects of Occupational Asthma*. London: HMSO, 1991.

28 Chan-Yeung M. Occupational asthma. *Chest* 1994; **98**: 24–61S.

29 The National Collaborating Centre for Chronic Conditions. Chronic Obstructive Pulmonary Disease. National clinical guidelines on management of chronic obstructive pulmonary disease in adults in primary and secondary care. *Thorax* 2004; **59** (Suppl. 1).

30 Chapman KR, Bowie DM, Goldstein RS, *et al.* Guidelines for the assessment and management of chronic obstructive pulmonary disease. Canadian Thoracic Society Workshop Group. *Can Med Assoc J* 1992; **147**: 420–8.

31 US Department of Labor. *Selected characteristics of occupations defined in the Dictionary of Occupational Titles*. Washington, DC: US Government Printing Office, 1981.

32 Cotes JE, Zejda J, King B. Lung function impairment as a guide to exercise limitation in work-related lung disorders. *Am Rev Respir Dis* 1988; **137**: 1089–93.

33 Williams SJ, Bury MR. Impairment, disability and handicap in chronic respiratory illness. *Soc Sci Med* 1989; **29**: 609–16.

34 Harber P. Respiratory disability: the uncoupling of oxygen consumption and disability. *Clin Chest Med* 1992; **13**: 367–76.

35 Gross NJ. Ipratropium bromide. *N Engl J Med* 1988; **319**: 486–94.

36 Tashkin DP, Ashutosh K, Bleecker ER, *et al.* Comparison of the anticholinergic bronchodilator ipratropium bromide with metaproterenol in chronic obstructive airway disease. *Am J Med* 1986; **81**: 81–90.

37 West R, M'Neill A, Raw M. Smoking cessation guidelines for health professionals: an update. *Thorax* 2000; **50**: 987–99.

38 Kearon MC, Summers E, Jones NL. Effort and dyspnoea during work of varying intensity and duration. *Eur Respir J* 1991; **4**: 917–25.

39 Becklake MR, Liddell FDK, Manfreda J, McDonald JC. Radiological changes after withdrawal from asbestos exposure. *Br J Ind Med* 1979; **36**: 23–8.

40 Steenland NK, Brown D. Silicosis among gold miners: exposure-reponse analysis and risk assessment. *Am J Public Health* 1995; **85**: 1372–7.

41 Health and Safety Executive. *Approved Code of Practice: The Control of Asbestos at Work Regulations 1987*, pp. 21–2. London: HMSO, 1988.

42 Wagner GR. *Screening and surveillance of workers exposed to mineral dusts*. Geneva: WHO, 1996.

43 Health and Safety Executive. *Crystalline silica*, p. 4. London: HMSO, 1992.

44 International Labour Office. *Guidelines for the use of ILO international classification of radiographs of pneumoconioses*. Geneva: ILO, 1980.

45 Report of the Joint Working Group of the Royal Colleges of Physicians, Psychiatrists and General Practitioners. *Chronic fatigue syndrome*. London: RCP, 1996.

46 Research Committee of the British Thoracic Association. A study of a standardised contact procedure in tuberculosis. *Tubercle* 1978; **59**: 245–59.

47 The National Collaborating Centre for Chronic Conditions. Tuberculosis: Clinical diagnosis and management of tuberculosis, and measures for its prevention and control. London: Royal College of Physicians, 2006, pp 1–215.

48 British Thoracic Society Standards of Care Committee. Statement on malignant mesothelioma in the United Kingdom. *Thorax* 2001; **56**: 250–65.

49 Royal College of Physicians. *Tobacco smoke pollution: the hard facts. 10 reasons to make public places smoke free.* London: Royal College of Physicians, 2004.

50 Bennett PB, Elliott DH. *The physiology and medicine of diving*, (4th edn). London: WB Saunders, 1993.

51 Hopkirk JAC, Denison DM. Areospace medicine. In: *The Oxford textbook of medicine* (eds Weatherall DJ, Ledingham JGG, Warrell DA). Oxford: Oxford University Press, 1995.

52 *Diving operations at work regulations.* London: HMSO, 1981.

53 Association of Local Authority Medical Advisers. Respiratory conditions. In: *Medical aspects of fitness for firefighting.* London: ALAMA, 1983.

Chapter 19

Renal and urological disease

J. Hobson and E. A. Brown

Introduction

The kidney has the vital function of excretion, and controls acid–base, fluid, and electrolyte balance. It also acts as an endocrine organ. Renal failure, with severe impairment of these functions, results from a number of different processes, most of which are acquired, although some may be inherited. Glomerulonephritis, which presents with proteinuria, haematuria, or both, may be accompanied by hypertension and impaired renal function. Pyelonephritis with renal scarring is the end result of infective disorders. Additionally, systemic diseases such as diabetes, hypertension, and collagen disorders can affect the kidney. Polycystic kidney disease is the commonest inherited disorder leading to renal failure. Chronic renal failure implies permanent renal damage, which is likely to be progressive and will eventually require renal replacement therapy.

Advances in the treatment of end-stage renal failure using haemodialysis (HD) and peritoneal dialysis (PD), and the success of kidney transplantation, have improved the quality of life for patients and mean that many can expect to return to normal lives including work. Better management of urinary infections and calculi, prostatic obstruction, incontinence, and other complications of urinary tract disease enable the attending physician or surgeon to predict less time lost from work and better capability for doing it.

The impact of renal and urinary tract disorders on work attendance and performance has been scantily reported in the literature. National data show that disease of the genitourinary tract accounts for less than 2% of absence but much of this occurs in people of working age. Women have twice as many episodes of absence as men but account for only a quarter of total lost time. There are, however, few overall contraindications to undertaking gainful employment for those suffering from renal or urological disorders, and now plenty of opportunity for encouraging both an early return to work and continuing in the same job.

Reintegration of patients into the workforce following transplantation or dialysis offers an exciting and rewarding challenge to the wider health team.

Prevalence and morbidity

The 2003 UK Renal Registry report[1] shows that in the UK, the 2002 annual acceptance rate for new patients starting on **renal replacement therapy (RRT)** is about 110/million population. This varies from 98/million in England to 120/million in Scotland. The type of patient has changed, with a dramatic increase in the age-specific rate of new patients over 65 years old and in the number of diabetics. In 1980, diabetes accounted for 2% of patients starting RRT, but now accounts for almost 20% of patients accepted for treatment in the UK. Crude annual acceptance rates vary from 52/million population to 165/million in different parts of the country. Acceptance ratios, standardized for age and gender of the population served, correlate significantly with both social deprivation and with ethnicity; the number of patients requiring RRT increases in areas with high numbers of ethnic minorities. The 2003 report also shows that the number of patients on RRT in the UK in 2002 was 626/million population with 34% aged over 65; the annual increase in prevalent RRT patients is 4%. The median age for HD, PD, and transplant patients, respectively, was 64.5, 58.3, and 49.6 years and 46% of RRT patients had a functioning transplant.

Chronic kidney disease (CKD) is common with only a minority developing end-stage renal disease (ESRD) requiring RRT. In the USA, the Third National Health and Nutrition Survey (Nhanes III)[2] has shown that 4.3% of the population has CKD with a glomerular filtration rate (GFR) of 30–59 ml/min per /1.73m^2 and 0.2% has CKD with a GFR <15–29 ml/min per 1.73m^2. In the UK, screening for renal disease by retrospective surveys of plasma creatinine measurements from chemical pathology laboratories serving defined populations has shown a similar prevalence of more severe CKD (0.2–0.5% general population).

In terms of claims for incapacity benefit, diseases of the genitourinary tract (ICD10 N00–N99) make up a small proportion of claimants nationally. In May 2004 approximately 0.6% of claims were for diseases of the genitourinary tract in men (8000 claimants) and 1.0% in women (9 000 claimants).[3] Certified incapacity due to sickness from genitourinary causes accounts for less than 1% of all lost time. In men most time is lost in those aged 60–64, whereas in women, most days are lost in those aged 30–39.[4]

Although many **urinary tract infections** are asymptomatic, there is much morbidity from this condition. The size of the problem is difficult to ascertain. Up to 50% of females have symptoms at some stage in their lives. Occurrence is much less frequent in males but rises sharply after the age of 60 due to lower urinary tract conditions, especially prostatic problems. It has been estimated that between 12 to 60 per 1000 consultations in general practice are for symptoms suggesting a urinary tract infection while an estimated 45 days per hundred persons each year are lost from work from this cause.[5]

Urolithiasis of the upper urinary tract is a fairly common condition in the UK, with a prevalence of 3.5–4 per hundred, but the incidence appears to be on the increase. The peak incidence in males occurs at the age of 35 years. Renal stones cause much morbidity, but with the widespread availability of lithotripsy, extensive renal surgery can be avoided in most cases and as a consequence time off work is considerably reduced.

Papilloma of the bladder is the only occupational cancer to reach double figures for annual disability benefit awards in England and Wales, apart from asbestos-related lung cancer.[6] In the 10 years between 1994 and 2003 there were 290 new cases assessed for disablement as Prescribed Disease C23 (papilloma of the bladder).

Benign prostatic hyperplasia (BPH) is the commonest prostatic problem after the fourth decade; 50% of men have BPH when they are 51–60 years old. At the age of 55, 25% notice some decrease in force of their urinary stream. At age 40 (surviving to 80) there is a cumulative incidence of 29% for prostatectomy.

Mortality

The majority of patients with renal disease will die from cardiovascular disease before they require RRT. A recent analysis of causes of death from 1996 to 2000 in over a million adults enrolled in the Kaiser Permamente of Northern California showed that risk of death from any cause increased sharply as the estimated GFR declined, ranging from a 17% increase in risk with an estimated GFR of 45–59 ml/min per 1.73 m^2 to a 343% increase with an estimated GFR <15 ml/min per 1.73 m^2.[7] There was a similar increase in cardiovascular events and hospitalization.

Table 19.1 Five-year survival rates for England and Wales

	Bladder (1986–90)	Kidney (1986–90)	Prostate (1992–94)
Males	62%	38%	55%
Females	57%	35%	

The age-adjusted mortality rate for an estimated GFR of 15–29 ml/min per 1.73 m^2 was strikingly high at 11.4/100 person-years, which is similar to those on RRT.

In the UK in 2002, there were 1536 male and 1526 female deaths (all ages) from renal failure, (ICD-10, N17–19).[8] Even though 90% occur over retirement age, much of the associated morbidity is incurred during the working years. These totals represent about 40% of all deaths from diseases of the urinary system (ICD-10 N00–N39).

In England and Wales during 2002 bladder cancer (ICD-10 C67) killed twice as many men (2919) as women (1501) in all age groups. About 87% of deaths occur in those over the age of 65 years. As a cause of death it was the fifth most common tumour for men (4% of male cancer deaths) and the eleventh for women (2% of female cancer deaths). Malignant neoplasms of urinary tract (C64–C68) accounted for 4782 male deaths and 2592 female deaths in 2002. Prostate cancer (C61) accounted for 8973 male deaths.

Presentation

Renal disease is easily missed. Early disease can often be asymptomatic and present as urinary abnormalities on routine urine testing, hypertension or as biochemical abnormalities. Unless GFR is calculated or measured, significant renal impairment can be present even when the plasma creatinine is in the normal range. The discovery of asymptomatic haematuria, whether macroscopic or microscopic, and not related to urinary tract infection, requires further investigation. If positive, dipstick testing should always be repeated. One + of blood or protein is probably of no pathological significance but repeated 2+ or more of blood should be followed up with an MSU. Red cells lyse in dilute urine so blood on dipstick may indicate free haemoglobin from normal amounts of red cells in urine. Repeated protein on dipstick can be followed up with spot urine protein/creatinine ratio to detect overt proteinuria, which is simpler than doing 24-hour urine tests.

In one study, **microscopic haematuria** was detected by the strip technique in 3.5% of 2100 men over the age of 40 systematically examined at their place of work.[9] Thirty-two men agreed to undergo further investigations of whom a quarter (0.4% of the initial group) were found to have urinary tract disease, including stones, prostatic adenoma, vesical diverticulum, and two bladder tumours. It was necessary to perform intravenous urography and cystoscopy to detect all these abnormalities. The conclusion was that even a single episode of microscopic haematuria in a man over 40 should be investigated with intravenous urography. If the results are normal and the subject is a smoker or has an occupational or familial risk of cancer, cytology and vesical echography should be performed and then cystoscopy if these are negative. A long-term prospective follow up study of 90 patients with asymptomatic isolated microscopic haematuria found that at least 19% developed at least one adverse event after a mean of 42 months, including one transitional cell carcinoma of the bladder and one chronic renal failure the remainder being hypertension or proteinuria.[10]

Proteinuria detected by urine dipstick is more suggestive of intrinsic renal disease. The urinary protein excretion needs to be quantified and plasma urea and creatinine should be checked; if proteinuria is more than 0.3 g/24 hour, or if the renal function is abnormal, the patient should be referred to a renal clinic.

Hypertension both causes renal disease and is a common complication of renal disease inducing a vicious cycle with further renal damage.

Diabetes is now the most common cause of ESRD, accounting for 20% of patients starting dialysis in the UK in 2002 and 40% in the USA. The natural history is the development of microalbuminuria, progressing to overt proteinuria with hypertension and subsequent decline in renal function. In young patients with insulin-dependent diabetes, this process does not commence until at least 10 years after the onset of diabetes. This is not true for non-insulin-dependent diabetes when the onset of the disease is less clear-cut; it is not uncommon for patients to have proteinuria or even significant renal disease at the time of diagnosis. The majority of patients with diabetic renal disease will also have diabetic retinopathy with its associated problems.

Complications and sequelae of renal disease

Hypertension

Most patients with renal disease will eventually develop hypertension. This needs aggressive treatment as tight blood pressure control, aiming for levels as low as 125/75, has been shown to significantly slow down the rate of progression of renal damage in the majority of renal disease. This usually requires multiple drugs, which may themselves cause side-effects. Monitoring of blood pressure is clearly important requiring frequent visits to medical or nurse-led clinics, though patients are increasingly being encouraged to monitor their own blood pressure at home as this correlates better with 24-hour blood pressure monitoring and avoids the white coat effect.

Cardiovascular disease

Cardiovascular disease is the major cause of death in patients with renal failure, but even mild renal disease is associated with increased cardiovascular risk. Patients with cardiovascular disease have a worse outcome if they have even mild renal disease.[11]

Renal failure

The early symptoms of renal failure are fatigue with poor exercise tolerance. These can develop when the GFR is high as 30 ml/min and can be exacerbated by the presence of anaemia, which can occur with GFRs of 30–40 ml/min. As renal function deteriorates further, appetite diminishes with subsequent loss of weight, fluid retention with associated symptoms (ankle swelling, shortness of breath on exercise), loss of libido, and nocturia (due to polyuria from osmotic diuresis) can occur. Many of these symptoms improve when the anaemia is corrected with appropriate use of erythropoietin and iron supplements, although haemoglobin is usually maintained at 11–12 g/dl as there is still no evidence about improvement in quality of life or survival with a haemoglobin closer to normal. The level of symptoms should determine the start of dialysis rather than blood tests or GFR measurements. It is more important that a patient remains relatively well and in employment (if working) than waiting (at home) to become really ill and then require a long period of rehabilitation.

Box 19.1 Treatment modalities for ESRD

- ◆ Haemodialysis (HD)
  - • Centre
  - • Satellite
  - • Home
- ◆ Peritoneal dialysis (PD)
  - • CAPD (continuous ambulatory PD)
  - • APD (automated PD)
- ◆ Transplantation
  - • Cadaver
  - • Living donor (related or unrelated)
- ◆ Conservative management
  - • Best supportive care

End-stage renal disease

The aims of RRT are not simply correction of blood abnormalities and maintenance of fluid balance. Patients can live on RRT for decades so the aims are for them to live as normal a life as possible. It is therefore important that they utilize a mode of RRT that they tolerate well and therefore comply with, that provides physical well-being and allows social and employment rehabilitation. There are now many treatment modalities for the treatment of end-stage renal disease (ESRD) as shown in the Box 19.1.

Dialysis

Patients with ESRD can now expect a reasonable survival and quality of life on dialysis. The 2003 UK renal registry report shows that the annual survival rate for patients <65 years old is 92% for non-diabetics and 82% for diabetics. For patients who can use any modality, the choice of HD or PD will depend on individual patient preference, nephrologist bias, and local resources. For instance approximately 20% of patients start PD in the USA compared with 40% in the UK and 90% in Hong Kong. Even within the same city there can be marked variation and 35% of new patients start PD in one London hospital compared with 10% in another 3 miles away. Dialysis affects all aspects of life including diet, family life, holidays, work, and travel. From the patient perspective, perceived quality of life on a given modality is the principal reason for choosing the dialysis modality they want to use. As shown in Box 19.2, the main differences of HD and PD stem from the fact that HD is a hospital-based treatment (although a few patients do carry out their HD at home), and PD is a home-based treatment.

A recent study of 1347 patients commencing dialysis in the Netherlands showed that of the 864 patients who chose their dialysis modality, 36% of the 416 patients starting PD were employed compared with only 16% of patients starting HD.[12]

Box 19.2 Quality of life and modality of dialysis

Haemodialysis

- ◆ Hospital-based treatment
  - • Suitable for dependent patients
  - • Provides social structure for frail elderly patients
  - • Requires transport time
  - • Interferes with work
- ◆ Increased hospitalization for vascular access problems
- ◆ Difficult to travel for holiday or work

Peritoneal dialysis

- ◆ Home-based treatment
  - • Patient independence
  - • Fits in with work
  - • Can be done by carer at home
  - • Less visits to hospital
- ◆ Easier to travel and go on holiday

Work and dialysis

The median age of starting dialysis is now over 65 years, so many patients will not be working. Many younger patients do continue to work, though it is often difficult to continue to do so full-time. The well-being of someone on dialysis depends on many factors, both physical and psychological. The physical symptoms that some continue to experience will depend on adequacy of dialysis and compliance with treatment. It is not surprising that there are many psychological factors that both cause symptoms and interfere with treatment; these include depression, anxiety, denial of illness, all of which can contribute to poor compliance. Family and social support is also important, helping individuals to cope with the rigours of treatment and providing emotional support needed to cope. Some of the complexities faced in helping an individual remain at work are illustrated by the case below.

> Mr C is a 50-year-old man from Hong Kong who had had a successful career as an accountant in a large firm. At age 45 he developed angina, required coronary bypass surgery and was found to be diabetic with renal impairment. As his renal function slowly declined, he was very anxious about his future. He found it hard to discuss things with his family (wife, who is a nurse, and two teenage children who do well at school and progress to university). He found his job stressful so left his firm and took on short-term contracts. He would not admit that he had any symptoms from his renal failure but was eventually persuaded to start dialysis in 2002 when his plasma creatinine was 950 μmol/l. He chose automated PD as this left him free during the day. He initially did very well, continuing to work full time. However, after a year he announced that he had given up work and was now spending all his time at home. Blood tests showed that he was not receiving enough dialysis; he was also anaemic. At a meeting with him, his wife, and members of the healthcare team (renal consultant, PD nurse, renal

counsellor), it became apparent that compliance was poor—he was often not putting himself on dialysis at night and was missing erythropoietin injections; he had lost self-esteem and felt a burden on his family. He accepted some counselling, compliance improved and he felt better. He has again taken on some short-term contracts though continues to need encouragement from the medical team to do so.

Many individuals do continue to work in all sorts of professions. They can be enabled to do so with the aid of the occupational health team at the place of work, or if the employer has some understanding of the flexibility required in the working day. It is also important for the dialysis team caring for the patient to adapt the treatment round the needs of the patient, e.g. arranging HD in the evening if the patient works during the day, flexibility with clinic appointments, etc. It is often easier to fit RRT round work if treatment is carried out at home, whether HD or PD. Specific problems related to working for patients on dialysis are shown in Box 19.3.

Box 19.3 Employment and dialysis

Haemodialysis

- Rigid timing—usually 4 hours three times a week plus transport to and from dialysis unit
- HD units usually have two to three shifts a day with little flexibility of timing for patients on shift work
- Difficult to arrange treatments at other units, particularly at short notice, making travel difficult
- Intermittent treatment so dietary and fluid restrictions
- Patients often feel washed out after dialysis and can be relatively hypotensive
- Presence of arteriovenous fistula in arm—needs to avoid heavy lifting with that arm
- If patient opts for home HD, some weeks dialysing at hospital needed to accustom patient to dialysis, and to train patient to needle their own fistula and manage machine

Peritoneal dialysis

- Home-based treatment allowing flexibility round work routine
- Travel relatively easy—patient can transport own fluid for short trips or fluid can be delivered to many parts of the world
- Can be difficult to fit in four exchanges a day if on CAPD and working, but some patients can arrange clean and private place at work to do an exchange
- More freedom during day if patient on APD—at most, one bag exchange is needed and this can be done at a time convenient for patient
- Continuous treatment, so no 'swings' in well-being of patient
- Heavy lifting should be avoided because of increased risk of abdominal hernias and fluid leaks
- PD usually started 2 weeks after catheter insertion with a training period of 1 week

Transplantation

Successful transplantation not only provides the best quality of life for patients with ESRD but also prolongs life expectancy compared with patients fit enough to be on a transplant list but who do not receive a transplant. The median wait for a cadaveric kidney in the UK has increased from 407 days in 1990–92 to 579 days in 1996–97 (data from UK Transplant). Patients who are blood group B have the longest wait (median wait of 912 days) compared with 317 days for blood group A. This is of particular importance for Indo-Asian patients who have a higher prevalence of blood group B than the indigenous Caucasian population. Patients who are on the waiting list for cadaveric transplantation need to come to the transplant unit as soon as they receive their call. The initial inpatient stay is usually 1–2 weeks and for the first 3–4 months frequent blood tests are needed, several times a week in the first instance and then weekly. Up to a third of transplants are from living donors, both related and unrelated. Living donor transplantation can be timed to suit the patient, e.g. during the school holidays for a teacher.

Patients can lead a normal life after successful transplantation, but they do need to continue daily immunosuppressive therapy. The actual immunosuppressive regimen will vary from unit to unit, as many different agents are now available (prednisolone, azathioprine, cyclosporin, tacrolimus, sirolimus, mycophenylate). Transplant patients are therefore at increased risk of infections and have a slightly increased risk of developing malignancy. Skin malignancies are among the most common, so patients should be advised to avoid sun exposure. If doing work outside, they should either wear clothing which covers arms, legs, etc., or use sun block creams. There are complications related to specific immunosuppressive drugs such as hirsutism with cyclosporine or diabetes with tacrolimus. Many patients also remain hypertensive after transplantation. Cardiovascular disease remains a major cause of morbidity and mortality but less so than patients on dialysis.

Long-term follow-up studies are encouraging. A study of 57 adult survivors from childhood transplantation showed a high level of employment (82%) and 95% reported their health as fair or good.[13] This was despite a high retransplantation rate and significant morbidity such as hypertension, bone and joint symptoms, fractures, hypercholesterolaemia, and cataracts. Nearly half of all respondents were severely short and 27% were obese. A study of 267 Japanese transplant recipients with a minimum follow-up of 10 years found actual patient and graft survival rates of 80% and 51% at 10 years and 56% and 33% at 20 years.[14] Dominant causes of death in patients with graft surviving for over 10 years were hepatic failure due to viral hepatitis and malignancies. In 15 patients with grafts surviving beyond 20 years malignancy occurred in five, viral hepatitis in three, aseptic necrosis in three, and diabetes mellitus in one patient but 11 of the 15 remained in full-time employment.

Renal failure and employment

Successful transplant patients should be capable of virtually any normal work and a useful simple guide for employers, patients, and their doctors has been published.[15] The work situation should carry no undue risk of blows or trauma to the lower abdomen and likewise the arteriovenous fistula at the wrist should be protected from injury by sharp projections or tools. In the USA differences have also been found in vocational rehabilitation in end-stage renal therapy patients[16] summarized in Table 19.2.

Various follow-up studies have found employment rates of 28% (Spain), 43% (USA), and 45% (Canada) with employment being predicted by employment before, and time following, transplantation.[17–19] Patient and physician expectation with regard to employment appear to be important to employment in both dialysis and following transplantation but can be modified.[18, 20]

Table 19.2 Vocational rehabilitation in patients with ESRD from the USA

	Male	Female
Transplant	70%	33%
CAPD	35%	15%
Hospital haemodialysis	19%	11%

The main problems surround those on dialysis. Loss of work is an important issue in both pre-dialysis and dialysis patients. A joint study from the Manchester and Oxford renal units found that there was a sharp decline in the percentage of those working some 6–12 months after the start of CAPD (44% from 73%), or of HD (42% from 83%).[21,22] A Croatian study of 161 HD patients found that starting HD was associated with leaving full-time employment and 50% of those in full or part-time employment were retired within 2 years of starting HD.[23]

A prospective study of over 4000 new US dialysis patients over their first year on dialysis revealed a decreasing number of working individuals over time, from 42% before the initiation of dialysis to 21% at initiation, and under 7% a year later.[24]

A Dutch study assessed employment status in 659 new ESRD patients at the start of dialysis and after 1 year.[25] At the start of dialysis, 35% of patients were employed, in contrast to 61% of the general population. Within 1 year, the proportion of employed patients decreased from 31% to 25% of HD patients, and from 48% to 40% of PD patients. Independent risk factors for loss of work were impaired physical and psychosocial functioning and therefore improvements in physical and psychosocial functioning are potentially preventive of loss of work in patients who are employed when they start dialysis.

A US study of 359 chronic dialysis patients (85 employed and 274 unemployed) found education to be a significant correlate of employment but neither mode of dialysis, length of time on dialysis, number of co-morbid conditions, nor cause of renal failure (e.g. diabetes) were associated with employment status.[26] Measures of functional status were positively associated with employment but patients' perceptions that their health limited the type and amount of work that they could do were negatively associated with employment. Patients who themselves believed that dialysis patients should work and had this notion reinforced by others were more likely to be employed. Twenty-one per cent of unemployed patients reported that they were both able to work and wanted to return to work. Other factors affecting employment in dialysis patients include selection of fitter patients for transplantation, availability of disability benefits and health insurances, education and employer attitudes.[27–29] However, pre-dialysis intervention in assisting workers with end-stage renal failure has been shown to be of benefit; in a study from California, those who had social worker assessment, patient education and counselling and renal unit orientation to the dialysis were 2.8 times more likely to continue work after starting HD.[30]

Fitness for work and renal failure

With flexibility, adaptation, careful planning and support, and a change of attitude on the part of employers, many more dialysis patients could work successfully. The aim should be to adapt both ways—the work to the patient's needs and the patient's treatment regimen to the work, whichever direction best achieves a satisfactory outcome. Many employers, although sympathetic, misunderstand what can be achieved by patients with chronic renal failure, and this by itself may preclude successful employment. There is thus a real need first to educate both doctors and employers about the work capabilities of such people, and to encourage a positive attitude in the patients themselves. The close co-operation of all concerned (the patient, the renal unit, the general practitioner, occupational health staff, and the employer) is often needed to effect a successful placement. The occupational physician is usually best placed to catalyse the necessary adjustments but it is necessary to actively seek out ways and means whereby a successful job placement can be achieved, rather than just looking for the contraindications. If reasonable adaptation in the workplace cannot be made, a special rehabilitation programme should be considered in conjunction with the social worker and the Disability Employment Adviser (DEA). Further details of help with return to work through the Employment Service are given in Chapter 4.

Restrictions and contraindications

The essential and relative employment contraindications for dialysis patients are shown in Table 19.3.

Patients in irreversible renal failure are unsuited for work as firemen, police on the beat, rescue personnel, or the armed forces on active service, because of the high energy demands, extended hours, and the flexibility required for emergency duty imposed by these jobs. Similar restrictions

Table 19.3 Haemodialysis and continuous ambulatory peritoneal dialysis and types of employment

1 Contraindications (unsuitable)	2 Relative contraindications (possible)	3 No contraindications (suitable)
Armed Forces (active service)	Catering trades*	Accountancy
Chemical exposure to renal toxins	Farm labouring*	Clerical/secretarial
Construction/building/scaffolding	Heavy goods vehicle driving*	Driving
Diving	Horticultural work	Law
Firefighters	Motor repair (care with fistula in HD patients)	Light assembly
Furnace/smelting	Nursing*	Light maintenance/repair
Heavy labouring	Painting and decorating*	Light manufacturing industry
Heavy manual work	Printing*	Medicine
Mining	Refuse collection*	Middle and senior management
Police (on the beat)	Shiftwork	Packing
Work in very hot environments	Welding*	Receptionist
		Retail trade
		Sales
		Supervising
		Teaching

*Not contraindicated in HD.

For patients on HD, shiftwork and extended hours may present problems requiring greater adaptation. Some patients have learnt to dialyse while asleep using the built-in warning devices on the machine.

Should occupations in column 2 entail much heavy lifting, or manual work, they may be unsuitable.

may apply to particularly stressful jobs demanding a very high degree of vigilance (e.g. air traffic controllers). Jobs combining both a high radiant heat burden and high physical activity may also be contraindicated. Patients in end-stage renal failure on dialysis are not suitable for underground working, for diving or other work in hyperbaric conditions such as tunnelling under pressure. They are also unlikely to meet the standards required for Merchant Shipping, which may require lengthy periods at sea and in tropical and subtropical climates.[31] Additionally, most seafarers nowadays will need to join and leave ships by air travel.

Although air travel is not contraindicated for those undertaking continuous ambulatory PD regimens, it imposes extra difficulties and the added inconvenience of carrying supplies of the dialysate solution. Also in the context of travel abroad, the reduced dosage required for drug prophylaxis against malaria for those in renal failure should be recognized.

It is essential for those on PD to avoid work in dirty or dusty environments, and also work that requires heavy lifting or constant bending. Tight or restrictive clothing should not be worn. Patients also need a clean area for performing their midday fluid exchange, as it is essential to prevent infection. The suitability, both of the type of work and of an area at the workplace for the exchange, should preferably be assessed on site by the renal unit specialist nurse, in conjunction with the occupational health staff and the employer.

Patients on HD need to be within easy reach of a dialysis facility, so work involving much distant travel and frequent periods away from home may not be suitable.

If there are canteen facilities, it can be helpful to ensure that the necessary low salt and high/low protein foodstuffs are readily available.

Usually there are no restrictions to employment for persons with only one kidney that functions well.

Holidays

Most patients on PD can take a holiday without restrictions, but HD patients either need to make special arrangements for a dialysis facility at the holiday centre, or arrange for the use of portable machines. Such provisions need to be planned well beforehand.

Shiftwork

Shiftworking is not generally contraindicated for patients with renal or urinary tract disorders or necessarily for dialysis patients if their treatment can be rescheduled to fit in with a regular shift rota. Rapidly rotating shift systems can be more difficult to accommodate because of their constantly changing patterns, especially for patients on HD.

Drivers

For vocational driving in PD or HD issue of Group 1 licence is dependent on medical enquiries but normally there is no restriction on holding a Till 70 licence unless the individual is subject to significant symptoms such as sudden disabling attacks of giddiness or fainting, or impaired psychomotor or cognitive function.[32] For Group 2 licences, drivers with these disabilities are assessed individually by the DVLA Medical Unit. However, driving goods vehicles may be precluded due to prolonged absences from home, fatigue, and hours spent at the driving wheel. The physical demands of loading and unloading vehicles may preclude similar work in transportation such as removals, warehouse storage, or dockyard labouring.

Patients on PD could seek an exemption under the Motor Vehicle (Wearing of Seat Belt) Regulations 1982, SI: 1982 Regulation 5, or under the Motor Vehicles (Wearing of Seat Belts in Rear Seats by Adults) Regulations 1991, SI: 1991 No. 1255, by obtaining a valid medical certificate from a registered medical practitioner. However, the hazards of not wearing a seat belt must be weighed against any relatively minor inconvenience and restrictions. Adaptations to seat belt mountings can often solve any problems.

Urinary tract infections

Symptoms that relate to urinary infection are very common, but of serious importance only when there is an underlying anatomical abnormality. A small percentage of women suffer from repeated infections and remain symptomatic in spite of antibiotic therapy. Anatomical abnormalities (such as ureterovesical reflux, or obstruction) are associated with repeated infection, which can eventually lead to chronic renal failure later in life. Tuberculous infection of the urinary tract is being seen again more often, but employment can continue because therapy is usually administered as an out-patient procedure.

Urinary incontinence and retention

Better incontinence devices, more thorough investigation and improved therapy with anticholinergic drugs have greatly assisted sufferers to stay at work, although incontinence remains an unrecognized problem at work. The Specialist Continence Nurse Adviser can help to improve work attendance by giving advice, reassurance, practical help, and support. The value of intermittent self-catheterization for helping patients with poor bladder emptying, urinary retention and incontinence, or even voiding difficulties, often associated with a neuropathic or hypotonic bladder, is underestimated.[33] The technique is still much under-used but, as awareness grows, it will be more frequently applied at the place of work. Those who learn the technique can become dry, gain more social acceptance and by establishing effective drainage, protect their kidneys from the effects of back pressure and urinary infection.

Urinary diversion procedures for incontinence are becoming more acceptable; the most acceptable one is the Mitrofanoff operation. The patient's bladder is left intact, although the bladder neck may be closed off in certain, but not all, situations. The right ureter is divided at its mid-point and joined to the left ureter, and the lower disconnected right ureter is brought out as a stoma in the right groin, above the inguinal ligament. Through this the patient catheterize with Lofric catheters. This is a form of continent diversion that is really quite acceptable for those who are unable to empty their bladder and get fed-up with self-administered intermittent catheterization, or alternatively, those who are totally incontinent and whose bladder necks are closed off surgically.

While male disabled patients in wheelchairs learn to catheterize themselves, and so improve their morale, quality of life, and increase their ability to attend at their place of work, it is very difficult, perhaps impossible, for female disabled patients to self-catheterize. Clean and private provisions at the workplace will enable the technique to be properly and hygienically undertaken.

Those with incontinence, repeated urinary infections, ileal conduits, or catheterization need good toilet facilities and nearby access. Ileostomy bags may be compressed by low benches, or desks, or the sides of bins or boxes. Excess bending, crouching, or poor seating may inhibit the free flow of urine in the bag, or damage it, causing leakage. Mining, tunnelling, quarrying, or foundry work is contraindicated for these patients including those using intermittent self-catheterization because a clean and private place is required to effect catheter changes, or bag emptying. Most other jobs, however, can accommodate this requirement.

Symptoms in men with BPH, are measured using the validated International Prostate Symptom Score (IPSS), which includes seven questions measuring symptoms on an overall scale from 0 to 35, with higher scores representing more frequent symptoms. Rates of acute urinary retention range from 1–2% a year. Systematic reviews and randomized controlled trials show that α-blockers and transurethral resection of the prostate are effective treatments. Surgery does not increase the risk of erectile dysfunction or incontinence. Transurethral incision, electrical vaporization, and visual laser ablation also appear to be effective treatments but the latter may be associated with a higher risk of blood transfusion.[34]

Urinary tract calculi

Kidney stones affect up to 5% of the population, with a lifetime risk of passing a kidney stone of about 8–10%.[35] The predominant composition of idiopathic renal calculi is calcium oxalate. Increased incidence of kidney stones in the industrialized world is associated with improved standards of living and is strongly associated with race or ethnicity and region of residence. A seasonal variation is also seen, with high urinary calcium oxalate saturation in men during summer and in women during early winter. Stones form twice as often in men as women. The peak age in men is 30 years; women have a bimodal age distribution, with peaks at 35 and 55 years. Once a kidney stone forms, the probability that a second stone will form within 5–7 years is approximately 50%. Risk factors include family history, insulin-resistant states, a history of hypertension, primary hyperparathyroidism, a history of gout, chronic metabolic acidosis, surgical menopause, and anatomical abnormality leading to urinary stasis. Occupational factors such as a high ambient temperature, chronic dehydration, and physical inactivity because of sedentary work are also implicated.

Stone formation is more frequent in male marathon runners, lifeguards in Israel, hot metal workers, and some British navy personnel. An Italian study of machinists at a glass plant found a prevalence of renal stone of 8.5% in those exposed to heat stress against 2.4% in controls working in normal temperature.[36] In those exposed to heat stress, 39% of stones were uric acid and such workers were found to have significantly higher and raised serum uric acid concentrations.

Those with a strong history of stone formation should be encouraged to increase their fluid intake liberally if they want to accept overseas postings in tropical climates and to maintain a high intake during their stay, especially when undertaking strenuous outdoor work. Fitness for furnace or other very hot work must be carefully assessed because of the relative dehydration and increased tendency for stone recurrence, which should be easily prevented by increased fluid intake.[37] Patients need to be warned about becoming dehydrated on long-haul journeys (>4 hours). Airline pilots have to drink 600ml/hour while they are in the cockpit.

About 10–20% of all kidney stones need radiological or surgical intervention to remove the stone. For proximal ureteric stones, shock wave lithotripsy is useful if the stone is less than 1 cm in size, and ureteroscopy is more successful for stones larger than 1 cm. Ureteroscopy is less expensive than shock wave lithotripsy, but is more time consuming and technically demanding. Extracorporeal shock-wave lithotripsy offers the prospect of dramatically improving the previous picture of long periods off work and poor attendance. This is entirely an out-patient procedure, with minimal postoperative discomfort, and generally a resumption of normal activity within a day or so.[38] All patients should be advised to follow general treatment recommendations for prevention of stone recurrence, and specific treatment should be advised to patients with specific problems or with frequent recurrences (a stone at least every 3 years). Medical prophylaxis is effective in up to 80% of patients with recurrent calcium stones.

Tumours of the renal tract

Adenocarcinoma of the kidney is the commonest adult renal tumour. In the bladder more than 95% of tumours are urothelial in origin. Only about 4–5% are occupational in origin from former association with the chemical, dye-stuffs, rubber, cable and other industries, or from occupations where exposure to carcinogenic aromatic amines or polycyclic aromatic hydrocarbons has occurred.

Employees in certain industries with historic exposure to known bladder carcinogens, may be required to provide regular samples for urine cytology. This is usually every 6 months and can be carried out by post if employees leave or retire. Routine urine cytology is also suggested for those exposed to 4,4'-methylene *bis*(2-chloroaniline) (MbOCA). In those who have had tumours an early warning of cytological change can herald recurrence and thus allow early treatment.

Advisory services

The staff of renal units, general practitioners, occupational health services, the Employment Services' Disability Employment Advisers, and the Employment Medical Advisory Service should variously be able to advise on all employment matters. The approach is usually spearheaded by members of the renal unit team; physician, specialist nurse, social worker, home dialysis administrator, and transplant co-ordinator. An occupational physician or nurse is uniquely qualified to assess the suitability of a patient with renal or urinary tract disease for a particular job, as well as on the ways and means to adapt it. The advice, guidance, and contacts of the social worker attached to renal units will be indispensable. Several associations offer useful advice and support, and their addresses and phone numbers are given in Appendix 7.

Existing legislation: seafarers

Restrictions on the employment of persons suffering from diseases of the genitourinary tract are imposed by the Merchant Shipping (Medical Examination Regulations) 2002 Statutory Instrument 2002 No. 2055, which require a statutory examination for fitness to work. (See Appendix 2.) The medical standards are not met by those with acute urinary tract infections or urinary incontinence if recurrent or with untreatable underlying cause, recurrent stone formation (less than 5 years), prostatic enlargement with urinary obstruction if unremediable, or for new entrants in distant water or tropics with only one kidney.

Conclusions and recommendations

Because of the great advances in dialysis and the good results of renal transplantation, most people with renal failure can now achieve significant rehabilitation, and often a degree of independence and quality of life sufficient to allow useful, gainful, and active employment.

Employment is predicted by being in employment before onset of renal failure and by preconceptions of the patient and their doctor. Employers must be actively encouraged to take on those with renal tract disease who are quite fit for work, but who may otherwise experience minor inconveniences (like catheterization) or experience more frequent short absences from work. Occasionally patients will experience difficulty in arranging associated life insurance cover, or joining superannuation schemes and this may be given as the reason for not employing someone in end-stage renal failure but apart from the renal condition itself those with renal failure should be regarded in the same way as everybody else. A successful transplant restores the recipient to full health with the same capability as his/her contemporaries.

Selected references

1 UK Renal Registry Report 2003, UK Renal Registry, Bristol, UK.

2 Coresh J, Astor BC, Greene T, Eknoyan G, Levey AS. Prevalence of chronic kidney disease and decreased renal function in the adult US population: Third National Health and Nutrition Examination Survey. *Am J Kidney Dis* 2003; **41**: 1–12.

3 National Statistics 2004. www.nationalstatistics.gov.uk

4 Department of Social Security. Social Security Statistics 1991. Tables D1. 11–16 pp. 153–70. London: HMSO, 1992.

5 Cattell WR. Lower and upper urinary tract infections in the adult. In: *Oxford textbook of clinical nephrology*, Vol 3 (eds Cameron S *et al.*), pp. 1676–99. Oxford University Press, 1992.

6 Health and Safety Commission: Health and Safety Statistics. 1995/96. Tables 2.1, 2.2, 2.8. Government Statistical Service.

7 Go AS, Chertow GM, Fan D, McCulloch CE, Hsu C. Chronic kidney disease and the risks of death, cardiovascular events, and hospitalisation. *N Engl J Med* 2004; **351**: 1296–305.

8 Mortality Statistics: Cause. Review of the Registrar General on deaths by cause, sex and age, in England and Wales 2002. Series DH2 no. 29. London: Office for National Statistics, HMSO, 2002.

9 Vallancien G. Cadranel J. Jardin A. [What should be done in the presence of isolated microscopic hematuria in man in the work environment?]. [French] Original Title Que faire en présence d'une hematurie microscopique isolée chez l'homme en milieu de travail? *Presse Méd* 1985; **14**(23): 1279–81.

10 Chow KM, Kwan BC, Li PK, Szeto CC. Asymptomatic isolated microscopic haematuria: long term follow-up. *Q J Med* 2004; **97**: 739–45.

11 Anavekar NS, McMurray JJV, Velazquez EJ, Solomon SD, Kober L, Rouleau JL *et al*. Relation between renal dysfunction and cardiovascular outcomes after myocardial infarction. *N Engl J Med* 2004; **351**: 1285–95.

12 Jager KJ, Korevaar JC, Dekker FW, Krediet RT, Boeschoten EW. The effect of contraindications and patient preference on dialysis modality selection in ESRD patients in The Netherlands. *Am J Kidney Dis* 2004; **43**: 891–9.

13 Bartosh SM, Leverson G, Robillard D, Sollinger HW. Long-term outcomes in pediatric renal transplant recipients who survive into adulthood. *Transplantation* 2003; **76**(8): 1195–200.

14 Yasumura T, Oka T, Nakane Y, Ohmori Y, Aikawa I, Yoshimura N, Nakai I, Hamashima T, Nakajima H, Nakamura K. Long-term prognosis of renal transplant surviving for over 10 yr, and clinical, renal and rehabilitation features of 20-yr successes. *Clin Transplant* 1997; **11**(5 Pt 1): 387–94.

15 *MIMS: Pocket guide to chronic renal failure*. London: Haymarket Medical Publications, 1991.

16 Simmonds RG, Anderson CR, Abress LK. Quality of life and rehabilitation differences among four ESRD therapy groups. *Scand J Urol Nephrol* (Suppl.) 1990; **131**: 7–22.

17 Pertusa Pena C, Llarena Ibarguren R, Lecumberri Castanos D, Fernandez del Busto E. Relation between renal transplantation and work situation. *Arch Esp Urol* 1997; **50**(5): 489–94.

18 Markell MS, DiBenedetto A, Maursky V, Sumrani N, Hong JH, Distant DA, Miles AM, Sommer BG, Friedman EA. Unemployment in inner-city renal transplant recipients: predictive and sociodemographic factors. *Am J Kidney Dis* 1997; **29**(6): 881–7.

19 Laupacis A, Keown P, Pus N, Krueger H, Ferguson B, Wong C, Muirhead N. A study of the quality of life and cost-utility of renal transplantation. *Kidney Int* 1996; **50**: 235–42.

20 Newton SE. Renal transplant recipients' and their physicians' expectations regarding return to work posttransplant. *ANNA J* 1999; **26**(2): 227–32; discussion 234.

21 Auer J, Gokal R, Stout JP *et al*. The Oxford-Manchester study of dialysis patients. *Scand J Urol Nephrol* 1990; **131** (Suppl.): 31–7.

22 Gokal R. Quality of life in patients undergoing renal replacement therapy. *Kidney Int* 1993; **38** (Suppl. 40): S23–7.

23 Orlic L, Matic-Glazar D, Sladoje Martinovic B, Vlahovic A. Work capacity in patients on hemodialysis. *Acta Med Croatica* 2004; **58**: 67–71.

24 Tappe K, Turkelson C, Doggett D, Coates V. Disability under Social Security for patients with ESRD: an evidence-based review. *Disabil Rehabil* 2001; **23**(5): 177–85.

25 van Manen JG, Korevaar JC, Dekker FW, Reuselaars MC, Boeschoten EW, Krediet RT; NECOSAD Study Group. Netherlands Cooperative Study on Adequacy of Dialysis. Changes in employment status in end-stage renal disease patients during their first year of dialysis. *Perit Dial Int* 2001; **21**(6): 595–601.

26 Curtin RB, Oberley ET, Sacksteder P, Friedman A. Differences between employed and non-employed dialysis patients. *Am J Kidney Dis* 1996; **27**(4): 533–40.

27 Raiz L. The transplant trap: The impact of health policy on employment status following renal transplantation. *J Nephrol Social Work* 1997; **17**: 79–94.

28 Friedman N, Rogers TF. Dialysis and the world of work. *Contemp Dial Nephrol* 1988; **19**: 16–19.

29 King K Vocational rehabilitation in maintenance dialysis patients. *Adv Renal Repla Ther* 1994; **1**: 228–39.

30 Rasgon S, Schwankovsky L, James-Rogers A, Widrow L, Glick J, Butts E. An intervention for Maintenance among blue-collar workers with End-Stage Renal Disease. *Am J Kidney Dis* 1993; **22**: 403–12.

31 Merchant Shipping Notice MSN 1765 (M); Seafarer Medical Examination System and Medical and Eyesight Standards; Application of the Merchant Shipping (Medical Examination) Regulations 2002.

32 *For Medical Practitioners: At a glance guide to the current medical standards of fitness to drive.* Issued by Drivers Medical Group, DVLA, Swansea. September, 2004.

33 Intermittent self catheterisation. Patient Guide. Nursing Standard 2002; **16**(29).

34 Interventions in benign prostatic hyperplasia. In: Clinical Evidence from the *British Medical Journal*. Available at: www.clinicalevidence.com.

35 Parmar MS. Kidney stones. *BMJ* 2004; **328**: 1420–4.

36 Borghi L, Meschi T, Amato F, Novarini A, Romanelli A, Cigala F. Hot occupation and nephrolithiasis. *J Urol* 1993; **150**(6): 1757–60.

37 Pin NT, Ling NY, Siang LH. Dehydration from outdoor work and urinary stones in a tropical environment. *Occup Med* 1992; **42**: 30–2.

38 Wickham JEA. Minimally invasive surgery. Treatment of urinary tract stones. *BMJ* 1993; **307**: 1414–17.

Women at work

S. E. L. Coomber and P. A. Harris

Introduction

The revision for this chapter coincided with the 75th anniversary of the Royal College of Obstetricians and Gynaecologists (RCOG) and the 25th anniversary of the Faculty of Occupational Medicine (FOM). When the FOM was established, the first IVF baby, Louise Brown was just 1 year old; by 2006 she is a working woman. Over the same time frame, the UK female employment rate rose from 42% to 70%.[1]

The title of this chapter is deliberately broad and we address much more than just pathology of the reproductive tract. Similarly, we cannot cover every eventuality, and the authors have advised on diverse scenarios: pregnant house officers running to cardiac arrests, pregnant jockeys at risk of falling off horses, cabin crew organizing their progesterone-only contraceptive pill schedules, and more unusual problems such as male-to-female transgender surgery.

Overall assessment of fitness to work may need to take some consideration of the domestic responsibilities: the 2001 OPCS survey confirmed that even a full-time working woman spends more time caring for their children than the man.[1] The working woman has considerable legal protection against discrimination and complicated rights during and after pregnancy. As these are legal and not medical issues they are covered elsewhere (see Chapter 2). Similarly, breast disorders are covered in Chapter 21.

Diagnosis and declaration of pregnancy

Home pregnancy testing kits which detect human chorionic gonadotrophin (hCG) release can now confirm pregnancy as early as 7 days postovulation. False negatives may result from testing too early, depending on the sensitivity of the test (20–100 mIU/ml). However, false positives are rare. Earlier awareness of pregnancy affects apparent miscarriage rates:

- From conception: probably 50%
- From biochemical confirmation of pregnancy: 30%
- Once fetal heart seen on ultrasound scan: 5%
- After 12 weeks since last menstrual period: 2%
- After 16 weeks since last menstrual period: 1%

Declaration to employer

The timing of the decision to inform the employer will vary with individual circumstances, including the pregnant worker's own perception of the associated risks. The organization may have a policy precluding certain duties, shifts or work for pregnant employees. Making an early declaration may be helpful at a time when the female worker is feeling tired and nauseated, but with no other obvious physical signs. Declaration may be after the first ultrasound scan or the

12th week when the risk of spontaneous miscarriage reduces. Screening tests for major fetal abnormalities, e.g. nuchal fold thickness from 11 weeks or 'triple test' from 14 weeks, where a decision to terminate the pregnancy may result, could be another consideration. Similarly, she may decide to delay declaration further if there is a perceived financial disadvantage to stopping certain duties, shifts or work. There may also be a perception that job offers and promotion may be adversely affected, although this is unlawful. (See Chapter 2.)

Pregnancy and related problems

There are two separate questions to consider when assessing a pregnant worker's fitness to work

1. What are the workplace hazards for the pregnant worker?
   - Can the risk be assessed reasonably accurately?
   - How can she and the fetus best be protected while at work?
2. What aspects of pregnancy may affect her fitness to work?

   - Common relevant symptoms and specific complications
   - What adaptations/change in duties should result from this?

Workplace hazards to the pregnant worker

Medical assessment takes place within an employer's legal framework of risk assessment for 'new and expectant mothers' (i.e. those who are pregnant, have given birth within 6 months or are breastfeeding).[2] As with any risk assessment, there is a need to consider systematically the workplace hazards and the likelihood of their causing harm to the health or safety of the mother and/or fetus. The Health & Safety Executive provides a useful guide for employers on this[3] that considers in turn physical, chemical, and biological agents. We follow the same format with our examples below.

This section concludes with a discussion of the more complicated issues in physically/psychologically demanding work.

Physical hazards

Ionizing radiation Ionizing radiation is a relatively well understood fetal risk. It is known to interfere with cell proliferation and the embryo and fetus are therefore highly radiosensitive. Detailed evidence exists from human and animal studies on the specific effects of irradiation at different stages of development:[4]

- Preimplantation (<10 days postconception): lethal chromosomal damage likely
- Major organogenesis (3–7 weeks): malformations
- Brain development (8–15 weeks): reduced IQ, mental retardation
- Throughout pregnancy: increased lifetime cancer risk.

The International Commission for Radiation Protection 2002 review[4] supported the current limits for an effective dose of 1 mSv for the duration of declared pregnancy set by the Ionizing Radiation Regulations 1999. The non-pregnant woman has the same level of protection as the man. A 1996 report on the health of children born to medical radiographers reassuringly showed normal results for 9208 pregnancies, though it could not examine any dose–response relationship.[5]

Natural radiation can account for, on average, an additional 1 mSv to the fetus during pregnancy. Cosmic radiation can account for 0.25 mSv per year at ground level but up to 2 mSv to aircrew[6] and pregnant aircrew may therefore be grounded for the duration of the pregnancy.

In 2003, a study of birth outcomes in the offspring of Norwegian pilots and cabin crew concluded that there were no increased adverse risks.[7]

Non-ionizing radiation By contrast, electromagnetic radiation at lower (non-ionizing) frequencies has been less vigorously studied but there is no current evidence of any significant reproductive hazard and there are no gender-specific occupational limits.[8]

A 1993 case–control study of 280 pregnancies in female clinical magnetic resonance facility workers across the USA showed no significant increase in common adverse outcomes.[9]

However, staff working with magnetic resonance imaging scanners may on occasion volunteer to be scanned themselves and National Radiological Protection Board (NRPB) guidance suggests the risk from heating by radiofrequency radiation should be avoided in the first trimester of pregnancy.[10]

VDUs Concern about the possible effect of weak electromagnetic fields from VDUs has been studied since as early as 1979. There is no substantial evidence of any consistent adverse effect: a 1993 meta-analysis of nine reports based on 9000 spontaneous miscarriages, 1500 low birth weights, 2000 congenital malformations, and 50 000 controls provided reassuring conclusions.[11]

Extreme heat Pregnant women are normally advised to avoid saunas and prolonged hot baths as a core temperature of over 38.9°C presents a theoretical teratogenic risk. Few jobs pose a risk of hyperthermia,[12] but environments not enough to cause faintness in late pregnancy are more numerous and more problematic.

Slips, trips, and falls A recent survey in Cincinnati suggests falls during pregnancy are common.[13] Of 2847 employed women who had given birth, 27% had a fall, 6% at work. Slippery floors, hurrying, and carrying an object accounted for two-thirds of these events, many of which are preventable.

Violence in the workplace The risk of violence to a pregnant worker may be a significant concern, both in the woman's ability to do her job and the potential harm to the fetus.

Studies of violence and trauma in pregnancy tend to be non-work related. A 2003 study of self reported physical violence in 7105 pregnant women in Saudi Arabia[14] showed a positive association with placental abruption, prematurity, fetal distress, and caesarean section. However, an earlier literature review found no consistent association between violence during pregnancy and poor outcome.[15] Deceleration during a road traffic accident can cause fetal death even in the absence of major abdominal injury.[16]

Electric shock An electric shock to the fetus could theoretically be fatal, but only a small number of case reports exist to assess the risk. A 1997 Toronto prospective study of 31 pregnant women exposed to domestic electric shock, mostly of 110 volts, showed no higher rate of spontaneous abortion or other adverse outcome than matched controls.[17] The article suggests that the risk is lower if voltage is low, the woman is not wet, and if the current passes hand to hand (instead of hand to foot and potentially across the uterus).

Chemical hazards

When assessing risk from chemicals, existing occupational exposure standards take into account information available on reproductive toxicity.[18] Similarly, risk phrases required on a safety data sheet (Chemicals (Hazard Information and Packaging for Supply) Regulations 2002) may identify a specific reproductive concern:

◆ R60 and R62 (fertility)

◆ R61 and R63 (development)

◆ R64 (may cause harm to breast-fed babies).

or a more general carcinogenic hazard: R40, R45, R49, R68. Where information is not available on a substance, absence of these identifiers is not a guarantee that the substance is safe for the fertile female.

Lead Lead is an example of a reproductive toxin where legislation and reliable biological monitoring over many years has produced explicit guidance. Lead is known to cross the placenta and have adverse effects on the fetus, including miscarriage, neural tube defects, and low birth weight. It therefore carries the risk phrases R61 and R62 among others. The Control Of Lead at Work Regulations (CLAW) (3rd edn) places restrictions on 'women of reproductive capacity' (those medically and physically capable of becoming pregnant unless sterilized, posthysterectomy, or postmenopausal, regardless of other circumstances). Such women are prohibited from certain work, e.g. in lead smelting/refining processes and lead battery manufacture (Schedule 1 of CLAW) The blood lead limits for health surveillance initiation (20 µg/dl), action (25 µg/dl), and suspension (30 µg/dl) are also lower.

Once pregnancy is declared, CLAW guidance states that the woman should be removed from any work where exposure to lead is 'liable to be significant'.

In a workplace where CLAW does not apply formally, normal risk assessment may still identify a significant lead hazard for the female worker.

Anaesthetic gases Common anaesthetic agents (e.g. halothane, isoflurane, nitrous oxide) currently carry occupational exposure standards, but no risk phrases. Historically, they have been associated with concerns about miscarriage, although more recent studies have not supported this: the advent of active scavenging systems has minimized the exposure in operating theatres. However, in paediatric anaesthesia the anaesthetist may be less well protected: more gaseous induction is used, higher flow rates may be required and scavenging is technically more difficult. A recent American study showed a higher prevalence of spontaneous abortion in anaesthetists doing more than 75% paediatric, as opposed to adult anaesthesia.[19]

Nitrous oxide may be used in less controlled environments (e.g. delivery rooms, Accident & Emergency and dental surgeries) and there is some evidence that this may cause impaired fertility,[20] increased spontaneous abortion,[21] and low birth weight,[22] although no other evidence of teratogenicity. Air monitoring and adequate scavenging or ventilation should be considered where exposure may be prolonged.

Carbon monoxide Carbon monoxide crosses the placenta and acute exposure can cause fetal death or malformations. It binds strongly with haemoglobin and acts as a chemical asphyxiant. In acute exposure, fetal outcome is related to both maternal carboxyhaemoglobin level and maternal toxicity.[23]

Low level exposure can occur from environmental tobacco smoke and traffic fumes though there is no direct evidence of harmful effects.[20]

Dichloromethane, a solvent used for paint removal, is readily absorbed through the skin and lungs producing carbon monoxide as a metabolite and presents a similar risk to the pregnant worker. It currently has a maximum exposure limit, but no relevant risk phrase on safety data sheets.

Organic solvents Workers exposed to organic solvents in laboratories, electronics production and dry cleaning work have consistently shown a higher risk of spontaneous abortion.[24–26] A 1999 Canadian study of 125 women occupationally exposed to solvents in the first trimester showed increased risk of major malformations, especially where solvent exposure causes symptoms in the mother.[27]

Cytotoxic drugs In therapeutic doses, the health risks of these drugs are well known. The risk to employees in their manufacture, reconstitution, and clinical administration on the ward will vary considerably. Consideration of frequency of exposure, level of protection, and practical issues of avoiding exposure when trying to conceive should guide the risk assessment.

A 1993 study of 734 pregnancies in French operating theatre staff and nurses recorded chemical exposures in the first trimester and found ectopic pregnancy to be associated with antineoplastic drugs, though the numbers were very small.[28]

Environmental tobacco smoke Exposure of pregnant non-smokers to environmental tobacco smoke increases the risk of intrauterine growth retardation and low birth weight[29] perhaps by directly increasing the vascular resistance of the placenta. There is also some evidence of delayed conception[30] and an increased risk of central nervous system tumours in the children of passive smoking mothers.[31]

Much of the research on this is based on non-occupational environmental tobacco smoke (e.g. partner who smokes at home). The Health Act 2006 requires 'enclosed and substantially enclosed public places and shared workplaces' to be smoke free by 2007 so there may be few workplaces where this risk arises.

Biological hazards

Pregnant women are theoretically in an immunocompromised state, but in practice they are no more likely to become infected and the risk to the mother is not significantly increased.[32] However, many infections cross the placenta and therefore have important implications for the fetus.

Exposures from humans Pregnant women who work in healthcare, teaching, or childcare may be closely exposed to greater numbers of potentially infectious children and adults. The authors are not aware of any routine exclusion of susceptible pregnant women from these occupations, but where cases or outbreaks of some infections occur, restrictions may then apply. In the authors' experience, the commonest enquiries are about rubella, varicella zoster, parvovirus, and cytomegalovirus.

Rubella, or German measles, has an incubation period of 14–21 days. Patients are infectious from 1 week before the onset of the rash until 4 days afterwards. The risk to a fetus is highest in the first trimester when a maternal rubella infection results in fetal damage in up to 90% of infants.

Evidence of immunity should be sought in all women of reproductive age. A history is unreliable. Rubella vaccine is a live preparation and contraindicated in pregnancy; however, in a series of over 500 pregnant women who required the vaccine no case of congenital rubella syndrome was found.[33]

Varicella zoster, or chickenpox, has an incubation period of 10–21 days. Patients are infectious from 2 days before the onset of rash until the last vesicle has crusted over.[34] The more prolonged the exposure, the worse the infection. In 1–2% of maternal varicella zoster infections that occur before 20 weeks, fetal varicella syndrome ensues with skin scarring, eye defects, and neurological abnormalities. From 20 to 36 weeks there appears to be no adverse outcome. After 36 weeks, there is a risk of varicella infection of the newborn.[34]

The maternal risks are no greater than those of a non-pregnant adult. A history of chickenpox is a fairly reliable indicator of natural immunity: over 90% of adults in the UK are immune.[35] However, with the advent of a varicella zoster vaccine, many occupational health units are testing healthcare workers for immunity regardless of history, before offering vaccination. A non-immune pregnant worker should be aware of the risk and seek medical advice if exposed. There is debate on what currently constitutes significant exposure: some consider it face-to-face contact for at least 5 minutes for non-household exposure. The Royal College of Obstetricians and Gynaecologists provides up-to-date advice on post-exposure prophylaxis.[34]

Parvovirus infections are asymptomatic in 50% of adult cases. Viraemia occurs 6–8 days after exposure. It is transmitted by respiratory droplets. The patient is no longer infectious when the rash appears on day 16. The rash classically has a 'slapped face' appearance and may be confused with rubella. A suspected maternal infection needs serological confirmation. Maternal infection requires obstetric referral as there is a risk of fetal hydrops and fetal death. There are no vaccines available. Some 30–50% of pregnant women are already immune.

A Pennsylvanian prospective study of 618 pregnant women exposed to parvovirus B19 showed that 17% contracted the infection and one-third of those were asymptomatic. In this study there was no instance of fetal deaths or hydrops. There was no link to occupation and the main risk of infection was from other children within the household.[36]

Cytomegalovirus (CMV) is commonly asymptomatic in adults, but may cause symptoms similar to glandular fever. Primary infection occurs in 2% of pregnant women. CMV is found in 1% of all newborn infants with about 5–10% clinically symptomatic. The prognosis is generally good. CMV is shed in body fluids including urine. Those involved in the care of young children such as nursery workers should pay scrupulous attention to hygiene including hand-washing, especially when changing nappies. There are no vaccines available. About 50% of pregnant women are already immune.

Zoonoses There are case reports of small numbers of zoonotic infections during pregnancy from farm animals and occupational exposure to contaminated raw meat and unpasteurized dairy products, including toxoplasmosis, chlamydiosis, brucellosis, listeriosis, and Q fever (*Coxiella burnetii*). Scrupulous hand hygiene is the main method of protection for the worker.

In farming communities, pregnant women are routinely advised that they should not help to lamb or milk ewes; should avoid contact with aborted or newborn lambs or with the afterbirth; and should also avoid handling clothing, boots, etc. that have come into contact with ewes or lambs.

Pregnant women whose work involves handling cat litter or faeces should also be aware of the risk of toxoplasmosis. Oocysts are not infectious until 24 hours after shedding[37] so changing cat litter daily is the safest option.

Physical demands

While recreational physical exercise is known to be beneficial, physically demanding work may have significant adverse effects on intra-abdominal pressure, uterine blood flow and possibly nutritional status and hormone levels.[38] A meta-analysis of 29 studies[39] confirmed modestly increased risks of preterm birth, small for gestational age babies, maternal hypertension, and pre-eclampsia. Prolonged standing (6–7 hours a day) and high cumulative work fatigue were linked to increased risk of preterm birth. Long hours of work in isolation and manual handling were not found to be important risk factors.

There is limited evidence elsewhere associating noise and whole body vibration with adverse pregnancy outcomes.[40] Congenital cardiac malformations have recently been studied and no link has been made with physical demands or thermal stresses at work.[41]

Social classes 4 and 5 (where many of these workplace hazards are more likely to occur) is widely accepted as an independent risk factor for poor obstetric outcomes, e.g. low birth weight, premature labour, and miscarriage.

Shift work

There is evidence from a number of large studies that shift workers are at increased risk of miscarriage, low birth weight, and preterm birth.[42] Irregular menstruation has also been associated with shift work and a recent small study suggests that sleep disturbance may be the cause.[43] Congenital malformations and shift work have not been studied to date.

Stress and pregnancy

The authors find it hard to give a definitive view in such a complex area. Simply being pregnant may introduce a number of psychological stressors: uncertainty, fears, loss of control, physical discomforts, poor sleep. Stressful life events may occur during pregnancy, and perceptions of work-related stress may alter. Recall bias in the event of an adverse outcome may blur evidence.

However, when someone is failing to cope and says that stress is the cause, this subjective view is hard to challenge. Where work is perceived to be more stressful than home life, giving time off may be pragmatic. However, for working women with small children at home, coming to work may be less demanding than 'rest' at home.

There is a substantial amount of literature showing that stress is associated with an adverse pregnancy outcome, whether the source of the stress is work or life events. These poor outcomes have included:

- hypertension
- preterm delivery
- low birth weight
- miscarriage.

There are no data on stopping work as an intervention, and there are almost as many studies showing no adverse effect for the same outcomes. However a study of mothers who were living within 2 miles of the World Trade Centre disaster on 9 September 2001 showed that they delivered babies who were significantly lighter and shorter in length than those who delivered at the same hospitals but lived further away.[44]

Pregnancy changes that affect fitness to work

The risk assessment should consider continuing practical and safety issues as the shape, physiology, and mobility of the pregnant worker change. Assessment will vary with both the individual pregnancy and the particular job. A medical opinion may not be required in a normal pregnancy, but issues to consider include:

- need to urinate more frequently/urgently
- nausea and need for frequent meals/snacks/increased fluid intake
- intolerance of strong odours
- liability to faint
- tiredness, poor tolerance of shift work
- susceptibility to occupational stressors
- reduced ability to run: effects of heavily pregnant abdomen, joint laxity, and/or ankle oedema (especially in the third trimester)
- centre of gravity changes, affecting risk of falls, work at heights
- heat intolerance
- comfort and efficacy of protective clothing and equipment
- work in confined spaces, access via emergency exits.

Other issues

Travel in pregnancy

Both fitness for the travel itself and the destination need to be considered. The normal discomforts of travel by car, train, or plane may be less well tolerated by a pregnant woman but there are a few specific risks to consider. The risk of deep vein thrombosis is increased in pregnancy and more so when flying. In 'high-risk' pregnancies the obstetrician should be consulted about fitness to fly. Under IATA (International Air Transport Association) guidelines, pregnant women are allowed to fly in weeks 36–38 if the flying time does not exceed 4 hours. However, many airlines will not carry pregnant women after 36 weeks. Written confirmation from the airline is advisable and the final responsibility for passengers always lies with the captain of the aircraft.

Considerations for foreign travel include availability of safe food and medical care, requirement for malaria prophylaxis and other infectious diseases.

Driving

Occupational driving in pregnancy requires a common sense approach for the management of most pregnancy symptoms, e.g. tiredness, feeling faint, backache, and limited space behind the steering wheel in the third trimester. Seatbelt wearing is still compulsory and the Royal Society for the Prevention of Accidents provides advice on this (see Box 20.1).

Two infrequent complications require DVLA notification:[45] eclamptic fits and gestational diabetes (grouped as 'temporary insulin treatment') may both be bars to group 2 entitlement. A group 1 driver must stop driving if experiencing disabling hypoglycaemia. Eclamptic seizures are not thought to represent continuing liability to future seizures, and are dealt with by the DVLA as 'provoked seizures', on an individual basis.

Prescribing at work

Occupational immunization and post-exposure prophylaxis (e.g. for blood-borne viruses, sharps injuries, varicella zoster contact, and human or animal bites) are the only routine situations where the occupational physician or adviser may be required to advise on prescribing during pregnancy and breastfeeding and individual decisions must be made based on risk/benefits. All live vaccines are contraindicated in pregnancy. The BNF (British National Formulary) on-line[46] provides up-to-date information on known risks.

Box 20.1 Seatbelt wearing in pregnancy: advice from the Royal Society for the Prevention of Accidents

All pregnant women must wear seat belts by law when travelling in cars. This applies to both front and back seats and pregnancy does not in itself provide exemption from the law.

The safest way to wear a seat belt is to place the shoulder strap between the breasts (over the breastbone) and the lap belt flat on the thighs, fitting comfortably beneath the enlarged abdomen. In this way the forces applied in a sudden impact can be absorbed by the body's frame.

Mother and unborn child are both safer in a collision if a lap and diagonal seat belt is being worn correctly, as opposed to a lap only belt.

Time off work during pregnancy

Increased sickness absence is more likely during pregnancy, although a 1989 Norwegian study showed that job adjustment may be able to reduce this.[47] However, if a woman raises a request for time off work, the threshold for agreeing tends to be low. On trying to untangle the basis for this, the authors believe there are a number of influences:

- a public perception that pregnancy should be treated as an illness and work may be intrinsically harmful
- a view that absence from work during pregnancy is short-term and therefore a minor problem
- a reluctance to affect patient rapport by seeming unsupportive
- such decisions tend to go unchallenged.

Complications of pregnancy

Miscarriage

Miscarriage is defined as pregnancy loss before 24 weeks. The term 'abortion' is still correct but usually confined to termination of pregnancy. Most cases arise in the first trimester (before 13 weeks) and some of the late second trimester miscarriages may be referred to as an intrauterine death (IUD). The risk to the mother of heavy bleeding is small but does increase with gestation.

An ultrasound scan earlier than 6 weeks from the last menstrual period is not particularly helpful. With a threatened miscarriage (a live intrauterine pregnancy with a history of bleeding) rest is usually recommended. With an incomplete or missed miscarriage management includes either a surgical evacuation of retained products or a conservative approach (medical or expectant). Return to work is often based on an assessment of emotional more than physical recovery.

Occasionally miscarriage will be due to a molar pregnancy (partial or complete hydatidiform mole). This requires follow-up surveillance of urine and blood hCG levels. This is co-ordinated by three centres at Charing Cross, Sheffield, and Dundee. Instructions are sent directly to the patient but an occupational health service could offer to take the blood samples if GP access is difficult. In an uncomplicated partial mole, follow-up is usually over 6 months.

Recurrent miscarriage and work

Recurrent miscarriage is defined as the loss of three or more pregnancies. The incidence is 1% of all women and maternal age and a previous number of miscarriages are known risk factors.[48] Very little has been published about the effect of work and, in clinical practice, the gynaecologist may routinely enquire about the type of employment but tend not to enquire further. A cause is only found in a small number of cases (e.g. polycystic ovary syndrome, antiphospholipid syndrome, and congenital abnormalities of the uterus).

Standing at work for more than 7 hours per day has been shown to be associated with a significantly increased risk of a further miscarriage in women who had already had two or more spontaneous miscarriages.[49]

Ectopic pregnancy

Maternal death from ectopic pregnancy accounted for 11 maternal deaths in the UK over 3 years.[50] The risk of an ectopic pregnancy is 1 in 400. When a previous ectopic has occurred, the risk rises to 1 in 10 and an early scan at 6–7 weeks is undertaken. Risk factors are intrauterine devices and previous tubal surgery or chlamydial infection. An ectopic pregnancy may require a laparoscopy with or without a laparotomy, with estimated return to work dates of 1 and 6 weeks. A small case-referent study of 140 French nurses found no association between exposure to chemical or physical agents at work and ectopic pregnancy rates.[51]

'High risk' pregnancy

Clinical risk assessment of the pregnancy is routinely used by the obstetric team during antenatal care. Designation of 'high' or 'low' risk depends on factors including problems identified at booking and those that develop through the pregnancy.

In practice, many co-factors may be involved in a high-risk pregnancy: she may have a poor obstetric history, smoke, have a poor diet, or work in a manual job. Assessing the extent of risk associated with work is hard to separate out but ideally decisions on restriction of duties in a high-risk pregnancy should be made jointly between the obstetrician and the occupational physician.

Surgery and invasive investigations during pregnancy

Amniocentesis and chorionic villus sampling Amniocentesis and chorionic villus sampling are invasive tests carried out under ultrasound control. The most common indication is to carry out fetal karyotyping (chromosome analysis) following a high-risk result from a screening test. Such procedures are associated with an increased miscarriage rate of less than 1% against a background miscarriage rate of approximately 2% at 12 weeks and 1% at 16 weeks. It is a minor procedure but it would be unreasonable to expect a patient to return to work the same day.

Caesarean section The Caesarean section rate in England is 20%.[52] Most of these are performed through a transverse suprapubic incision. Early return to work may need to be deferred in the event of a section, as lifting and driving may be a problem, comparable with other types of surgery, such as abdominal hysterectomy.

'Minor disorders of pregnancy'

An obstetrician may refer to many of the unpleasant symptoms of pregnancy as 'minor disorders of pregnancy' as they have a minor effect on the pregnancy outcome. However, these may have a significant effect on the pregnant employee and her ability to work. These are often worse in women with a multiple pregnancy.

Musculoskeletal problems are common in pregnancy. This is partly due to a rise in relaxin levels that relax connective tissue and increase joint mobility. There is an increase in body mass as well as a redistribution of the load, plus a reluctance to prescribe or to take analgesia. There are a number of braces and splints that can give symptomatic relief and seeing a physiotherapist or chiropractor is often more helpful than an obstetrician.

Up to 75% of women report having **backache** at some time in pregnancy and 30% find it a severe problem. It is often worse in the third trimester. It has been suggested that many of the symptoms are similar to overuse disorders and that restriction of activity is more useful than the progressive strengthening programmes used in non-pregnant back pain management

Carpal tunnel syndrome occurs in up to 20% of pregnancies particularly in the second half. Compression of the median nerve results in pain, numbness, and weakness. Initial treatment is by rest and wrist splinting.

Symphysis pubis dysfunction involves painful mobility of the symphysis pubis. It can present at any stage, gradually or suddenly (even immediately postnatally) and is common in the last trimester. Symptoms include localized pain, provoked by getting up from a chair, lifting, walking, or climbing stairs, which is relieved by rest.[53]

The exact cause remains unclear, and it tends to be under-recognized. The amount of discomfort and disability is variable, some patients can barely walk, even with a Zimmer frame. Recovery following delivery is also variable: the majority improve rapidly after delivery but one-quarter still have symphysis pubis dysfunction pain up to 6 months postnatally; 85% recur in a subsequent pregnancy.[53] Referral to an obstetric physiotherapist for assessment and treatment is advised, and time off work may be necessary.

Tiredness and emotional lability These symptoms may be significant in the first trimester, even before the pregnancy is declared. It may affect work performance but usually improves as pregnancy progresses.

Hyperemesis

Seventy-five per cent of all pregnant women experience nausea and in 10% the condition persists beyond the first trimester. Although rest and dietary advice is common it has not been evaluated in randomized trials.[54] Small amounts of carbohydrate may be helpful and if retained may provide some nutrition. Proven treatment includes antiemetics such as antihistamines, vitamin B6, ginger, and acupressure, e.g. wrist bands used for travel sickness, which apply pressure to the Neiguan acupuncture point.[55]

Heartburn Heartburn affects 70% of all women at some stage in their pregnancy and may be aggravated by stooping or bending. Management involves avoiding fatty or spicy food and minimizing bending or lying flat after eating. Antacids are often sufficient but H_2 blockers are sometimes justified though the manufacturers' advice is to 'avoid unless essential' in pregnancy.

Hypertension A diastolic pressure of >90 mmHg requires urinalysis and referral for further assessment. Rest is often recommended for non-proteinuric hypertension. Despite three controlled trials the value of bed rest is still not clear[54] and time off work may not be necessary. Methyl dopa is commonly used to treat hypertension in pregnant women, and can affect concentration and alertness.

Cognitive function While pregnant women frequently report impairments in memory and attention, there is sparse and conflicting evidence whether this is an objective mild cognitive impairment or only a perceived one, possibly related to low mood in pregnancy.[56] Reduced learning and retrieval in early pregnancy has been reported in a cross-sectional study of 71 pregnant women and matched controls.[57] There may be work situations where such subtle changes can be noticeable, but the woman is likely to be aware and compensate for it. Problems in late pregnancy and the immediate postnatal period have been reported but are unlikely to be relevant to work.

Postnatal issues

Return to work

Return to work postnatally tends to be dictated by socio-economic issues, e.g. duration of paid or unpaid maternity leave, childcare arrangements. Medical reasons for delayed return to work include:

- complications of wound healing, usually infection (perineal or caesarean section)
- musculoskeletal problems
- psychological well-being
- ill health in the baby.

Breastfeeding and work

There are few contraindications to return to work while breastfeeding, but some practicalities to consider:

◆ To what extent are they breastfeeding? The assessment may differ where a baby is dependent on the mother for much of its nutrition, or simply has a night-time comfort feed.

◆ What facilities are available at work if she needs to feed or express milk during working hours? It is good practice and there are legal requirements to support this.

◆ Are there potential hazardous substances (risk phrase R64) in the workplace that could be absorbed and secreted in breast milk? Examples include highly fat-soluble compounds such as organic solvents, organochlorine pesticides, and polychlorinated biphenyls. There have been case reports of maternal hydrogen fluoride exposure causing dental fluorosis in her children and tetrachloroethylene causing jaundice in a baby.[58] Mercury excreted in breast milk may be up to 5% of blood levels.[59]

Some employers simply take the view that breastfeeding is not compatible with certain front-line jobs, e.g. armed forces, fire, and police services. Reasons for this may be multiple: potential for uncontrolled workplace exposures, physical fitness, unpredictable working hours incompatible with feeding or expressing demands, impact of serious injury on the dependent baby.

Postnatal depression

During the first 6 months after delivery, the prevalence of major depression is estimated at 12–13%. Postnatal depression is thought to be generally underdiagnosed and most patients can be treated in primary care settings. There is an effective screening tool available: the 10-item Edinburgh Postnatal Depression Scale[60] and a score of 12 or more out of 30 indicates the likelihood of depression but not its severity. (See Box 20.2.)

Box 20.2 Edinburgh Post Natal Depression Scale (EPDS)*

Name   EPDS score

Assessment date   Assessor

As you have recently had a baby, we would like to know how you are feeling.

Please underline the answer which comes closest to how you have felt in the past 7 days—Not just how you feel today. Here is an example, already completed:

I have felt happy:

Yes, all the time

Yes, most of the time

No, not very often

No, not at all

This would mean 'I have felt happy most of the time during the past week'. Please answer the following 10 questions by placing a tick in the appropriate box. Thank you.

In the past 7 days:

1. I have been able to laugh and see the funny side of things:

As much as I always could

Not quite so much now

Box 20.2 Edinburgh Post Natal Depression Scale (EPDS) (continued)

Definitely not so much now

Not at all

2. I have looked forward with enjoyment to things:

As much as I ever did

Rather less than I used to

Definitely less than I used to

Hardly at all

3. I have blamed myself unnecessarily when things went wrong

Yes, most of the time

Yes, some of the time

Not very often

No, never

4. I have been anxious or worried for no good reason

No, not at all

Hardly ever

Yes, sometimes

Yes, very often

5. I have felt scared or panicky for no good reason

Yes, quite a lot

Yes, sometimes

No, not much

No, not at all

6. Things have been getting on top of me

Yes, most of the time I haven't been able to cope at all

Yes, sometimes I haven't been coping as well as usual

No, most of the time I have coped quite well

No, I have been coping as well as ever

7. I have been so unhappy that I have had difficulty sleeping

Yes, most of the time

Yes, sometimes

Not very often

No, not at all

8. I have felt sad or miserable

Yes, most of the time

Yes, quite often

Not very often

No, not at all

Continued

Box 20.2 Edinburgh Post Natal Depression Scale (EPDS) *(continued)*

9. I have been so unhappy that I have been crying

Yes, most of the time

Yes, quite often

Only occasionally

No, never

10. The thought of harming myself has occurred to me

Yes, quite often

Sometimes

Hardly ever

Never

Edinburgh Post Natal Depression Scale (EPDS)—Guidelines for raters

Response categories are scored 0,1,2, and 3 according to increased severity of the symptom. Questions 3,5,6,7,8,9,10 are reverse scored (i.e., 3,2,1,0).

Individual items are totalled to give an overall score. A score of 12+ indicates the likelihood of depression, but not its severity. A score just below the cut-off should not be taken to indicate an absence of depression as the EPDS Score is designed to assist, not replace clinical judgement.

*Reproduced from reference 60 with permission from The Royal College of Psychiatrists.

Several studies have reported that antidepressants can be used safely by nursing mothers of healthy full-term infants. However, women's choice of treatment may be non-pharmacological and cognitive behaviour therapy has been demonstrated to be comparably effective for non-psychotic depression.[61] There is little evidence available about prognostic factors.

Gynaecological problems

This section mainly addresses the impact of gynaecological disorders on both attendance and performance at work. There is very little evidence of relevant occupational hazards.

Fertility issues

In vitro fertilization

In vitro fertilization involves hyperstimulation of the ovaries to produce a number of eggs, egg collection (usually transvaginally under ultrasound control), fertilization, and incubation for a couple of days before embryo transfer. Additional embryos may be frozen and used in subsequent cycles. The overall success rate is 20% but varies with personal factors. In the UK 80% of treatment cycles are privately funded. The National Institute for Clinical Excellence (NICE) is set to recommend greater availability of treatment on the NHS.

The length of treatment is hard to anticipate as patients vary in their response and so do treatment protocols between units. Predicting time off work is difficult: treatment schedules change at short notice and patients may travel considerable distances to receive it. Work performance may also be affected by emotional lability associated with the drugs. Complications can include ovarian hyper stimulation syndrome (OHSS) where hospital admission may be required.

What interferes with conception?

Patients with subfertility (failure to conceive after a year) may be concerned about the impact of occupational stress and night work. There is some evidence these can increase prolactin levels,[62] which in turn may inhibit ovulation. A Danish study of 297 couples found more reduced fertility in women with high-strain jobs.[63] We would recommend consulting the woman's gynaecologist before making individual recommendations about work.

Menstrual disorders

Problems of the menstrual cycle include heavy bleeding, pain, and mood changes. A few days each month of absence and/or reduced performance soon adds up to cause a considerable impact on work. Medical management in primary care should be able to control many of the debilitating symptoms but there may be a reluctance to take regular medication, e.g. a combined pill for non-contraceptive reasons.

Menorrhagia is a common problem: each year 5% of women aged 30–49 years consult their GP with heavy periods that may disrupt work and home life. In practice objective measurements of menstrual blood loss are not helpful.[64] Initial management includes a range of drug treatments that should be offered before specialist referral. Surgical treatment includes endometrial ablation and hysterectomy (see below).

Dysmenorrhoea can be physiological or associated with menorrhagia, fibroids, or endometriosis, which may require treatment of the underlying cause. Pain management includes simple analgesia and non-steroidal anti-inflammatory drugs such as mefenamic acid.

In **premenstrual syndrome** symptoms occur typically in the luteal phase of the menstrual cycle in the 7–10 days before the period, though other patterns can occur. The variety of symptoms is enormous (up to 88 have been described), but in this context the relevant ones will be those that affect attendance and performance at work (e.g. irritability, lability, forgetfulness, and even violence). In practice there is no quantifiable assessment tool and for significant symptoms a detailed history should be documented. Many women will have self-diagnosed premenstrual syndrome. A wide range of self-help and some medical treatments can be tried: none are universally effective.

Endometriosis is another highly variable condition. The amount of disease seen at laparoscopy does not correlate with the level of symptoms. Classically, the pain is cyclical but may be continuous. Treatment includes controlling pain, hormonal manipulation, and surgery.

Menopause

In the UK, 70% of women between 45 and 59 are employed, potentially working through and beyond the menopause. The average age of the menopause is 51 and up to 75 symptoms have been attributed to it. A high FSH level may support the diagnosis of menopause but is not helpful in predicting when the symptoms will stop.

In the authors' experience it has not presented as a common fitness for work issue. However, a TUC survey reported in 2003 that over a third of workers felt embarrassment or difficulties in discussing the menopause with their employers and that hot flushes, headaches, tiredness, and lack of energy were the symptoms most likely to be perceived to be made worse by work.[65]

Work may be affected by sleep deprivation, hot flushes, mood alteration, memory, or concentration difficulties. Vasomotor instability may be helped by clonidine. HRT may help some symptoms but needs careful assessment of the risks and benefits by the GP or gynaecologist. Recent large UK studies have shown an association between HRT and increased relative risk of breast cancer, stroke, venous thromboembolism, and possible small increases in coronary heart disease and endometrial and ovarian cancer.[66] Alternative therapies are gaining in popularity. Postmenopausal osteoporosis may be a longer term outcome affecting ability to work.

Gynaecological cancers

Historically association has been shown between ovarian cancer and asbestos exposure,[67] but in general gynaecological cancers are not occupational in origin. Anticipating time off work is difficult to predict as the management depends on the staging of the disease. This may not be clear with the initial diagnosis but may depend on operative findings, imaging, or histology. Management may include radical surgery, radiotherapy, chemotherapy, or a combination of these approaches.

Urogynaecology

Urinary problems are common in women but often unreported. In practice patients often have mixed symptoms of stress incontinence and overactive bladder symptoms. In cases where diagnostic studies have been performed, the nomenclature has recently been changed by the International Continence Society to 'urodynamically proven stress incontinence' or 'detrusor overactivity'. Urodynamic assessment is not essential in the initial management.

Work that entails lifting, bending and even brisk walking may exacerbate **stress incontinence** symptoms but not alter the course of the condition. Initial management should include pelvic floor physiotherapy with a 40% reported cure rate. The drug Duloxetine was licensed in 2004 for stress incontinence. Open surgery such as a Burch colposuspension or sling involves a suprapubic or Pfannensteil incision and has an 80–90% cure rate with a return to work date of 6–12 weeks. The tension-free vaginal tape (TVT™) is a popular minimal access operation with similar cure rate to open surgery and in practice has a return to work date of 3–4 weeks.[68]

Overactive bladder symptoms vary from frequency and urgency to urge incontinence all of which may interrupt work. A urinary tract infection should be excluded. The GP should have access to a continence advisor who has a lot to offer including teaching bladder drill. Some anticholinergic medications have centrally acting side-effects such as drowsiness.

Gynaecological surgery and work

Generic timescales for return to work after different procedures are inevitably of limited value. Different authorities quote different intervals and individual and work factors are highly variable. Table 20.1 gives the Department of Health statistics for waiting lists and mean duration of hospital stay for three common gynaecological procedures, alongside what the authors view as typical advice on return to 'light' or 'heavy' work.

However, early return to work is not usually associated with adverse wound outcomes and the pain and tiredness are more limiting than wound integrity.

For example, a self-employed accountant successfully returned to her office just 4 days after an uncomplicated abdominal hysterectomy, albeit on limited hours. The Department for Work and Pensions, who also give indicative timescales for some procedures, estimate her return to full activity would take 7 weeks.[69]

Table 20.1 Department of Health statistics for three Gynaecological Operations, NHS Hospitals, England 2003/4[73] plus typical estimates for duration of return to work

Operation	No. performed 2003/4	Mean NHS waiting list time (days)	Mean length of hospital stay (days)	Estimated return to light work	Estimated return to heavy work
Repair of vaginal prolapse	20 240	160	4.7	6 weeks	12 weeks
Hysterectomy	40 276	99	5.9	Abdominal: 6 weeks	Abdominal: 12 weeks
				Laparoscopic: 3 weeks	Laparoscopic: 6 weeks
Laparoscopic sterilization	23 876	107	1.1	3 days	1 week

Major abdominal surgery

Most open gynaecological surgery is performed though a transverse suprapubic or Pfannensteil incision. This includes abdominal hysterectomy, myomectomy, salpingo-oopherectomy, and Burch colposuspension. Estimated return to work is 6 weeks, or 12 weeks for heavy lifting work. Mid-line incisions are performed for ovarian malignancy or when better access is required such as removing a large fibroid. Patients with mid-line incisions take longer to recover and are more prone to complications. Patients with a vaginal hysterectomy tend to recover quicker.

Laparoscopic surgery

In the last 10 years this has replaced open surgery for many disorders. Recovery and return to work is quicker, but still variable for different procedures: after laparoscopic sterilization it may only be 2–3 days but after extensive ablation of endometriosis it may take 2–3 weeks for pain to settle.

Hysteroscopic procedures

Diagnostic hysteroscopy is sometimes performed as an outpatient procedure. There is a risk of fainting from vagal stimulation that can last beyond the procedure. Most units do not advise driving immediately afterwards. Hysteroscopic surgery, e.g. resection of fibroids, usually requires a general anaesthetic and return to work after a few days.

Termination of pregnancy

As a procedure this can be done medically or surgically and the patient should normally be physically fit almost immediately. Medical termination usually involves oral mifepristone followed 48 hours later by oral or vaginal misoprostol. Psychological fitness may be less predictable, depending on circumstances. Complications include retained products of conception that may require further intervention.

Cervical smears and colposcopic treatment

As a result of the effective screening programme for cervical cancer, some women may require colposcopic assessment. Outcomes may vary from examination only to loop excision but rarely require more than a day or so off work unless complications arise.

Working women: other issues

Work-life balance In the authors' experience in assessing women's fitness to work there needs to be some knowledge of the woman's commitments and responsibilities outside of work. There is good evidence that differences in sickness absence rates between men and women reflect the need to manage other, immediate and domestic responsibilities. Therefore taking a social history along with a medical and occupational one is important (arguably for both sexes) including:

- who is at home and other dependants
- supportive/difficult relationships
- practical domestic support, e.g. childcare, cleaning
- the woman's proportion of the family income
- other paid and unpaid jobs she may have.

Understanding the work-life balance is particularly important in planning return to work after major illness. Domestic responsibilities rarely reduce on return to work and a phased start can be highly successful, e.g. working mornings only at first and increasing back to full duties within 4–6 weeks. This allows for increased afternoon rest while adapting back to work both physically and psychologically.

Domestic violence It is worth remembering that one in four women (and one in six men) will be a victim of domestic violence in their lifetime. One of the difficulties is that the woman may be very reluctant to declare the problem at the time. Almost a third of domestic violence starts during pregnancy and existing violence often escalates during it.

Ergonomic issues It is obvious that not only are there male–female differences in body size and function but that there is considerable variation and overlap. For example, according to Stephen Pheasant[70] women on average have 61% of male muscle strength but there is still a 10% 'Chance Encounter of Female Exceeding Male' strength (% CEFEM). Joint flexibility, however, has been shown to be 5–15% greater in females.

On average, women are smaller in all dimensions except hip breadth: 13 cm shorter in stature, 5 cm lower eye height when sitting. Grip reach is 15 cm less when standing, 10 cm sitting, and 7 cm less for forward reach.[70] These anthropometric differences affect a woman's ability to use equipment designed for men (and vice versa), especially where there is a mechanical advantage from both height and strength (e.g. pushing and pulling).

This can be illustrated with Royal Air Force air crew anthropometric limits,[71] which require, among others, a minimum sitting height of 865 mm and functional reach (or arm length) of 720 mm in order that crew can fly a wide range of aircraft. Using standard anthropometric data[70] it can be shown that more men than women will meet these current criteria. Table 20.2 gives details of 5th, 50th, and 95th centiles by gender for these two measurements.

Physical fitness and injury In a post requiring a high level of physical fitness (e.g. armed forces or fire service), any standard will need to apply to the demands of the job, not the gender of the applicant. The British armed forces has published data from 1985 to 2000 showing that female medical discharge rates for musculoskeletal disease are more than three times that for males.[72]

Undertaking the Army Phase 1 basic fitness training (which is 'gender free'), males may be typically exercising at 30–40% of capacity and females at 80–90%. Females are less likely to complete the training and are known to be more prone to stress fractures during Phase 1. Continuous high

Table 20.2. Comparison of RAF recruitment standards and Pheasant's anthropometric data: examples of gender difference for sitting and arm length.

RAF limits	Anthropometric measurements		5th centile	50th centile	95th centile
Minimum 865 mm	Sitting height	Males	850 mm	910 mm	965 mm
		Females	795 mm	850 mm	910 mm
Minimum 720 mm	Arm length	Males	720 mm	780 mm	840 mm
		Females	655 mm	705 mm	760 mm

impact exercise with inadequate recovery disturbs bone remodelling: bone resorption is accelerated faster than bone formation. Inadequate diet and the popularity of depot medroxyprogesterone contraception (DMPA) may both reduce bone density and increase the risk of stress fracture in this particular occupational group.[73]

Conclusions

The 2005 Labour Force Survey[1] showed that, with increasing numbers of women at work, both sexes now undertake about 13.3 million jobs in the UK. There are notable differences in employment, though. The careers they follow differ: relatively few women work in 'skilled trades' and 'process, plant and machine operatives' and over one fifth works in 'administrative and secretarial' jobs. Half of women but only one in six men work part-time.

Rates of sickness absence (measured as days off due to sickness in the week before the survey) remained slightly higher for women than men (2.1% and 1.4% respectively). Higher rates were found for disabled women, lone mothers, and mothers with the youngest dependent child aged 5–10 years: socioeconomic factors may be just as relevant as health ones.

The authors have summarized the available medical evidence, guidelines, and clinical consensus affecting the health issues for women at work—including fertility, declaration of pregnancy, workplace hazards, complications of pregnancy, common gynaecological issues, and briefly looked at non-reproductive topics. The risk management issues for women at work remain far from clear-cut.

References

1 National Statistics Online. *Work and family*. www.statistics.gov.uk

2 Health & Safety Executive. *Management of health and safety at work regulations 1999*. London: HMSO, 2000.

3 Health & Safety Executive. *New and expectant mothers at work. A guide for employers*. London: HMSO, 2002.

4 Streffer C *et al*. Biological effects after prenatal irradiation (embryo and fetus). A report of the International Commission on Radiological Protection. *Ann ICRP* 2003; **33:** 5–206.

5 Roman E *et al*. Health to children born to medical radiographers. *Occup Environ Med* 1996; **53** (2): 73–9.

6 Gibson TM. Flying. In: *Hunter's diseases of occupations*, (9th edn) (eds Baxter PJ, Adams PH, Aw T-C, Cockcroft A, Harrington JM), p. 374. London: Arnold, 2000.

7 Irgens A *et al*. Pregnancy outcome among offspring of airline pilots and cabin attendants. *Scand J Work Environ Health* 2003; **29**(2): 94–9.

8 Kheifets LI. Extremely low frequency electric and magnetic fields. In: *Hunter's diseases of occupations*, (9th edn) (eds Baxter PJ, Adams PH, Aw T-C, Cockcroft A, Harrington JM), pp. 439–50. London: Arnold, 2000.

9 Kanal E. Survey of reproductive health among female MR workers. *Radiology* 1993; **187**(2): 395–9.

10 NRPB (National Radiological Protection Board) 2004. Limits on patient and volunteer exposure during clinical magnetic resonance diagnostic procedures: Recommendations for the practical application of the Board's statement. 2004. On NRPB website www.hpa.org.uk/radiation/publications

11 Parazzini F *et al.* Video display terminal use and reproductive outcome – a meta-analysis. *Journal Epidemiol Community Health* 1993; **47**(4): 265–8.

12 Office of The Deputy Prime Minister. *Medical and occupational evidence for recruitment and retention in the fire and rescue service*, pp. 11-1–11-10. London: HMSO, 2004.

13 Dunning K *et al.* Falls in workers during pregnancy: risk factors, job hazards and high risk occupations. *Am J Ind Med* 2003; **44**(6): 664–72.

14 Rachana C *et al.* Prevalence and complications of physical violence during pregnancy. *Eur J Obstet Gynaecol Reprod Biol* 2002; **103**: 26–9.

15 Peterson R *et al.* Violence and adverse pregnancy outcomes: a review of the literature and directions for future research. *Am J Prevent Med* 1997; **13**(5): 366–73.

16 Theodorou DA *et al.* Fetal death after trauma in pregnancy. *Am Surg* 2000; **66**(9): 809–12.

17 Einarson, ARN *et al.* Accidental electric shock in pregnancy: a prospective cohort study. *Am J Obstet Gynaecol* 1997; **176**(3): 768–81.

18 Health & Safety Executive. *EH64 Summary Criteria for Occupational Exposure Limits*. London: HMSO, 2002.

19 Gauger VT *et al.* A survey of obstetric complications and pregnancy outcomes in paediatric and non-paediatric anaesthesiologists. *Paediatr Anaesth* 2003; **13**(6): 490–5.

20 Baxter PJ. Gases. In: *Hunter's diseases of occupations*, (9th edn) (eds Baxter PJ, Adams PH, Aw T-C, Cockcroft A, Harrington JM), pp. 123–78. London: Arnold, 2000.

21 Rowland AS *et al.* Nitrous oxide and spontaneous abortion in female dental assistants. *Am J Epidemiol* 1995; **141**(6): 531–8.

22 Bodin L. The association of shift work and nitrous oxide exposure in pregnancy with birth weight and gestational age. *Epidemiology* 1999; **10**(4): 429–36.

23 Norman CA, Halton DM. Is carbon monoxide a workplace teratogen? A review and evaluation of the literature. *Ann Occup Hyg* 1990; **34**(4): 335–47.

24 Taskinen H *et al.* Laboratory work and pregnancy outcome. *J Occup Med* 1994; **36**(3): 311–19.

25 Comb JA *et al.* Pregnancy outcomes in women potentially exposed to occupational solvents and women working in the electronics industry. *J Occup Med* 1991; **33**(5): 597–604.

26 Doyle, P *et al.* Spontaneous abortion in dry cleaning workers potentially exposed to perchlorethylene. *Occup Environ Med* 1997; **54**(12): 848–53.

27 Khattak S *et al.* Pregnancy outcome following gestational exposure to organic solvents: a prospective controlled study. *JAMA* 1999; **281**(12): 1106–9.

28 Saurel-Cubizolles MJ, Job-Spira N, Estryn-Behar M. Ectopic pregnancy and occupational exposure to antineoplastic drugs. *Lancet* 1993; **341**(8854): 1169–71.

29 Misra DP, Nguyen RH. Environmental tobacco smoke and low birth weight: a hazard in the workplace? *Environ Health Perspect* 1999; **107**(6): 897–904.

30 Hull MG. Delayed conception and active and passive smoking. The Avon longitudinal study of pregnancy and childhood study team. *Fertil Steril* 2000; **74**(4) 725–33.

31 Fillippini G, Farinotti M, Ferrarini M. Active and passive smoking during pregnancy and risk of central nervous system tumours in children. *Paediatr Perinat Epidemiol* 2000; **14**: 78–84.

32 Health & Safety Executive. *Infection risks to new and expectant mothers in the workplace: a guide for employers*. London: HMSO, 1997.

33 Centers for Disease Control. Rubella vaccination during pregnancy—United States, 1971–1988. *MMWR Morb Mortal Wkly Rep* 1989; **38**: 289–291.

34 Royal College of Obstetricians & Gynaecologists. *Chickenpox in pregnancy*. Guideline No. 13.2001, 2001. On RCOG website www.rcog.org.uk.

35 MacMahan E *et al*. Identification of potential candidates for varicella vaccination by history: questionnaire and seroprevalence study. *BMJ* 2004; **329**: 551–2.

36 Harger JH *et al*. Prospective evaluation of 618 pregnant women exposed to Parvovirus B19: risks and symptoms. *Obstet Gynaecol* 1998; **91**(3): 413–20.

37 Newton LH, Hall SM. A survey of health education material for the primary prevention of congenital Toxoplasmosis. *Commun Dis Rep* 1995; **5**(2): R13–20.

38 Ahlborg G. Physical work load and pregnancy outcome. *J Occup Environ Med* 1995; **37**(8): 941–4.

39 Mozurkewich EL. Working conditions and adverse pregnancy outcome: a meta-analysis. *Obstet Gynaecol* 2000; **95**(4): 623–35.

40 Barlow S, Dayan AD, Stabile IK. Workplace exposures and reproductive effects. In: *Hunter's diseases of occupation*, (9th edn) (eds Baxter PJ, Adams PH, Aw T-C, Cockcroft A, Harrington JM), pp. 823–40. London: Arnold, 2000.

41 Judge CM. Physical exposures during pregnancy and congenital cardiovascular malformations. *Paediatr Perinat Epidemiol* 2004; **18** (5): 352–60.

42 Knutsson A. Health disorders of shift workers. *Occup Med* 2003; **53**: 103–8.

43 Labyak S *et al*. Effects of shiftwork on sleep and menstrual function in nurses. *Health Care Women Int* 2002; **23**(6–7): 703–14.

44 Lederman SA *et al*. The effects of the World Trade Centre event on birth outcomes among term deliveries at three lower Manhattan hospitals. *Environ Health Perspect* 2004; **112**(17): 1772–8.

45 DVLA website www.dvla.uk/at_a_glance.

46 British National Formulary online www.bnf.org.

47 Strand K, Wergeland E, Bjerkedal T. Job adjustment as a means to reduce sickness absence during pregnancy. *Scand J Work Environ Health* 1997; **23**(5): 378–84.

48 Royal College of Obstetricians and Gynaecologists. *Guideline No 17: The investigation and treatment of couples with recurrent miscarriage*. On www.rcog.org.uk.

49 Fenster L *et al*. A prospective study of work related physiological exertion and spontaneous abortion. *Epidemiology* 1997; **8**: 66–74.

50 *Why Mothers Die 2000–2002—Report on confidential enquiries into maternal deaths in the United Kingdom*. On The Confidential Enquiry into Maternal and Child Health website *www.cemach.org.uk*.

51 Bouyer J *et al*. Ectopic pregnancy and occupational exposure of hospital personnel. *Scand J Work Environ Health* 1998; **24**(2): 98–103.

52 Thomas J, Paranjothy S. Royal College of Obstetricians and Gynaecologists Clinical Support Unit. *National Sentinel Caesarean Section Audit Report*. London: RCOG Press, 2001.

53 Leadbetter RE, Mawer D, Lindow SW. Symphysis pubis dysfunction: a review of the literature. *J Matern Fetal Neonat Med* 2004; **16**, 349–54.

54 Enkin M *et al*. *A guide to effective care in pregnancy and childbirth*, (3rd edn). Oxford: Oxford University Press, 2000.

55 Rosen T *et al*. A randomized controlled trial of nerve stimulation for relief of nausea and vomiting in pregnancy. *Obstet Gynaecol* 2003; **102**: 129–35.

56 Crawley RA, Dennison K, Carter C. Cognition in pregnancy and the first year post-partum. *Psychol Psychother* 2003; **76**: 69–85.

57 De Groot RHM *et al*. Memory performance, but not processing speed, may be reduced during early pregnancy. *J Clin Exp Neuropsychol* 2003; **25**(4): 482–8.

58 Levy LS. Aliphatic chemicals. In: *Hunter's diseases of occupations*, (9th edn) (eds Baxter PJ, Adams PH, Aw T-C, Cockcroft A, Harrington JM), p. 833. London: Arnold, 2000.

59 Morgan L, Scott A. Metals. In: *Hunter's diseases of occupations*, (9th edn) (eds Baxter PJ, Adams PH, Aw T-C, Cockcroft A, Harrington JM), p. 91. London: Arnold, 2000.

60 Cox JL, Holden JM, Sagovsky R. Detection of postnatal depression. Development of the 10-item Edinburgh Postnatal Depression Scale. *British J Psychiatry* 1987; **150**: 782–6.

61 Hendrick V. Treatment of postnatal depression. *BMJ* 2003; **327**: 1003–4.

62 Wallace M. National Occupational Health & Safety Commission. Review: The effects of shiftwork on health. On Australian Government website www.nohsc.gov.au/ResearchCoordination/researchreports.

63 Hjollund NHI *et al.* Job strain and time to pregnancy. *Scand J Work Environ Health* 1998; **24**(5): 344–50.

64 Royal College of Obstetricians & Gynaecologists. *The initial management of menorrhagia*. 2001. On RCOG website www.rcog.org.uk.

65 Paul J (2003). *Working though the change*. London: TUC Publication, 2003.

66 Committee on Safety of Medicines. Review of the evidence regarding long-term safety of HRT. *Curr Prob Pharmacovil*, **30**, pp. 4–7.

67 Wignall BK, Fox AJ. Mortality of female gas mask assemblers. *Br J Ind Med* 1982; **39**: 34–38.

68 Ward K, Hilton P. Prospective multicentre randomised trial of tension-free vaginal tape and colposuspension as primary treatment for stress incontinence. *BMJ* 2002; **325**: 67–74.

69 On Department for Work and Pensions website www.dwp.gov.uk/medical/hot.asp.

70 Pheasant S. *Bodyspace. Anthropometry, ergonomics and the design of work*. London: Taylor & Francis, 1996.

71 AP1269A. *Royal Air Force manual of medical fitness*, Section 5, (3rd edn). 1998.

72 Geary KG, Irvine D, Croft AM. Does military service damage females? An analysis of medical discharge data in the British Armed Forces. *Occup Med* 2002; **52**(2): 85–90.

73 Greeves JP, Bishop A, Morgan CK. The effect of depot-medroxyprogesterone acetate on bone health and stress fracture risk during British Army Phase-1 Training. QinetiQ report for the MoD (QinetiQ/K1/CHS/TR0315359 December 2003). Farnborough, Hampshire: QinetiQ Ltd, 2003.

74 On Department of Health website www.dh.gov.uk/PublicationsAndStatistics/Statistics/HospitalEpisodeStatistics

Chapter 21

Fitness for work after surgery

A. M. Samuel and J. Mc K. Wellwood

Occupation

The duration of convalescence after a surgical operation will vary with the type of work to which the patient will be returning. Whereas an uncomplicated 'open' cholecystectomy may result in a period of 2–3 weeks away from office work, 4–6 weeks will be required before the patient can return to heavy manual work. In a recent randomized study, return to a non-manual job after laparoscopic inguinal hernia repair was a median of 10 days and after open hernia repair was 14 days; return to work for those with manual occupations was a median of 17 days after laparoscopic hernia repair and 21 days after open hernia repair.[1]

Several studies have shown that self-employed patients return to work sooner than others.[2] An important factor affecting the speed of return to work is the individual patient's motivation. Unless advised otherwise, patients may stay away from their work until they 'feel like' returning. They should therefore be advised before the surgical procedure how long they are likely to be in hospital and how long it is likely to be before they will be fit to go back to work after their operation.

Severity of disease and complications of surgery

The severity of the disease for which a surgical procedure was undertaken may affect the timing of return to work. Whereas an elective laparoscopic cholecystectomy for uncomplicated biliary colic may permit return to light work within a week, a patient undergoing the same operation for acute gangrenous cholecystitis will require a longer convalescence. Patients who have undergone emergency laparotomy for a life-threatening condition such as faecal peritonitis, a ruptured aortic aneurysm or ruptured viscera following trauma may have a long hospital stay and be absent from work for several months.

Surgical complications such as wound infection, intra-abdominal abscess, pulmonary atelectasis or bronchopneumonia, deep vein thrombosis and pulmonary emboli may lengthen a hospital stay and delay a return to work. Pathological persistence of wound pain is also an occasional cause of delayed return to work.

Treatment advances

Improvements in surgical technique and advances in medical management have improved the outcome of treatment for many patients. The increasing use of Day Care Units (DCU) for surgical operations has increased the efficiency with which patients can be treated in the National Health Service. Many surgical and anaesthetic advances have reduced the morbidity of surgical operations and hence reduced the need for prolonged convalescence prior to return to work.

'Keyhole surgery'

Muhe[3] was the first surgeon to describe cholecystectomy 'through the laparoscope' and in 1987 the French Surgeon, Philippe Mouret from Lyon, demonstrated removal of the gall bladder using minimal access surgery. Others soon followed,[4,5] and laparoscopic cholecystectomy is now the undisputed operation of first choice for the treatment of symptomatic gallstones and is increasingly performed in the DCU. The role of laparoscopy has since expanded in several specialities including general surgery, gynaecology, and urology, and large painful surgical wounds have been replaced with small, relatively painless, 'keyhole' incisions, facilitating more rapid postoperative recovery for many patients. The small wounds of laparoscopic surgery are also less prone to complications such as wound infection than the larger laparotomy wounds. Furthermore, the handling of the intestine and the fluid loss involved in abdominal procedures performed through laparotomy wounds is largely eliminated by laparoscopic techniques. Postoperative ileus and pulmonary and thromboembolic complications are less frequent after laparoscopic surgery. Laparoscopic techniques thus promote early recovery and enable quicker return to work after surgery. Other minimally invasive procedures such as arthroscopy and thoracoscopy similarly contribute to earlier recovery after orthopaedic and chest surgery respectively.

'Day surgery'

The proportion of operations performed in DCUs has increased as surgical and anaesthetic techniques have evolved to cause less postoperative pain and to enable a quicker recovery. The use of local anaesthetic for operations such as hernia repair has also increased the use of the DCU. As no 'in-patient' bed is required, the risk of cancellation of a surgical operation booked for the DCU is greatly reduced. Even with the annual 'winter bed crisis', day surgery should continue as normal, and delays waiting for elective surgical procedures should be reduced. Day surgery is conducive to a 'diary system' so that the patient is given a date for surgery well in advance. This not only reduces the likelihood of patient default but also allows for reliably planning absence from work.

The report of the Royal College of Surgeons of England in 1992[6] envisaged a time when 50% of all elective surgical procedures would be performed in the DCU. Subsequently, the Audit Commission reported on the use of the DCU for different surgical procedures during 1999/2000.[7] The figures show a wide variation in the use of day surgery between different Trusts in the use of day surgery. For example, a Trust at the lower quartile for 'day case' inguinal hernia repair carried out 33% of hernia repairs in the DCU, whereas the same figure for a Trust at the 95th percentile was 65%. Subsequently the NHS plan predicated that 75% of elective surgery would be undertaken in DCUs by 2002.[8] Day case rates for England 2003/2004 are show in Table 21.1.

It is now recognized that the majority of inguinal hernias can be repaired in the DCU unless the patient's social circumstances make returning home on the same day as the operation unsafe or impractical. Patients in the DCU can be treated by open mesh repair using a local or general anaesthetic or by laparoscopic hernia repair, which requires a general anaesthetic.[1] Increasingly laparoscopic cholecystectomy is being performed in the DCU. Typically, the operation is performed in the morning and the patient is fit to return home, if accompanied, by mid afternoon of the same day.

Other treatment advances

The development of 'keyhole' surgery has been an important but not the only recent treatment advance. Other changes in surgical technique have contributed to shorter convalescence before a return to work. For example, the use of 'tension-free' mesh in the repair of groin hernias whether placed laparoscopically[9,10] or through an open groin incision,[11] has reduced the pain after hernia repair and speeded up the return to normal activity.

Table 21.1 Day case rates for common surgical procedures in English Acute Provider Trials 2003/2004

Operations	Day case (%)
Repair inguinal hernia	47.9
Laparoscopic cholecystectomy	4.3
Haemorrhoidectomy	19.9
Surgery of anal fissure	65.7
Stripping or ligation of varicose veins	55.4
Excision of breast lumps	62.0

Department of Health Hospital Episode Statistics, NHS Hospitals, England 2003/2004. Reproduced under the terms of the click-use licence.

Advances in medicine have improved the management of certain conditions such as peptic ulcer as a result of the development and availability of highly effective pharmacological agents. These drugs enable a patient with an active peptic ulcer to rapidly control the symptoms and to avoid surgical operation. Elective surgery for peptic ulcer is now very uncommon and is generally only necessary for complications such as perforation or haemorrhage.

Operations involving laparotomy incisions

Standard 'open' abdominal wounds are still required when a laparoscopic procedure (e.g. cholecystectomy) proves technically impossible or dangerous, and for many major abdominal operations such as those on the pancreas and those for abdominal aortic aneurysm, colorectal resections, etc. The major abdominal wound involved in laparotomy as opposed to laparoscopy is a cause of considerable postoperative pain and morbidity.

Most abdominal wounds are now closed with non-absorbable or slowly absorbable materials rather than the rapidly absorbed cat gut used by many surgeons in the past. As a result of the improved suture techniques the incidence of wound dehiscence is reduced and early return to non-manual work should not increase the risk of the development of an incisional hernia. Heavy manual work, however, will not normally be undertaken for 6–8 weeks after a major laparotomy wound. The length of convalescence after a laparotomy will be affected not only by the type and size of wound but also by the procedure performed and the occurrence of complications in the postoperative period. A subcostal incision for removal of the gall bladder (if laparoscopic access has been unsuccessful) is less traumatic for the patient than a full-length vertical abdominal incision, as is commonly needed for colonic or vascular procedures. Whereas the former may result in a hospital stay of 2–5 days and a quick return to work, most patients with a long vertical abdominal wound will remain in hospital for 1–2 weeks if there are no procedural or wound-related complications and absence from work will be longer.

Complications of laparotomy wounds include wound infection and wound dehiscence and, at a later date, the development of an incisional hernia. Occasional consequences of laparotomy, for whatever cause, include small bowel obstruction due to ileus in the immediate postoperative period or due to adhesions at a later date.

Individual procedures

Table 21.2 shows the incidence of common general surgical procedures in the NHS in England for the year 2003/2004.[12]

Table 21.2 Common surgical operations performed in English NHS Hospitals

Operations	No.	Mean hospital stay (days)
Repair inguinal hernia	81 175	2.2
Repair femoral, umbilical, incisional hernias	33 028	4.0
Cholecystectomy	49 288	3.9
Operations for gastric reflux	2936	4.7
Partial/total gastrectomy	1807	19.4
Appendicectomy	40 455	4.0
Colectomy	18 942	16.5
Excision of rectum	12 414	17.7
Haemorrhoidectomy	23 567	2.5
Other anal/perianal operations	74 272	2.3
Excision of varicose veins	42 484	1.5
Repair of aortic aneurysm	1663 (emergency)	14.2*
	3856 (elective)	14.7
Thyroidectomy	7566	3.8
Excision of salivary glands	4303	2.6–4.5
Operations on lung	9997	7.0–10.5
Oesophagectomy	1754	21.6
Mastectomy	16 552 (total)	5.8
	35 567 (partial)	3.1

Department of Health Hospital Episode Statistics, NHS Hospitals, England 2003/2004. Reproduced under the terms of the click-use licence. *Skewed by early deaths.

Inguinal hernias

The number of operations performed on inguinal hernias on the NHS in England during the year 2003/2004 was 81 175.[12] Forty-five per cent were repaired in a DCU, commonly using a non-absorbable mesh to 'patch' the defect in the groin. These mesh repairs are much better than earlier stitched methods of repair as the mesh does not create tension and causes relatively little pain. There is a much lower recurrence rate (as low as 1%) and early vigorous activity does not compromise the integrity of the repair. The synthetic mesh may be inserted through a standard groin incision under a local or general anaesthetic. Alternatively the mesh may be put in laparoscopically using general anaesthesia. Whichever method is chosen the majority of patients will be able to leave hospital on the same day as their surgical procedure.

Whether the mesh should be placed laparoscopically or through an open groin incision is controversial.[1,9,10,13–15] It is now agreed that recovery is quicker and pain reduced if the laparoscopic route is used. Initially, the National Institute for Clinical Excellence (NICE) recommended that laparoscopic repair be reserved for bilateral groin hernias and recurrent groin hernias in view of the rare but occasional major complications reported after laparoscopic hernia repair.[16] However, the guidelines were reviewed in 2004 and NICE now proposes that the technique may be used for 'first time' unilateral hernia repair (provided the surgeon is skilled at the technique).[16] Bilateral hernias should be repaired during one operation particularly if the procedure is laparoscopic. If open procedures are planned, some surgeons prefer to treat one side at a time, although others will repair both sides using either local or general anaesthetic.

Patients should be advised to walk about as soon as they have recovered from the anaesthetic and to resume normal activities as soon as pain permits. Patients should be advised that nothing that they can do will result in a recurrence of the hernia. Advice to refrain from lifting is poor advice and slows recovery. The recurrence rate should be less than 1% and is dependent on surgical technique and not how quickly the patient returns to full and vigorous activity. It may be advisable for the patient to refrain from driving a motor car for approximately a week in case the ability to put the brake on in an emergency is compromised by pain.

Return to work following unilateral hernia repair (first time or recurrent) should only be a few days for non-manual occupations and 2–4 weeks for manual occupations, as manual handling activities are more likely to result in painful symptoms but not a recurrence. If bilateral hernias are repaired at the same operation, recovery will tend to be approximately 1 week slower than that following unilateral hernia repair.[1]

Factors that may delay a return to work include wound infection, wound haematomas, and persistent groin pain. The latter is less common after laparoscopic repair.

Femoral hernias, umbilical hernias, epigastric hernias, and incisional hernias

Operations for the above conditions accounted for 33 028 procedures in the NHS in England during 2003/2004. Thirty-two per cent were performed in a DCU.[12]

Various techniques may be used to repair femoral or small umbilical hernias both of which are suitable for treatment in a DCU. Simple suture techniques are still used for both. Alternatively, rolls of mesh may be used as a plug to cure femoral hernias and a flat mesh, which can be placed through an open incision or laparoscopically, may be used to treat a large umbilical defect. Return to normal activity in a non-manual capacity should be possible within a few days. Employees with manual jobs may require 2–3 weeks before pain permits full activities.

Patients with epigastric hernias are treated using a small incision placed in the region of the hernia and one or two non-absorbable sutures are used to close the defect. A non-manual worker should be able to return to work within a few days. A further week or two of convalescence may be required for a manual worker.

For large umbilical hernias and for most incisional hernias the surgical placement of a mesh to repair the defect will be required. In most hospitals these operations will be performed via a skin incision and a flat mesh will be placed deep to the rectus abdominus muscle but superficial to the posterior rectus sheath and peritoneum. When these operations are performed using an 'open' technique, the patient will normally be hospitalized for a period of days after the operation, the length of stay in hospital being determined by the extent of the dissection necessary to place the large mesh and the absence of complications such as infection. A minority of surgeons now treat large umbilical hernias and some incisional hernias laparoscopically. The patient requires a general anaesthetic and three small wounds for the trocars are placed at the lateral margin of the abdomen. Dissection is usually required to reduce the contents of the incisional or umbilical hernia. A flat mesh is then placed into the abdominal cavity through a laparoscopic port and is stapled in position to cover the defect on the inside. Meshes with a low tendency to adhere to the intra-abdominal contents are now available and may be preferred to conventional polypropylene meshes. Recovery after a laparoscopically placed mesh for large umbilical or incisional hernias may require several days in hospital after the procedure. Thereafter, return to non-manual occupations should be possible within 2–3 weeks. Open as opposed to laparoscopic repair of a large umbilical or incisional hernia using a flat mesh may require 3–5 weeks of convalescence.

Cholecystectomy

Cholecystectomy was performed 49 288 times in English NHS hospitals in the year 2003/2004.[12] Although some surgeons perform the majority of these operations in a DCU, the national figure is only 3%.

Laparoscopic cholecystectomy is the treatment of choice for symptomatic gallstones. However, a proportion of these patients will have their laparoscopic procedures converted into the standard open cholecystectomy if undue difficulty performing the laparoscopic procedure is encountered. Most experienced laparoscopic surgeons will need to convert 2–5% of laparoscopic cholecystectomy operations into open cholecystectomy procedures.

Patients with symptomatic gallstones will be absent from work during attacks of pain or cholecystitis and may continue to miss work intermittently until cholecystectomy is performed. Patients with symptomatic gallstones may, therefore, have a number of periods away from work, the final period being that to allow recovery from cholecystectomy. A more efficient management of acute gallstone disease involves proceeding to urgent laparoscopic cholecystectomy during the initial hospitalization. This leads to fewer unplanned absences from work.[18]

Most patients who have undergone elective laparoscopic cholecystectomy should be fit for non-manual work 1–2 weeks after surgery and for manual work after 2–4 weeks. Those patients who undergo urgent laparoscopic cholecystectomy for acute cholecystitis may require a longer period of recovery due to the debilitating effect of the cholecystitis rather than the effect of laparoscopic cholecystectomy.

Stomach, duodenum, liver, and pancreas

Surgical operations for gastro-oesophageal reflux disease (GORD)

There were 2936 operations for gastro-oesophageal reflux in English NHS hospitals for the years 2003/2004.[12]

The majority of patients who suffer from regular symptomatic acid reflux are satisfactorily treated by antacids or by H2-blocking agents or proton pump inhibitors. Open surgical procedures to reduce reflux have been available for many years, but became unpopular due to complications and slow recovery. The effectiveness of modern drugs reduced the attraction of such open surgical interventions. However, laparoscopic antireflux operations have now superseded the older 'open' procedures. Geagea[19] and Dalmaigne et al.[20] introduced the laparoscopic version of a Nissen fundoplication in 1991. Since then there has been increasing use of this minimally invasive surgical operation when either medical management fails to control symptoms or they rapidly recur on cessation of medical agents.[21] The operation is performed under general anaesthetic using five 10-mm incisions that accommodate five 1-cm diameter operating ports. The oesophagogastric junction is mobilized and the oesophageal crura are sutured together behind the oesophagus to form a snug (but not tight) passage for the oesophagus through the diaphragm. The mobilized fundus of the stomach is then pulled behind and around the oesophagus and is stitched to the left side of the upper part of the body of the fundus, thus forming a collar of stomach or 'wrap' encircling the lower oesophagus. Other forms of fundoplication in which the stomach is not brought 360 degrees around the oesophagus (partial fundoplication) are used particularly when there is some concern about oesophageal dysmotility.

The patient will typically leave hospital on the second or third postoperative day after laparoscopic fundoplication or partial fundoplication. Subsequent recovery may be rapid with the patient able to resume non-manual work at between 10 days and 2 weeks and manual work at 3 or 4 weeks. However, difficulty swallowing solid food may occur after surgery in up to 30% of patients for up to 3 months. The dysphagia usually resolves spontaneously without treatment, although occasionally further intervention is necessary. Despite dysphagia, a patient will be able to return to non-manual work on a liquid or soft solid diet 10 days–2 weeks after surgery. However, a patient will probably not be fit for heavy manual work until a solid meal can be eaten. The period of convalescence for each patient following a laparoscopic fundoplication will need to be tailored individually to take account of any postoperative symptoms.

Operations on the stomach and duodenum

During the year 2002/2003, partial or total gastrectomy was performed 1807 times in the English NHS. The mean stay in hospital was 19.4 days.[12] Gastrectomy for benign disease is now an uncommon procedure, being seldom required except for bleeding or occasionally perforation of a peptic ulcer. However, radical gastric resection remains the cornerstone of the treatment of gastric cancer. The hospital stay and duration of convalescence will depend on the nature of the operative procedure and the disease for which it is being performed. Gastrectomy will normally require a hospital stay of 10–14 days followed by a 6–8-week recovery period before return to non-manual work. Return to manual work may be more delayed, particularly if the patient has to adjust to a radical change in his diet. Patients who undergo radical gastrectomy or oesophagogastrectomy for malignant disease are often very weakened prior to surgery and may require a longer convalescence. A patient who has undergone a successful radical gastrectomy or oesophagogastrectomy will probably be fit for non-manual work at 2–3 months. Patients may not, however, be able to return to manual work particularly if the malignant process recurs.

Some patients will develop 'dumping syndrome' after gastric resection and these symptoms may delay return to work. The symptoms of 'early dumping' occur soon after a meal and consist of epigastric fullness, sweating, a sensation of warmth, tachycardia, intestinal colic, and diarrhoea. These symptoms will tend to subside with time. Meals in general should be small in bulk and dry. The patient may find that lying down gives relief, whereas further food intake aggravates the symptoms. Alternatively, patients may suffer a late dumping syndrome, almost certainly due to low blood sugar occurring about 2 hours after meals. Chief symptoms are tremor, faintness, epigastric emptiness, and nausea; relief may be obtained by eating more food or glucose. Weight loss and a variety of nutritional disturbances may occur after gastrectomy. These may limit the patient's capacity to return to previous working activities and alternative employment may be desirable.

Duodenal surgery is now uncommon and is most frequently required when duodenal ulcers perforate or bleed. Patients in whom a duodenotomy with under running of a bleeding ulcer is required as an emergency, or patients in whom a perforated duodenal ulcer requires suture will have a laparotomy wound and may remain in hospital for 10 days or more. Return to non-manual work will probably be possible at 4–6 weeks and to manual work at 6–8 weeks. These figures will vary depending on the general health of the patient prior to the procedure. Dumping syndromes and diarrhoea may occur after vagotomy.

Operations on the liver and pancreas

Surgical procedures on the above organs, although uncommon, are frequently major in extent. Patients will have to be assessed individually with regard to return to work and modification of work when, and if, they do return to work.

Colorectal

Appendicectomy

Appendicectomy was performed 40 455 times in the English NHS during the year 2003/2004.

Return to work following appendicectomy will be influenced by the presence or absence of pelvic abscess or generalized peritonitis. Recovery from a simple early appendicitis without any pelvic or peritoneal sepsis will be much quicker than recovery following serious intra-abdominal sepsis.

The appendix is removed under general anaesthesia, either through a standard 'grid-iron' incision in the right iliac fossa, 6–9 cm in length, or, increasingly, via a laparoscopic approach involving three small incisions. Debate continues about the relative merits of each approach. However, early appendicitis treated laparoscopically should result in a hospital stay of no more than 2 or 3 days followed by a return to non-manual work at 7 days and manual work at 2–3 weeks. 'Open' appendicectomy performed for early appendicitis will involve a hospital stay of under a week followed by a return to work for non-manual workers 2 weeks after surgery and for manual workers 3–4 weeks after surgery. Appendicitis complicated by pelvic abscess, peritonitis, or severe wound infection will require convalescence tailored to the individual's circumstances.

Operations on the colon

The number of 'finished episodes' involving colonic operations in England in 2003/2004 was 18 942 and the mean hospital stay was 16.5 days.[12] The figure for excision of the rectum was 12 414 'finished episodes'. The mean in-patient stay for operations on the rectum was 17.7 days.[12]

Experience with the laparoscopic resection of the colon and rectum is being increasingly reported but the 'open' surgical approach remains the norm.

Right hemicolectomy is most commonly performed for malignant disease, but may also be required for Crohn's or other diseases. The procedure is generally straightforward with an end to end anastomosis and no stoma. Assuming rapid recovery without complication, the patient can usually leave hospital 5–10 days after surgery and should be able to return to non-manual work 3–6 weeks after operation. Return to manual work would probably take 4–8 weeks in the majority of patients.

The operations of left hemicolectomy or anterior resection of the rectum are generally performed for malignant disease or for diverticular disease. If the operation is straightforward and an end-to-end anastomosis is done without a colostomy, hospital stay will usually be 7–14 days. Return to non-manual work would take 4–6 weeks and return to manual work 6–10 weeks. If a temporary diverting colostomy or ileostomy has been necessary, the patient may be reluctant to return to work until the stoma has been closed. Learning how to manage a stoma will delay the initial discharge from hospital and return to work. Surgeons vary in the timing of colostomy or ileostomy closure, which depends on satisfactory healing of the anastomosis. However, a defunctioning stoma is commonly closed 3–6 months after the initial resection. The period of convalescence after the closure of the stoma will be tailored to the individual who may not return to work for 3–4 weeks after a stoma has been closed.

Abdominoperineal excision of the rectum is most commonly performed for malignant disease of the lower third of the rectum. The patient will have a permanent left iliac fossa colostomy. Hospital stay may be 2–4 weeks in order to allow the patient to recover from surgery and to enable him to learn to manage the colostomy. Micturition and sexual functioning may be adversely affected in the male as a result of denervation of the pelvic organs associated with the radical excision of the rectum. The operation can be debilitating and patients may require 2–3 months of convalescence before returning to non-manual employment. Return to manual work may take longer or may not occur. Any return should be individually tailored to the patient's ability to cope with the changed anatomy and permanent colostomy.

Pan-proctocolectomy is usually undertaken when medical management fails to control the diseases ulcerative colitis or Crohn's colitis. In this operation the anus, rectum, and the colon are excised. The patient will be left with a permanent ileostomy and must learn to manage it. Many of these patients are unwell before operation as a result of their chronic or acute inflammatory bowel disease. For these reasons, such patients may require anything between 3 and 4 weeks in hospital even in the absence of any postoperative complications. Months of convalescence may follow. In some patients, excision of the rectum and colon for refractory ulcerative colitis may be combined with the preservation of the anal sphincters and the formation of a 'new rectum' from small bowel. The resultant 'pouch' replaces the excised rectum and is anastomosed to the upper cut end of the anal canal (restorative proctocolectomy). In this way some patients will maintain continence and will avoid a permanent stoma, although many patients will find it necessary to pass a catheter several times per 24 hours through the anus into the pelvic pouch in order to empty the pouch. Restorative proctocolectomy is particularly indicated in young people who are sexually active and wish to avoid a permanent ileostomy. A temporary defunctioning ileostomy will subsequently be closed assuming satisfactory healing of the small bowel pouch in the pelvis and the anastomosis to the anal canal. Restorative proctocolectomy may be complicated by pelvic sepsis and small bowel obstruction and any patient undergoing restorative proctocolectomy will almost certainly be away from work for several months.

Anal region and pilonidal sinus

There were 23 567 operations for haemorrhoids in England during 2003/2004.[12] Other operations on the anal and perianal region accounted for 74 272 episodes during the same period.[12]

Haemorrhoids

By far the commonest presentation of internal haemorrhoids is painless, fresh rectal bleeding. This is normally dealt with in the out-patient clinic by attention to diet and injection or banding of the internal haemorrhoids. Time away from work should not be necessary apart from attendance at the out-patient clinic.

Anal verge haematomas, otherwise known as thrombosed external piles, present as a painful blue lump at the anal verge. The lump is skin covered and is not produced by prolapse of an internal haemorrhoid. Such patients are simply treated with analgesics and stool softeners, although in some cases the patient may require 2 or 3 days away from work due to pain. This lesion is not a haemorrhoid and is thought to occur when a subcutaneous vein at the anal verge ruptures to produce a haematoma immediately deep to the skin.

Internal haemorrhoids may enlarge, prolapse and thrombose, and present as an acutely painful swelling at the anal verge, which may involve the whole circumference of the anal verge or may involve only part of it. The patient may need to be away from work for up to 2 weeks in severe cases. Normally resolution occurs spontaneously with bed rest, analgesia, and aperients. Rarely this acute condition persists and haemorrhoidectomy is required. The recovery from haemorrhoidectomy under these circumstances is similar to that from a planned haemorrhoidectomy for chronically prolapsing haemorrhoids.

Elective haemorrhoidectomy is most commonly performed for chronically prolapsing haemorrhoids. Conventional haemorrhoidectomy leaves three anal wounds, which are allowed to close slowly by second intention. Attempts have been made to speed recovery by various suturing procedures but these have not gained universal use. Following conventional haemorrhoidectomy patients may remain in hospital until they have had a bowel movement, although increasingly such patients may go home the same day as surgery. The wounds will be painful for a few days but then the pain will be noticed mainly after bowel movements. This pain will subside over a period of 2 weeks and most patients will be fit to return to work, either non-manual or manual, after 2–3 weeks. Complete healing of the anal wounds, however, may not occur for 5 or 6 weeks after surgery and the patient should have access to washing facilities at work.

Recent developments include 'stapled haemorrhoidectomy'. This is designed to reduce postoperative pain and speed recovery and return to work. A circumferential segment of the mucosa above the anal canal is resected and the edges stapled together. This operation draws the haemorrhoids back up into the anal canal to their normal position rather than excising them. The procedure is performed using a stapling device, which both resects the mucosa and staples the cut edges. Although gaining in popularity, this technique has not yet replaced conventional haemorrhoidectomy.

Perianal sepsis

Drainage of ischiorectal or perianal abscesses may be performed under local or general anaesthetic. Rapid relief of pain and swelling will ensue and provided there are facilities for bathing and dressing the area at work most patients should be able to return within a week. Occasionally a large neglected ischiorectal abscess requires a prolonged hospital stay with analgesics and return to work will be more delayed.

Many ischiorectal or perianal abscesses will be found to be associated with a fistula-in-ano and will recur unless such a fistula is treated. Treatment for fistula-in-ano consists of laying open or excising the track. In the majority of cases the fistula will be low down in the anal canal. Healing may take several weeks and return to work will depend on the size of the ensuing wound. For a very short, low level anal fistula, little dressing is required and the return to work can be correspondingly rapid, usually in 1 week or less. The patient may be spared major surgery when a high-level anal fistula is managed by the use of a seton to avoid injury to the continence mechanism. However, hospital attendances will be needed to supervise the management of the seton. A seton comprises a non-absorbable suture, which is passed into the anal fistula via the external opening and then is passed out via the internal opening. The ends are tied together externally. Thus the surgeon does not 'lay open' the fistula as, by so doing, he might cause a reduced level of continence due to division of the sphincter muscles. Rather, the seton will slowly cut through the sphincter muscles over several months allowing healing to occur above the seton and avoiding disruption of the continence mechanism. The surgeon may choose to tighten the seton from time to time to hasten the process. When the seton has converted a high fistula (whose laying open would risk incontinence) to a low fistula the latter may easily and safely be laid open. Surgical procedure for extensive fistulas will result in bigger wounds and dressings may be difficult and painful and attention by a qualified nurse may be necessary. This may preclude return to work for several weeks. Each case will require individual assessment. As soon as the dressings can be performed without great pain by the patients themselves, it should be possible for the patient to return to some form of work, provided suitable washing facilities are available. Alternatively, it may be possible for dressings to be performed before or after work by a district nurse.

Anal fissure

An anal fissure is a tear in the lining of the anal canal. The fissure causes pain and bleeding after defecation. Anal fissures are treated by the application locally of glyceryl trinitrate or diltiazem ointment to the perianal skin two or three times a day. These creams have superseded the use of intra-anal local anaesthetic gel. When, however, treatment is not successful, the surgical procedure of choice remains lateral internal sphincterotomy. Although this is a minor procedure it carries with it a small risk of reduced continence. The procedure is carried out generally as a day case and the patient should be able to return to work 1 or 2 days later.

Pilonidal sinus

The presence of a pilonidal sinus is indicated by an abscess or a discharging sinus either to one side of the midline or in the midline of the natal cleft. An abscess should be drained and simple drainage will result in a few days away from work. When the inflammation has resolved, the pilonidal sinus itself must be excised. A variety of different procedures are available for the treatment of pilonidal sinuses, underlining the fact that none are 100% successful. The basic operation is an excision of the skin and subcutaneous tissues of the natal cleft including all sinuses down to the fascia over the back of the sacrum. This wound may be left open to heal slowly by second intention, which may take 6–8 weeks. Alternatively an attempt may be made to close the defect primarily using various suturing techniques. If the pilonidal wound heals following primary suture, the patient will be fit to return to non-manual work at 2–4 weeks and to return to manual work at 3–6 weeks. When the pilonidal sinus has been excised and the wound left open, healing will take 6–8 weeks and it will be possible to return to work before this period only if arrangements for satisfactory dressing of the open wound can be made at work or by arrangement with the patient's local general medical practice and the district nursing service.

Vascular system

Varicose veins

Operations for varicose veins in the leg occurred 42 484 times in the English NHS during 2003/2004.[12]

Most operations for varicose veins involve disconnecting the long saphenous vein from the femoral vein and/or the short saphenous vein from the popliteal vein ('high tie'). The long saphenous vein may still require to be stripped, although it is not usual to strip the short saphenous vein. Surgery for varicose veins is increasingly being performed in DCUs. Individual surgeons differ in the postoperative management of patients who have undergone varicose vein surgery. Bandaging is now often used for 24 hours only and is then replaced by thromboembolic deterrent (TED), above-knee stockings for a period of 2 weeks. Patients should be able to return to light work 7–10 days after unilateral surgery for varicose veins and to manual work after 2–3 weeks. When procedures have been performed on both legs, patients will probably need up to 2 weeks away from light work and up to 4 weeks away from manual work. New techniques to replace stripping of veins are being evaluated. These include endovenous LASER ablation of the long saphenous vein. Such procedures are not yet standard but may in the future reduce the period away from work after varicose vein surgery.

Abdominal aortic aneurysm

There were 1663 emergency operations and 3856 other operations for abdominal aortic aneurysm in England for the year 2003/2004.[12]

Patients with an abdominal aortic aneurysm of 5 cm or greater will normally be advised to undergo elective grafting of the aneurysm to prevent rupture in the future. The majority of these patients will have already retired from work. Ultrasound screening of the population for aneurysms may reduce the age and increase the number of such patients. Aneurysmal rupture will be treated by emergency grafting provided the patient survives to reach hospital. Patients who do not reach hospital in time will die and a proportion of those who undergo emergency grafting for a ruptured aneurysm will also die. Emergency repair of a ruptured aortic aneurysm may be followed by a variety of major complications including acute renal failure, ischaemia of the limbs and intestinal ileus. Those few patients in work who survive emergency grafting of a ruptured aneurysm and those patients who undergo successful elective resection of an aortic aneurysm, will not usually return to work for 2–3 months or more and may never return to heavy manual work.

Minimally invasive endovascular placement of grafts within an aneurysm to prevent aortic aneurysm rupture may provide an alternative to major open surgery[23,24]. Such procedures currently account for less than 10% of operations for aortic aneurysm in the United Kingdom. Not all patients are suitable but technology is developing rapidly. Although perhaps up to 50% of elective procedures for aortic aneurysm may currently be possible using endovascular placement of grafts in specialist units, more patients may become suitable for this minimally invasive treatment as technology develops in the future. In-patient stay after minimally invasive endovascular placement of grafts for an abdominal aortic aneurysm is between 1 and 5 days. Patients should be able to return to a light job within a week and a manual job in 2–4 weeks if the endovascular procedure has been trouble-free. Currently, however, endovascular placement of grafts requires endoluminal re-intervention in up to 30% of patients and 5% may need a secondary open operative procedure. Regular surveillance of endovascular grafts is carried out every 2–3 months by computed tomography scan for 18 months. Complications include the leakage of blood following graft fracture or migration of the graft into the old abdominal aortic aneurysm sac.

Aorto-iliac and aorto-bifemoral grafting

Open surgical procedures for aorto-iliac and aorto-bifemoral atheroma are becoming less common due to the decreasing incidence of severe atheromatous disease and the alternatives to open surgery, namely peripheral vascular angioplasty with or without stenting. Patients who do undergo open aorto-iliac or aorto-bifemoral grafting will require 2–3 months away from work if their job is non-manual. For manual workers, return to work will be longer and they may be unable to return to heavy manual work.

Peripheral vessel angioplasty with or without stenting has reduced the need for open vascular bypass for aorto-iliac and more distal disease. The indications for angioplasty with or without stenting include a short stenosis measuring less than 10 cm and occluding the iliac, femoral, or popliteal arteries. The morbidity is lower than for open surgery and the return to full ambulatory activity and work is quicker. Angioplasty with or without stenting is normally performed by interventional radiologists, although occasionally vascular surgeons perform the technique.

A puncture wound is made in the skin of the groin for insertion of the balloon catheter into the femoral artery. There is no other wound. Occasionally a haematoma or rarely a false aneurysm may develop in the groin at the site of arterial puncture. Normally, however, patients should be able to return to light work at 1–2 weeks after angioplasty with or without stenting and there is no reason why manual workers should not return to work 2–3 weeks after the procedure.

Femoro-popliteal and femoro-distal grafts

These 'open' surgical procedures for more distal peripheral vascular disease are usually performed using an autologous long saphenous vein, which is either reversed so that the flow of blood is not held back by the valves or used *in situ* as a bypass after valve lysis. Patients with ischaemic limbs may avoid amputation by such procedures. Such patients are almost all in the older age group having retired from work. The results of surgery are not as good as the results of surgery involving the larger arteries.

Carotid stenosis

Patients undergoing carotid endarterectomy for carotid stenosis due to atheroma are seldom less than 60 years of age. A successful procedure should permit the patient to leave hospital 2–3 days after surgery and return to work 2–3 weeks later providing that there is no pre-existing neurological deficiency that would prevent this. Stroke is an occasional undesired sequel of such operations.

Adjuvant treatment after cardiovascular surgery

Some cardiac patients will require long-term anticoagulation with drugs such as warfarin or may be advised to take prophylactic aspirin in the long-term. Those with peripheral vascular disease will usually be asked to take an antiplatelet agent such as aspirin. Anticoagulation treatment is compatible with most types of work but a risk assessment should be carried out to ensure that any necessary control measures are instituted and any reasonable adjustments made to minimize the risk of trauma. Time off work should be factored in for attendance at haematology appointments for monitoring an adjustment of dosage.

Abdominal trauma

Blunt abdominal injury may occur in a road accident or following a fall. One classical example is the fall off a bicycle when a handlebar causes blunt injury to the spleen. Penetrating abdominal injuries may occur in road and other accidents or more typically as a result of assault with a weapon such as a knife or gun.

Assessment in hospital will determine whether or not the patient requires a laparotomy. Diagnostic laparoscopy may be of value. Intra-abdominal injuries may include trauma to the solid organs such as the spleen or liver with profuse and possibly life-threatening haemorrhage. Hollow viscera such as the gut may be ruptured or incised with resulting leak of faecal contents into the abdominal cavity. Penetrating injury either by a knife, a shard of glass or a gun, may cause widespread damage to several viscera and to the large vessels within the abdomen and pelvis.

Laparotomy will reveal the extent of the injuries occasioned by blunt or penetrating trauma. A badly injured spleen will require removal, although efforts may be made to preserve the spleen in order not to reduce the body's resistance to sepsis. Should splenectomy be necessary, the patient will normally be given pneumococcal vaccine and asked to take penicillin daily for life. Injuries to the liver may be managed by suture or packing or even partial resection. Severe bleeding from a kidney may require nephrectomy. Injuries to the bladder will be repaired and a catheter left in position. Injuries to the gut will be repaired and in some circumstances a temporary stoma may be required. Pancreatic injuries may be amenable to conservative management unless, for example, the gland has been transected by blunt injury when it may be advisable to remove the distal portion. The great vessels within the abdomen or pelvis may require repair.

In many cases, patients will have multiple injuries in addition to their abdominal trauma. In such cases, severe head injuries or extensive orthopaedic injuries may determine the patient's length of hospital stay and duration of convalescence before returning to work.

When abdominal trauma is the only injury, the duration of stay in hospital and the length of convalescence required, will depend on the patient's condition prior to resuscitation, the success of resuscitation, the severity and nature of the intra-abdominal injuries and the surgery required to deal with them. The laparotomy alone will necessitate a period of convalescence. The individual patient will need assessment in the light of his condition on discharge from hospital and the intra-abdominal surgery which has been necessary.

Head and neck

Thyroidectomy

Partial or complete thyroidectomy was undertaken 7566 times in NHS hospitals in England during the year 2003/2004.[12] The main indications for thyroidectomy include carcinoma of the thyroid gland, the presence of some solitary thyroid nodules, and some selected patients with multinodular goitre.

Hemi-thyroidectomy for a solitary thyroid nodule is a relatively minor procedure requiring 1 or 2 days in hospital and permitting a return to non-manual work within 1–2 weeks and heavy manual work at 2–4 weeks.

Subtotal thyroidectomy for multinodular goitre will require a longer convalescence and a patient may legitimately be away from non-manual work for 2–4 weeks, or from heavy manual work for 4–6 weeks. Calcium metabolism may be disordered if parathyroid glands are removed inadvertently or injured during surgical operation.

Follicular or papillary carcinoma of the thyroid is usually treated by total thyroidectomy. Being a more radical procedure than partial thyroidectomy, the risk of parathyroid deficiency in the postoperative period is increased. The risk of temporary or permanent damage to a recurrent laryngeal nerve is also increased. The patient will normally be in hospital for 1–2 weeks and return to non-manual work will not be earlier than 3 or 4 weeks after surgery. Heavy manual work will normally not be undertaken for 4–6 weeks. Time away from work may be required if any form of adjuvant treatment such as the administration of radioactive iodine is given.

Operations on salivary glands

There were 4303 recorded operations to remove salivary glands in NHS hospitals in England during the year 2003/2004.[12]

Removal of the superficial and/or deep lobe of the parotid gland preserving the facial nerve may be required for a number of benign conditions, the commonest of which is pleomorphic adenoma (mixed parotid tumour). The surgery is likely to involve 2–5 days stay in hospital with return to non-manual work being possible at 2 weeks. Heavy manual work might involve a longer convalescence. Cancer of the parotid gland will often require radical surgery with sacrifice of the facial nerve and adjuvant treatment. A patient who has suffered from this condition will need an individualized plan for return to any working activities.

The removal of a stone from the submandibular duct in the floor of the mouth is a day case procedure and the patient should be able to return to work within 1 or 2 days. Removal of the submandibular gland for sepsis with stone formation may involve a hospital stay of several days and a period away from non-manual work of 7–14 days. The delay before return to heavy manual work may be longer, perhaps 2 or 3 weeks.

Thorax

The advent of thoracoscopy as part of the minimal access revolution has resulted in a reduction in the number of procedures for which a full thoracotomy used to be mandatory. The minimal access procedure brings with it the benefits of less pain and a quicker return to normal activity.

The procedures that can be performed using minimal access thoracoscopic techniques include cervical sympathectomy for hyperhidrosis, biopsy of intrathoracic tumours, and surgery for pneumothorax. Resection of peripheral lung lesions may also be performed thoracoscopically.[25] Even major pulmonary resections can be performed thoracoscopically.[26] With the exception of patients who have had a major thoracoscopic pulmonary resection, most patients should recover from thoracoscopy and return to non manual duties within a fortnight and to full manual work within 4 weeks, depending on the nature of the underlying disease and any further treatment that may be required.

Partial and total pneumonectomy

There were 9997 operations on the lung recorded in English NHS hospitals during the year 2003/2004.[12]

Usually a thoracotomy wound is required for these procedures, although, recently, recovery after surgery has been shown to be faster when thoracoscopic techniques have been used to perform pulmonary resections.[25,26] Following partial or total pneumonectomy, exercise tolerance will be reduced. This will be the case particularly in those whose pulmonary reserve has already been compromised by smoking or by pulmonary disease.

Patients who have undergone thoracotomy and major lung resection will be unlikely to resume non-manual work without a convalescent period of 2–3 months. Heavy manual work will not be possible following pneumonectomy and less strenuous work will be required. Partial pneumonectomy may result in less dyspnoea and return to a sedentary job should be possible in approximately 6 weeks. It should also be possible for some patients to return to light manual work depending on their respiratory function.

The disease for which the lung or part of the lung was removed may affect the time of return to work. If, for example, chemotherapy or radiotherapy are to be used as an adjuvant treatment to partial or total pneumonectomy, return to work will be correspondingly delayed and it may be many months, if at all, before the patient can return to light duties at work.

Carcinoma of the oesophagus

Partial or total excision of the oesophagus was recorded 1754 times in the NHS in England during 2003/2004.[12] The main indication for oesophagectomy is carcinoma of the oesophagus.

Carcinoma of the oesophagus, when operable, requires major incisions and extensive dissection. Surgeons may choose different procedures. For cancers of the oesophagogastric junction, a left thoraco-abdominal incision may be employed to enable a removal of the proximal stomach and lower oesophagus. For tumours of the lower or mid oesophagus, an abdominal laparotomy to mobilize the stomach may be followed by a right thoracotomy pulling the stomach up to the chest, resecting the oesophagus, and joining the oesophagus to the mobilized stomach now resident in the chest. Finally some surgeons will practise total oesophagectomy. Having mobilized the stomach or colon in the abdomen and then the oesophagus in the chest via a thoracotomy, the oesophagus will be resected and removed through a cervical incision when intestinal continuity will be restored by joining the divided end of the upper oesophagus to the mobilized stomach or colon. A patient undergoing oesophagectomy is very unlikely to return to manual work. Non-manual work may, however, be practical. There will be a considerable period of convalescence perhaps 3 months or longer during which the patient will recover from the major procedure and re-establish normal swallowing and eating. Adjuvant radiotherapy or chemotherapy may be required for malignant disease and such treatments will further delay return to work. Unfortunately the cure rate, even for resectable carcinoma of the oesophagus, is low.

Spontaneous pneumothorax

This is commonly seen in young adults and is usually due to rupture of pulmonary bullae, especially in the upper lobe. Chest aspiration or drainage by an intracostal tube may be sufficient treatment. Surgery is not indicated for a first episode, although special consideration would have to be given if the employee was a diver or hyperbaric worker (see Appendix 4). Following a first episode of spontaneous pneumothorax, prolonged absence from light work will probably not be necessary but an interval of several weeks to enable healing would be required for an employee in a heavy manual job.

If a second episode occurs, the chances of a further pneumothorax exceed 50% and investigation and surgery is warranted. Surgery is also warranted if there is a persistent air leak with failure of the lung to expand within 5 days even after a first episode. The surgical procedure aims to close the air leak and create pleural adhesions to prevent further collapse of the lung (pleurodesis). A small lateral thoracotomy or a muscle sparing thoracotomy in the axilla may be used but thoracoscopic pneumothorax surgery with resection of bullae and pleurodesis is perhaps the best solution.[25]

Pneumothorax may be associated with chest pain. It is important to warn patients that even when their lung has fully expanded, they may experience atypical chest pain after pleurodesis. Return to light work is possible when the patient has recovered, perhaps 2 or 3 weeks after surgery. Return to heavy work may be longer.

Thoracic trauma

As with abdominal trauma, patients may suffer blunt or penetrating injuries. Blunt injury, which is common in road traffic accidents, may lead to fractured ribs, pneumothorax, and intrathoracic bleeding. The lung may be bruised or lacerated. In very severe trauma, the heart and great vessels may be seriously injured and survival is unlikely in these patients. Penetrating injuries by a knife, shards of glass, or a bullet may produce injury to the intrathoracic viscera, including one or both lungs, the heart, the great vessels, and the oesophagus.

Depending on the degree of trauma, the patient may only require a simple pleural drain to treat the pneumothorax and drain the haemothorax. Analgesia will be given for pain. Severe bleeding may indicate the need for a formal thoracotomy. Severely crushed ribs, particularly if a flail segment has been produced, may make prolonged ventilation of the patient necessary even if thoracotomy is not required. The surgery of severe trauma within the chest should ideally be in a specialist unit where pulmonary resection and reconstruction of vascular injuries including injury to the heart may be undertaken. The duration of stay in hospital and indeed survival will depend on the seriousness of the injuries caused by blunt or penetrating trauma. The duration of convalescence required may vary from a few days for undisplaced rib fractures to many months for serious intrathoracic injury. Assessment of the patient after discharge from hospital will give an indication of each individual's convalescent needs and their ability to return to non-manual or manual work. Chest pain and reduced exercise tolerance may limit the work that can be done. The younger the patient the more likely it is that they will be able to return to full activities at work in due course.

Breast

Removal of the whole breast was performed in the NHS in England for the year 2003/2004 on 16 552 occasions. Similarly partial excision of the breast is recorded as occurring on 35 567 occasions.[12]

Most breast cysts are benign, are aspirated in the out-patient department and require no protracted absence from work. Diagnosis of a benign lump may be confirmed by fine needle aspirate cytology or core biopsy. Removal if necessary is done in the DCU usually under a general anaesthetic. The patient should be able to return to work within 24 or 48 hours of an uncomplicated removal of a benign breast lump.

Breast cancer is normally diagnosed without resort to open surgery. The standard practice is termed 'triple assessment' and this involves a clinical and radiological assessment, and fine needle aspiration for cytology and/or core biopsy for histology. Thus the diagnosis of breast cancer should be made either after one or two hospital out-patient visits.

The treatment of a patient with breast cancer depends on the patient's preferences and the size, type, grade, and site of the tumour. The presence or absence of metastases will also affect treatment. Cancers of up to 4 cm in size may be treated by wide local excision, although this will depend on the relative size of the tumour and the breast. Total mastectomy is likely to be the treatment of choice for women with multifocal or large resectable cancers. A small number of women with breast cancer will express a preference for a total mastectomy with or without reconstruction of the breast rather than wide local excision of the breast cancer.

In addition to wide local excision or total mastectomy, the glands in the ipsilateral axilla will be excised or, alternatively, a sentinel node biopsy will be performed. Sentinel node biopsy is likely to become routine practice in the UK during the next year or two and automatic axillary dissection for breast cancer is likely to be abandoned. If the sentinel node contains metastatic tumour, axillary clearance will usually follow a few days later. However, when the sentinel node does not show any tumour, axillary dissection is not undertaken and the patient avoids the morbidity of axillary dissection which includes a stiff shoulder and lymphoedema of the arm. Adjuvant treatments for breast cancer currently include radiotherapy, chemotherapy, and the use of various drugs that work by hormonal manipulation.

Patients who undergo radical surgical treatment for breast cancer, which includes either a wide local excision of the tumour in the breast with axillary clearance or total mastectomy with axillary clearance, will usually remain in hospital for 4 or 5 days after the procedure unless a well developed domiciliary service is available when specialist nurses visit the patient at home and remove any drains 3–5 days after surgery. When breast surgery combined with sentinel node biopsy has been performed the patient may be able to leave hospital very quickly, perhaps after 24 or 48 hours. No further admission will be required if the pathologist reports that there is no evidence of metastasis in the sentinel lymph nodes but the patient will be re-admitted and axillary clearance performed if the sentinel node shows tumour.

Radiotherapy to the chest wall may be unnecessary if a full mastectomy has been performed, but radiotherapy to the remaining breast is usually given when only part of the breast has been removed. Chemotherapy is generally administered when there is evidence of involvement of the axillary lymph nodes with tumour. Adjuvant tamoxifen or other similar agent is currently given daily in the form of a tablet for 5 years if the cancer is 'oestrogen receptor positive'.

Women treated for breast cancer will be emotionally as well as physically affected. Early return to work may be helpful for some but too stressful for others. Return to work following treatment for breast cancer will also depend on the nature of the operative procedure undertaken, the presence or absence of adjuvant radiotherapy following surgery and the need for adjuvant chemotherapy. For those patients in whom adjuvant radiotherapy and chemotherapy are not required, return to work will depend on the nature of the surgical procedure undertaken. If the axilla has been dissected, the patient will not return to work until the ipsilateral shoulder is relatively pain-free and mobile and the surgical wound healed. This may take several weeks. Adjuvant radiotherapy may be undertaken during a 4–6-week period and during this time patients do not have time to return to full-time work, although half days are often possible. However, patients are often absent for the duration of radiotherapy treatment. Chemotherapy may be given monthly over a 6-month period and this will involve intermittent absences from work, particularly when the patient is admitted for intravenous chemotherapy and in the days afterwards when the patient may be feeling unwell. Reaction to chemotherapy varies and absence will be for a variable period depending on individual patients. Some will not be able to return to work until after completion of both radiotherapy and chemotherapy. Hair loss associated with chemotherapy may cause considerable personal anguish and, even with the provision of a wig, this may delay the patient's reintegration into the workplace.

Although the majority of women undergoing surgery for breast cancer will not have heavy manual jobs, return to a variety of jobs may occasionally be compromised by persistent stiffness of the shoulder and reduced function in the arm on the side of the axillary clearance. The advantage of sentinel node biopsy is that it will enable a number of patients to avoid axillary gland clearance and therefore avoid the morbidity associated with this procedure. Such women should be able to return to their previous job whether it be non-manual or manual.

References

1 Wellwood J, Sculpher MJ, Stoker D, Nicholls GJ, Geddes C, Whitehead A, Singh R, Spiegelhalter D. Randomised controlled trial of laparoscopic versus open mesh repair for inguinal hernia. *BMJ* 1998; **317**: 103–10.

2 Salcedo-Wasicek MC, Thirlby RC. Post-operative course after inguinal herniorrhaphy. A case-controlled comparison of patients receiving workers' compensation vs patients with commercial insurance. *Arch Surg* 1995; **130**: 29–32.

3 Muhe E. The first cholecystectomy through the laparoscope. *Langenbecks Arch Chir* 1986; **369**: 804.

4 Dubois F, Berthelot G, Levard H. Cholecystectomy par coelioscopy. *Nouv Presse Med* 1989; **18**: 980.

5 Reddick EJ, Olsen DO. Laparoscopic laser cholecystectomy. *Surg Endosc* 1989; **3**: 131.

6 The Royal College of Surgeons of England. *Guidelines for day case surgery*. London: Royal College of Surgeons of England, 1992.

7 Day Surgery Audit Commission. *Day Surgery: Review of National Findings: Acute Hospital Portfolio*, No. 4, 2001.

8 Department of Health. *Day surgery: operational guide*, 2002.

9 Corbitt JB. Transabdominal preperitoneal herniorrhaphy. *Surg Laparosc Endosc* 1993; **3**: 328–32.

10 Stoker DL, Spiegelhalter DJ, Wellwood JM. Laparoscopic versus open inguinal hernia repair: randomised prospective trial. *Lancet* 1994; **343**: 1243–5.

11 Amid PK, Shulman AG, Lichtenstein IL. Critical scrutiny of the open 'tension-free' hernioplasty. *Am J Surg* 1993; **165**: 369–71.

12 Department of Health. *Hospital episode statistics, NHS hospitals, England, 2003/2004*.

13 Collaboration EH. Laparoscopic compared with open methods of groin hernia repair: systematic review of randomized controlled trials. *Br J Surg* 2000; **87**: 860–7.

14 Collaboration EH. Mesh compared with nonmesh methods of open groin hernia repair: systematic review of randomized controlled trials. *Br J Surg* 2000; **87**: 854–9.

15 Collaboration EHT. Repair of groin hernia with synthetic mesh: meta-analysis of randonmized controlled trials. *Ann Surg* 2002; **235**: 322–32.

16 National Institute for Clinical Excellence. *Guidance on the use of laparoscopic surgery for inguinal hernia*. NICE technology appraisal guidance No. 18. London: NICE, 2001.

17 National Institute for Clinical Excellence. *Final appraisal determination on laparoscopic surgery*. NICE technology appraisal guideline (Review of existing guidance 18). London: NICE, 2004.

18 Mercer SJ, Knight JS, Toh SKC, Walters AM, Sadek SA, Somers SS. Implementation of a specialist-led service for the management of acute gallstone disease. *Br J Surg* 2004; **91**: 504–8.

19 Geagea T. Laparoscopic Nissen's fundoplication: preliminary report on 10 cases. *Surg Endosc* 1991; **5**: 170–3.

20 Dallemagne B, Weerts JM, Jehaes C, Markiewicz S. Lombard R. Laparoscopic Nissen fundoplication: preliminary report. *Surg Laparosc Endosc* 1991; **1**: 138–43.

21 Watson DI. Laparoscopic treatment of gastro-oesophageal reflux disease. *Best Pract Res Clin Gastroenterol* 2004; **18**: 19–35.

22 Lan WL, Chu KW, Tung HM. Early outcomes of 100 patients with laparoscopic resection for rectal neoplasm. *Surg Endosc* 2004; **18**: 1592–6.

23 Dehn T. Controversial Topics in Surgery. Endovascular report (EVAR) of abdominal aortic aneurysms: the case for and against. *Ann R Coll Surg Engl* 2004; **86**: 377–80.

24 Graham TJ, Taylor J, Raptis S. Endovascular treatment of abdominal aortic aneurysms. *Br J Surg* 2004; **91**: 815–27.

25 Sedrakyan A, van der Meulen J, Lewsey J, Treasure T. Variation in use of video assisted thoracic surgery in the United Kingdom. *BMJ* 2004; **329**: 1011–12.

26 Roviaro G, Varoli F, Vergani C, Maciocco M, Nucca O, Pagano C. Video assisted thoracoscopic major pulmonary resections. *Surg Endosc* 2004; **18**: 1551–8.

Chapter 22

Dermatology

U. T. Ferriday and I. S. Foulds

The skin acts as a protective barrier against a number of hazards within our environment. These hazards can be: **chemical**, e.g. acids, alkalis, solvents, cutting, or soluble oils; **biological**, e.g. bacteria, plant allergens, or raw food; or **physical**, e.g. ultraviolet light, or mechanical shearing forces. In some situations the defensive properties of the skin are exceeded resulting in cuts, grazes, inflammation, ulceration, infection, and occasionally malignant change.

The risk factors for breakdown of skin defences can be categorized as occupational (common at risk groups are: cleaners, food handlers, hairdressers, and workers in contact with cutting fluid), and non-occupational (where genetic predisposition to skin disorders is an important factor).

Workers with non-occupational skin disorders can be disadvantaged in certain workplaces where the environment may be hot and humid or extremely cold or dry and exacerbations of their underlying dermatological condition can occur.

Prevalence

It is estimated that approximately 20% of the UK population suffers with some form of skin disease at a given time, with eczema, acne, and infectious disorders (e.g. athlete's foot) being the most commonly presenting complaints to general practitioners and dermatologists. Approximately 15–20% of a GP's workload and 6% of hospital outpatient referrals are for skin problems.

The 2001/2002 Self-reported, Work-related Illness survey estimated some 39 000 cases of work-related skin disease in Great Britain. The Industrial Injuries scheme, which compensates workers who have been disabled by a prescribed disease, has seen a fall in the numbers receiving benefit for occupational dermatitis from 400 in the early 1990s to 200 in 2002/2003.

EPIDERM is a voluntary surveillance scheme for occupational skin disease run by the University of Manchester. Approximately 240 members of the British Association of Dermatologists report to the scheme. Data collected from EPIDERM and by OPRA—a similar reporting system for occupational physicians, have established that skin disease accounts for 20% of all reported work-related disease, the incidence of occupational contact dermatitis being approximately 12.9 per 100 000 workers.[1]

A breakdown of occupational dermatoses from EPIDERM showed that contact dermatitis represented 83%, skin cancer 10%, infective causes 4%, and contact urticaria 3% of cases reported.[2] The majority of occupational dermatitis is due to irritant contact factors. In the UK approximately four million working days a year may be lost due to work-related skin disease.[3]

Data from EPIDERM have shown that three factors affect time off work for contact dermatitis: age, allergic dermatitis, and medico-legal assessments.[4] Other interesting observations include the fact that cases of latex-attributable contact urticaria have been in decline since 1996 and that the majority of occupational skin cancers are attributed to ultraviolet radiation.[5]

The incidence of occupational skin disease reported through the surveillance schemes appears roughly constant at 2700 to 3400 new reports per year. These schemes only register the more serious cases of dermatitis, and do not for example, reflect the incidence of skin disease amongst small and medium size enterprises; thus there be a degree of under-reporting.

In 2001–2003 the *occupations* most commonly reported to EPIDERM by dermatologists were: floral arrangers/florists; hairdressers and barbers; beauticians and related occupations; printers; assemblers of vehicles and metal goods; chemical and related process operatives; bakers; and dental nurses.

The most common *agents* cited by dermatologists and occupational physicians as causes of skin disease were rubber chemicals/materials, followed by wet work and soaps and detergents.

Pre-employment assessments

At pre-employment, in some occupations where the prevalence of skin disorders is high, health assessments may focus on existing or previous skin problems and, if appropriate, redirecting individuals with pre-existing skin problems to different employment.

In cases were there is a history of dermatitis, patch testing is sometimes necessary.[6]

Each case, however, needs to be considered on an individual basis, with the prospective future employee being made fully aware of the potential risks of the work, and advice should be sought from an occupational physician and/or a dermatologist before a final decision is made regarding employability in a specific job.

Eczema

Atopic eczema affects one in five children and can render a potential employee more susceptible to the effects of irritants in contact with the skin. If the condition was severe in childhood, and particularly if the hands were involved, then the risk for developing dermatitis in employment with irritants is significant.[7] Atopics with a history only of asthma or hay fever do not have an increased susceptibility. There is no evidence that atopics are at increased risk of developing allergic contact reactions, and clinical experience suggests that they are less likely to develop sensitization to potential contact allergens than non-atopics. However, all atopics are more likely to develop contact urticaria, asthma, and anaphylaxis from natural rubber latex, and preventative measures need to be considered.[8] Many establishments, particularly those employing healthcare workers, now have policies on the wearing of gloves at work for specific tasks, including guidelines on the type of glove to select.

Several jobs should be considered an absolute contraindication for atopics with a history of severe childhood disease and hand involvement: hairdressing (shampoos), catering (wet work and detergents), and machine engineering (metal-working fluids).

Caution is also needed in placing nursing and healthcare workers. Ideally, occupational health advice should begin with the parents of children who have severe atopic eczema, to avoid careers with a risk of high irritant exposures. Unfortunately this seldom occurs. When faced with an enthusiastic candidate for shortage employment areas such as nursing, dilemmas can ensue. Historically, when nursing involved early ward training and frequent hand washing those who could not survive the irritant assault on their hands were quickly identified. Now in the UK, with the move to undergraduate nursing teaching, exposure is delayed until 3 years of training have been completed. The requirement for hand washing between patients has increased, to reduce methicillin-resistant *Staphylococcus aureus* infections (MRSA), and this has raised the risk of flare-ups of dermatitis in atopics with a past history of hand eczema. Risk is further enhanced by demands for alcohol cleansers at every bedside in UK hospitals; alcoholic preparations are poorly tolerated by those with a history of atopic skin disease, with up to 15% of all nurses experiencing intolerance or non-compliance with such products. On balance this suggests a need to discourage those with active skin involvement or a past history of severe eczema from entering nursing. Those who do proceed should join a carefully supervised programme of hand care and should be followed up in case of further difficulty.

Other occupations that carry a significant risk from irritant contact exposure are domestic cleaning, bar work, construction work, motor vehicle maintenance, horticulture and agriculture. Extremes of temperature and humidity can also aggravate atopic eczema.

In certain occupations hand involvement can also pose a risk of bacterial contamination. Eczematous skin is more prone than normal skin to be colonized with *Staphylococcus aureus*, and sometimes with *Streptococcus pyogenes*. Densities of *S. aureus* may exceed $10^6/cm^2$, leading to clinically apparent infection (impetigo); non-involved skin is colonized in up to 90% of individuals.[9] Any organism that colonizes or contaminates the skin surface is dispersed into the environment on naturally shed skin scales. This has major implications in healthcare (patient infection), catering (food poisoning), and the pharmaceutical industry (product contamination). Hospitals where MRSA strains can be found need to be vigilant in case staff members carry staphylococcus in their nasal passages. Active eczema in these occupations therefore carries a risk of infective spread and requires individual assessment.

It has been shown[10] that, even where the occupation provides no apparent recognizable hazard to the skin, around half of those with a previous history of atopic eczema may develop hand eczema *de novo* or exacerbations of pre-existing hand eczema. When hand eczema develops in an atopic exposed to a potential skin irritant, it is often difficult for the patient, their trade union, or their insurers to accept that the condition may not be occupational. In claims for compensation, industrial injury assessors and expert witnesses will often allow patients the benefit of the doubt.

Seborrhoeic eczema may be aggravated by exposure to chemical irritants, but hot environments will contribute most to potential flare-ups of the disease. As the hands are not affected, restrictions are not needed for occupations involving wet work. The main problem is shedding of scales from facial, scalp, skin, or otitis externa with risks of bacterial contamination akin to those found in atopics.

Stasis (varicose) eczema, which may be associated with varicose ulceration, can be aggravated by prolonged standing. Management requires extra support compression of the legs and encouragement to walk regularly, to increase venous pressure. Leg elevation may be required during rest periods.

Discoid (nummular) eczema carries few implications for employment, as it is treatable with appropriate topical therapies and rarely aggravated by the work environment. It can sometimes present as a feature of chromate dermatitis and soluble oil dermatitis, but in this situation it is usually associated with coexisting hand dermatitis.

Asteototic eczema (eczema craquelé) is a type of eczema that is caused by drying out of the skin. It commonly affects the lower limbs. Low humidity (air conditioning, car and lorry heaters), frequent showering, and use of degreasing chemicals (soaps, shampoos) will cause the skin to dry and crack. It can be prevented and treated by minimizing the causative factors.

Other non-cancerous skin disorders

Chronic urticaria can be aggravated by temperature (heat and rarely cold) and emotional stresses at work. Cholinergic urticaria is specifically triggered by exercise. Most forms of urticaria can be controlled by adequate doses (sometimes greater than the licensed amount) of non-sedating antihistamines during the daytime, and may also require the addition of sedative antihistamines at night. If sedative antihistamines are used then short-acting ones should be considered (e.g. chlorpheniramine) so that no sedative after-effects ensue. Sedative antihistamines are contraindicated where alertness is required, particularly to operate machinery or drive vehicles. Where urticaria is associated with natural rubber latex, the provision of a latex-free environment will be needed to prevent anaphylaxis.

Photosensitive dermatoses and, to a lesser extent, **vitiligo** may make outdoor work inadvisable. Up to 80% of available ultraviolet light penetrates through cloud cover. Sufficient protection in the form of clothing and high factor sunscreens will be needed. The latter should be applied frequently around the middle of the day (e.g. 10 a.m., noon, and 2 p.m.). Many medications (e.g. tetracyclines, amiodorone) can increase the risk of photosensitivity.

Acne, if severe and nodulocystic, can be a contraindication to working in hot, humid, steamy environments as severe exacerbations can occur. There is no evidence that pre-existing acne increases the risk of oil-induced acne, which is caused by occlusion and blockage of the pilosebaceous units in the skin. Acne is responsive (albeit slowly) to treatment, and even the most resistant cases can be treated with systemic isotretinoins. There is a higher prevalence of acne in the unemployed and a risk of unfair discrimination on the grounds of appearance at the recruitment stage.[11] To avoid this, all acne should be treated effectively.

Viral warts have a predilection for the hands and are a source of cosmetic embarrassment. Most viral warts involute spontaneously over time. They pose little risk to fellow workers as adults typically acquire immunity in childhood and become protected. In occupations involving food handling, patient care and contact with the public, a pressure often exists to actively treat the condition with cryotherapy and other therapeutic modalities. Butchers and abattoir workers are at special risk of hand warts, as the causative papillomavirus can infect meat and poultry. These occupations are associated with repeated minor trauma to the skin of the hands, so spread and cross-contamination can easily occur. Active treatment is therefore justified for these groups. Verrucas, which are also papillomaviruses, pose little risk to other people. No restrictions need to be placed upon swimming pool attendants, divers and workers sharing showering facilities.

Fungal skin infections are common. The antifungal action of sebum in post-puberty tends to discourage fungal growth in adults. Therefore ringworm in the scalp (tinea capitis) from cats and dogs (*Microsporum canis*) is rare in adults. More aggressive fungi, as found on cattle and hedgehogs, can grow in the presence of sebum, leading to potentially causing hair loss (alopecia) and secondary bacterial infections (kerion).

In warm and moist body locations (e.g. in between the toes and in the groin) the common fungus *Trichophyton rubrum* thrives (tinea pedis, tinea cruris). It is easily spread in occupations that require communal showering or the use of occlusive footwear. Infected individuals should not be excluded from work, but diagnosis and treatment should be initiated. Athletes' foot (tinea pedis) is commonly misdiagnosed. One-third of suspected cases arise from other causes. Unresponsive cases may actually be due to occlusive maceration between the toes, with overgrowth of commensal bacteria (*Staph. pyogenes*). This disorder can be treated with appropriate footwear, wedging toes apart with cotton wool rolls and adequate drying. Ringworm on the body (tinea corporis) is overdiagnosed and confused with other skin conditions (psoriasis, granuloma annulare, etc.). It is associated with immunosuppression and responds well to treatment.

Although zoonoses can be acquired by humans from animals, they cannot be transferred between humans and so no restrictions are required for infected employees.

Bacterial skin infections are potentially transmissible to other employees. Impetigo, which is the commonest, is usually caused by *Staph. aureus* and requires prompt local treatment.

For widespread infections, temporary debarment from work may be required, although the risk of cross-contamination becomes minimal after 2 days of treatment. Boils (carbuncles) are also usually caused by *Staph. aureus*, but the potential for contamination is less than for impetigo. Staphylococci can grow in foods and release endotoxins that cause serious food poisoning. Thus, in occupations involving food handling, exclusion is required until clinical resolution occurs.

Hyperhidrosis that affects the hands may cause problems in engineering, as sweat can corrode ferrous metalwork pieces (these employees are known as 'rusters'). Hyperhidrosis may also be a disadvantage in public facing work and sales or public relations jobs that require frequent hand shaking. Although historically treatment was limited (aluminium salts, iontophoresis, chemical or surgical sympathectomy), the use of botulinum toxin has revolutionized treatment.

Psoriasis is present in 1 in 20 persons, but most cases are minor and not apparent even to the sufferer. Psoriasis may be aggravated occupationally by physical or chemical trauma (Köebner phenomenon). The commonest presentation is with psoriatic knuckle pads.

The disease can be unpredictable, with sudden active and extensive flare-ups. Rarely this can involve the entire body surface. Although psoriasis typically develops in early teens and twenties it can start at any age. The absence of psoriasis at pre-employment does not guarantee subsequent freedom from the condition. With adequate treatment it is possible to clear and control most cases of active psoriasis, although only with adequate compliance and motivation. Psoriasis may also undergo spontaneous remission. In practice, individuals with psoriasis from early childhood and with more than 40% of the surface skin affected are the most difficult to control.

Within the workplace psoriasis that affects the palms and soles can be particularly troublesome. Affected individuals are unable to wear protective shoes and have difficulty with work involving heavy manual handling, and that in the construction and service industries. Embarrassment because of visible psoriatic patches on hands or scalp can compromise emotional and social well-being.[12,13]

Some chemicals and solvents can cause existing psoriasis to flare up. Solvents such as trichloroethylene will degrease the skin, causing drying, and cracking, which then köebnerizes the psoriasis. Other everyday products such as soap, detergents, washing-up liquids, and shampoos also have a similar degreasing effect. The effect of chemicals is minimal compared with the effects of friction, which is the main perpetuating factor in the hands and feet. Demanding and stressful work has also been associated with exacerbations of the disease.

Psoriatic arthropathy can affect mobility, while the associated pain can increase sickness absence. Although infection of psoriatic lesions can occur, work in catering or nursing is generally tolerated and helped by regular monitoring by the occupational health department.

Alopecia is seen quite often in skin clinics. Hair loss, particularly in women, can lead to a degree of mental anguish that makes attendance at work difficult. Treatable causes such as endocrine disorders, drugs, or iron deficiency need to be excluded. The wearing of a wig will sometimes aid return to work.

Disorders of pigmentation particularly if on the face, i.e. vitiligo or hyperpigmentation can cause embarrassment, especially in Asians and individuals of African descent. Specialists in cosmetic camouflage can help such cases.

Skin cancer

There are about 40 000 new registrations for skin cancer in UK annually. Few are due to occupational causes, but 1608 work-related cases were reported to EPIDERM in a 6-year period. Epithelioma of the scrotum due to contact with mineral oils is hardly ever seen these days, although cases have been reported at other anatomical sites such as arms and hands. Ultraviolet radiation from excessive exposure to sunlight is one of today's main causes of skin cancer.[14] Other causes include X-rays, arsenic, tar products, and industrial burns. Ultraviolet radiation from welding is a potential risk factor in non-melanotic skin cancer among welders.[15]

Basal cell carcinoma, or rodent ulcer, is the commonest skin cancer. It is frequently found on the face and is associated with exposure to sunlight. Fair-skinned expatriates working in sunny climates are a group at special risk. However, an excess of risk has not been consistently demonstrated in surveys of outdoor and indoor workers.[16,17]

Squamous cell carcinomas commonly occur on hands, ears, and lips. Sunlight, chronic trauma, and chronic inflammation are aetiological factors.

Malignant melanoma is one of the most aggressive skin cancers. Its incidence has increased dramatically over the last couple of decades, probably due to peoples' greater exposure to sunlight. Recent reports indicate a higher prevalence of malignant melanomas in aircrew, possibly because of cosmic radiation. A higher than average sunlight exposure may also contribute.[18]

Common primary cancers that can metastasize to skin are breast, lung, and leukaemia.

Surgical excision is the most effective and preferred treatment for primary skin cancer. A return to work is normally possible after excision and wound healing. A poor cosmetic result occasionally affects the outcome.

Skin and the psyche

There are many myths and folklore surrounding skin disorders. One of the commonest of these is that eczema is in some way contagious. Bacterial contamination can occur in some cases but the risk to work colleagues is considered small and restrictions are only relevant in selected occupations such as food handlers or healthcare workers. However, concerns within the workplace this can sometimes lead to individuals being shunned and excluded from communal and social activities. There is a clear need to ensure that health education is undertaken and that the supervisor or line manager understands the nature of the skin condition.

Skin ailments are sometimes a feature of sick building syndrome. Symptomatology tends to vary, ranging from dryness of the skin to skin rashes. It is important to rule out underlying causes such as infections, scabies, or irritant dermatitis from an occupational hazard. Not infrequently, however, the presenting skin conditions of the workforce are not related to the work or the workplace.

Cases of scabies, athletes' foot, psoriasis, constitutional eczema, symptomatic dermographism, and rosacea are some of the commoner skin diseases falsely attributed to a dermatitis outbreak. If unions are involved, or new work practices have been introduced then an emotionally charged situation can develop which requires skills to resolve. Intervention by an occupational physician or a dermatologist may reduce the heightened concern of affected staff.

Investigation

Patch testing has a vital role to play in the investigation of persistent dermatitis, and will identify hidden causes of delayed Type IV hypersensitivity. No employee should be advised to give up their work without the benefit of detailed patch test investigations at a regional centre. Patch testing will identify causes of acquired sensitization and allow avoidance and substitution regimens to be planned, permitting continuing employment for the majority. However, it will not identify those individuals who may subsequently become sensitized, and therefore has no role to play as part of routine pre-employment screening. The only exception to this is when prior to employment a case of dermatitis (present or previous) has not been properly investigated.

Although patch testing appears to be a simple procedure to undertake, there are many pitfalls and relatively few specialists undertake it well. In practice a minimum of 6 months training is required to undertake even the most basic patch test investigations, with more experience required to investigate complex cases of occupationally acquired dermatitis.

Prick testing prior to employment has little value apart from confirming an atopic constitution. It can now be replaced by IgE and RadioAllergoSobentTest (RAST) blood tests, which seek specific allergens to confirm an atopic tendency. However, as it is only those with active atopic eczema (past or present) that carry a risk of developing dermatitis from irritants, these investigations really have no additional benefit to a good personal history and examination. RAST tests are not 100% specific. In particular, some atopics will have a strong positive reaction to latex and yet can handle latex with impunity, whereas others have negative antibodies but develop anaphylaxis with minimal latex exposure. A prick test in this situation can be more reliable, but in view of the risk of anaphylaxis it should never be carried out without having full resuscitation equipment to hand.

Rehabilitation

Rehabilitation of employees with skin ailments can usually be undertaken without too much difficulty. This is even true in cases where the skin problem is occupational dermatitis and the employee is working with a known irritant or sensitizer. If temporary employment can be found away from the offending agent, a return to work can usually be effected prior to the complete resolution of the skin condition.

Flexible working and working from home have allowed workers with significant skin disfigurements to continue in employment without affecting their psychosocial well-being or sense of rejection and social stigmatization.

However, some safety critical occupations may be considered unsuitable. For example, public health considerations relating to secondary skin infection may preclude employment in healthcare, food handling, and in the pharmaceutical industry.

Individuals with widespread skin lesions may not be suitable for work in some industries because of a heightened risk to themselves. For example, in the nuclear industry a reduction in the protective barrier of the skin may provide a portal of entry, and decontamination may be rendered more difficult; in the sewage or waste disposal industry there is a greater risk of exposure to infection.

Close collaboration between the occupational physician, the dermatologist, the GP, the employer, and the employee may be needed to effect a successful rehabilitation and return to work. The assessment of alternative skills through the Employment Rehabilitation Centre can help in difficult cases.

Skin care

Skin care at work should be part of a positive but pragmatic managerial response to healthcare. Good housekeeping, adequate washing facilities, attention to maintenance programmes, and cleanliness within the working environment can lead to positive behaviours by individual employees (e.g. more frequent to overall changing and hand washing).

Good **occupational hygiene** practice requires less irritant or sensitive alternatives to be substituted where possible, and for technical control measures (e.g. enclosure of the process or automation) to be maximized to avoid skin problems.

Emollients or moisturizers have now gained a place in the secondary prevention of dermatitis. Their frequent use during the working day helps to overcome excessive degreasing of the skin.

Barrier creams often contain lanolin, paraffin, silicones, or polyethylene glycols. These constituents can in themselves occasionally cause sensitization. Some barrier creams are also highly fragranced and may contain detergents to aid cleansing, which are potentially irritant to already damaged skin. It is also not uncommon to find that the most effective cleansers are also the most irritant.

Studies of alcohol handrubs that contain skin emollients versus soap, show that healthcare workers have accepted this method of reducing hand contamination and complaints of dry skin are fewer than with other hand hygiene products.[19]

Protective clothing can be provided in the form of gloves, aprons, overalls, hats, masks, safety boots, etc. Commonly the hands and arms are most at risk. Protective gloves can be made from many different materials, and the characteristics of permeability and durability need to be considered in selecting the correct type. Further information is available from the British Standard specification for Industrial gloves. HSE has also provided guidance for the selection of gloves.[20] However, the use of gloves should be the last solution in reducing harm, as compliance is often a problem.

When powders such as cement dust or paper dust are being handled, the operator may not be aware of possible entry under the cuff. This can be prevented by the wearing of gauntlets or armbands, or by tucking sleeves underneath the cuff. Extract ventilation may help with dust exposure and subsequent irritant and allergic skin reactions. Regular washing or changing of gloves will help to reduce contamination from the surface.

Legal considerations

The Control of Substances Hazardous to Health (COSHH) and the Management of Health and Safety at Work Regulations require that all employers offer appropriate information, instruction, and training to employees with regard to substances that can damage the skin. The training should include characteristic signs and symptoms of the particular dermatoses and arrangements should be in place to identify any cases of skin disorder. Employees should therefore be encouraged to examine their own skin and report all changes. It should also be borne in mind that the true risk of irritation or sensitization may not be stated explicitly on many health and safety data sheets.

Chronic skin disorders in those cases that can be described as having a substantial and long-term adverse affect on the individual's ability to carry out normal day to day activities will be covered by the Disability Discrimination Act 1995 (DDA). Severe disfigurement such as facial scarring is also a qualifying condition. Employers need to be aware that in such cases discrimination within the employment setting is unlawful.

Final comments

Most skin conditions in the workplace are neither infectious nor contagious. The opinion of a dermatologist is essential in order to be able to make a sound decision based on medical facts as to whether an employee should change jobs because of a skin condition. Redeployment within a company should be the first option if a job change is inevitable and many individuals can now be kept at work with a chronic skin disorder.

With the development of research into the genetic basis of skin disease it may be expected that treatments will become more specific to the underlying hereditary abnormality, rather than reactive to symptoms, as now. Thus, options for effective management may grow over time.

References

1 Meyer JD *et al.* Occupational contact dermatitis in the UK: a surveillance report from EPIDERM and OPRA. *Occup Med* 2000; **50**(4): 265–73.

2 Cherry NM, et al. Surveillance of work related diseases by occupational physicians in the UK: OPRA 1996–1999. *Occup Med* 2000; **50**(7): 496–503.

3 Cherry NM, McDonald JC. The incidence of work-related disease reported by occupational health physicians, 1996–2001. *Occup Med* 2002; **52**: 407–11.

4 Adisesh A, Meyer J D, Cherry N M. Prognosis and work absence due to occupational contact dermatitis. Outcome of cases reported to EPIDERM. *Contact Dermatitis* 2002; **46**(5): 273–9.

5 Cherry N, et al. Surveillance of occupational skin disease: EPIDERM and OPRA. *Br J Dermatol* 2000; **142**(6): 1128–34.

6 Milkovic-Kraus S Macan J. Can pre-employment patch testing help to prevent occupational contact allergy? *Contact Dermatitis* 1996; 35: 226–228.

7 Rystedt I. Factors influencing the occurrence of hand eczema in adults with a history of atopic dermatitis in childhood. *Contact Dermatitis* 1985; **12**: 185–91.

8 Posch A, Chen Z, Raulf-Heimsoth M, Baur X. Latex allergens. *Clin Exp Allergy* 1998; **28**: 134–40.

9 Noble WC. *Microbiology of human skin*, p. 325. London: Lloyd Luke, 1981.

10 Rystedt I. Work related hand eczema in atopics. *Contact Dermatitis* 1985; **12**: 164–71.

11 Cunliffe WJ. Acne and unemployment. *Br J Dermatol* 1986; **115**: 386.

12 Krueger G, Koo J, Lebwohl M et al. The impact of psoriasis on quality of life: results of a National Psoriasis Foundation patient-membership survey. *Arch Dermatol* 2001; **137**(3): 280–4.

13 Ginsburg IH, Link BG. Psychosocial consequences of rejection and stigma feelings in psoriasis patients. *Int J Dermatol* 1993; **32**(8): 587–91.

14 Snashall D (ed). *ABC of work related disorders*. London: BMJ Publishing Group, 1997.

15 Currie CL, Monk BE. Welding and non melanoma skin cancer. *Clin Exp Dermatol* 2000; **22**: 259–67.

16 Freedman DM, Zahn SH, Dosemeci M. Residential and occupational exposure to sunlight and mortality from non-Hodgkin's lymphoma: composite (threefold) case control study. *BMJ* 1997; **314**: 1451–5.

17 Green A et al. Skin cancer in a subtropical Australian population: incidence and lack of association with occupation. *Am J Epidemiol* 1996; **144**: 1034–40.

18 Rafusson V, Hrafnkelsson J, Tulinius H. Incidence of cancer among commercial airline pilots. *Scand J Work Environ Med* 2000; **57**: 175–9.

19 Ojajarvi J. Finnish experience shows that alcohol rubs are good for hands. *BMJ* 2003; **326**: 50.

20 HSE. *Selecting protective gloves for working with chemicals: guidance for employers and health and safety specialists*. Leaflet INDG3 30. London: HSE Books, 2000.

Further reading

Adams RM. *Occupational skin disease*, (3rd edn). Philadelphia: WB Saunders, 1999.

Kanerva L, Elsner P, Wahlberg JE, Maibach KI. *Handbook of occupational dermatology*. Berlin: Springer, 2000.

Rietschel RL, Fowler JF. *Fischers contact dermatitis*, (5th edn). Philadelphia: Lippincott Williams and Wilkins, 2000.

Chapter 23

Human immunodeficiency virus (HIV)

S. Williams and B. G. Gazzard

Introduction

By the end of 2003 there were an estimated 53 000 people living with HIV in the UK. The majority of these are of working age, reflecting the main mode of transmission which is through sex.[1]

In many developing countries where antenatal testing and treatment are rare, HIV is also a disease of infancy, transmitted vertically from mother to child during childbirth or breastfeeding.

The development in the 1990s of highly active antiretroviral treatment (HAART) with two or three antiretroviral drugs used in combination has greatly improved disease-free survival in developed countries. This has increased the potential for those of working age to remain in, or return to, work following their diagnosis. While antiretroviral treatment (ART) has increased survival, many HIV-infected people remain symptomatic, either through drug side-effects, HIV-related illnesses or the psychological morbidity associated with the diagnosis and disease. All of these factors can have a significant effect on an individual's ability to find, and remain in, work. In addition an employer's approach to those with chronic illness, and HIV in particular, can have a major influence on the workplace support received by infected workers.

As the epidemiology, treatment and drug resistance of HIV infection is evolving so rapidly, it is difficult to predict what the future holds for HIV-infected individuals of working age. The picture may be very different two decades from now.

This chapter reviews the current epidemiology and clinical picture of HIV, barriers to work and available support for overcoming them, legal and ethical considerations, occupational risks for HIV-infected workers and the risk of acquiring HIV through work. Particular attention is given to HIV in healthcare workers, which raises some specific issues.

Epidemiology of HIV in the UK

In 2003, approximately 7000 new cases of HIV were diagnosed in the UK. This compares with 6017 newly diagnosed cases in 2002 and 3088 new cases in 1999. Twenty-seven per cent of those with HIV in 2003 were unaware that they were infected.

As well as this significant increase in incidence and prevalence, the demography of HIV has changed substantially over the last 10 years. In the 1990s HIV was more prevalent in males. In the UK it remains more prevalent in males, however, the greater *rise* is now in females. In some parts of the world, particularly sub-Saharan Africa, infected females now outnumber infected males.

In the UK about a quarter of the 2003 diagnoses were in men who have sex with men, who despite accounting for fewer of these newly diagnosed infections are still the highest risk group for acquiring HIV in the UK. Over half of newly diagnosed cases of HIV in 2003 were in heterosexual men and women. About three-quarters of these heterosexually acquired HIV infections were probably acquired in Africa.[1]

Table 23.1 United Kingdom[1] data cumulative to end December 2004: HIV infected individuals[2] by exposure category and latest reported stage

Table will include some records of (a) the same individuals which are unmatchable because of differences in the information supplied and (b) of individuals who left the country at some date after diagnosis

How HIV infection was probably acquired	Infection reported only		AIDS but not death reported		Latest reported stage Death in reported AIDS cases[3]		Death without reported AIDS		Total[4]
	Males	Females	Males	Females	Males	Females	Males	Females	
Sex between men[5]	19329		3678		8909		1121		33037
Sex between men & women	7128	12276	1524	1794	1173	1024	312	290	25528
Injecting drug users	1582	800	232	94	636	250	456	152	4202
Blood factor	398	5	64	1	616	5	269	2	1360
Blood/tissue transfer	105	103	23	36	47	74	19	18	428
Mother to infant[6]	313	317	194	202	102	84	8	11	1235
Other/Undetermined	1333	768	74	12	148	14	284	104	2766
Total	30188	14269	5789	2139	11631	1485	2469	577	68556

[1] Includes reports of 81 individuals first reported from the Channel Islands or the Isle of Man.

[2] Individuals with laboratory reports of infection plus those with AIDS or death reports for whom no matching laboratory report has been received.

[3] Excludes 151 AIDS cases lost to follow up and presumed to have died.

[4] Includes reports of 43 individuals with sex not stated.

[5] 747 individuals exposed to infection through both sex between men and injecting drug use.

[6] Includes individuals diagnosed as adults (aged 15 or above).

Reproduced with permission from Communicable Disease Surveillance Centre (HIV & STI Department), Health Protection Agency Centre For Infections, and Scottish Centre for Infection & Environmental Health. Unpublished Quarterly Surveillance Tables No. 65, 04/4 table 1.

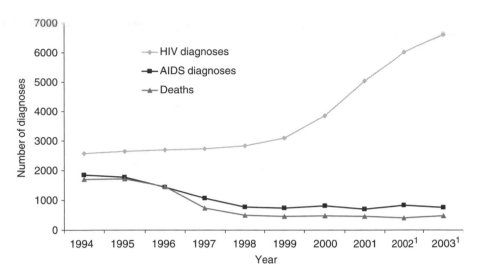

[1]Numbers will rise for recent years as further reports are received.

Fig. 23.1 Reproduced with permission from The UK Collaborative Group for HIV and STI Surveillance. *Focus on Prevention. HIV and other Sexually Transmitted Infections in the United Kingdom in 2003*. London: Health Protection Agency Centre for Infections. November 2004.

Despite the increased incidence of HIV infection, the incidence of AIDS has decreased significantly due to effective and earlier treatment.[2]

It is likely that the epidemiology of HIV and AIDS will continue to change in future decades, driven by the science of drug development, viral mutation, drug resistance, and socio-demographic variables such as migration and routes of transmission.

Natural history of HIV infection

Patients develop an AIDS-defining illness on average 10 years after acquiring HIV infection.

Within 2–3 weeks of being infected, there is a burst of HIV viraemia with several million copies of virus in the plasma. This level falls over the succeeding few weeks. Within 6 months of infection, the plasma viral load settles at a relatively stable value and subsequently changes little over a number of years. Both the CD4 (a T-cell-helper subset) count at this time and the viral load are predictive factors for the rate at which the first opportunistic infection will develop. In addition the degree of activation of the immune system, measured by the levels of CD38 (an activation marker) on either CD4 or CD8 cells, provides an additional prognostic marker to determine the speed at which AIDS is likely to develop.

Factors influencing the rate of progression to AIDS

1. *Age*: this has a marked influence on the rate of development of opportunistic infections. The rate increases with older age.
2. *Social and educational factors*: the less privileged and the less well educated develop opportunistic infections at a faster rate.
3. *Genetic factors*: two groups of genes affect the rate of progression to AIDS. Individuals with a specific haplotype progress more slowly, while individuals with a specific deletion rarely become HIV-infected (homozygous) or progress at slower rates (heterozygous).

4. *Treatment*: the most important influence on progression rates in the twenty-first century is access to effective antiretroviral treatment. This has revolutionised care in the developed world. Many would now predict that patients who have developed HIV infection recently will never develop an opportunistic infection providing they take the drugs on a regular basis.

There is no evidence that means of acquisition, life-style issues such as smoking, nutrition, or stress-related illnesses have any impact on the rate of progression towards AIDS. However, the life expectancy of individuals who continue intravenous drug use is reduced.

Markers of HIV infection and their clinical relevance

Two laboratory markers are commonly used to chart the progress of individuals with HIV infection and determine their needs for treatment. While both the CD4 count and viral load have an independent prognostic value for determining the rate of progression to AIDS, in recent years the CD4 count has become the important measure for determining the timing of treatment. Opportunistic infections are relatively rare with a CD4 count above 200 cells/mm^3 and reconstitution of the immune system following the introduction of ART is relatively complete. Most international guidelines now recommend that treatment should be started once the CD4 count has fallen to about 200 cells/mm^3. The viral load is chiefly used to assess how rapidly the CD4 count is likely to fall in an individual patient. Relatively low viral loads (less than 50 000 copies per ml) are associated with a low annual fall rate of CD4 count of about 40 cells. A high viral load (above 100 000 copies per ml) is associated with a much more rapid annual fall of CD4 count of 80 cells or more per year. The relative importance of the CD4 count and viral load measurements are reversed following initiation of therapy. The main aim of ART is to stop viral replication as completely as possible and thus prevent the development of viral resistance. Thus the most important monitor of success of ART is regular measurement of the plasma viral load, which if at all possible should be kept below the detection limit of a highly sensitive assay (usually less than 50 copies per ml).

Patients' symptoms and signs are also of considerable importance as markers of both progression of known HIV infection and also of alerting the physician or patient to the possibility of an underlying HIV diagnosis. Between 30% and 50% of individuals who are eventually diagnosed as HIV positive have previously come into contact with the medical profession with conditions that retrospectively should have led to an earlier diagnosis. The most important of these are skin and mucosal manifestations. However, all the opportunistic infections discussed below and non-specific symptoms such as weight loss, diarrhoea, or fever of unknown cause also may also lead to a diagnosis being suspected. Suspicions would be further aroused if these symptoms and signs occurred in individuals in high risk groups.

Symptoms

Symptoms in HIV-infected individuals may be due to the disease process itself or the potent drug treatment (see Table 23.2).

Seroconversion illness

About 75% of all individuals who become HIV-infected develop an illness within 2–3 weeks. This illness is often non-specific, but frequently there is a macular papular rash and there may be prominent cervical lymphadenopathy and abnormal liver function tests. Occasionally there are neurological symptoms and, uncommonly, opportunistic infections may occur during this period because of a precipitous decline in the CD4 count. Patients with a symptomatic illness at

Table 23.2 Common symptoms in HIV disease*

Symptoms	Cause
Due to HIV	
Pain in limbs	Neuropathy
Disfiguring skin lesions	Kaposi's sarcoma, seborrhoeic dermatitis, molluscum contagiosum
Nausea, vomiting	GI infections, intracranial pathology
Diarrhoea	HIV, cryptosporidiosis, MAI, salmonella
Abdominal pain	Sclerosing cholangitis, MAI, lymphadenopathy, TB peritonitis
Breathlessness	Pneumocystis pneumonia, other chest infections, TB lung, Kaposi's sarcoma, lymphoid interstitial pneumonitis in children
Headache	Cerebral lymphoma, toxoplasma, TB
Lymphadenopathy	HIV, lymphoma, TB
Drenching sweats	HIV, TB, lymphoma
Blindness	Cytomegalovirus, toxoplasma, progressive multifocal leucoencephalopathy
Mouth discomfort	Candida, herpes simplex, herpes zoster, aphthous ulcers, gingivitis, peridontitis, malignancy, Kaposi's sarcoma
Tiredness	HIV, anaemia due to HIV
Due to therapy	
Neuropathy	Nucleoside analogues, especially ddI, ddC, d4T
Pancreatitis	Nucleoside analogues
Lactic acidosis, liver failure	Nucleoside analogues
Diarrhoea	ddI, ritonavir, nelfinavir
Nausea	ddI, ritonavir, 3TC, ZDV
Anaemia	ZDV
Rash	Nevirapine, abacavir
Agitation, euphoria	Efavirenz
Lipodystrophy	Protease inhibitors, d4T
Renal colic	Indinavir

DDC=dideoxycytosine; DDI=dideoxyinosine; MAI=*Mycobacterium avium intracellulare*; ZDV=zidovudine

*Reproduced with permission from Easterbrook P. The changing epidemiology of HIV infection: new challenges for HIV palliative care. *J R Soc Med* 2001; **94**: 442—8.

seroconversion progress to AIDS more rapidly. Diagnosis of seroconversion is important as those patients with a high viral load are particularly likely to transmit infection to others. It is also theoretically possible that treatment at this early stage with ART may have an effect on long-term outcome.

Latent period

Following a seroconversion illness, most patients are relatively well for a period of some years. However, most are not asymptomatic and the course of their disease is punctuated by a number of illnesses. Perhaps the commonest of these are skin conditions caused by infections that are particularly florid in HIV-infected individuals. Examples are seborrhoeic dermatitis, bacterial skin infections, tinea pedis, and molluscum contagiosum. Of particular importance is herpes zoster infection. While shingles is a relatively common disease, multiple dermatome infection should strongly suggest the possibility of HIV-related immunosuppression. In the case of somebody who is known to be HIV-infected, herpes zoster infection indicates a high likelihood of development of AIDS in the next 2 years. Herpes simplex is commoner in HIV-infected individuals and frequently recurrent with severe attacks. One of the commonest manifestations of an underlying immune deficiency during this latent period is mucocutaneous candidiasis. Oral thrush always strongly suggests the possibility of underlying immunosuppression and leads to relevant questioning about potential risk factors for HIV. In those known to be HIV positive, 50% will develop full blown AIDS within 18 months of having an episode of thrush. Another oral manifestation is hairy leucoplakia, which is thought to be a reaction to opportunistic infection with Epstein–Barr virus. Again this is strongly predictive of HIV infection.

Unexplained weight loss, diarrhoea, and fever are also features of this latent period although with careful investigation, an infectious cause other than HIV *per se* is usually revealed.

Opportunistic infections

There are many opportunistic infections associated with HIV, some of which may be encountered through work. The commoner ones are listed in Table 23.3.

Table 23.3 Common opportunistic infections associated with HIV infection

Pneumocystis carinii pneumonia (PCP)
Toxoplasmic encephalitis
Cryptosporidiosis
Microsporidiosis
Tuberculosis
Disseminated MAC (*Mycobacterium avium* complex) infection
Bacterial respiratory infections
Bacterial enteric infections
Bartonellosis
Candidiasis
Cryptococcosis
Histoplasmosis
Coccydioidomycosis
Cytomegalovirus disease
Herpes simplex virus disease
Varicella zoster virus disease
HHV-8 infection (Kaposi sarcoma-associated herpesvirus)
Human papillomavirus infection
Hepatitis C virus infection

Neurological presentations

Meningitis

A viral meningitic illness, thought to be related to HIV infection, can occur at seroconversion. But the most important cause of meningitis is cryptococcus, which is prevalent in communities that come into close contact with a natural bird host for this fungal infection. The diagnosis and treatment of cryptococcal meningitis is straight forward providing it is thought of. The most serious complication of cryptococcal meningitis is high pressure hydrocephalus that needs expert management.

Stroke-like syndromes

Other neurological conditions usually present with stroke-like syndromes with sudden onset of focal neurological defects or less commonly, a general dementing process.

Toxoplasma gondii is the commonest of these infections and leads to a toxoplasma abscess. In two-thirds of such individuals this is caused by activation of a previous acquired infection and in a quarter represents recent acquisition from a primary host (e.g. domestic cat). Scans show fairly characteristic lesions and the diagnosis is confirmed by an adequate response to antitoxoplasma treatment. A quarter of patients, however, have residual neurological defects, which arise because of neuronal damage prior to the disease being controlled.

Progressive multifocal leucoencephalopathy is caused by an opportunistic infection with the JC variant of the polyoma virus, which is extremely rare outside the context of HIV infection. The diagnosis is usually most readily made by a magnetic resonance scan. Although the prognosis of such patients might be improved by treatment with ART, there is no specific remedy of proven value for this disease, which is usually fatal.

Primary cerebral lymphoma is also much commoner in HIV-infected patients. Epstein–Barr virus can be detected in the cerebrospinal fluid by polymerase chain reaction. In contrast to non-HIV-infected patients, primary cerebral lymphoma, even in the era of HAART, has a very poor prognosis with an average survival of only 100 days.

Gastrointestinal manifestations

Oesophageal disease

Oesophageal candidiasis is a common AIDS-defining illness, which is usually inferred by the presence of candida in the mouth plus symptoms of pain on swallowing. Although this is straight-forward to treat with azole antifungals, it is an important marker of a severely compromised immune system. Cytomegalovirus (CMV) infection also causes an oesophagitis and aphthoid ulcers treatable with thalidomide or intralesional steroids.

Diarrhoea

There are a number of causes of diarrhoea in HIV-infected patients, which are markers of severe immunodeficiency and constitute an AIDS diagnosis. The three commonest of these are cryptosporidiosis, microsporidiosis, and CMV infection.

Both cryptosporidiosis and microsporidiosis are relatively common when the CD4 count falls below 200 cells/mm^3. They both produce diarrhoea with dehydration and massive weight loss. The outcome is frequently fatal without effective antiretroviral therapy.

CMV infection of the lower gut produces diarrhoea, which is often bloody. Untreated colonic CMV is a particularly serious condition and frequently leads to perforation, colonic dilatation, and massive bleeding. In the short term both lower and upper gut infections with CMV are treatable using antiviral agents. Prevention of recurrent infection is crucially dependent upon the ability to control HIV viral replication using highly effective ART.

Eye manifestations

An important AIDS-defining diagnosis that leads to loss of vision is CMV retinitis. This is rare with a CD4 count of more than 100 cells/mm³ and is treatable but the only way to control this disease in the long term is to provide effective ART.

Another rare condition that leads to rapid blindness is progressive outer retinal necrosis thought to be caused by a herpesvirus infection. Toxoplasmosis of the eye is also probably commoner in HIV-infected individuals.

Lung manifestations

The commonest AIDS-defining diagnosis, particularly in individuals previously not suspected to be HIV positive, is *Pneumocystis carinii* pneumonia (PCP). This fungal disease has previously been recognized to be a rare opportunistic infection in debilitated patients. The symptoms of PCP are predominantly those of breathlessness in an unwell patient who feels as though s/he has a virus infection. The standard treatment for this disease is high-dose cotrimoxazole. The mortality should be less than 10% for a first attack. Recurrent attacks can be prevented by the use of cotrimoxazole, which is also effective in those vulnerable because of a low CD4 count but who have not had PCP.

A number of other opportunistic infections involve the lung but are rare in the Western world. These include histoplasmosis, cryptococcosis, and coccidioidomycosis.

Tumours

A variety of tumours are commoner in HIV-infected individuals. Most of these result from unrestrained proliferation of opportunistic oncogenic viruses. A variety of tumours form the basis for an AIDS diagnosis but a much wider range of tumours is commoner in HIV disease, including Hodgkin's disease, T-cell lymphomas, carcinoma of the lung, and testicular tumours.

Kaposi's sarcoma

The hallmark tumour of the AIDS epidemic is Kaposi's sarcoma (KS), caused by a human herpesvirus[8] commonly known as KS associated **herpes**virus (KSHV). Although this virus causes KS in non-HIV-infected people, particularly those who are elderly in certain geographical distributions and those who are immunosuppressed for other reasons (e.g. transplantation), it is markedly commoner in those who are HIV infected. Men having sex with men are particularly likely to acquire KSHV. KS presents with classic purplish nodules, often in the flexural creases and affects the extremities. It can also be visceral and a marker for this is KS involving the palate. Tumours of the gut are often asymptomatic but may bleed and KS involving the lung is often rapidly fatal, producing symptoms of severe cough and shortness of breath. This unusual multicentric tumour does not metastasize and is rare in people who are well treated for HIV infection. In those who have never been treated for HIV who develop KS, the first step is the introduction of ART, which usually results in stopping KS progression. Chemotherapy is usually reserved for those with progressive disease despite the introduction of ART and those with KS of the lung.

Lymphoma

Non-Hodgkin's lymphoma is a common manifestation of HIV infection and is strongly related to the patient's nadir (lowest) CD4 count. If the patient's CD4 count has never fallen below 250 cells/mm³ the incidence of this tumour is no different to that of the general population. However, if the nadir CD4 count falls below this, the incidence is approximately 10-fold that in the general population. About half the cases of non-Hodgkin's lymphoma are associated with Epstein–Barr virus infection and the others with genetic abnormalities, which are commonly seen in non-Hodgkin's lymphoma unrelated to HIV disease. Two rare forms of lymphoma (primary effusion lymphoma and plasmacytoid multicentric Castleman's disease) are both thought to be associated with KSHV. The prognosis for the treatment of lymphoma has improved markedly with the introduction of ART such that in most patients who are virologically undetectable at the time of diagnosis, the overall prognosis is not dissimilar from that in the non-HIV-infected population, although more patients with HIV infection have widespread disease with symptoms.

Tumours associated with the papillomavirus

Cervical cancer and anal cancer, which is particularly common in HIV-infected homosexual men, indicate AIDS. Both are treated along standard lines.

Increased risk of virulent infections in HIV disease

HIV-infected patients are more liable to develop a variety of virulent infections throughout the course of their disease. Thus respiratory infections are a common cause of morbidity in the developed world and of mortality in the developing world with pneumococcal pneumonia being a particularly common cause of death.

Tuberculosis

The major pandemic of tuberculosis (TB) is intimately related to the HIV epidemic. More than 50% of people with TB in the developing world are co-infected with HIV. While the lifetime risk of developing TB in an immunocompetent patient who has had a primary infection is 10%, this risk rises to 10% per year for those who are infected with HIV. It is also likely that HIV-infected patients are more liable to acquire TB and develop progressive disease than the general population. There is evidence that even HIV-infected individuals with a 'normal' CD4 count above 400 have a twofold risk of TB compared with immunocompetent HIV-negative individuals. TB in the context of HIV infection has a number of differences compared with classical infection. These include a higher incidence of disseminated disease, a greater incidence of blood cultures for TB being positive but a lower chance of TB being detected on sputum smear. TB does, however, respond to standard antituberculous therapy and there is no need for more prolonged courses of treatment in HIV-infected individuals.

Psychiatric morbidity

Depression is common in HIV-positive individuals with the majority of studies reporting a prevalence between 15% and 40%. Depression may alter the course of HIV infection by impairing immune function or influencing behaviour such as non-adherence to therapy. The signs and symptoms of depression and effectiveness of therapy are similar in HIV-infected and non-infected patients.[3]

Treatment of HIV infection[4,5]

The prognosis of HIV infection has been transformed, at least in the short term, by the use of HAART. Currently four different classes of agents are available to inhibit viral replication. All four classes take advantage of the unique aspects of the viral replication cycle.

Commonly used drugs

Nucleoside analogue reverse transcriptase inhibitors (NRTI or NA)

Drugs from this group act to inhibit reverse transcription. Common adverse effects include peripheral neuropathy (stavudine and didanosine), pancreatitis (didanosine), and myopathy (zidovudine). Certain NAs, particularly when used in combination, lead to a potentially fatal complication—lactic acidosis (Table 23.2). This condition has become much rarer since stavudine and didanosine are no longer combined. A further drug, tenofovir, is also usually included within the NA group (although it is more correctly a nucleotide).

Non-nucleoside reverse transcriptase inhibitors (NNRTI)

Drugs from this group also act to inhibit reverse transcription. Two agents are currently in widespread use. Efavirenz is preferred by most clinicians. It has the disadvantage of a usually evanescent central nervous system toxicity in the early stages of treatment and a potential for teratogenicity. With nevirapine there is a small incidence of fatal hepatotoxicity and serious skin reactions including Stevens–Johnson syndrome.

Proteinase inhibitors (PI)

The other agents in widespread use are PIs. Most of the early PIs suffered from the disadvantages of frequent daily dosing because of short plasma half lives (mainly being metabolised by the cytochrome P450 system) and also highly variable pharmacokinetics, which led to difficulties of establishing optimal dosing. One new PI, atazanavir, is associated with a much longer plasma half life, allowing once daily doses. For the other PIs, most clinicians now would only use them in conjunction with an inhibitor of cytochrome P450 (low-dose ritonavir) which boosts plasma levels significantly allowing less frequent daily dosing.

Fusion inhibitors

Fuzeon T20 is a spectacular example of an agent developed as a result of basic understanding of the virology of HIV. The process by which HIV gains access to the cell, i.e. fusion, has been explored in detail and as a result a short peptide was developed that was predicted to inhibit this process. This has proved to be an effective antiretroviral agent that has to be administered twice daily by subcutaneous injection and so is mainly used in the so-called salvage setting.

Current consensus guidelines relating to HIV treatment

There is considerable agreement in the developed world that treatment should begin for HIV-infected individuals when the CD4 count lies somewhere between 350 and 200 cells/mm^3. However, up to a third of patients will be treated much later than this because they first present with an opportunistic infection and a very low CD4 count. One of the ways of improving outcome is to identify such groups earlier.

Standard treatment is a combination of two NAs and either an NNRTI or a PI (usually boosted with ritonavir). With such a wide array of drugs available, randomized controlled trials cannot be used to assess all potential combinations.

The choice between using an NNRTI or a boosted PI first as part of an initial regimen remains an area of controversy, although most believe that using an NNRTI first is beneficial because most of these drugs have particularly long half lives, which make them easy to combine as part of once a day regimens.

The metabolic syndrome—lipodystrophy—fat redistribution syndrome

One of the most important complications of treatment of HIV infection is the development of a metabolic syndrome. This comprises plasma lipid abnormalities, increased insulin resistance (causing frank diabetes in a small proportion of patients), and fat redistribution. There is increased visceral fat in the abdomen of men and in the breasts of women, and loss of subcutaneous fat, which can cause discomfort when it occurs around the buttocks and heels. The causes of this syndrome are not clear. It is more common in those with: advanced disease, PIs rather than NNRTIs, and older age. The stigmatizing effect of facial lipo-atrophy can lead to poor drug adherence. It is associated with certain NA combinations, particularly the use of stavudine. It may be that some of the newer NAs such as abacavir or tenofovir may not be associated with lipo-atrophy. Cohort data strongly suggest that the combination of insulin resistance and plasma lipid abnormalities is associated with an increased risk of cardiovascular disease. While this is not of sufficient magnitude to make patients reluctant to take ART, it is an area of concern and one of the main motivators for the development of new compounds where this risk is lessened.

Adherence issues

Adherence is the single most important factor in determining the ability of ART to suppress HIV replication in the long term and therefore produce a sustained improvement in prognosis. Adherence has been much studied in the context of HIV infection and there are a number of demographic factors, life-style issues, and belief systems that have profound effects on adherence but are difficult to modify with behavioural intervention.

Other issues related to adherence are more amenable to pharmaceutical manipulation. These include total pill burden, frequency of dosing, freedom from strict food requirements in relationship to dosing, short-term drug toxicities, and fears of long-term toxicities. Present standard regimens of first-line therapy can usually now be given once a day with a pill burden of two tablets a day. Careful attention to gastrointestinal side-effects is important in the initial stages of therapy giving treatment to prevent these wherever possible. Careful explanation of the evanescent nature of the CNS toxicities associated with Efavirenz help adherence in the early stages. Most clinicians would now avoid stavudine as part of an initial regimen and so they can reassure the patient that the regimen chosen is that least likely to cause lipoatrophy.

Drug interactions

Other factors that influence the success of ART include pharmacokinetic variability and perhaps particularly unexpected pharmacological interactions when other drugs are given in conjunction with antiviral agents. The list of potential interactions is very long and clinicians prescribing any drugs to patients known to be taking antiretrovirals are strongly advised to consult an expert to ensure that the treatment they are proposing to give with the antiretroviral regimen is safe.

Second-line regimens

The choice of an optimum second line regimen is usually straight forward and is aided by tests now available to detect drug resistance. Usually a new combination of nucleoside analogues is coupled with a boosted PI if an NNRTI has been used as part of the initial regimen.

'Salvage therapy'

This term refers to therapy where achieving complete virological undetectability is unlikely. In this group of patients the risk of death is closely related to the CD4 count and is low providing this can be kept above 50 cells/mm^3. The CD4 count is preserved better providing ART is continued, perhaps because virus with drug-resistant mutations is relatively disabled and is less destructive of CD4 cells For long-term survival, these patients will be dependent on the development of new drugs, which can be combined in such a way as to completely inhibit viral replication. This is a highly specialized area of treatment and such patients need to be referred to experienced centres.

Employment status and barriers to employment

The widespread use of ART has had a profound impact on HIV-related morbidity and mortality. Over a 6-year period in the 1990s during which highly active ART was introduced, new AIDS diagnoses in the UK halved.[6]

Yet the dramatic reduction in mortality and morbidity does not appear to have been followed by a corresponding increase in employment in this group. There is some evidence that the introduction of ART increases the probability of remaining employed.[7] However, a prospective cohort study showed that despite improved health, most men who were unemployed at the study baseline in 1995 remained unemployed 2½ years later.[8] This phenomenon is not unique to HIV: social security data in the UK and other countries show that the proportion of people disabled by illness who then return to work is very small. In the UK, once a person has been on an incapacity benefit for a year they have only a 20% chance of returning to work within 5 years.[9] For HIV, studies have consistently identified common factors associated with unemployment and perceived barriers to return to work. These are: loss of disability income benefits; past or current mood disorders; impairment in some areas of cognitive functioning; physical limitations; work-related ill health; limited job skills, and discrimination.[8,10–13]

There is evidence that some HIV-related symptoms are associated with worse quality of life and more disability days. In such patients, targeting specific symptoms may improve health-related quality of life and reduce disability.[14]

However, in general, and again consistent with studies of non-HIV sufferers with chronic illness, the HIV literature suggests that change in health status accounts for only a minority of changes in employment status.[15]

Interestingly, while the number of people in the UK living with HIV is steadily increasing year on year, the number claiming incapacity benefit for HIV disease is growing more slowly (Figure 23.2). Many factors may be contributing to this picture. An optimistic interpretation would be that employers are more aware of their need to accommodate staff with HIV and that infected individuals are remaining well for longer.

Vocational support and rehabilitation

The UK Government Department for Work and Pensions (DWP) provides support for disabled people via its national network of JobCentre plus offices. Each office has a disability employment advisor who provides specialist advice to disabled people in finding and keeping a job. Job applicants and employees disabled because of HIV can apply via the disability employment advisor to the 'access to work' scheme for help (advisory and financial) in overcoming the problems resulting from disability. Equipment or support needs identified within 6 weeks of the employee starting work are eligible for 100% funding. After 6 weeks the employer has to bear the first £300 of the cost and the scheme will pay 80% of the remaining cost. (http://www.jobcentreplus.gov.uk).

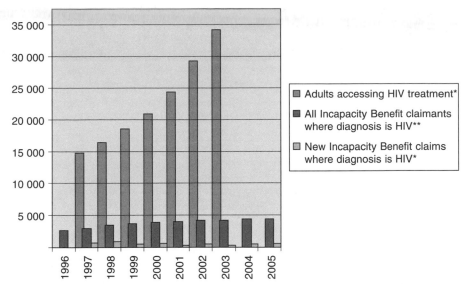

Fig. 23.2 Annual numbers of adults claiming Incapacity Benefit where the diagnosis is HIV compared with total number of adults being treated for HIV in the UK. *Number of adults (aged 15 years and over) accessing NHS HIV-related treatment and care services in England, Wales and Northern Ireland between 1997 and 2003. (Source: Health Protection Agency Centre for Infections, Survey of Prevalent HIV Infections Diagnosed (SOPHID), 1997–2003). **Number of adults (age 16 years and over) claiming incapacity benefit and Severe Disablement Allowance with a diagnosis of HIV in England, Wales and Scotland between 1996 and 2005 (source: 5% samples from February data annually, Statistics Directorate, Department for Work and Pensions).

For the common disabilities experienced by HIV-infected workers, the type of support required might include:

- voice-activated computer (neuropathy)
- installation of home office (tiredness, diarrhoea)
- taxi to work (tiredness, diarrhoea, neuropathy).

Funding under the 'Access to Work' scheme is available when *additional* costs are incurred because of a disability. It cannot be used to provide support usually provided by employers or required under legislation for all their employees. In addition it does not necessarily absolve the employer of its duty under the Disability Discrimination Act 2005 (DDA). The employer still has to make reasonable adjustments to reduce or remove any substantial disadvantage that a physical feature of the work premises or employment arrangements causes a disabled employee or job applicant compared with a non-disabled person.

UK AIDS charities

In addition there are many charitable organizations that provide specific advice and support for HIV-infected individuals. Some of these provide comprehensive advice on employment issues. For example Positive Futures Partnership (PFP) is a coalition of several HIV charities working together in partnership to support people with HIV. PFP offers employment advice to individuals with HIV. It also provides a service to employers that includes advice, training, and seminars.

Box 23.1 Employment advice booklets published by Positive Futures Partnership

- *Thinking about the future*
- *Positive about work: a guide to your rights*
- *Positive about work: a practical guide to finding employment*

In particular it produces a series of practical booklets for HIV-infected individuals with advice on various employment issues (Box 23.1). Several other large national HIV charities provide employment advice (Box 23.2).

Legal and ethical framework for assessing work fitness

The Disability Discrimination Act and the Human Rights Act now give much greater scope for people to challenge what appears to be HIV-related discrimination in the workplace.

The Disability Discrimination Act

The major piece of UK legislation offering employment protection for people with HIV is the Disability Discrimination Act 2005[16] (DDA). This Act covers progressive conditions, where impairments are likely to become substantial. The previous 1995 Act covered people with HIV from the moment that there was a noticeable effect on normal day-to-day activities, however slight. The 2005 amendments to the 1995 Act extend the definition of disability so that HIV infection now counts as a disability from the time at which it is diagnosed (Box 23.2).

Box 23.2 Examples of UK HIV charities that provide employment advice

The Terrence Higgins Trust: THT, 52–54 Grays Inn Road, London WC1X 8JU. Tel.: 020 78310330; website:www.tht.org.uk

UK coalition of people living with HIV and AIDS (UKC): UKC 250, Kennington Lane, London SE11 5RD. Tel.: 0207 564 2180; website: www.ukcoalition.org

Positively Women: PW, 347–349 City Road, London EC. Tel.: 020 7713 0444; website: www.positivelywomen.org.uk

The National AIDS Trust (NAT): NAT New City Cloisters, 196 Old Street, London EC1V 9FR. Tel.: 0207 814 6767; website: www.nat.org.uk

National Aidsmap (NAM): NAM, Lincoln House, 1 Brixton Road, London SW9 6DE. Tel.: 0207 840 0500; website: www.aidsmap.com

Positive Futures Partnership: PFP, 250 Kennington Lane London SE11 5RD. Tel.: 0207 564 2188; website: www.positive-futures.org

Box 23.3 Current and previous provisions of the Disability Discrimination Act relevant to HIV and employment

Legislation	*What it says*
Current	
Disability Discrimination Act 2005: amendments relevant to HIV came into force on 5 December 2005	'a person who has cancer, HIV infection or multiple sclerosis is to be deemed to have a disability, and hence to be a disabled person.' 'HIV infection means infection by a virus capable of causing the Acquired Immune Deficiency Syndrome.'
Previous	
The Disability Discrimination Act 1995: Code of Practice for the elimination of discrimination in the field of employment against disabled persons or persons who have had a disability	Progressive conditions are conditions which are likely to change and develop over time. Examples given in the Act are cancer, multiple sclerosis, muscular dystrophy, and HIV infection. Where a person has a progressive condition s/he will be covered by the Act from the moment the condition leads to an impairment which has some effect on ability to carry out normal day-to-day activities, even though not a substantial effect, if that impairment is likely eventually to have a substantial adverse effect on such ability. (Medical diagnosis of the condition is not by itself enough.)

Reasonable adjustments

The purpose of the DDA is to protect disabled people from discrimination in the field of employment. As part of this protection employers may have to make 'reasonable adjustments' if their employment arrangements or premises place disabled people at a substantial disadvantage compared with non-disabled people. Reasonable adjustments for employees infected with HIV might be:

- to accommodate more sickness absence than they would in someone without the illness;
- to allow time off to attend treatment (may include psychological treatment if psychological illness is a direct result of diagnosis);
- to make arrangements for home working where symptoms of HIV interfere with ability to attend work;
- in the healthcare setting, to make arrangements for protection from infectious diseases to which they have increased susceptibility, such as TB.

Pre-employment screening, HIV testing, and the DDA

There are very few circumstances where an individual's HIV status is directly relevant to their employability. In the UK, healthcare workers who are HIV positive are not allowed to perform exposure-prone procedures (see Box 23.4). Even then the onus is on the individual to assess their own risk and to come forward for testing if they believe they are at risk of HIV.[17] At the time of writing there is no requirement for compulsory pre-employment or in-employment HIV testing

---

Box 23.4 Definition of exposure-prone procedures

Exposure-prone procedures

Procedures in which injury to the healthcare worker could result in the worker's blood contaminating the patient's open tissue.

---

of this group of healthcare workers, although the Department of Health is reviewing the situation and is expected to publish its advice in 2006.

Another group are those whose employment will take them to countries where an HIV test is a requirement of entry. In this instance it could be argued that a pre-employment HIV test, along with other tests required for travel, is necessary to assess fitness to work abroad.

There is no law specifically addressing the legality of pre-employment HIV testing. However, there are several pieces of legislation, including the DDA 2005, the Data Protection Act 1998 and the Human Rights Act 1998, which would make it difficult for employers to justify such testing. To comply with antidiscrimination law the test would have to be applied equally to all groups, otherwise it could be construed as direct or indirect discrimination (e.g. sex discrimination if only men are tested). Any test must be 'adequate, relevant and not excessive in relation to the purpose for which it is being processed' under the DPA.

With the recent advances in drug treatment, HIV-positive individuals can remain well for many years. Therefore screening could be deemed irrelevant. In addition such screening would be inequitable unless screening for a whole range of diseases with comparable natural histories was undertaken.

There are ethical and other criticisms of pre-employment HIV screening. The test may be negative for up to 3 months after infection and tested employees may become infected after employment. Occupational physicians and nurses asked to arrange such tests must satisfy themselves that there is a justifiable reason for requesting an HIV test. For testing in any circumstances, they must ensure that explicit, informed consent has been obtained and an adequate pre- and post-test discussions held.

HIV and the pre-employment health questionnaire

All job applicants should be advised to complete their pre-employment health questionnaire honestly. The UK Department of Health issues specific guidance for HIV-positive healthcare workers recommending that 'HIV-infected healthcare workers applying for new posts should complete health questionnaires honestly'.[17] And the General Medical Council (GMC) in its booklet 'Serious Communicable Diseases 1997' expands this to say that 'if you apply for a new post you must complete health questionnaires honestly *and fully*[18] (see Box 23.5).

Ethical framework

The occupational physician, just like any other doctor, is bound by the ethical code of the GMC. In addition the Faculty of Occupational Medicine of the Royal College of Physicians publishes its interpretation of the GMC generic guidance.[19] Other healthcare professionals must follow similar guidance produced by their relevant regulatory body.

Healthcare workers

The ethical position for HIV-infected doctors and doctors of HIV-infected patients is addressed explicitly by the GMC. Its document *Serious Communicable Diseases: Guidance to Doctors*,

Box 23.5 Responsibilities of doctors who have been exposed to a serious communicable disease

29. If you have any reason to believe that you have been exposed to a serious communicable disease you must seek and follow professional advice without delay on whether you should undergo testing and, if so, which tests are appropriate. Further guidance on your responsibilities if your health may put patients at risk is included in our booklet *Good Medical Practice.*

30. If you acquire a serious communicable disease you must promptly seek and follow advice from a suitably qualified colleague—such as a consultant in occupational health, infectious diseases or public health on:

♦ Whether, and in what ways, you should modify your professional practice.

♦ Whether you should inform your current employer, your previous employers or any prospective employer, about your condition.

31. You must not rely on your own assessment of the risks you pose to patients.

32. If you have a serious communicable disease and continue in professional practice you must have appropriate medical supervision.

33. If you apply for a new post, you must complete health questionnaires honestly and fully.

Extract from: *Serious communicable diseases: guidance to doctors,* October 1997 General Medical Council[18]

October 1997 provides guidance to doctors who have been exposed to a serious communicable disease (Box 23.5), defining this as 'infections such as human immunodeficiency virus (HIV), tuberculosis and hepatitis B and C.' The guidance also lays out the responsibilities of doctors who are treating colleagues with serious communicable diseases (Box 23.6).[18]

Box 23.6 Treating colleagues with serious communicable diseases

34. If you are treating a doctor or other health care worker with a serious communicable disease you must provide the confidentiality and support to which every patient is entitled.

35. If you know, or have good reason to believe, that a medical colleague or health care worker who has or may have a serious communicable disease, is practicing, or has practiced, in a way which places patients at risk, you must inform an appropriate person in the health care worker's employing authority, for example an occupational health physician, or where appropriate, the relevant regulatory body. Such cases are likely to arise very rarely. Wherever possible you should inform the health care worker concerned before passing information to an employer or regulatory body.

Extract from: *Serious communicable diseases: guidance to doctors,* October 1997 General Medical Council[18]

Box 23.7 Guidance for nurses

8   As a registered nurse, midwife or specialist community public health nurse, you must act to identify and minimise the risk to patients and clients

8.1   You must work with other members of the team to promote health care environments that are conducive to safe, therapeutic and ethical practice.

8.2   You must act quickly to protect patients and clients from risk if you have good reason to believe that you or a colleague, from your own or another profession, may not be fit to practice for reasons of conduct, health or competence. You should be aware of the terms of legislation that offer protection for people who raise concerns about health and safety issues.

Extract from: *Code of professional conduct: standards for conduct, performance and ethics*, December 2004, Nursing and Midwifery Council

Similar guidance is produced for nurses (Box 23.7) and dentists (Box 23.8) by their registration bodies.

Additional guidance is published by the UK Department of Health regarding HIV-positive healthcare workers.[17] This addresses both the infected healthcare worker and the healthcare worker aware of an infected colleague (Box 23.9).

Box 23.8 Guidance for dentists

4.1   It is unethical for a dentist to refuse to treat a patient solely on the grounds that the person has a blood borne virus or any other transmissible disease or infection.

4.2   A dentist who is aware of being infected with a blood borne virus or any other transmissible disease or infection which might jeopardise the wellbeing of patients and takes no action is behaving unethically. The Council would take the same view if a dentist took no action when having reason to believe that such infection may be present.

It is the responsibility of the dentist in either situation to obtain medical advice which may result in appropriate testing and, if a dentist is found to be infected, regular medical supervision. The medical advice may include the necessity to cease the practice of dentistry altogether, to exclude exposure prone procedures or to modify practice in some other way.

Failure to obtain such advice or to act upon it would almost certainly lead to a charge of serious professional misconduct.

Extract from: *Maintaining standards. Guidance to dentists on professional and personal conduct*, November 1997, General Dental Council

---

Box 23.9 HIV-infected healthcare workers

4.7 A health care worker who has any reason to believe they may have been exposed to infection with HIV, in whatever circumstances, must promptly seek and follow confidential professional advice on whether they should be tested for HIV. Failure to do so may breach the duty of care to patients.

4.16 Health care workers who know or have good reason to believe (having taken steps to confirm the facts as far as practicable) that an HIV infected worker is performing exposure prone procedures or has done so in the past, must inform an appropriate person in the health care worker's employing authority (e.g. an occupational health physician) or, where appropriate, the relevant regulatory body. The DPH should also be informed in confidence. UKAP* can be asked to advise when the need for such notification is unclear. Such cases are likely to arise very rarely. Wherever possible, the health care worker should be informed before information is passed to an employer or regulatory body.

Extract from: *HIV-infected healthcare workers: guidance on management and patient notification*, July 2005, Department of Health, UK[17]

*UK Advisory Panel for Healthcare Workers Infected with Blood-borne Viruses. (UKAP was set up originally under the aegis of the UK Health Departments' Expert Advisory Group on AIDS in 1991, and in 1993 its remit was extended to cover healthcare workers infected with all blood-borne viruses. UKAP advises physicians of healthcare workers infected with blood-borne viruses, occupational physicians, professional bodies, individual healthcare workers or their advocates; and directors of public health on patient notification exercises.)

Occupational risks for HIV-infected workers

Potential occupational exposures to opportunistic infection

Healthcare work

Studies early in the twentieth century established that healthcare workers were at increased risk of TB. This risk appeared largely to disappear with the advent of effective chemotherapy. However, in the 1990s about a twofold increased risk of TB was found among UK healthcare workers suggesting continuing occupational risk.[20] For HIV-positive healthcare workers the risk is likely to be even higher and the consequences of infection with TB greater. In view of this, every effort should be made to protect an HIV-positive healthcare worker from exposure to infectious TB patients and material. The British Thoracic Society guidelines *Control and prevention of tuberculosis in the UK: code of practice 2000* specifically addresses the case of HIV-positive job applicants and those diagnosed with HIV while in post. The guidance states that:[21]

> if HIV-infected healthcare workers choose to care for HIV-infected patients, they should understand that they should not care for patients with infectious TB as they put themselves at risk and may then put others at risk should they themselves become infected. ... Since so many HIV-infected patients are admitted with respiratory symptoms, this will raise practical issues such as implications for staffing and difficulties in maintaining confidentiality.

Decisions about risk should take into account the patient's specific duties in the workplace, the prevalence of TB in the local community and the degree to which precautions designed to prevent the transmission of TB are taken in the workplace. The estimate of risk will affect how and in what capacity the HIV-infected worker should be employed and the frequency with which the worker should be screened for TB. In the UK the employer owes a higher duty of care to any particularly vulnerable employee with a known, pre-existing medical condition (the 'eggshell skull principle'). (See Chapter 3.) So, in practice, an HIV-infected healthcare worker may need to be restricted from working in areas such as HIV, infectious diseases, and respiratory medicine.

Regardless of potential risk of exposure to TB-infected patients or material, *all* HIV-positive healthcare workers should be alerted to the symptoms of TB, the need to avoid patients and material suspected or known to be infected with TB and to seek medical advice immediately if they develop any symptoms suggestive of TB.

HIV and occupational health specialists advising HIV-positive healthcare workers should refer to the British Thoracic Society code of practice[21] for further guidance.

Other occupations

In 2002 the US Public Health Service and Infectious Diseases Society published evidence-based recommendations for preventing opportunistic infections among HIV-infected persons.[22] The guidance referring to different occupations is summarized below.

Work in prisons and with the homeless There is evidence that TB is more common in the prison population than the general population in the USA and several European countries and this is likely to be the case in the UK. Accurate estimates of TB in the UK homeless are difficult to obtain but all available studies point to TB being a particular problem in this group. HIV-positive prison officers and workers in homeless shelters are likely therefore to be at increased risk of TB.

As for healthcare workers above, similar principles of risk reduction should apply.

Child-care providers HIV-positive child-care providers are at increased risk for acquiring CMV infection, cryptosporidiosis, and other infections such as hepatitis A and giardiasis from children. The risk for acquiring infection can be diminished by optimal hygiene practices such as hand-washing after faecal contact (e.g. during nappy changing) and after contact with urine or saliva.

Occupations involving contact with animals (e.g. veterinary work and employment in pet shops, farms, or abattoirs) Workers in the above occupations could be at risk of cryptosporidiosis, toxoplasmosis, salmonellosis, campylobacteriosis, or *Bartonella* infection. However, available data are insufficient to justify a recommendation against HIV-infected persons working in such settings. Optimal hygiene practices should be adhered to.

Working overseas

There are a few particular considerations for the HIV-positive overseas worker. Little additional care need be taken for the day trip abroad to an urban office in a developed city. Of more concern is an overseas posting for many months or even years to a remote area of a developing country. Consideration needs to be given to:

- immigration requirements of country being visited
- risk of exposure to opportunistic pathogens

- speed of access to and adequacy of healthcare facilities
- repatriation arrangements.

Travel to developing countries might result in substantial risks for the exposure of HIV-infected persons to opportunistic pathogens, particularly for patients who are severely immunosuppressed. Consultation with healthcare providers or specialists in travel medicine should help patients plan itineraries.

HIV-infected travellers are at a higher risk for food-borne and water-borne infections than they are in the UK. The usual hygiene precautions recommended for all travellers should be strictly adhered to by those who are infected with HIV. These include steaming hot foods, peeling own fruit, drinking only bottled beverages or boiled water. They should avoid direct contact of the skin with soil or sand (e.g. by wearing shoes and protective clothing and by using towels on beaches) in areas where faecal contamination of soil is likely.

Antimicrobial prophylaxis for traveller's diarrhoea is not recommended routinely for HIV-infected persons travelling to developing countries. Such preventive therapy can have adverse effects and can promote the emergence of drug-resistant organisms. All HIV-infected travellers to developing countries should carry a sufficient supply of an antimicrobial agent, to be taken empirically if diarrhoea occurs. One appropriate regimen is 500 mg of ciprofloxacin twice daily for 3–7 days.

In general live-virus vaccines should be avoided. There are some exceptions and expert advice should be sought from a travel clinic and the worker's HIV specialist.

Countries requiring an entry HIV test

An increasing number of countries require foreigners to be tested for HIV prior to entry. It is usually required as part of a medical examination for long-term visitors, and this includes workers. Table 23.4 shows a list of 60 countries that have some test requirements, although not necessarily applicable to all types of workers. For example, Saudi Arabia and Taiwan require all applicants for work permits to be tested while Canada will test 'any foreigner suspected of being HIV positive'. The table reflects information available as of March 2003 (Human Immunodeficiency Virus (HIV) Testing requirements for entry into foreign countries (http://travel.state.gov/law/info/info 621.html.) and is subject to change. Before accepting a post abroad it would be prudent to check with the embassy of that country for more detail and if HIV status is required or unknown, to arrange testing.

Occupational immunizations

The majority of occupational vaccines are given to healthcare and laboratory workers and those travelling overseas. As a general rule HIV-positive workers should avoid live vaccines; however, some are not absolutely contraindicated. Most of the safe vaccines can be given according to the usual schedule in the 'green book'[23] (see below) however an HIV-infected individual may not mount a good immune response.

The list below includes some of the commoner occupational vaccines. This list is based on information from the Department of Health's Immunization Against Infectious Disease 1996 'The green book'[23] and the advice should always be checked on their website for updates. It would also be sensible to check safety with the individual's HIV specialist.

Varicella zoster virus, BCG, and yellow fever are all live vaccines and should not be given to HIV-positive individuals. **MMR** contains live attenuated measles, mumps, and rubella virus but may be given safely provided there are no contraindications. An inactivated **polio** vaccine (IPV) is now available and can be given. Oral **typhoid** is live attenuated vaccine so is contraindicated in

Table 23.4 HIV testing requirements for entry into foreign countries

Country	Test required for
Aruba	Intending immigrants
Australia	All applicants for permanent residence over age 15 (all other applicants who require medical examinations are tested if it is indicated on clinical grounds)
Bahrain	Individuals employed in jobs involving food handling, and patient or child care
Belarus	All persons staying longer than 3 months
Belize	All persons applying for residency permits
Brunei	All persons applying for work permits
Bulgaria	All intending immigrants (and may be required for foreigners staying longer than 1 month for purposes of study or work)
Canada	Any foreigner suspected of being HIV-positive (HIV testing is not mandatory for entry)
Central African Republic	Anyone seeking residence, work and student permits must submit to a medical exam (which includes an HIV test)
China, People's Republic of	Foreigners planning to stay for more than 6 months (testing is not required for entry or residency in Hong Kong or Macau)
Colombia	Anyone suspected of being HIV-positive (HIV-positive persons are not admitted without a waiver from a Colombian consulate in the USA)
Cuba	Anyone staying over 90 days, excluding diplomats
Cyprus	All foreigners working or studying are tested after entry
Dominican Republic	Foreigners planning to reside, study or work
Egypt	Foreigners applying for study, training or work permits (spouses of applicants are exempt)
El Salvador	Anyone age 15 and older applying for temporary and permanent residency
Georgia	All foreigners staying longer than 1 month
Greece	Prostitutes (as defined by Greek law)
Hungary	Anyone staying over 1 year, and all intending immigrants (some employers may require workers to be tested)
India	All students over 18, anyone between the ages of 18 and 70 with a visa valid for 1 year or more, and anyone extending a stay to a year or more, excluding accredited journalists and those working in foreign missions
Iraq	All foreigners (except diplomats, Muslim pilgrims transiting through Iraq, children under 14 who do not suffer from haemophilia, men over 60 and women over 50 years of age) will be tested upon entry and are required to pay a $50 (US) fee for the test (persons possessing a current medical certificate confirming that they do not suffer from AIDS may also be exempt from being tested.)

Table 23.4 HIV testing requirements for entry into foreign countries—cont'd

Country	Test required for
Jordan	Anyone staying longer than 3 months
Kazakstan	All visitors staying more then 1 month must present a certificate of an HIV test within 10 days of their arrival
Korea, Republic of	Foreigners working as entertainers staying over 90 days
Kuwait	Those seeking to obtain a residence permit
Kyrgyzstan	All foreigners, excluding diplomats, staying more than 1 month
Latvia	Anyone seeking a residency permit
Lebanon	Those planning to reside or work (universities may require testing of foreign students)
Libya	Those seeking residency permits, excluding official visitors
Lithuania	Applicants for permanent residence permits
Malaysia	Foreigners seeking work permits as unskilled labourers
Marshall Islands, Republic of the	Temporary visitors staying more than 30 days, and applicants for residence and work permits
Mauritius	Foreigners planning to work or seek permanent residence (testing performed upon arrival in Mauritius)
Micronesia, (Federated States of)	Anyone applying for a permit needs to obtain a medical clearance, which may include an HIV test
Moldova	Anyone staying more than 3 months
Montserrat	University students and applicants for work and residency
Oman	Those newly employed by private sector companies and upon renewal of work permit
Panama	Women intending to work in prostitution and anyone who adjusts visa status once in Panama
Papua New Guinea	Applicants seeking work or residency visas and their dependents
Paraguay	Applicants seeking temporary or permanent residency status
Qatar	Applicants seeking work or residency visas and visitors staying more than 1 month
Russia	All foreign visitors staying longer than 3 months
Saudi Arabia	Applicants for residency/work permits
St Vincent	Applicants seeking temporary and permanent residency visas
St Kitts and Nevis	Students, intending immigrants and anyone seeking employment
Seychelles	Foreigners planning to work must under go a medical exam, which includes an HIV test, upon arrival
Singapore	Workers who earn less than $1250 per month and applicants for permanent resident status (except spouses and children of Singapore citizens)
Slovakia	Applicants for long-term or permanent residency visas

Continued

Table 23.4 HIV testing requirements for entry into foreign countries—cont'd

Country	Test required for
South Africa	All mine workers (irrespective of their positions)
Spain	Anyone seeking residence, work and student permits must submit to a medical exam (which may include an AIDS test)
Syria	All foreigners (ages 15–60 years) staying more than 15 days
Taiwan	Applicants for residency and work permits (testing is also required for anyone staying over 90 days)
Tajikistan	Anyone staying more than 90 days (pending legislation)
Turkmenistan	All foreigners staying longer than 3 months
Turks and Caicos	Foreign workers (HIV testing is part of the medical exam that is required for work permits)
Ukraine	Anyone staying longer than 3 months
United Arab Emirates	Applicants for work or residence permits except those under age 18
United Kingdom	Anyone who does not appear to be in good health may be required to undergo a medical exam (including an HIV test) prior to being granted or denied entry
Uzbekistan	Anyone staying more than 15 days (long-term visitors must renew HIV certificate after the first 3 months in Uzbekistan and annually thereafter)
Yemen	Applicants seeking permanent residence including work or study (students over age 16), all foreigners staying longer than 1 month, and foreign spouses of Yemeni nationals (excludes experts, teachers, and foreign missions who are required to work in Yemen)

HIV. The parenteral typhoid vaccine is not live so may be given in the absence of other contraindications. **Diphtheria** containing vaccines should be given according to the usual schedule in the Green Book. **Influenza** vaccine contains inactivated virus. It may be given to HIV-infected individuals and is specifically recommended for healthcare workers and for those with immunosuppression including HIV. **Hepatitis B** vaccine contains hepatitis B surface antigen and **hepatitis A** is an inactivated vaccine. Both are safe in HIV disease.

Risk of transmitting HIV at work

Transmission from worker to client/patient

Sex workers

The route of transmission of HIV means that the only two occupations with potential for transmission of HIV from an infected worker during the normal course of their work are sex work and healthcare. Sex workers in the UK are unregulated. Both they and their client group are difficult to access for routine data collection and research purposes. Therefore little is known about transmission rates from sex workers to their clients.

Healthcare workers

The situation in healthcare in developed countries, and in particular in the UK, is very different. The healthcare industry is regulated and it is possible to investigate both the healthcare workers and their patients in the case of a potential HIV transmission.

Evidence of transmission of HIV from healthcare worker to patient

Worldwide, there have been two reports of probable transmission of HIV from infected health-care workers performing exposure-prone procedures to patients: Both cases were reported in the literature in the 1990s. The first report was of a Florida dentist with AIDS who transmitted HIV to six patients.[24] The second case involved a French orthopaedic surgeon who transmitted HIV to an elderly woman during a surgical procedure.[25] In both cases molecular analysis indicated that the viral sequences obtained from the surgeons and their HIV-infected patients were closely related. In 1995 the American Centre for Disease Control and Prevention summarized the results of all published and unpublished investigations. Of over 22 000 patients tested who were treated by 51 HIV-positive infected healthcare workers, 113 HIV-positive patients were reported, but epidemiological and laboratory follow-up did not show any healthcare worker to have been a source of HIV for any of the patients tested.[26] Many lookback exercises undertaken in the UK, USA, and elsewhere since that study have failed to identify further cases.

Occupational restrictions placed on HIV-positive healthcare workers

In the UK HIV-positive healthcare workers (including students in training) must not perform exposure-prone procedures (Box 23.4).[17] In practice these restrictions apply mainly to those carrying out surgical procedures, such as surgeons, dentists, and midwives.

At present there is no requirement for HIV screening of any occupational group within healthcare, although the Department of Health requires 'a healthcare worker who has any reason to believe they may have been exposed to HIV to promptly seek and follow confidential professional advice on whether they should be tested for HIV. Failure to do so may breach the duty of care to patients'. This guidance is reiterated in various regulatory bodies' statements on professional responsibilities (see Boxes 23.5, 23.7–23.9).

Draft guidance from the Department of Health (*Health clearance for serious communicable diseases: new healthcare workers. Draft guidance for consultation*. Department of Health, January 2003) requires compulsory HIV testing for healthcare workers moving into training or posts involving exposure-prone procedures for the first time. It is likely that this guidance will be implemented shortly.[27]

Patient notification exercise

HIV-positive healthcare workers who are newly diagnosed and have been performing exposure-prone procedures may be subject to a 'lookback' exercise. It is not necessary to notify automatically every patient who has undergone any exposure-prone procedure by an HIV-infected healthcare worker as the overall risk of transmission is very low. The Director of Public Health has responsibility for deciding on the need for a lookback and which patients to include. S/he may seek advice from the UK Advisory Panel if there is doubt.[17]

Care of the HIV-infected healthcare worker

The management of workers with HIV and AIDS should be consistent with the policy and procedure developed for people affected by other serious and potentially progressive medical conditions. The occupational physician has an important advisory role. This is particularly central in the management of HIV-infected healthcare workers, as emphasized in the government guidance on this issue.[17] If limitation of practice is necessary, the occupational physician should advise management accordingly but without revealing any clinical information and with the agreement of the individual concerned. Where possible, redeployment without loss of income should be pursued. This will require a sympathetic approach by management.

The Department of Health guidance also requires all HIV-infected healthcare workers who provide clinical care to patients (even if they have not been involved in performing exposure-prone procedures) to remain under regular medical and occupational health supervision. They are required to follow appropriate occupational health advice, especially if their circumstances change.

No other restrictions are placed on HIV-positive healthcare workers except at local level where their condition would be managed with the same approach used for other chronic illnesses with potential for immunosuppression.

Confidentiality

Confidentiality is of great importance when dealing with HIV infection. Healthcare workers have the same rights of confidentiality as anyone else. Patients can be reassured that the routine precautions taken in their care protect them from the tiny risk of infection from their carers.

For healthcare workers involved in exposure-prone procedures, the possibility of a patient notification exercise is likely to be extremely emotive. Assurances should be given about measures to protect their identity, including seeking an injunction if necessary to prevent publication of their name. Advice on the need to modify their practice can be sought from a specialist occupational physician. The Trust's Director of Human Resources and/or the Regional Postgraduate Dean should be approached for advice on retraining and redeployment issues or alternative careers.

Other than the special case of HIV-infected healthcare workers performing exposure-prone procedures, modification of working practices are not necessary to protect others from infection.

Risk of acquiring HIV through work

There are very few occupations and work tasks that have the potential for transmission of HIV to the worker. The two main ones are:

1. Sex work, although there is evidence that in Western Europe the route of transmission is more likely to be through needle sharing in drug addicted sex workers rather than directly through unprotected sex in the course of their work.[28]

2. Healthcare work where the worker is exposed to the blood and other body fluids of HIV-infected patients through percutaneous injury or blood splash on to mucous membranes or non-intact skin.

Unlike sex workers, serosurveys of healthcare workers have not shown a higher prevalence of HIV. However, we know that HIV can be transmitted in the healthcare setting from patient to worker. Large prospective studies have found that the risk of transmission of HIV from an infected patient to a healthcare worker, after a single infected needlestick, is about 0.3%.[29]

Table 23.5 Occupational transmission of HIV up to end December 2002*

	USA	UK	Rest of Europe	Rest of world	Total
Documented seroconversions (specific exposure incident)	57	5	30	14	106
Possible occupational infection (no life-style risks)	139	14	71	14	238

*Reproduced with permission of the Health Protection Agency. Occupational Transmission of HIV—summary of published reports. March 2005 edition (data to the end of December 2002). London: Health Protection Agency, March 2005.

Since 1984 five cases of occupationally acquired HIV infections in UK healthcare workers have been documented. In one case the healthcare worker seroconverted despite receiving PEP with triple therapy. A further 14 healthcare workers with probable occupational acquisition have been diagnosed in the UK. These had no risk factor other than an occupational exposure but they did not have a baseline HIV negative test; 13 of these healthcare workers worked in countries of high HIV prevalence.[30]

Some of the cases in Table 23.5 were reported to voluntary national surveillance schemes. Others were case reports from a variety of other sources. It is likely that the table underestimates the actual number of occupational infections, particularly in those developing countries with poor infection control practices and reporting systems, but a high prevalence of HIV in the general population.

Despite awareness of the risk among UK healthcare workers, accidental exposure to blood continues to occur. Over a recent 7-year period 150 centres participating in a national voluntary surveillance scheme reported 551 occupational exposures to HIV with one seroconversion.[31] Such exposures can cause great anxiety to employees. Procedures for reporting and managing blood exposure incidents should be set up and publicized widely within the workplace.

Postexposure prophylaxis

There is evidence from a case-referent study that a reduction in the rate of HIV seroconversion after HIV positive needlestick injury occurs when zidovudine is given.[32] Since 1997 UK guidance, produced by the government's Expert Advisory Group on AIDS (EAGA), has recommended the use of three antiretroviral drugs as postexposure prophylaxis. At the time of writing the recommended three are: zidovudine, lamivudine, and nelfinavir.[33] These should be given within an hour of exposure if possible, but may be given up to 2 weeks after the incident. They should be given for 4 weeks, with follow-up HIV antibody testing at 6 weeks, 12 weeks, and 6 months to check for seroconversion. The regimen has significant side-effects and reports suggest that many people discontinue the treatment because of these. In the author's experience a large proportion require a period of sickness absence and this is supported by the literature.[34]

There is no requirement for exposed healthcare workers to stop exposure-prone procedures during the treatment or follow-up period, as the risk of seroconversion is so small (0.3% and lessened by suitable PEP).[33]

The latest EAGA guidance covers the question of healthcare workers and students who travel to work in countries where the prevalence of HIV is much higher than in the UK and antiretroviral drugs are not commonly available. The guidance suggests taking a 7-day starter pack of zidovudine and lamivudine with arrangements for expert phone advice on the need to continue and urgent repatriation.

RIDDOR reporting

In the UK accidental occupational exposure to HIV is reportable to the Health and Safety Executive under the Reporting of Injuries, Diseases and Dangerous Occurrences regulations 1995 (RIDDOR) as a dangerous occurrence (accidental release of biological agent likely to cause serious human illness) or injury (if three or more days off work). Reporting may be done by telephone, post or online.

Compensation for HIV infection contracted at work

Industrial injuries disablement benefit

HIV is not a prescribed disease under the Social Security Acts. However, healthcare workers who have acquired HIV because of accidental occupational exposure, e.g. needlestick, may be able to claim.[17]

NHS injury benefits scheme

The NHS injury benefits scheme provides temporary or permanent injury benefits for all NHS employees who lose remuneration because of an injury or disease attributable to their NHS employment. The scheme is also available to general medical and dental practitioners working in the NHS. Under the terms of the scheme it must be established whether, on the balance of probabilities, the injury or disease was acquired during the course of NHS work.[17]

These potential benefits support the reporting of *all* accidental blood exposures, as documentation and appropriate blood tests on both the source patient and injured staff member will not only allow access to postexposure prophylaxis and where necessary HIV treatment, but also eligibility for injury benefit schemes.

Prevention of occupational HIV transmission

Control of Substances Hazardous to Health (COSHH) Regulations

HIV, and the other blood-borne viruses, are covered by the Control of Substances Hazardous to Health (COSHH) Regulations 2002, as 'biological agent(s) ... which may cause infection'. Therefore the hierarchy of control measures applies. Of particular relevance is the COSHH principle: *Design and operate processes and activities to minimize emission, release and spread of substances hazardous to health.* Applied to HIV in the healthcare setting this can be interpreted as a need to:

* reduce invasive techniques
* use safe systems for clinical procedures
* consider safer needles
* perform laboratory work at an appropriate containment level (e.g. safety cabinets, eliminate aerosols, eliminate sharps).

Standard precautions

In the healthcare setting prevention relies on safe practice to avoid exposure to blood and body fluids. A 'standard precautions' approach should be adopted. This means that all blood is considered infectious. Precautions, to avoid needlesticks and skin or mucous membrane exposures to blood, are taken with all patients and with all blood and tissue samples. Local guidelines should be drawn up for safe practice in all situations where contact with blood or body fluids is possible. All employees who may have contact with blood or body fluids should be trained in these practices and adherence to practice guidelines should be regularly reviewed. Protective equipment and clothing, such as gloves, gowns, and eye protection should be provided as necessary. Such an approach will reduce the risk of transmission of HIV (and other blood-borne viruses such as hepatitis B and C) in both directions.

Summary

Despite a dramatic increase in disease-free survival, there has not been a corresponding increase in employment for those infected with HIV. It is likely that drug side-effects, psychological barriers, and continuing (but lessening) prejudice among employers contribute.

Occupational physicians require specialist knowledge of guidelines governing the management of HIV-infected healthcare workers. In nearly all other industries HIV-infected individuals can be managed in the same fashion as any other worker with a chronic, immunosuppressive disease.

If the development of novel drugs outstrips viral resistance, and the disabling side-effects of effective treatment reduce, the employment prospects for HIV-infected individuals, at least in developed countries, should continue to improve.

References

1 The UK Collaborative Group for HIV and STI Surveillance. *Focus on prevention. HIV and other sexually transmitted infections in the United Kingdom in 2003*. London: Health Protection Agency Centre for Infections, 2004.

2 Meheus A. Epidemiology of sexually transmitted infections and HIV in Europe. *Int J STD AIDS* 2002; **13** (Suppl. 1): 1–2.

3 Penzak SR, Reddy YS, Grimsley SR. Depression in patients with HIV infection. *Am J Health-System Pharmacy* 2000; **57**: 376–89.

4 Yeni PG *et al.* Treatment for Adult HIV Infection: 2004 Recommendations of the International AIDS Society-USA Panel. *JAMA* 2004; **292**: 251–65.

5 *British HIV Association (BHIVA) guidelines for the treatment of HIV-infected adults with antiretroviral therapy: an update*. April 2005 BHIVA Writing Committee on behalf of the BHIVA Executive Committee, 2005.

6 Communicable Diseases Surveillance Centre. AIDS and HIV infection in the United Kingdom; monthly report. The effect of highly active antiretroviral therapy (HAART) on progression to AIDS. *Commun Dis Rep (CDR) Wkly* 2000; **10**: 123–4.

7 Goldman DP, Bao Y. Effective HIV treatment and the employment of HIV +ve adults. *Health Serv Res* 2004; **39**: 1691–712.

8 Rabkin JG *et al.* (2004). Predictors of employment of men with HIV/AIDS: a longitudinal study. *Psychosomatic Med* 2004; **66:** 72–8.

9 Department for Work and Pensions. *Pathways to work: helping people into employment.* White paper November 2002. London: The Stationery Office, 2002.

10 Martin DJ *et al.* Perceived employment barriers and their relation to workforce-entry intent among people with HIV/AIDS. *J Occup Health Psychol* 2003; **8:** 181–94.

11 Dray-spira R *et al.* Socio-economic conditions, health status and employment among persons living with HIV/AIDS in France in 2001. *AIDS Care* 2003; **15**: 739–48.

12 Brooks RA *et al.* Perceived barriers to employment among persons living with HIV/AIDS. *AIDS Care* 2004; **16**: 756–66.

13 Schlecter ES. Work while receiving disability insurance benefits: additional findings from the New Beneficiary Follow up Survey. *Soc Security Bull* 1997; **60**: 3–17.

14 Lorenz KA. Associations of symptoms and health-related quality of life:Findings from a national study of persons with HIV infection. *Ann Intern Med* 2001; **134**: 854–60.

15 Pattani S, Constantinovici N, Williams S. Predictors of re-employment and quality of life in NHS staff one year after early retirement because of ill health; a national prospective study. *Occup Environ Med* 2004; **61**: 572–6.

16 *The Disability Discrimination Act 2005*. London: The Stationery Office Limited, 2005.

17 Department of Health. *HIV infected health care workers: guidance on management and patient notification*. London: UK Health Departments, 2005.

18 General Medical Council (GMC). Serious communicable diseases. London: GMC, 1997.

19 The Faculty of Occupational Medicine. *Guidance on ethics for occupational physicians*, (6th edn). London: Faculty of Occupational Medicine, 2006.

20 Meredith S *et al.* Are healthcare workers in England and Wales at increased risk of tuberculosis? *BMJ* 1996; **313**: 522–5.

21 Joint Tuberculosis Committee of the British Thoracic Society. Control and prevention of tuberculosis in the United Kingdom: Code of Practice 2000. *Thorax* 2000; **55**: 887–901.

22 Masur H, Kaplan JE, Holmes KK. Guidelines for Preventing Opportunistic Infections among HIV-Infected Persons—2002: Recommendations of the US Public Health Service and the Infectious Diseases Society of America. *Ann Intern Med* 2002; **137** (5 Pt 2; Suppl.): 435–77.

23 Department of Health. *Immunisation against infectious disease 1996—'The green book'*. London: Department of Health, 2005.

24 Hillis DM, Huelsenbeck JP. Support for dental HIV transmission. *Nature* 1994; **369**: 25–5.

25 Lot F *et al.* Probable transmission of HIV from an orthopedic surgeon to a patient in France. *Ann Intern Med* 1999; **130**: 1–6.

26 Laurie M *et al.* (1995). Investigation of patients of health care workers infected with HIV: the Centers for Disease Control and Prevention database. *Ann Intern Med* 1995; **122**: 653–7.

27 Health clearance for serious communicable diseases: new health care workers. Draft guidance for consultation. Department of Health January 2003.

28 Belza MJ. Prevalence of HIV, HTLV-I and HTLV-II among female sex workers in Spain, 2000–2001. *Eur J Epidemiol* 2004; **19**: 279–82.

29 Occupational Transmission of HIV. Summary of published reports, Dec 1999, PHLS AIDS and STD Centre at the CDSC and Collaborators. Public Health Laboratory Service, London, 1999.

30 Health Protection Agency. Occupational Transmission of HIV—summary of published reports. March 2005 edition (data to the end of December 2002). London: Health Protection Agency, March 2005.

31 Health Protection Agency Centre for Infection, National Public Health Service for Wales, CDSC Northern Ireland. *Eye of the needle. Surveillance of significant occupational exposure to bloodborne viruses in healthcare workers, seven-year report.* January 2005.

32 Cardo DM *et al.* A case-control study of HIV seroconversion in health care workers after percutaneous exposure. *N Engl J Med* 1997; **337**, 1485–90.

33 *HIV Post-exposure prophylaxis: guidance from the UK chief medical officers' expert advisory group on AIDS*. London: Department of Health, February 2004.

34 Parkin, J M *et al.* Tolerability and side-effects of post-exposure prophylaxis for HIV infection. *Lancet* 2000; **355**: 722–3.

Further reading

Natural history of HIV infection. In: *Clinical Virology*, (2nd edn) (eds Richman DD, Whitley RJ, Hayden FG). Washington DC: ASMPress, 2002.

Chapter 24

Alcohol and drugs misuse

O. H. Carlton and C. C. H. Cook

Misuse of alcohol and other drugs is of concern both to employers and to occupational physicians because it can produce an adverse effect in the workplace, be it in terms of output and performance or behaviour, such as interaction with colleagues. It also has an important impact on the health and well-being of employees and carries significant legal implications for both employees and employers. The possession of alcohol is not illegal but the possession of drugs of abuse is, and employers may be vicariously liable if employees have drugs in the workplace.

Prevalence

The largest drug abuse problem in the UK relates to the legal drug alcohol. Over 90% of adults in Britain consume alcohol. Almost 1 in 3 men and 1 in 5 women consume more than 21 and 14 units a week respectively. There are an estimated 1.2 million incidents per year of alcohol-related violence and 85 000 cases of drink driving. Alcohol-related disease accounts for 1 in 26 NHS bed days; up to 40% of all A&E admissions are alcohol-related and up to 150 000 hospital admissions per year are related to alcohol misuse.[1]

Information on the pattern of drug use for drugs other than alcohol in the general and working UK population is poor.

The British Crime Survey (BCS) is the only major source of population drug misuse information. The BCS of 2002/3 shows that it is mainly young adults who declare use of illicit drugs— 30% of 16–24 year olds and 15% of 25–24 year olds declared using illicit drugs in the previous year. This equates to approximately 12% of the working population having used illicit drugs in the previous year if the proportion of drug users in the general population of the UK (the population surveyed) is much the same as the proportion of drug users in the working population.[2] Recent research undertaken for the HSE found 13% of working respondents reporting drug use in the previous year, with an age profile of use similar to that found by BCS.[3] Cannabis is by far the most commonly used 'illicit' drug. Its use in the general population appears to be fivefold higher than any other illicit substance.[2]

A 1995 report of OPCS surveys of psychiatric morbidity[4] suggested a prevalence of drug dependency of 1.5% among workers. This was much lower than that in the unemployed (8.3%).

Impact

The use and misuse of drugs and alcohol at work is said to have an unfavourable impact on productivity, quality, and safety. The evidence to support this is variable, as discussed below.

Alcohol

The risk of causing a driving accident increases three-, 10-, and 40-fold if the blood alcohol exceeds 80, 100, or 150 mg/100 ml respectively. In fact many skills and cognitive processes begin to decline at much lower blood alcohol concentrations (BAC). In the US armed forces a blood alcohol level of 50 mg/100 ml or above indicates unfitness for duty and such a level merits disciplinary action. At this level memory transfer from immediate recall to permanent storage may be disturbed, causing impairment of long-term recall. Companies operating oil and gas rigs offshore ban alcohol completely and refuse access to the work site to anyone reporting for duty under the influence of alcohol. Studies of pilots in flight simulators indicate that performance is impaired at a BAC as low as 11 mg/100 ml, the equivalent of consuming only one standard drink.[5]

It has been shown that driving at levels below the prescribed blood alcohol level introduced in the Road Traffic Act 1967 (80 mg/100 ml) is not free from hazards. Even 'safe' levels of alcohol may be associated with significant impairment of driving ability. Drivers who have consumed moderate doses of alcohol and have BACs of 30–60 mg/100 ml have impaired ability to negotiate a test course with artificial hazards. Furthermore, it has been shown that the combination of alcohol and cannabis (see below), even at low levels, has a hazardous effect on the driving task. The impairment created by the combination of these two drugs is much greater than that created by either drug alone.

A strong association has been demonstrated between a raised gamma-glutamyl transferase (GGT) and road traffic accidents in drivers aged over 30, indicating that many of these accidents may be caused by problem drinkers. Of even greater concern is that a high prevalence of raised liver enzyme activity has also been demonstrated in those over the age of 30 who apply for licences as drivers of large goods vehicles (LGVs) and passenger carrying vehicles (PCVs).

The findings of a major review of the international literature[6] of the relationship between alcohol and occupational and work related injuries are shown in Table 24.1.

Drugs

The knowledge base of how drug impairment affects safety in the workplace remains relatively small.

Recent questionnaire research in the UK undertaken for the HSE by Cardiff University concluded that there is no association between drug use and workplace accidents. The authors argue, however, that the known effects of illegal drugs on cognitive functions such as reaction times, concentration, and memory are such that they may reduce performance, efficiency and safety at work.[3]

Two major literature reviews have concluded that there is no clear evidence of the deleterious effects of drugs, with the exception of alcohol, on safety and other job performance indicators.[2] In practice, many occupational health practitioners will be able to cite specific cases of the unfavourable impact of drug misuse by an employee on both work performance and safety, but this experience is not yet supported by published well designed studies.

Table 24.1 Relationship between alcohol and work-related injuries (from Zwerling[6] as summarized by Coomber[2])

- Acute alcohol impairment is present in about 10% of fatal occupational injuries

- Acute alcohol impairment is present in about 5% of non-transport, non-fatal, work-related injuries

- A history of alcohol abuse may be weakly associated with occupational injuries (odds ratios ranging from 1.0 to 2.58)

- The wide variety of methodological difficulties in the various studies of the association of a history of alcohol abuse and occupational injures should make the reader cautious about drawing conclusions about the data

One study reported in the Francis review of the literature drew upon data of injuries and illnesses per 100 workers by industrial classification in the years 1989–91 across 40 US States. The authors state that the 'evidence strongly suggests that the most overwhelming determinant of occupational injury is the industry of employment ... neither the legal environment of the State nor any of its demographic characteristics had any significant statistical effect on injuries'.[7]

Cannabis

There is an extensive literature on human performance under the influence of cannabis and effects on memory, attention span, and perception have been demonstrated. This has implications not only for operating complicated, heavy equipment but also for aircraft pilots, air traffic controllers, train drivers, and signalmen.

Cannabis can have an adverse effect on any complex learnt psychomotor task involving memory, skill, concentration, sense of time, orientation in three-dimensional space, and on the performance of multiple complex tasks. Cannabis impairs judgement, performance, and immediate recall, whereas alcohol tends to affect the transfer process from short- to long-term memory stores. There is no cerebellar dysfunction (slurred speech and ataxia) due to cannabis, but there is impairment of glare recovery, peripheral vision, and sense of time. Visual hallucinations and the intrusion of inappropriate memories can also occur.

Cannabis can cause temporal disorganization with disruption of the correct sequencing of events in time and work requiring a high level of cognitive integration is adversely affected. A single 'joint' of cannabis can cause measurable impairment of skills for more than 10 hours. This cognitive impairment lasts for long after the euphoria has disappeared. Psychophysiological activities impaired by cannabis include tracking ability, complex reaction time, hand steadiness, complicated signal interpretation, and attention span. There are therefore deficiencies in perception, memory, and cognition. Cannabis has a particularly deleterious effect on pilots who have to orientate themselves in three-dimensional space, which is particularly crucial for helicopter pilots.[8,9]

In the intoxicated state cannabis, like alcohol, impairs short-term memory in proportion to the dose. However, unlike alcohol, moderate cannabis use is associated with selective short-term memory deficits that persist following a period of several weeks of abstinence.

A recent review for the Department of Transport has concluded that the actual effect of cannabis on real driving performance rather than the effects measured in the laboratory are not as pronounced as would be predicted. Four to 12% of accident fatalities have detectable levels of cannabis but the majority of these cases also have detectable levels of alcohol as well. There is not sufficient knowledge concerning detectable levels of cannabis in non-fatal cases to identify a baseline for comparison. The combination of alcohol and cannabis increases impairment, accident rate, and accident responsibility and the same is true for alcohol alone.[10]

Prescribed medication

Sedative psychoactive medication, like alcohol, reduces the overall level of alertness of the central nervous system. Certain antidepressants, anxiolytics, and hypnotics have side-effects that reduce skilled performance, concentration, memory, information processing ability, and motor activity as demonstrated in both volunteers and patient populations. All these effects increase the risk of driving accidents. It is for this reason that airline pilots are prohibited from flying while taking prescribed psychotropic medication. It is also known that the use of both prescribed and illicit drugs is associated with an increased liability to road traffic accidents.[11]

The relative contributions of mental illness and psychotropic drug use as causes of accidents have not been analysed in many studies. It is possible that some mentally disturbed patients would pose a greater danger without treatment. On the other hand, after taking their drugs in normal therapeutic doses, these individuals may still present a risk to road safety. Laboratory studies on the effects of psychotropic drugs on driving-related skills of patients on long-term medication are rare. However, it has been demonstrated that patients receiving diazepam perform more poorly, exhibiting impaired visual perception and impaired anticipation of dangerous events when driving.

Laboratory assessments of the effects of psychotropic drugs on sensory and motor skills, steering, brake reaction time, divided attention, and vigilance have shown specific impairment following the administration of minor tranquillizers and tricyclic antidepressants. Similar effects have been found to persist in the morning after taking benzodiazepine hypnotics. Data from the Netherlands have shown that hypnotics, minor tranquillizers, and tricyclic antidepressants cause driving errors in real-life conditions on the open road, including a tendency to wander across the carriageway. Even fairly low doses of psychoactive drugs have a detrimental effect on the performance of car-driving tests and related measures of psychomotor ability.[12]

These detrimental effects have been demonstrated with the hypnotic nitrazepam in a dose as low as 5 mg, and with other psychotropic agents including flurazepam (30 mg), amitriptyline (50 mg), mianserin (10 mg), lorazepam (1 mg), diazepam (5 mg), and chlordiazepoxide (10 mg). The hypnotics were assessed for their residual activity the morning after night-time sedation, whereas the effects of the antidepressants and anxiolytics were measured during the day. The amnesic effect of some benzodiazepines is such that drivers fail to remember routines and cannot read maps competently.

The sleep disturbance caused by jet lag might lead pilots or other people whose work requires vigilance, motor skill, and a high level of decision-making to take a hypnotic. A benzodiazepine with a short half-life might appear to be an attractive option because of the reduction of daytime sedation, but amnesia may persist after the sedation has disappeared. For sedatives or hypnotics, the available data show that their use could more than double the risk of road accidents.

Whereas both amitriptyline and dothiepin impair performance on laboratory analogues of car-driving and related skills, the serotonin reuptake inhibitor fluoxetine, in a dose of 40 mg, showed a lack of cognitive and psychomotor effects when administered in an acute dose to volunteers. However, fluoxetine has a long half-life and may, if administered to patients over a therapeutic period, cause some impairment of skill performance and car-handling ability.

Accidents

In the USA there were several critical accidents involving drugs or alcohol during the 1980s and early 1990s, which are thought to have played a part in bringing in workplace testing in safety critical industries. In May 1981 a naval aircraft crashed on an aircraft carrier. Nine of the fourteen dead had cannabinoids at autopsy testing and the pilot was identified as having taken prescribed antihistamines. In January 1987 there was a rail crash in Maryland that resulted in 16 deaths and 174 people injured. The engineer and brakeman tested positive for marijuana. As a result, testing was brought in for several types of transport workers in USA. In 1989 the grounding of the Exxon Valdez oil tanker was linked to alcohol misuse. This led to billions of dollars' worth of property and environmental damage. In 1991 a subway train in New York City derailed, killing five people. The driver had been using alcohol (see Francis et al.,[7] p. 24).

In the official report of a railway accident in Scotland (March 1974, Glasgow Central Station) it was concluded that the use of diazepam by the train driver was a contributory cause; and Scandinavian researchers have found that serum concentrations of benzodiazepines are significantly greater in drivers involved in road traffic accidents than in control groups.

Absenteeism

There is strong evidence that alcohol problems affect absenteeism. Problem drinkers have a rate of absence between two and eight times as high as non-problem drinkers.[13] The UK Government estimates that up to 17 million days are lost annually due to alcohol-related absence, costing up to £6.4 bn.[1] The Whitehall II study found that alcohol consumption, even at moderate levels, leads to increased risk for absence due to injury, but with a much weaker relationship to all other absences.[14]

Belief

The research evidence may be limited, but the belief that there are clear-cut deleterious effects of drugs and alcohol on work is very strongly held. Many employers consider that both alcohol and drug use are major causes of absenteeism. Occupational health practitioners will be able to bring cases to mind where drug misuse by an employee had a major effect on their safe working or productivity.

In a survey of drug misuse undertaken in 30 companies by Personnel Today:

- 27% reported problems of some kind
- 31% reported a negative impact on attendance
- 27% reported poor employee performance
- 3% reported damage to their business
- 3% reported accidents at work.

Drug and alcohol at work policies

Alcohol and drugs policies are introduced in order to:

- reduce the adverse effect of alcohol on the health and well-being of employees and to encourage safer and more sensible drinking
- minimize problems at work
- make employees aware of the problems
- identify employees with problems
- ensure fair and even-handed treatment
- offer early advice and access to help
- make staff aware of their responsibilities.

Even if there is no formal policy, certain things will be obvious simply by observing what is acceptable in the workplace. Taking alcohol as an example, attitudes range from permitting alcohol to be consumed at work through to a zero tolerance policy that expects employees to have no alcohol in their system during working hours. Some employers may ban alcohol at work but be tolerant of people coming to work regularly with a hangover. The employer may have a differential policy according to the type of work that the employee does. For example, employees in a large company who work closely with the media or who entertain clients may be permitted to drink while involved in this type of work whereas employees involved in work that has an impact on safe working or product safety may not be permitted to drink at work at all.

Where safety is of paramount importance to the organization it is not uncommon for a zero alcohol policy to be in place, at least for those directly involved in activities which may affect safe working or product safety.

The common elements of an alcohol policy are shown in Table 24.2.

Drugs at work policy

A policy on drugs and the workplace will be similar in many ways to the alcohol policy but will also include information on prescribed and over-the-counter drugs as well as illegal drugs. It is likely to include requirements about:

◆ Consumption, possession, storage, and selling of illegal drugs on company premises.

It may also include:

◆ a requirement not to come to work under the influence of illegal drugs;

◆ a requirement not to bring the company into disrepute by being involved in activities related to illegal drugs out of work;

◆ a requirement to find out about the side-effects of legal medication and declare the medication to the occupational health practitioner (or manager) if the side-effects could affect performance, safety, the safety of others, or the quality of the product;

◆ specific arrangements relating to young people working for the company in view of their known vulnerability in terms of likelihood of taking illegal drugs;

◆ the company's procedures as they relate to solvents, gases, glues, and aerosols.

Supplier companies of drug testing services (e.g. urine collection, breath testing, and laboratory analysis) offer help in developing such policies. It is useful to bear in mind that their policies are likely to include drug testing, which may or may not be appropriate.

Table 24.2 Common elements of an alcohol at work policy

◆ An explanation of why there is a policy

◆ The scope of the policy—who it applies to, including whether or not it applies to contractors, consultants and agencies

◆ The required code of conduct. This is likely to cover:

• consumption of alcohol while at work

• consumption of alcohol during meal breaks

and may include requirements on the following:

• consumption of alcohol while in uniform

• arrival to work (zero alcohol, hangovers)

• if testing is used, then some reference to that including the action taken when an employee has a positive test

◆ The consequences if the policy is breached

◆ Any support that the company offers to someone prepared to address an alcohol problem

◆ The responsibilities of all relevant parties

◆ The policy may also contain reference to the use of alcohol in relation to company cars and the procedure for employees who have been banned from driving due to alcohol

Implementation of a new policy

Implementation of a new alcohol and drug policy requires a careful prior assessment of the financial and other implications, and clear agreement on who will be responsible for drawing it up. The workforce should be educated about the content and the implementation of the policy, which should be carefully monitored and reviewed. In setting up company alcohol and drug policies it is essential that wide consultation is held at the draft stages, particularly with staff associations or trade unions. Their acceptance and co-operation is crucial to success and so they should be well-briefed.

Training for managers

As part of the people management training that managers are given, it is useful if training or information on awareness of drug and alcohol related issues is included. This would usually include information about the company's policy, how to recognize potential problems (see Table 24.3 below), how to arrange testing if this is available, and what support is available.

Referral to occupational health

This section assumes that the manager has access to occupational health advice. This is often not the case but this section reviews the process where it does exist.

Ideally managers will identify the warning signs described above, discuss their suspicions with the individual and refer them for assessment by occupational health.

It is common for managers who suspect a problem to find it very difficult to discuss these openly and honestly with the person concerned. Most occupational health practitioners will be familiar with the scenario in which a manager contacts them, describes behaviour that is strongly suggestive of a problem, and then suggests that they refer the person to occupational health on a pretext 'so that you can just ask about drug use or alcohol use in passing'. This is a recipe for an unsuccessful consultation.

It can be helpful to explain this. Inexperienced managers or those who are not used to having difficult conversations with their employees struggle in this type of situation. Bear this in mind and offer as much support as possible. It is helpful if the manager has had training or has access to support, perhaps from the human resource specialist, if they work for a large company. The occupational health or human resources team may have written materials to educate the manager. The manager needs to be aware that the individual may deny everything, become very

Table 24.3 Possible signs of drug and alcohol misuse

- Short-term sickness absence, especially recurrent Mondays
- Lateness
- Unkempt appearance
- Involvement in accidents and assaults
- Inappropriately aggressive behaviour
- Worsening performance
- Unreliability in someone previously reliable
- Smelling of alcohol
- Shaking/tremor/sweating
- Pinpoint or very large pupils
- Inability to concentrate

angry, make many explanations for what has been observed, accuse the manager of bullying, discrimination, etc.

In some companies there is a contractual requirement for employees to attend the occupational health department if their managers refer them. In such companies it is essential for the manager to explain to the individual what they have observed and why they are making a referral, and then confirm this in writing. Even where this occurs in an unequivocal way, the employee may deny it and state that they have no idea why they have been referred. If the manager can only request that the employee attend occupational health, and the employee refuses, the manager will need to document this and then take action without the benefit of an occupational health assessment.

Assessment for drug or alcohol misuse and addiction

The assessment is twofold, as is the case for nearly all occupational health assessments. The first part is to identify whether the employee has a significant drug or alcohol problem. The second part is to advise the employee and their manager whether they are fit to work, whether adjustments are needed or whether they are unfit to work.

These assessments are among the most challenging in occupational health practice. This is because the condition of alcohol or drug addiction is usually characterized by denial, is associated with feelings of shame and is a condition in which difficult and painful feelings are avoided, sometimes at any cost.

The assessment by the occupational health adviser usually includes taking a full history of drug or alcohol use and an examination. A variety of questionnaires may be useful—see Table 24.4. For alcohol, blood tests may assist (GGT, alanine transferase (ALT), mean corpuscular volume (MCV)) but are rarely diagnostic on their own and may be normal in employees who subsequently admit to a serious problem. Where drug and alcohol testing are available, this can also assist assessment.

In one occupational health centre that employs addiction specialists, assessment is undertaken over a period of 3 weeks, using questionnaires, assessment in a series of groups and in one to one enquiry, liver function blood tests, and breath or urine testing for alcohol and/or drugs. This is an unusually thorough provision, but gives an idea of the complexity of this area of diagnosis.[15]

The degree of alcohol and drug use and misuse lies on a spectrum, from social use not associated with harm through harmful use to dependence.

Box 24.1 Dependence syndrome[19]—seven elements of this biopsychosocial state

1 Narrowing of repertoire of drinking behaviour (so that eventually one day becomes much like another).

2 Salience of drinking behaviour over other priorities in life.

3 Tolerance to alcohol.

4 Repeated withdrawal symptoms.

5 Drinking to relieve withdrawal symptoms.

6 Rapid reinstatement of dependent drinking after a period of abstinence.

7 Subjective experience of 'compulsion' to drink.

Table 24.4 Some of the tests available for identification of alcohol or drug misuse[16–18]

◆ Substance Abuse Subtle Screening Inventory (SASSI)

◆ Michigan Alcoholism Screening Test (MAST)

◆ The Alcohol Use Disorders Identification Test (AUDIT)

◆ Diagnostic interviewing techniques

Features of denial

Alcohol or drug-dependent patients often engage in denial of the nature or extent of their problems, especially when first confronted. Such denial must be dealt with firmly but sensitively. It is rarely productive to engage in directly confrontational arguments about whether or not someone is addicted. However, carefully considered confrontation by experienced clinicians can be helpful. Such confrontation should focus on the evidence available, and on the realities of the workplace. Thus, to say 'the problem is that you have lost 12 hours work over the last month due to lateness on Monday mornings' is preferable to 'the problem is that you are obviously an alcoholic'. The former can lead to constructive discussion, which may eventually lead to admission of the underlying cause of the problem. The latter is likely to lead to outright denial, anger, and breakdown of trust.

Assessment of fitness to work

It may not be possible for the occupational health adviser to come to a conclusion in their assessment. They may need to refer the individual to an addiction specialist, or to provide pragmatic advice to the manager and individual. Where the person admits a problem and believes that they can address it, a return to full or adjusted duties may be appropriate under regular review. If the person works in a safety critical role, it may be necessary for them to be placed in a non-safety critical role or even to go off sick for the duration of assessment and treatment if it is provided. These decisions involve an assessment of risk, and the involvement of the manager and a health and safety adviser will assist the process. The permission of the individual is, of course, required to reveal the nature of the risk, but will usually be given if it means they are likely to get back to work.

Treatment of dependence

The principles of treatment are initially detoxification, followed by psychological support to enable the individual to admit they have a problem and then develop the skills to address it. Treatment may be residential in the first instance. The '12-Step' philosophy of Alcoholics Anonymous and Narcotics Anonymous is the basis of many treatment programmes. This is based on abstinence and the ongoing support of peers, through mutual help groups. However, this is not the only approach available, and is more prevalent in North America than in the UK. Professional treatment programmes, based upon psychological and medical approaches to treatment, are also available and should be considered as potentially valuable alternative resources. Matching individual patients to particular treatment philosophies is a controversial subject and research evidence provides little information upon which to base such decisions. Patient preference, and availability of treatment programmes with proven results, should therefore dictate the choice.

Return to work

It is often possible to support an employee in their return to work after treatment for addiction. In safety-related jobs this may need ongoing testing, at least for an agreed period of time.

A signed 'contract' between the manager and the employee can be helpful, giving written details of expected behaviour. It is very helpful to have the co-operation of the manager, who is usually in a position to identify signs of relapse. London Underground has a return to work programme with these ingredients. The rehabilitation programme has a success rate of 75% for employees whose condition is serious enough to merit residential treatment still at work at 1 year, and 65% are still at work 3 years later.[15] A report by the Health and Safety Laboratory cites a Civil Aviation Authority estimate that about 85% of professional pilots whose medical certification of fitness has been withdrawn for drug and alcohol problems and have undergone treatment and rehabilitation could be returned to flying.[20]

Drug and alcohol testing at work

Drug and alcohol testing in the workplace is still relatively rare in the UK but is becoming more common. A comprehensive review of the issues is given in the Independent Inquiry into Drug Testing at Work (IIDTW) published in 2004.[13]

Studies in the USA have reported that 40–50% of organizations employ some kind of testing with 85% of major firms doing so.[20] In the USA there is a government body, Substance Abuse and Mental Health Services Administration (SAMHSA), which provides guidance and regulation for the drug testing of federal employees. In Europe there is a European Workplace Drug Testing Society (EWDTS). In the UK there is the UK Workplace Drug Testing Forum, which currently has a membership almost exclusively of laboratories who undertake drug testing.

In the European Union (EU) and in particular in the UK, testing is most common in industries where at least some employees' jobs are defined as being safety critical. The IIDTW commissioned two surveys of workplace alcohol and drug testing with different findings. In a CBI study 30% of 50 firms conducted tests, whereas just 4% of the 204 firms polled by MORI did so.

Drug and alcohol testing should always form a part of a workplace alcohol and drug policy, rather than being in lieu of a policy. It follows that the decision to test, and then how to test, should be made following a risk analysis, looking at the company in question, its activities, and any legislation that may apply.

Francis et al.[7] mention the criteria which Parrott developed for employers to consider when assessing whether a programme of testing is appropriate:

- drug use poses a significant workplace problem
- testing will solve this problem
- the benefits of testing will outweigh the costs
- the response to a positive test is legally and ethically acceptable.

Evidence that testing is effective

The effectiveness of drug testing programmes depends on why they are being implemented. The usual reasons are legislative requirement (more relevant in the USA than the UK), reduction of workplace accidents and injuries, and reduction in loss through absenteeism and other forms of reduced productivity. In the USA, drug testing programmes are also considered to contribute to a societal aim for a drug-free society.

In general the evidence of benefit is inconclusive, but negative studies have often been criticized as being poorly designed. Those studies with very positive findings have been reviewed by Francis et al.[7] and some are described below.

It is argued that testing can have an impact on identifying, controlling, and suppressing corruption within police forces that deal with drug crime.

A review in the US construction industry concluded that companies undertaking testing were able to reduce injury rates by 50% over a 10-year period and that for the average company this reduction was achieved within 2 years of introducing the testing programme.

There is strong evidence of behaviour change in the US military as a result of introducing a drug testing programme. Between 1980 and 1990 the 1-month prevalence of reported drug use fell from 27.6% to 4.8% and the proportion of positive drug tests fell from 48% to 3%, although the criteria and techniques varied over this interval.

When to test?

Possible timings for testing are:

+ Pre-employment.

+ Post-accident or incident.

+ Prior to promotion or transfer. This is usual in safety critical industries when employees are first promoted or transferred into jobs with a safety critical element.

+ At random and without announcement. This is commonly used in safety critical industries, but is the most expensive and difficult testing schedule to organize. No prior warning is given to the individuals who are tested. Ideally testing is undertaken at the worksite. It usually requires a visit by a person or team acting as the collecting agent. One option is to test everyone in the workplace but it is more usual to test a sample of the workforce. This requires careful advanced planning, to ensure that the right facilities are available and it is clear who is to be tested. Usually at least one manager needs to be involved. Both staff and managers should be well informed of the procedures. An impartial method of selecting those to be tested is required. This type of testing is often known as 'random' testing, but in fact it may be semi-random, opportunistic, or systematic. Where there is a geographically dispersed workforce or it is too difficult to organize the testing on site, the employee may be advised to attend a centre and may be given a period of notice.

+ For cause or due cause—i.e. where the manager has reason to suspect that drugs or alcohol may be affecting performance or safety.

+ Voluntary testing can give an employee the opportunity to clear their name or confirm a problem for which help and support could be offered.

+ As part of an employee's rehabilitation programme in order to monitor their recovery and/or identify otherwise undisclosed relapse to drug use.

Each type of testing has its own practical and ethical issues, which need to be considered in the light of the company's overall alcohol and drugs policy.

Types of test

Alcohol screening

This can be conducted in various biological media:

+ *Breath*. This methodology is similar to that employed for roadside testing of drivers by the police, and uses validated instruments. The breath measurements can be directly related to blood measurements, which themselves can be directly related to the likely degree of impairment of performance.

+ *Urine*. Urine testing for alcohol is sometimes used for convenience if drug testing is also undertaken on a urine sample. The disadvantage is that it does not directly reflect the level of alcohol in the blood at the time of testing, but the delayed excretion of alcohol through the renal system.

◆ *Blood*. This represents the definitive measure of alcohol level and can be directly related to likely degree of impairment of performance. It is not usually used in a workplace context though, as it is too invasive.

Drug testing

Several common methods exist for drug testing:

◆ *Urine*. This is the most common and convenient form of sample collection for the purposes of drug testing in the UK.

Other approaches are less intrusive but, when testing was first introduced in the UK, there was insufficient evidence of their reliability.

◆ *Oral fluid*. This consists of a combination of secretions from salivary glands, transudates across mucosal membranes, plasma exudates, and cellular and other oral debris. It is some-times called mixed saliva. Some investigators also call the fluid collected by an absorptive instrument in the mouth oral fluid, and the fluid collected by spitting mixed saliva, but this appears to be an arbitrary distinction.

Drugs pass into oral fluid in three main ways:

• Diffusion through cells

• Ultra-filtration via pores in cell junctions

• From blood exudates via the crevice between gum and tooth

For certain drugs different metabolites are present in oral fluid compared to urine (e.g. cocaine).

The test is undertaken by either asking the employee to spit into a receptacle, or using an absorptive instrument to extract fluid from the mouth. There is evidence that some people find spitting objectionable.

◆ *Hair*. Hair samples are useful for assessing past drug use (over a period of months). They can-not detect alcohol. Hair grows at a rate of about 1 cm a month. In the workplace context it is sometimes used for monitoring abstinence during rehabilitation, but is not appropriate oth-erwise, because it is often not considered defensible to have a policy based upon an absolute ban of drug use that would include an individual's leisure time.

◆ *Sweat testing*. Patches or swipes can be used. The police have tried swipes, but did not find them to work well.

For urine, oral fluid, sweat, and hair an initial screening of the sample is undertaken using an immunoassay screening kit, looking for the presence of drug groups or specific drugs. It may be possible to obtain on-site results for urine and oral fluid; positive results must be confirmed to legal standards by laboratory testing based on mass spectrometry.

Table 24.5 summarizes the key types of drug testing and provides details of detection times and reliability.

Which method to use

A review of drug testing methods, undertaken for the Railway Safety and Standards Board by the Health and Safety Laboratory,[20] concludes that in addition to urine testing there is a justifiable case for testing oral fluids and hair. The choice of test depends on convenience cost and the aim of the testing programme.

Table 24.5 Key types of drug testing with detection times and reliability[21]

Type of test	Detection time*	Reliability
Urine	2/3 days	Most researched; has been around for 20 years; best test for cannabis use; sample needs to be stored and preserved properly; most open to fraud (substitution of samples); positive result needs laboratory confirmation.
Oral fluid	24 hours	Good for recent drug use (cannabis and opiates in particular) but a mouthwash would defeat on-site detection; samples may need refrigeration; dipsticks can be used for on-site results (e.g. can test saliva at the road side); positive tests need to be confirmed.
Sweat	24 hours to 2/3 days	Drug patches used mainly for monitoring; when worn, can detect up to a week; drug swipes can detect other use (last 24 hours) but not very reliably.
Blood	Up to 31 hours	Vulnerable to fraud; sample needs careful storage and preservation; needs laboratory analysis; on-site results not available.
Hair	1 week–18 months	Cannot detect alcohol; needs laboratory analysis.

*length of time test remains positive following drug use.

What to test for

Testing programmes in the UK usually cover amphetamines, barbiturates, benzodiazepines, cannabis, cocaine, opiates (including a specific test for heroin), methadone, and propoxyphene. The specific profile should be reviewed regularly to reflect drugs in local use. Testing laboratories and toxicologists with an interest in drug misuse can provide useful advice.

LSD is only found in the urine for 12 hours after use. Heroin is not normally identified more than 24 hours after use. Cocaine and amphetamines can be found in the urine for between 2 and 4 days after use. Cannabis can be found up to 5 days after use in a casual occasional user but can be found up to 30 days after discontinuation of use in a former heavy user. Benzodiazepines are found for 3 days after short-term use, but up to 6 weeks after long-term chronic use.

Cut-off levels

The cut-off levels for positivity differ between international authorities. For example, in the USA SAMHSA has set a much higher cut off-level for opiates in urine (2000 ng/ml) than is set in Europe (300 ng/ml). (This is to allow for the possibility of poppy seed in the diet).

Chain of custody

One key aspect of drug testing is to maintain the 'chain of custody'. This is a process that ensures results can indisputably be connected with the person who produced the test sample. It includes the requirement for secure storage of samples. The procedures are based on those used for handling forensic samples.

Medical Review Officer

The Medical Review Officer (MRO) is a doctor who can issue a negative report for a positive analytical result.[20] Where a drug test is classified as positive following laboratory analysis, good practice requires that medical review is arranged. The purpose of this is to tell the individual of the result and confirm that the positive result came from a drug, usually an illicit drug, which was not prescribed by the GP or other specialist. This advice is based on consultation with the individual, their GP, the laboratory toxicologist, and any information provided at the time the test was undertaken.

This stage is an important check. Codeine use for example often results in a positive analytical test but a negative report following MRO review.

The experience, skills, and knowledge to undertake the MRO role are covered by US guidelines; as yet these are not well defined in Europe. Training courses on medical review are available in the UK, usually provided by laboratories that undertake the analysis for drug testing.

Interpretation of results

The interpretation of results for drug tests cannot usually be taken further than confirmation that the drug was taken. Unlike alcohol, it is not usually possible to relate the result to a quantitative estimate of the degree of impairment of performance at the time at which testing was conducted. A positive result may indicate a large dose taken some time ago or a small dose taken recently, and often it is not possible to establish which of these is the case. One of the underlying objections to the use of drug testing in the workplace is the problem of interpretation.

One of the arguments for using oral fluid testing for drugs, rather than urine testing, is that the tests remain positive for a much shorter time and are therefore more likely to be associated with actual impairment in the workplace.

Management of a positive result

The consequences of a positive result, confirmed by the MRO, will depend on the policy of the employer. It can range from no action being taken, through the provision of assistance in addressing an alcohol or drug problem to disciplinary action leading to loss of job. **It is important that the employer has decided and communicated to employees the consequences of a positive drug test before drug testing is introduced.**

Role of occupational health departments in a drug and alcohol testing programme

There is debate in Europe as to whether occupational health teams should be involved in drug and alcohol testing in the workplace. There is a school of thought that acting in a policing capacity may compromise the team's position of trust. On the other hand, the occupational health team is well placed to ensure that the process is undertaken in a fair way and to acceptable professional standards.

Drug screening programmes require medical involvement and if the occupational health team is involved the following points should be considered.

In pre-employment screening, which can be done at the same time as the standard new entrant medical assessment, the drug screening process should be regarded as a management responsibility, delegated to the occupational health department. Separation of function can be achieved by separately reporting results so that the drug screening test is not perceived as part of the clinical procedure. It is then possible for a candidate to meet the medical fitness requirements of the post applied for, but fail to be offered the job by management because of a positive drug screening test.

However, the distinction from other aspects of medical assessment for work fitness may be regarded as artificial.

In 'for cause' and unannounced or random screening, the role of the occupational health department should, ideally, be more detached. Both might be considered as 'policing' activities that could compromise the rehabilitation role of the occupational health department in cases of alcohol and drug misuse. The best means of overcoming this objection is for the collection of samples to be undertaken by a separate organization, possibly external to the company. The occupational physician can help to select the contractor and set up the necessary procedures for sample collection. However, after this, it is often best that the only direct involvement of the occupational health department is to receive the screening results and report them to the employees and to line managers. In this way the occupational health department will be more securely placed to implement an appropriate rehabilitation programme in accordance with company policy.

In addition to the need to maintain strict impartiality in the implementation of the alcohol and drugs policy, the occupational physician also has an active part to play in reporting results, if they provide the MRO role. This role is crucially important as discussed earlier.

Cost of drug screening programmes

In one federal testing programme in the USA, only 0.53% of 30 000 employees tested positive in a programme that cost $11.7 million. So the average cost to identify each positive case was $77 000.[7]

Table 24.6 Helpful hints for occupational practitioners advising an employer on 'random' drug testing

- Consult current guidance from the UK Faculty of Occupational Medicine
- Refer to, or advise the need for, a company workplace alcohol and drug policy
- Consider whether or not unannounced testing supports the policy
- If so, decide who will be subject to testing
- Involve trade union representatives in the decision-making process at an early stage
- Consider the legal and personnel implications, including the need to change employment contracts
- Discuss relevant issues with testing laboratories
- Decide how to conduct the testing and who will undertake testing (some laboratories provide on-site testing teams)
- Consider how to organize the chain of custody
- Agree who holds the records, how to manage confidentiality, who communicates the results to managers, e.g.:
  - managed through the occupational health department
  - managed through human resources
  - results go straight from laboratory to manager
- Sort out medical review arrangements for positive drug tests
- Agree with the business how to manage positive test results (will the employee be subject to disciplinary action, offered help, or some other action?)
- Agree what communications and training will be provided and ensure that this is carefully managed
- Consider what, if any, support will be given to those who have problems and how to provide it

Testing for impairment

As discussed above, breathalyser testing for alcohol can be related to impaired performance, but the same is not true of the results of most other types of testing for drugs in the workplace. Direct tests of impairment would be more acceptable, and could be followed up with a drug test if impairment were demonstrated. The IIDTW gives examples of tests currently being trialled in the USA:

- A computer test of judgement and response time.
- A test of the response of a controlled dose of light to the eye against an established baseline for that person.
- A computer reaction test, used before every shift against an established baseline for that person.

In view of the robust views of the Information Commissioner that drug and alcohol testing must always be justified and that the least invasive method must be used to achieve the aims, (see section on Data Protection Act below) tests of impairment may well become more common in the UK.

Summary of IIDTW findings

A UK-based Independent Inquiry into Drug Testing at Work was set up by the Joseph Rowntree Foundation and the Network of European Foundations.[13] Sixteen commissioners considered evidence from a wide range of professionals and experts during a period of 18 months of work. The report was published in 2004. The key findings and recommendations are given below. Many will look familiar because much of this chapter has been informed by the comprehensive literature reviews that were commissioned for the report.

Key findings

- There is inconclusive evidence on links between drug use and accidents at work/absenteeism/low productivity/poor performance.
- There is a lack of evidence for a strong link between drug use and accidents in safety critical industries.
- Evidence suggests alcohol is a greater cause for concern in the workplace than illicit drugs.
- There is no clear evidence that drug testing at work has a deterrent effect on drug use.
- Drug testing is not a measure of current intoxication.
- Empowering employers to investigate private behaviour actively (especially where there are no safety issues) is in conflict with liberal values.
- The legal position on drug testing at work is confused and possibly vulnerable to challenges under the Human Rights Act 1998 and the Data Protection Act 1998.
- Little is known about the extent of drug testing at work in the UK. A small survey by the Inquiry showed 4% of companies surveyed currently conducting drug tests and 9% intended to introduce drug tests.
- Drug testing is costly.

Recommendations

- Employers have a legitimate interest in drug and alcohol use among employees only where:
  - Illegal activities are being engaged in at work or where engagement in illegal activity outside of work would affect suitability for employment in a particular capacity (e.g. in the police force).
  - Employees are intoxicated at work.

- Drug and/or alcohol use is having a demonstrable and unacceptable impact on performance.
- Where the nature of the work requires strict avoidance of accidents (e.g. aviation).
- Where the public might reasonably expect and be entitled to assurance that employees are not using drugs (e.g. aviation, medical personnel, PSV and HGV drivers, train drivers, nuclear power station workers, etc.).

- There is a need for continued research, monitoring, and analysis of the impact of drug testing at work.
- Improvements are needed in systems of laboratory accreditation.
- Government guidance is needed.
- If employees have drug and alcohol problems, this should not be an automatic trigger for dismissal.
- Workplace drugs and alcohol policies should only be introduced after proper consultation with staff.
- For most businesses, investment in management training and systems is likely to have more impact on safety, performance, and productivity than introducing drug testing at work.

Data Protection Act

Part 4 of the Data Protection Act's employment practices data protection code provides recommendations on how organizations can meet the requirements of the Data Protection Act through the adoption of good practice when obtaining and handling information about workers' health.[22] These recommendations are based on the ethical principles of autonomy, integrity, beneficence, fairness and justice.

The key recommendations are given below:

- Before obtaining information through drug or alcohol testing, ensure that the benefits justify any adverse impact, unless the testing is required by law.
- Minimize the amount of personal information obtained through drug and alcohol testing.
- Ensure the criteria used for selecting workers for testing are justified, properly documented, adhered to and are communicated to workers.
- Restrict random testing to those workers who are employed to work in safety critical activities.
- Focus on safety at work, rather than the illegal use of substances in a worker's private life.
- Ensure that workers are fully aware that drug or alcohol testing is taking place, and of the possible consequences of being tested.
- Ensure that information is only obtained through drug and alcohol testing that is:
  - of sufficient technical quality to support any decisions or opinions that are derived from it;
  - subject to rigorous integrity and quality control procedures; and
  - conducted under the direction of, with positive test results interpreted by, a person who is suitably qualified and competent in the field of drug testing.

Conclusions

The management of work-related drug and alcohol problems and misuse requires careful consideration, a high level of people management skills and up to date knowledge of what is good practice. It is an area where even the most experienced managers, occupational health specialists, and addiction specialists sometimes struggle. It is important that processes are carefully developed and then regularly reviewed with full involvement of all stakeholders.

Resources

Publications

There are several recent significant publications of note:

- Independent Inquiry and the two literature reviews.[2,7,13]
- Review of Drug Testing Methodologies by HSL, commissioned by RSSB.[20]
- Proposed guidelines for USA federal employee testing from SAMSHA.[23]
- Information Commissioners' guidance on Employment Practices Data Protection Code, specifically dealing with information about workers' health.[22]

Drug and alcohol policy development

Guidance on workplace drugs and alcohol policy development can be found in HSE[24] and HSL[25] publications and on the websites of the Northern Ireland DHSS (www.dhsspsni.gov.uk) and the Drugs and Alcohol Workplace Service (www.alcoholconcern.org.uk). An international perspective is given by the International Labour Organization, which provides information on resources and reports about workplace drug policies (www.ilo.org).

For information on recognizing the effects and risks of drugs, consult the National Drugs Helpline tel.: 0800 77 66 00. Websites: www.ndh.org.uk or www.trashed.co.uk

References

1 UK Government Strategy Unit National Harm Reduction Strategy—Interim Analysis Executive Summary *http://www.number-10.gov.uk/output/Page77.asp* 2003

2 Coomber R. *A literature review for the independent inquiry into drug testing at work* (IIDTW.) Available from Drugscope, 2003.

3 Smith A, Wadsworth E, Moss S, Simpson S. The scale and impact of illegal drug use by workers. *HSE Res Rep 293*. 2004.

4 Melzer H, Gill B, Pettigrew M, Hinds K. *OPCS surveys of psychiatric morbidity in Great Britain. Report 1 the prevalence of psychiatric morbidity among adults living in private households*. HMSO: London, 1995.

5 Davenport M, Harris D. The effect of low blood alcohol levels on pilot performance in a series of simulated approach and landing trials. *Int J Aviat Psychol* 1992; **2**: 271–280.

6 Zwerling C. *Current practice and experience on drug and alcohol testing in the workplace*. Geneva: International Labor Office, 1993.

7 Francis P, Hanley N, Wray D. *A literature review on the international state of knowledge of drug testing at work, with particular reference to the US*. Available from Drugscope.

8 Calder IM, Ramsey J. A survey of cannabis use in offshore rig workers. *Br J Addict* 1987; **82**: 159–61.

9 Yesavage JA, Leirer VO, Denari M, Hollister LE. Carry-over effects of marijuana intoxication on aircraft pilot performance: a preliminary report. *Am J Psychiatry* 1985; **142**: 1325–9.

10 *Cannabis and driving: a review of the literature and commentary (12)*. Department for Transport Report (2003) available from www.dft.gov.uk

11 Skegg DCG, Richards SM, Doll R. Minor tranquillisers and road accidents. *BMJ* 1979; **1**: 917–19.

12 Hindmarch I. The effects of psychoactive drugs on car handling and related psychomotor ability. In: *Drugs and driving* (eds O'Hanlon JF, de Gier JJ), pp. 71–9. London: Taylor and Francis, 1986.

13 Report of Independent Inquiry into Drug Testing at Work, Joseph Rowntree Foundation Drug and alcohol research programme, 2004. pdf ISBN 1 85935 212 X available from www.jrf.org.uk; paperback ISBN 1 85935 211 1 Available from York Publishing Services Ltd.

14 Head J, Martikainen P, Kumari M, Kuper H, Marmot M. Work environment, alcohol consumption and ill-health The Whitehall II Study. *HSE Contract Res Rep 422*, 2002.

15 London Underground Drug and Alcohol Assessment and Treatment Service.

16 Miller FG. SASSI: application and assessment for substance-related problems. *J Substance Misuse* 2: 163–6.

17 Poorny AD, Miller BA, Kaplan HB. The brief MAST: a shortened version of the Michegan Alcoholism Screening Test. *Am J Psychiatry* 1972; **129**,: 342–5.

18 Babor TF, de la Fuente JR, Saunders J, Grant M. *AUDIT The Alcohol Use Disorders Identification Test. Guidelines for use in primary health care*. Geneva: World Health Organisation, 1992.

19 Edwards G, Gross MM. Alcohol dependence: provisional description of a clinical syndrome. *BMJ* 1976; **i**: 1058–61.

20 Akrill P, Mason H. Review of Drug Testing Methodologies, prepared for Railway Safety and Standards Board. Health and Safety Laboratory HE, 2005: 04/04.

21 Fact Sheet. *DrugLink* March/April 2004; **19**(2). Reproduced in the IIDTW.

22 Information Commissioner. *The Employment Practices Data Protection Code: Part 4 Information about Workers' Health*. Wilmslow Cheshire: Information Commissioner, 2004.

23 Substance Abuse and Mental Health Services Administration. Proposed revisions to mandatory guidelines for federal workplace drug testing programs. *Fed Reg* 2004: **69**(71): 19673–732.

24 HSE/*Drugs misuse at work: a guide for employers*. HSE INDG91 rev2 8/01 C100. Suffolk: HSE Books, 2001.

25 West NG, Stephens R. *Review of literature on developing a workplace substance misuse policy, in HSL reports*. Sheffield: Health and Safety Laboratory, 1999.

Chapter 25

Medication

I. G. Rennie and G. T. McInnes

Most people at work do not take regular medication. However, many people work while taking medication and many can only work because of their medication. Additionally, many people have to take medication because of their work, e.g. those who travel regularly to areas of the world where malaria is endemic.

The benefits of being at work must be balanced against the risks of side-effects and other consequences of taking medication, or the health consequences of omitting the medication altogether. There are very few studies that help in making such an assessment. Moreover, most treatments are ordered by general practitioners and hospital doctors who rarely have sufficient knowledge of the patients' work and working environment to assess the consequences of any incompatibility between medication and work.

The risks associated with alcohol and medication, particularly psychotropic drugs, impairing performance, skills, and memory have led to particular concerns for those taking such drugs[1] (see Chapter 24). As a consequence the World Health Organization (1983) gave advice and guidance in a booklet (*Drugs, driving and traffic safety*). This publication is concerned with drugs and driving; such advice is also relevant to those who fly aircraft, operate machinery or perform skilled tasks, and those who must remain vigilant at a workstation.

Frequency of use of medication in society

Use of medicines continues to rise in all developed countries. In 1963, the average number of prescriptions per head for UK National Health Service patients was 4.6; in 2002 it was estimated to be 12.1.[2] This estimate covers the entire population, however, and the extent of drug consumption among those at work has rarely been investigated. A study in the 1970s[3] indicated that 55% of a sample general population had taken or used some medication during the 24 hours before the interview, whereas a study by Rennie in 1984[4] indicated that 20% of a factory population were taking medication. A study by Swales[5] in 1999 reviewing medication taken by employees at a chemical plant found 21.9% had taken prescription only medication and 26.8% over-the-counter medication in the 2 weeks prior to the study.

The frequency of drug taking within a working population is dependent on a number of factors, in particular age and sex. Prescribing patterns have changed over the decades. In 1985, Lader[6] found that psychotropics were the most commonly taken drugs in a female working population. At the same time, in a mainly male population cardiovascular drugs, especially β-blockers, were commoner.[4] In the Swales[5] study, the most common prescription medications taken by 10.2% of the study group were antibiotics followed by β-blockers (9.1%) then non-opiod analgesics and angiotensin-converting enzyme (ACE) inhibitors (7.1%). For males β-blockers and antibiotics (10.1%) followed by ACE inhibitors (7.9%) were most common. For females oral contraceptives (33.3%) were most common. The study showed the number of prescription only medication drugs used increased with age. For over-the-counter medication, analgesics formed 50.1%, cold remedies 13.8% and indigestion remedies 10.8%. Over-the-counter medication use decreased with advancing age. Many of these drugs can affect performance adversely.

Age of the working population: impact on medication at work

Although 65 years is currently considered the normal retirement age, government predictions suggest increasing numbers of older individuals will need to remain in employment. Furthermore, many choose for a variety of reasons to continue working to supplement their pensions. Such a trend will inevitably lead to increasing numbers of people at work taking medication for a variety of conditions. In addition the Labour Force Survey[7] predicted that by 2001 the number of employees in the 45–59 age group would have increased by 900 000 on account of demographic changes, resulting in a group forming just under one-third of the total workforce. In contrast the population of employees in the 16–24 age group was predicted to fall from 23% in 1984 to 14% in 2001 primarily due to young people remaining longer in higher education. This change in working population with older people at work will result in more people at work taking medication.

Clinical aspects affecting work capacity

Unwanted effects of medication fall into two main categories: those that are predictable and usually dose-related, and those that are unpredictable and not usually dose-related.[8] In addition, unwanted effects may result from interactions with other drugs, with alcohol, and with other chemical substances which may be encountered at work. Of particular concern to the patient at work are effects on performance, especially for those who operate machinery, drive vehicles, or fly aircraft, or whose sound judgement or vigilance is imperative. Some drugs may produce particular problems for patients in specific jobs. Any doctor prescribing medication, or any occupational physician reviewing an individual returning to work, should consider whether there might be hazards to the patient from drug effects, e.g. slowing of reaction time, drowsiness, or altered thermoregulatory systems. In addition, because people differ in their response to drugs, particularly in reactions to psychoactive drugs, any potentially dangerous occupation should be avoided for at least a week after starting such therapy. Thereafter, treatment can be reviewed.

The Disability Discrimination Act 1995 and medication

To qualify within the scope of the Disability Discrimination Act 1995 (DDA), an employee must have, or have had, a physical or mental impairment causing a substantial and long-term adverse effect on their ability to carry out normal day to day activities. Long-term means that the impairment must have lasted for, or be likely to last for, 12 months or more.

The use of medication and the successful control of a disability by medication does not invalidate the protection afforded to such people by the DDA. Examples such as diabetes and epilepsy were considered during the committee stage of the Act. In addition, whereas drug addiction is normally excluded from the Act, any addiction that was originally the result of administration of medically prescribed drugs or other medical treatment is covered by the Act.

The DDA requires employers to make reasonable adjustments to enable qualifying employees to remain at work. Such adjustments may require alterations in working hours or type of work if the effects of the medication lead to problems at work. The employer needs to consider the requirement of the Health and Safety at Work Act etc. (HSAWA) in reviewing whether it is possible to make 'reasonable adjustments' to the job and not place the individuals taking the medication at risk to themselves or others.

General effects of medication on performance

Circadian rhythm

Changes in performance occur naturally as part of the circadian rhythm. Scores for most simple tasks rise during the day to a peak between 12.00 and 21.00 hours and fall to a trough between 03.00 and 06.00[9] correlating with body temperature. During the day increased arousal partly compensates for the effect of prolonged work, whereas at night the normal circadian decrease in alertness may aggravate the effect. Problems may occur in shiftwork, submarines, and aircraft and be aggravated by crossing time zones; the actions of drugs that affect performance may be additive in such circumstances.

There is also evidence that the absorption and elimination, as well as the pharmacological effect, of some drugs are influenced by circadian rhythms. For example, blood levels of amitriptyline are higher after a morning dose than an evening dose and this difference is associated with greater sedative and anticholinergic effects.[10] The mechanism is unknown, as is the relevance to shiftworkers.

In patients on long-term corticosteroid treatment, suppression of the hypothalamic–pituitary–adrenal axis can be minimized by giving the steroid as a single daily dose in the early morning, after the diurnal peak of adrenocorticotrophic hormone secretion, which occurs just prior to waking. In long-term night workers the diurnal rhythm is reversed, and the steroid should then be given in the evening, immediately on waking.

Testing drugs to assess their effect on performance

Drug testing is complex and time consuming. Tests fall into two main categories: those that measure the effects of drugs on individual components of psychomotor function, and those that measure their effects on activities of everyday life, such as car driving. Assessing the effects of drugs on real-life activities has many problems, but there is now much evidence that some laboratory tests of psychomotor function correlate well with, for example, driving ability. The components of psychomotor function measured by laboratory tests include cognitive information processing, short-term memory and learning, motor function, and activities involving sensory, central, and motor abilities. Such well-controlled psychopharmacological tests can now indicate with reasonable reliability those drugs that may affect regular activities such as driving and operating machinery.[11,12]

Laboratory testing in carefully placebo-controlled conditions has been used to assess the effects of various benzodiazepine hypnotics and antihypertensive drugs in airforce pilots. This has led to recommendations that are discussed in later sections. In theory, similar approaches could be used to screen workers taking essential long-term medication such as anticonvulsants in professions where safety is critical, e.g. train drivers, air traffic controllers, or even doctors, or where impaired cognitive function may have major commercial consequences, e.g. company executives or accountants. However, marked variability in responses between individuals greatly reduces the precision of such tests and only gross abnormalities are likely to be detected with confidence. Laboratory assessments therefore have a limited role in determining suitability for a particular employment.

Effects of environmental chemicals on drug response

Most drugs are inactivated by detoxification in the liver. Drug metabolism can be affected by factors that increase or reduce the activity of the responsible hepatic enzyme systems. Many environmental chemicals have been shown to be enzyme inducers, which increase the rate of metabolism of many drugs in animals. These include polycyclic aromatic hydrocarbons and organochlorine and other pesticides. Studies of workers engaged in pesticide manufacture have demonstrated enzyme induction,[13] but its practical importance is unknown. Organochlorine use is reduced but they continue to be used in the developing world.

In theory, any drug metabolized by the liver might be involved in such interactions but examples most likely to be relevant in the work environment include warfarin, sulphonylureas, and cyclosporin. The main danger arises when exposure to the enzyme-inducing agent is discontinued with the result that plasma concentrations increase and toxicity can occur.

Unlike organochlorine compounds the more widely used organophosphorus compounds inhibit enzymes, in particular the enzyme cholinesterase; exposure to such compounds may affect virtually all organ systems. Short-term depression of cholinesterase activity can be produced by a number of drugs, e.g. atropine, caffeine, codeine, morphine, theophylline, folic acid, and vitamin K.[14]

Effects on work capacity

Drugs that primarily affect the central nervous system (CNS) causing lethargy and drowsiness are likely to reduce work capacity. However, other commonly prescribed drugs, such as β-blockers, can also affect the capacity to work.

Effects on adaptation to extremes of temperature

The human body temperature is maintained within limits of ±0.5°C, despite wide ambient changes superimposed on the circadian rhythm, which is individually consistent.[15] Drugs that affect the control of body temperature may place patients at risk if they are working in an inhospitable environment. Drugs can influence body temperature either by interfering directly with effector pathways or through the central control of temperature.

Effector pathways

Sweating provides coarse control of heat loss; it is under cholinergic control and hence may be diminished by drugs with anticholinergic (antimuscarinic or atropine-like) properties. Thus antiparkinsonism agents, antihistamines, tricyclic antidepressants, and neuroleptics such as chlorpromazine can cause heat intolerance. However, as most of these drugs cross the blood–brain barrier their effects on body temperature may also involve central effects.

Cutaneous blood flow is responsible for the fine control of heat loss, and drugs that act on the peripheral sympathetic nervous system, e.g. α-adrenoreceptor antagonists such as doxazosin; and those that act on the vasculature, e.g. direct vasodilators such as hydralazine, and calcium antagonists such as nifedipine, may impair the vasomotor response to cold exposure. Normally, however, reflex mechanisms compensate for these effects.

The cutaneous vasoconstriction that occurs following administration of β-adrenoreceptor antagonists does not affect body temperature but may cause local signs and symptoms such as cold extremities, chilblains, and Reynaud's phenomenon. Those working in cold environments should be warned of potential side-effects, and the suitability of such work for individuals requiring β-blockers must be assessed.

Central mechanisms

Virtually all drugs with cerebral depressant properties may alter thermoregulation when given in sufficient doses. Body temperature is influenced by the surroundings. The mechanisms involved are complex. In therapeutic doses barbiturates, benzodiazepines, and neuroleptics may all impair central temperature regulation. Tricyclic antidepressants and monoamine oxidase inhibitors may precipitate hyperthermia both singly, and more commonly, in combination.

Effects due to occupational exposure to central nervous system depressants

Employees who work with solvents (e.g. in degreasing plants, printing, paint spraying, or with adhesives) and those who work in atmospheres where there may be a potential build-up of gases or fumes that can depress the CNS may be at risk; this risk may be potentiated if they also take medications which depress the CNS. Safe exposure levels at work are based on occupational exposure limits: these have been derived from animal experiments and experiments on humans who are not on medication. An interaction with the CNS depressant action of medication may place the treated worker at increased risk.

Hypnotics and sedatives

Hypnotic and sedative drugs are all CNS depressants and most have been shown to inhibit psychomotor function, retard responsiveness, and impair motor skills, co-ordination, and responses concerned with self-preservation. As a result, such drugs may affect the ability to drive or operate machinery. Moreover, the hangover effects of a night dose may impair driving and other skilled tasks the following day. The duration of effect after a single dose depends on the plasma half-life of the drug and on the dose, but most hypnotics produce residual effects the following morning. Effects on psychomotor function persist during long-term administration, although some tolerance or habituation occurs. These are more marked in elderly patients and are potentiated by alcohol.

Barbiturates have a greater effect on performance than benzodiazepines do and should not be used in patients who drive or operate machinery. Long-term barbiturates have a very limited role in modern therapeutics. These drugs are not recommended as hypnotics or anxiolytics.

The individual benzodiazepines differ in effects on psychomotor performance. When used as hypnotics, short-acting drugs such as temazepam and lormetazepam are less likely than nitrazepam, flunitrazepam, and flurazepam to produce effects the following morning. When used during the day as an anxiolytic, clobazam appears to have less effect on performance than other benzodiazepines. However, all these drugs can affect performance in susceptible patients and differences are of degree only. Benzodiazepines and newer hypnotics and anxiolytics such as zolpidem, zopiclone, and buspirone may cause dizziness, light-headedness, and vertigo, confusion, visual disturbances, and amnesic effects, which are to a certain extent independent of sedative actions. Lorazepam and diazepam severely affect performance in memory-based tests. Less is known about other benzodiazepines but some, e.g. clobazam, appear to have less effect on memory. Effects on memory are unlikely to produce problems when benzodiazepines are used as nocturnal hypnotics but the effects of daytime use on immediate memory could affect performance in a wide range of activities. Temazepam, because of its short activity time, is the only hypnotic approved by the Royal Air Force for use in pilots.

A study from Dundee[16] on the association of road traffic accidents with benzodiazepine use has proved useful guidance as to the risk of using such medication not only for drivers but also, potentially, for those working in other hazardous situations. This study found a significant increase in the risk of having a road traffic accident among those in the study population taking anxiolytic benzodiazepines; users of hypnotic benzodiazepines were not at increased risk (probably because they had little residual pharmacological effect the next day). However, the short-acting hypnotic zopiclone, included in the study because it acts on the same receptors as benzodiazepines even though it is a cyclopyrrolone rather than a benzodiazepine, did have residual effects that impaired car-driving. There was no increase in road traffic accident rates among users of tricyclic antidepressant medication or selective serotonin re-uptake inhibitors.

It is likely that anxiolytic benzodiazepine exposure is causally related to road traffic accidents and that those using long half-life anxiolytic benzodiazepines and zopiclone should be advised not to drive.

Particular problems can arise when these drugs are stopped. Benzodiazepine withdrawal can produce a characteristic syndrome of anxiety, sleeplessness, perpetual disturbances, depersonalization, and general malaise. When severe, these effects can markedly impair work performance.

Barbiturates can interfere with central thermoregulation, and this may occasionally be a problem with benzodiazepines.

Antipsychotics

The antipsychotics include: the phenothiazines, such as chlorpromazine; the butyrophenones, such as haloperidol; and similar drugs, such as pimozide and fluspirilene, which are used mainly to treat schizophrenia and other psychotic illnesses. Many of these drugs impair psychomotor performance and the degree to which they do so probably depends on the degree of sedation produced. Thus, flupenthixol and low doses of sulpiride, which have a predominantly alerting effect, may have less effect on performance than the more sedative phenothiazines such as chlorpromazine. Psychotic patients show impairment of psychomotor function even without drugs and in some this will be improved by treatment. This needs to be considered when advising such patients about the possible risks of working or driving while taking antipsychotic medication. Lithium probably has little effect on performance, though impairment of some laboratory tests of psychomotor functions has been described.

The extrapyramidal side-effects of antipsychotic drugs, particularly tremor, may interfere with precision work and affect driving. Lithium rarely produces extrapyramidal effects but commonly produces tremor. Postural hypotension may cause problems, particularly in hot environments. Patients taking lithium should maintain an adequate fluid consumption and avoid dietary changes which might alter sodium intake.

Interference with temperature regulation is more profound than with the hypnotic/sedative drugs. Neuroleptics interfere both with hypothalamic temperature regulation and with cholinergic control of sweating. Either hyperthermia or hypothermia can occur when environmental temperatures are extreme.

Chlorpromazine and thioridazine can cause visual disturbances through various mechanisms. The antimuscarinic effects of chlorpromazine may result in blurred vision; corneal and lens opacities may occur during chronic high-dose therapy. Pigmentary retinopathy with thioridazine is associated with reduced visual acuity.

Antidepressants

Many antidepressants produce sedation, especially at the start of treatment and this is markedly potentiated by alcohol. Psychomotor impairment has been demonstrated and seems to be related to the sedative effect. Of the tricyclic antidepressants, amitriptyline, doxepin, mianserin, trazodone, and trimipramine are the most sedative and imipramine, nortriptyline, protriptyline, and viloxazine the least. Monoamine oxidase inhibitors usually have a stimulant effect although phenelzine can sometimes be sedative. The newer serotonin reuptake inhibitors such as fluoxetine and paroxetine do not usually produce sedation and appear to have little effect on performance. As tolerance to the sedative effects develops, it seems sensible to advise patients not to drive or to undertake work that could be affected by sedation during the first few days of treatment with the more sedative agents.

Tremor due to antidepressants may be a problem in some types of work. Many antidepressants produce blurring of near vision, which may affect driving and the performance of other tasks. Those with anticholinergic (antimuscarinic) effects interfere with sweating and can also affect central temperature regulation. All can produce postural hypotension, but this is more likely to occur with the monoamine oxidase inhibitors and with imipramine and amitriptyline than with nortiptyline or some of the newer antidepressants, such as mianserin or maprotiline.

Antihistamines and anticholinergic (antimuscarinic) anti-emetics

The tendency of these drugs to cause blurred vision, sedative effects, and the potentiating effect of alcohol are well recognized. The effects vary, depending on individual susceptibility and the properties of the individual drugs. Antihistamines that produce less blurred vision and sedation, such as desloratidine and terfenadine, should be used where driving cannot be avoided as such more modern drugs tend to have less side-effects. Otherwise, patients should be warned that their ability to drive or operate machinery is likely to be impaired. Although it produces some sedation, hyoscine is thought to have less effect on driving skills than most antihistamines and is the anti-emetic of choice for drivers with travel sickness.

Stimulants and appetite suppressants

Amphetamines and other stimulants increase risk-taking behaviour and can be expected to diminish work performance and driving safety, especially if combined with alcohol. Fenfluramine produces sedation but its effects on psychomotor function are unknown.

It should be remembered that theophylline and related substances have stimulant properties. Tremor, dizziness, anxiety, agitation, insomnia, visual disturbances, and even seizures are well recognized side-effects of the theophylline and related substances.

Analgesics and anti-inflammatory drugs

The more powerful opioid analgesics, such as morphine, produce marked sedation, and patients requiring these drugs should not drive or undertake work likely to be affected adversely. Of the milder opioid analgesics codeine is known to affect driving-related skills and others, such as dextropropoxyphene, may also do so. Alcohol potentiates the effects of all these analgesics, even dextropropoxyphene.

Indomethacin has been reported to impair laboratory tests of driving-related skills. The effects of other anti-inflammatory analgesics are unknown. All non-steroidal anti-inflammatory drugs (NSAIDs) have caused nervous system effects and can cause dizziness and vertigo. Even over-the-counter preparations such as ibuprofen can uncommonly provoke symptoms of drowsiness, fatigue, and dizziness. These reactions can be hazardous in workers where safety is critical, e.g. train drivers, or lead to commercial loss in other occupations, e.g. management. Recognitions of such risks in advance is important because NSAIDs are widely self-prescribed for minor musculoskeletal injuries.

Anticonvulsants

Studies of cognitive function, both in normal volunteers and in patients on chronic anticonvulsant therapy, have shown impairment of concentration and sustained attention, and other aspects of psychomotor performance. Impairment is greater in patients on polytherapy than in those treated with a single drug, and there is some evidence that it is greater with phenytoin than with carbamazepine. However, patients on well controlled long-term monotherapy should have few side-effects but caution should be taken when adjusting doses. Driving must be temporarily suspended if treatment is changed until there has been a fit-free interval of 1 year (see Chapter 28).

Excessive doses of phenytoin, carbamazepine, and newer drugs such as lamotrigine or gabapentin produce drowsiness, tremor, ataxia, and double vision. Patients affected by drowsiness should not drive or operate machinery. It may be necessary to ensure that blood levels are within the therapeutic range in patients at work.

Anaesthetics

As a general rule patients should not drive or operate machinery for 24–48 hours after general anaesthesia for minor out-patient surgery, but this depends to some extent on the drug used, the duration of anaesthesia, and the response of the individual patient. Clear written instructions should be provided for the patient at the time of discharge from the day surgery centre.

Antihypertensive drugs

Most modern antihypertensive drugs (low dose thiazides, calcium channel blockers, α-blockers, ACE inhibitors, and angiotensin receptor blockers) do not have important central effects and do not appear to affect performance. Older drugs such as methyldopa, clonidine, guanethidine, bethanidine, debrisoquine, and indoramin produce sedation, and methyldopa has been shown to impair driving performance. The newly introduced imidazoline (I_1) receptor agonist moxonidine has sedative properties but these are less than those seen with clonidine.

Beta-blockers, especially the more lipophilic agents such as propranolol, can affect psychomotor functions which return to normal after about 3 weeks' administration. Aircrew are permitted by the Civil Aviation Authority to take specified β-blockers, but only after careful specialist evaluation and simulation after initiation testing. A period of ground duties should be undertaken after initiation to allow for stabilization and habituation.[17] (See also Appendix 1).

In a small proportion of patients β-blockers have other side-effects that could impair work capacity. These include general fatigue, malaise, tiredness, and muscle fatigue. Reduced exercise tolerance has been reported with all β-blockers and there is no good evidence that the cardioselective drugs such as metoprolol have lesser effects than those of non-selective drugs such as propranolol. Both types of β-blocker significantly increase the sense of fatigue during exercise compared with placebo, and a given workload appears subjectively more difficult to achieve. Fatigue has been reported in about 5% of patients on β-blockers but minor unreported symptoms are probably more common, and it is important to be aware of the potential effect of these drugs on work capacity.

β-blockers can produce bronchospasm in susceptible people, and this should be considered when they are prescribed for patients working in irritant atmospheres. α-blockers and β-blockers with α-blocking properties, such as carvedilol and labetalol, can cause postural hypotension, which may affect work performance.

All antihypertensive drugs may cause unexpected hypotension but the risks with modern drugs at current recommended doses have probably been exaggerated. Patients should not drive or operate machinery in the first few hours after beginning treatment or after a dose increment. Particular care should be taken if the patient works in a hot environment. Most antihypertensive drugs affect cutaneous blood flow and can impair the vasomotor response to cold exposure. Diuretics increase the risk of dehydration at high temperatures and are not the antihypertensive of choice for patients working in a hot environment.

Antidiabetic drugs

Loss of warning of hypoglycaemia is a common problem among insulin-treated patients and can be a serious hazard, especially for drivers. The cause is not known but very tight control of blood sugar appears to lower the threshold needed to trigger hypoglycaemic symptoms. Some patients have reported loss of warning of hypoglycaemia after transfer to human insulin. β-blockers can blunt hypoglycaemic awareness and delay recovery.

Car drivers and operators of machinery need to take particular care to avoid hypoglycaemia. Drivers should check blood sugar before starting and at intervals of approximately 2 hours on long journeys and they should ensure that a supply of sugar is always available. If hypoglycaemia occurs, the driver or operator should stop immediately and wait until recovery is complete. Driving is not allowed when hypoglycaemia awareness has been lost. (See also Chapter 28.)

Anticoagulants

Consideration must be given to the suitability for employment of people taking anticoagulants. Usually the underlying condition is the limiting factor. Should bleeding occur, the guidelines given in the *British National Formulary* should be followed. It is advisable for employees taking such medication to carry anticoagulant treatment cards, or other means to indicate that they are receiving this treatment (see Chapter 16).

Any occupation that involves potential hazards that significantly increase the risk of injury and bleeding should be reviewed for suitability while the individual is taking the anticoagulant. Such jobs might include, for example, fishing, mining, foundry working, and labouring activities. If such hazards are present it would be appropriate, where possible, for adjustments to be made to the job to reduce the risk; if that is not possible, alternative work should be recommended while the individual is taking the medication. Those individuals whose work involves foreign travel should not undertake such travel until their anticoagulant medication is stabilized; in addition they should remember to take sufficient medication with them on the trip. Once stabilized on the medication it is more likely to be the underlying medical condition or the available medical facilities in the countries to be visited that become the deciding factors as to whether travel is advised.

Specific jobs, because of safety or isolation issues, require particular consideration, e.g. flight crew prescribed anticoagulants must discuss with an Authorized Medical Examiner (AME) both the reason for taking the medication and the risks associated with taking it, because flight safety implications will require removal from operational activity until the AME believes it is safe to resume flight crew duties. Similarly, those prescribed anticoagulants are considered unsuitable for work offshore; in addition, because of the risks associated both with the underlying medical condition and the unsupervised taking of anticoagulants for long periods, it is considered inappropriate to undertake work as seafarers on long sea journeys—those working on shorter ferry crossings should seek the advise of a Department of Transport Medical Referee.

Anticancer medication

A significant number of employees remain at work while undergoing chemotherapy. Sometimes the patient needs admission to hospital for intravenous therapy but most frequently the medication is taken orally. Employees taking such medication require support and understanding from their employer in view of the potential side-effects. For instance, the widely used oestrogen receptor antagonist tamoxifen is associated with light-headedness and visual disturbances (corneal opacities, cataracts, and retinopathy). Frequently work patterns have to be adjusted, as the employee often feels temporarily unwell as a result of therapy, and will require support when such worrying side-effects as hair loss occur. Continuity of therapy is essential and must not be interrupted in those whose work takes them overseas, for example.

Continuous ambulatory infusion therapy

Some employees wish to return to work while receiving medication via continuous ambulatory infusion. In such circumstances a discussion between the employee's general practitioner or consultant and the occupational health adviser or the employer should identify the potential needs of the employee receiving the therapy to allow a risk assessment of the working environment and arrangements for changing of infusion bags in a safe environment.

Antimigraine drugs

The $5HT_1$ agonists naratriptan, sumatriptan, and zolmitriptan can cause drowsiness, which may affect performance of skilled tasks such as driving. Other drugs such as ergotamine, isometheptene (Midrid), pizotifen, clonidine, and methsergide are associated with dizziness, vertigo, and postural hypotension.

Drugs for parkinsonism

Hypotensive reactions with cabergoline, lysuride, pergolide, and ropinirole may be disturbing in some patients during the first few days of treatment and particular care should be exercised when driving or operating machinery. Troublesome hypotension may also be encountered with levodopa (and combinations with DOPA decarboxylase inhibitors) and selegiline. Blurred vision may complicate the use of most antiparkinsonism drugs, including amantadine and antimuscarinics such as benhexol, benzatropine, and orphenadrine.

Cardiovascular drugs

Most patients treated with amiodarone develop corneal microcrystals. Drivers may be dazzled by headlights at night. Visual disturbances also occur with disopyramide, flecainide, propafenone, and gemifibrozil. Fibrates, statins, and dipryidamole can cause myalgia or myositis, which can affect ability to perform physical work. Many cardiovascular drugs can cause dizziness and hypotension, e.g. disopyramide, flecainide, propafenone, nicorandil, dipyridamole, and nitrates.

Respiratory drugs

The anti-asthmatic drug ketotifen causes drowsiness, which can affect performance of skilled tasks such as driving. The fine tremor caused by β-agonists and ephedrine can cause difficulty with precise tasks.

Anti-infective agents

The antituberculosis drug ethambutol is associated with visual disturbances in the form of loss of acuity, colour blindness, and restriction of visual fields. Patients should be advised to discontinue therapy immediately if vision deteriorates.

The 4-quinolone antibiotics, such as ciprofloxacin, may affect performance of skilled tasks such as driving. The effect of alcohol is enhanced. The risk of convulsions is increased particularly if used with NSAIDs.

Many diverse antimicrobials can cause dizziness, which may affect performance. Examples include the cephalosporins, metronidazole, 4-quinolones, griseofulvin, and itraconazole.

Endocrine drugs

The dopamine receptor stimulants bromocriptine, cabergoline, and quinagolide can cause dizziness and postural hypotension. Hypotensive reactions with quinagolide may be disturbing during the first few days of treatment and after dose increments; particular care is needed with driving and operating machinery; tolerance is reduced by alcohol. High-dose steroids cause cataracts, which can affect performance of skilled tasks.

Other drugs

The muscle relaxants baclofen, dantrolene, and methocarbamol produce sedation and muscle weakness and make driving and operating machinery dangerous. Mydriatic eye-drops such as homatropine, atropine, and cyclopentolate paralyse accommodation and produce blurred vision. Blurred vision to antimuscarinic actions is also seen with oxybutynin and flavoxate for urinary incontinence and pilocarpine tablets used for dry mouth. With pilocarpine, blurred vision may affect the ability to drive, particularly at night, and to perform hazardous activities in reduced light. It should also be remembered that for those exposed to harmful effects of noise on the middle ear that the taking of ototoxic drugs such as gentamicin or salicylates, which, themselves may induce vestibular damage, may make the situation worse.

Malaria prophylaxis

Drugs used for prophylaxis of malaria can cause symptoms that may affect ability to work. Chloroquine is often associated with visual disturbances. Dizziness or disturbed sense of balance after taking mefloquine may affect performance of skilled tasks such as driving. Dizziness is to some extent dose-related but neuropsychiatric reactions can occur even during prophylactic use. The incidence of minor symptoms is 20–90%. Severe transient neuropsychiatric reactions are less common with an estimated frequency of 1 in 13 000 during prophylactic use but 1 in 215 with therapeutic use. Symptoms include non-cognition, disorientation, mental confusion, hallucinations, agitation, and decreased consciousness. A single dose can be all that is needed to evoke a mental reaction. Unpredictable reactions can be provoked by concomitant use of CNS-active drugs and alcohol. Because of these potential side-effects caution is required prior to prescription with a risk assessment comparing benefits with risk based on past medical history. In addition, it is good practice for individuals to commence taking this medication 2 weeks prior to travel rather than the usual 1 week so that any potential side-effects can be detected and alternative medication prescribed before leaving the UK.

Prospective travellers should consult their general practitioner or a specialist in tropical diseases who will determine the appropriate prophylactic drug and its dosage according to the area to be visited and the time to be spent away, also taking into consideration any drug contraindication. It is advisable to start medication a week before departure if the patient has not taken antimalarials before or 14 days in the case of mefloquine. The recommended prophylactic drug for malaria protection varies according to the type of malaria present in the area to be visited and the sensitivity of the parasites. The traveller's age and previous exposure to antimalarial drugs, the duration of stay, and other conditions will need to be taken into account.

Drug prophylaxis should begin, at the latest, on the day of travel to the endemic area and continue for at least 4 weeks after returning. Whether drugs are taken daily or weekly, it is advisable to take them at the same time each day, or the same day each week, with unfailing regularity to be fully effective. Drugs should be taken with liquids after a meal in order to reduce the occurrence of nausea and vomiting or mild gastrointestinal upsets, particularly if chloroquine is used.

See Appendix 5 for advice regarding medical care of overseas employees, and Appendix 8 for agencies from whom further information can be obtained.

Patient pack prescribing and provision of patient information leaflets

Since December 1998 patients have been provided with detailed written information about drugs that are dispensed to them,[18–20] bringing the UK into line with EU legislation. All drugs in the *British National Formulary* dispensed by general practitioners are now covered. The full scheme does not apply to medication dispensed through hospitals. Patients now receive packs of medicines containing an information sheet describing side-effects, interactions, etc. in simple terms. The wording on the pack and the leaflet must be approved by the Medicines Control Agency. These leaflets should provide patients with a better understanding of the risks of working with machines or driving. Patients who cannot read English or with poor sight will require risks to be explained, but in a study[5] of prescription medication used by employees at a chemical plant, 74% had read and understood information about possible side-effects, 17% had not understood this, and 6.5% had not consulted the information.[5] General practitioners had provided warnings about side-effects that could affect safety in only a minority. Of the 75% whose general practitioner had not warned of side-effects, 43% were taking medication where potential disabling side-effects could have arisen. Of those taking over-the-counter medication 80% had not read the information sheet and 15% had read but not understood it. This study also found that 11.4% of the study population had experienced side-effects that they felt could have affected their safety. Of those reporting side-effects 30% were working in high-risk duties and 25% moderate risk. For males, drowsiness was reported as the side-effect occurring most frequently in 29%, poor concentration in 18.4%, and dizziness in 11.7%. For females visual deterioration was the most common side-effect reported. Of those with adverse medication effects only 40% informed any medical personnel and only 22.5% had informed the occupational health department.

From these data it is clear that more explanation of potential risks of taking medication at work by the prescribing physician is appropriate and simple guidance for over-the-counter medication is required.

Special problems in specific occupations

Flying (see also Appendix 1)

All medication that affects performance is likely to be a hazard to aircrew. In addition, environmental factors such as pressure, gravity, and temperature may all affect the performance of those flying, together with the potential additive effects of the medication. The Civil Aviation Authority Aeronautical Information Circular 63/2002, *Modern Medical Practice and Flight Safety*, states that 'any regular use of medication' requires the advice of a CAA Authorised Medical Examiner (AME) before duty resumes—this applies to both flight crew and air traffic control officers. The following advice is taken from the Civil Aviation Authority Aeronautical Information Circular—AIC 58/2000, which gives guidance on medication, alcohol, and flying. The following widely used medications are normally incompatible with flying.

- **Antibiotics**: apart from any potential effects of the antibiotics, the effects from the infection will almost always mean that the pilot is not fit to fly.

- **Tranquillizers, antidepressants, and sedatives**: because of their effects on performance those who are required to fly must not take these drugs. In addition, the pilot's underlying mental state is almost certainly incompatible with flying.

- **Stimulants** (e.g. caffeine and amphetamine): the use of such 'pep' pills while flying cannot be permitted.

- **Antihistamines**: many cause drowsiness. In many cases the condition requiring treatment precludes flying and if treatment is necessary, expert advice should be sought.

- **Drugs for the control of high blood pressure**: if the blood pressure is such that drugs are needed, the pilot must be temporarily grounded. Any treatment instituted should be discussed with an expert in aviation medicine before returning to flying.

- **Analgesics**: the more potent analgesics may have marked effects on performance. In any case, the pain for which they are being taken is likely to indicate a condition, which is a bar to flying.

- **Anaesthetics**: following dental and other anaesthesia, at least 24 hours should elapse before return to flying after a local anaesthetic, and 48 hours after a general anaesthetic.

- **Other medication**: if there is any change in medication or dosage or if any other medication is taken, those flying are exhorted not to take such medication unless they are completely familiar with the effect on their own body. Those taking such medication should ask three questions:

  - Do I feel fit to fly?
  - Do I really need to take medicine at all?
  - Have I given this particular medication a personal trial on the ground for at least 24 hours before flying, to ensure it will not have any adverse effects on my ability to fly?

In certain selected cases, aircrew who are under the care of cardiologists and consultants in aviation medicine may be allowed β-blockers. Additionally, the use of temazepam as a hypnotic by aircrew in the Royal Air Force has been shown by Nicholson to have no residual effects on performance.[21] It is, however, most important that, before issuing hypnotics to aircrew, the cause for the requirement should be sought as this may be work-related and amenable to change, e.g. unusual work rosters. Similar advice is given by the CAA regarding medication and air traffic controllers.[22] In addition to avoiding medication as for pilots this guidance advises against the use of Sudafed used for nasal congestion because of reported side-effects of anxiety, tremor, rapid pulse, and headaches.

Note it is also an offence for a licensed maintenance engineer to be under the influence of drugs to such an extent to impair their capacity to work safely.

The position regarding cabin crew is different, as these staff are unlicensed and each company sets its own health standards. However, Air Navigation (No. 2) Order 1995: article 57(2) states:

> A person shall not, when acting as a member of the crew of any aircraft or being carried in any aircraft for the purpose of so acting, be under the influence of drink or a drug to such an extent as to impair his capacity so to act.

The question of risks from medication to cabin crew is less relevant than their health status. The same applies to those travelling as passengers as part of their job.

Merchant navy (see also Appendix 2)

The fitness of merchant seafarers to serve at sea is determined more by the underlying condition than any medication, but it is doubtful if it is ever wise to commence seafaring if the loss of an essential drug could cause a rapid deterioration of health. Where medication is acceptable for serving seafarers, arrangements should be made for a reserve stock of the prescribed drugs to be held in a safe place, with the agreement of the ship's master.

Diving (see also Appendix 4)

Any medication that may affect performance is a potential hazard to those who dive. Additionally, environmental temperature and pressure and the use of gas combinations, e.g. oxygen/helium, may cause further problems. Guidance is given on Form MA1 from the Employment Medical Advisory Service (EMAS) on the medical examination of divers where it is stated in Note 3: 'The diver should be asked specifically for details of any current medication'. In general, it is the medical condition rather than the medication that is the bar to diving.

The question of the effect and use of drugs in hyperbaric conditions is an interesting but practical problem for those who have to treat sick divers under pressure. Cox[23] lists drugs that have been used by divers; the depths to which they have been used; and whether there were any untoward effects.

Offshore workers (see also Appendix 3)

Guidance is given by the UK Offshore Operators Association in its *Guidance for medical aspects of fitness for offshore work*. Referring to medicine, it states the following:

- Individuals on anticoagulants, cytotoxic agents, insulin, anticonvulsants, immunosuppressants, and oral steroids are unacceptable for offshore work.

- Individuals on psychotropic medication, e.g. tranquillizers, antidepressants, narcotics, and hypnotics are also unacceptable. A previous history of such treatment will require further consideration.

- Individuals taking medication must ensure they have an adequate supply and must report any adverse drug reaction to the offshore medic.

Those who work in the Norwegian and Dutch sectors of the North Sea come within the similar legislation of those countries.

Driving

Ordinary driving licences

Section 4 of the Road Traffic Act 1988 does not differentiate between illicit or prescribed drugs. Hence, there is liability to prosecution if driving in an unfit condition.

The Poisons Rule (1972) requires a number of substances containing antihistamines to be labelled with the words 'Caution, may cause drowsiness, if affected do not drive or operate machinery'.

Advice from the Drivers Medical Unit of the Driver and Vehicle Licensing Agency (DVLA) for medical practitioners on medication[24] states:

- Driving while unfit through drugs provided or illicit is an offence and may lead to prosecution.

- All CNS-active drugs can impair alertness, concentration, and driving performance. This is particularly so within the first month of starting or increasing the dose. It is important to cease driving during this time if adversely affected.

- Benzodiazepines are the most likely psychotropic medication to impair driving performance, particularly the long-acting compounds. Alcohol will potentiate the effects.

- Antipsychotic drugs, including depot preparations, can cause motor or extapyramidal effects as well as sedation, or poor concentration, which may, either alone or in combination, be sufficient to impair driving. Careful clinical assessment is required.

- The older tricyclic antidepressants can have pronounced anticholinergic and antihistamine effects, which may impair driving. The more modern antidepressants may have fewer effects.
- The epileptogenic potential of psychotropic medication should be considered particularly when patients are professional drivers.
- Drivers with psychiatric illnesses are often safer when well and on regular psychotropic medication than when they are ill.
- Doctors have a duty of care to advise their patients of the potential dangers of adverse effects from medication and interactions with other substances, especially alcohol.

Drivers of LGVs, PCVs, and taxis

Much stricter criteria have to be applied to professional than to private drivers. As a class they have to drive for longer hours, so the risks of adverse drug reactions or interactions coinciding with a situation in which other road users could be injured by loss of control is far greater. Furthermore, it is not so easy for a professional driver to stop driving when feeling unwell as a result of adverse effects of drugs.

Where there is a need for long-term medication, the issue of whether it is safe for vocational driving to continue may not arise as the driver will often be excluded from holding an LGV or PCV licence as a result of the medical condition requiring treatment The DVLA publication—*At a Glance Guide to Current Medical Standards of Fitness to Drive—for Medical Practitioners*, gives guidance on the desirability or otherwise for Group 1 or Group 2 licence holders to drive dependent on medical condition or medication.

In the case of short-term medication, the safest course is to certify the driver as unfit to drive for an initial period if it seems at all likely that the treatment might impair his driving ability. If treatment has to continue, a decision about returning to work can then be taken in the light of any adverse reactions that may have occurred in the initial stage of treatment.

Conclusions and recommendations

Suggestions for advice to patients taking drugs which affect the CNS

- Do not exceed the stated dose.
- Do not drive, fly, or operate machinery until the nature and extent of any side-effects are known.
- Do not take any other medication or drugs unless prescribed for you.

General principles of prescribing for people at work

- Always enquire into the patient's occupation, and be aware of drug effects that can be hazardous in the work environment.
- Make sure the patient understands what to expect and what action to take.
- Be particularly careful with all drugs that act on the CNS and avoid polypharmacy as this may have unintended additive effects.
- Keep treatment regimens simple and, where possible, avoid more than two daily doses to increase compliance.
- If a hypnotic is required, use one with a short duration of effect.
- Avoid unsupervised use of drugs; give a minimum of repeat prescriptions and supervise regularly.

◆ Avoid the use of antihistamines in those who have to operate machinery, drive, or fly. Where they are essential, favour less-sedating agents.

◆ Reserves of medication must be carried by those whose occupations takes them abroad for long periods of time, e.g. those on board ship. Reserves should also be available for emergency use for those working in isolated or dangerous situations where evacuation may be delayed.

Selected references

1 Edwards F. Risks at work from medication. *J R Coll Phys Lond* 1978; **12**: 219–29.

2 Kirkness B (ed.) *Pharma facts and figures*. London: Association of the British Pharmaceutical Industry, 1997.

3 Dunnell K, Cartwright A. *Medicine takers, prescribers and hoarders*. London: Routledge and Kegan Paul, 1972.

4 Rennie IG. *Accidents at work—risks from medication*. Royal College of Physicians, Faculty of Occupational Medicine, MFOM Dissertation, 1985.

5 Swales CL. A study to determine the prevalence of adverse side effects arising from the use of prescription and non-prescription medication on a chemical manufacturing site. Royal College of Physcians, Faculty of Occupational Medicine, MFOM Dissertation, 1999.

6 Lader M. Benzodiazepines – long-term use and problems of withdrawal. MIMS Magazine 1985, March.

7 Social Trends 26. *1996 Labour Force Survey*. London: Central Statistical Office.

8 Rawlins MD, Thompson JW. In: *Textbook of adverse drug reactions*, (4th edn) (ed. Davies DM). Oxford: Oxford University Press, 1991.

9 Nicholson AM, Stone BM. Disturbance of circadian rhythms and sleep. *Proc R Soc Edin* 1985; **82BL**: 135–9.

10 Nakano S. Time of day effect on psychotherapeutic drug response and kinetics in man. In: *Towards chronopharmacology* (eds Takahashi R, Holberg F, Walker CA). *Adv Biosci* 1982; **41**: 51–9.

11 Hindmarch I. Psychomotor function and psychoactive drugs. *Br J Clin Pharmacol* 1980; **10**: 189–209.

12 Broadbent DE. Performance and its measurement. *Br J Clin Pharmacol* 1984; **18**: 5–9S.

13 Hunter J. Maxwell JS, Stewart DA. Increased hepatic microsomal enzyme activity from occupational exposure to certain organochlorine pesticides. *Nature* 1972; **237**: 399–401.

14 Ebert F, Harlison RD, Zerry C. In: *Textbook of occupational medicine principles and practical applications*, (2nd edn) (ed. Zerz, C). St. Louis: Mosby-Year Book Inc. 1988.

15 Blain PG, Rawlins MD. Drug-induced body temperature changes. *Prescribers J* 1981; **21**: 204.

16 Barbone F, McMahon AD, Davey PG *et al.* Association of road-traffic accidents with benzodiazepine use. *Lancet* 1998; **352**: 1331–6.

17 Second European Workshop in Aviation Cardiology. *Eur Health J* 1999; **1** (Suppl. D).

18 *The patient pack initiative*. London: Medicines Control Agency, 1995.

19 Council Directive 92/27 EEC. Official Journal of the European Community 1992 L113/8-/12.

20 *Medicines. The Medicine for Human Use (marketing authorisations, etc.) Regulations 1994*. Statutory Instrument No.30144. London: HMSO, 1994.

21 Nicholson AN. Long periods of work and disturbed sleep. *Ergonomics* 1984; **27**: 629–30.

22 *Medication and air traffic control*. Aeronautical Information Circular, United Kingdom Civil Aviation Authority AIC 143/1998.

23 Cox RAF (ed.) *Offshore medicine: medical care of employees in the offshore oil industry*, 2nd edn. Berlin: Springer-Verlag, 1987.

24 *At a glance guide to the current medical standards of fitness to drive*. Swansea: DVLA, 2004.

Chapter 26

The older worker

H. N. Goodall and J. Grimley Evans

Age will not be defied.

Francis Bacon (1561–1626) English Philosopher
Essays, 'Of Regiment of Health'*

Introduction

Throughout the world, populations are ageing, as birth rates fall and people live longer. This brings about a permanent change in population structure and an increase in the ratio of people traditionally regarded as being of 'retirement age' to those traditionally regarded as being of 'working age'. Both for the productivity of a population and for the funding of pensions and other social benefits, the whole trajectory of working life and the social structures that underpin it have to change to match labour resources to needs. In particular, people in the developed world must expect to continue working to later ages than in the past, a change that has implications both for the employed and for employers. Occupational physicians have an important role to play in making longer working lifetimes possible, productive, and pleasant.

The demographic background

Over the next 40 years there will be a permanent change in population structures in Europe and North America. It is estimated that by 2050, the number of people over the age of 60 in Europe will have doubled to 40% of the total population.

Other things remaining equal, a rise in life expectancy as has occurred in the UK throughout the twentieth century, increases the proportion of older people in a population. The proportion is also affected as a long-term consequence of changes in birth rate. As shown in Figure 26.1, populations that have not yet undergone full economic development show a broad-based rapidly tapering structure characteristic of high birth and infant mortality rates. Figure 26.1 also shows the very different pattern established in the developed world and, assuming no major global disasters, the future convergence of populations responding to the effects of economic advance in reducing birth rates and prolonging life.

Against these general trends in world populations, European nations, including the UK, are undergoing shorter-term changes due to the large numbers of children who were born between the mid-1940s and the mid-1960s—the 'baby boom' generation. They have proved less fertile than their parents and so as the baby boomers grow old over the next 30 years there will be a relative decline in the proportions of people of working age following on behind them (Figure 26.2). The 'age dependency ratio', that is the number of people past retirement age compared with the number of people of working age, will virtually double from about 1:3 to about 2:3.[1] This forms

*Reproduced with permission from Kiernan M (ed). *The Oxford Francis Bacon XV. The Essayes or counsels, Civill and Morall*. Oxford, Oxford University Press (2000).

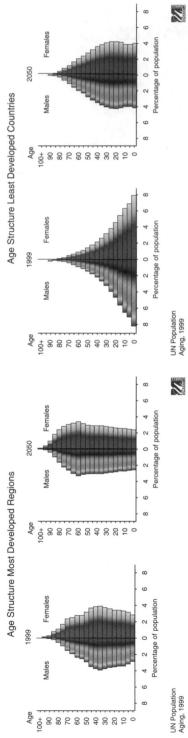

Fig. 26.1 The changing age structure of developed and developing countries. Reproduced with permission from Professor David Wegman, from the keynote speech, SOM ASM 2003.

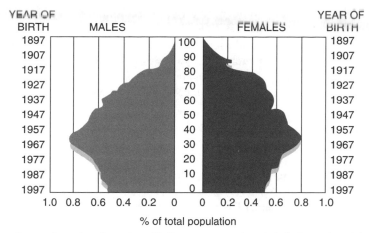

Fig. 26.2 How Europe is ageing (based on 11 European member states). Reproduced from europa.eu.int/comm/eurostat/

the basis of the so-called 'pensions crisis'. Mass immigration of younger workers is not a sensible response to this challenge, especially for a country, such as the UK, whose population has already outgrown its substructure and natural resources. Young workers grow old, so the problem is merely postponed, not solved. Hence the primary need is for all workers to increase their lifetime contribution to the funding of social substructure including pensions. This means working more productively—not necessarily harder—and longer, but not necessarily full-time. It also means increasing the opportunities for citizens under-represented in the current workforce, such as women and people with disabilities, to be productively employed.

The United Kingdom

In a position paper on Age and Employment, the Faculty of Occupational Medicine has drawn attention to particular issues in the UK:[2]

> The majority of non-working men (in the UK) aged between 50 and 65 are economically inactive (i.e. retired, sick or caring for others and unavailable for work) rather than unemployed (one in ten of this non-working age group). The number of people over 50 and on Incapacity Benefit has trebled in the last 20 years. Of those not seeking work, approximately half are on sickness or disability benefit (over 1 million people) and nearly half a million, mainly women, are full time carers. Individuals in this age group are more likely to experience low self-esteem, ill health and poverty. Thirty-seven per cent of 55–64 year olds say they have a limiting long-standing illness. Depression, social exclusion, and marital problems are also more common in this age group. Most of those not working have been out of employment for long periods, many having previously been in long standing jobs. Involvement in other activities (such as charitable work) is also declining in this age group.

However, this probably gives too gloomy a picture of the health and fitness of the population in middle age. Disability benefit is more generous than unemployment benefit and it is well documented that in places where traditional industries, such as steel making, have been closed down, redundant workers very sensibly seek status as disabled rather than unemployed. Few citizens would grudge them this benevolent 'bending' of the system. But the resulting statistics can mislead policy makers, when facing up to the need for socio-economic change, brought about by increased longevity and consequently, longer working lives.

In this chapter we review some of the implications of the employment of older workers, for occupational medicine. The first section outlines age-associated changes in health and function, the second deals with the adaptations in occupational health services and the third raises some broader issues relating to the organization of industries and companies.

General age-associated changes

Ageing

Ageing, in the sense of senescence, comprises a loss of adaptability of an individual organism over time. As we become older we become less able to respond adaptively to challenges from our external or internal environments. The homoeostatic responses on which survival depends become on average less sensitive, slower, weaker, and less well sustained. For most human beings, loss of adaptability may not be obvious until very late in life, as we live in non-challenging environments that rarely bring individuals to the limit of their functional capacity. None the less, as we grow older, many of us go about our work and daily life with diminishing functional reserves.

The loss of adaptability that characterizes ageing is due to the accumulation of un-repaired or only partially repaired damage to body systems, organs, tissues, cells, and intracellular organelles. The longevity of a species is determined by the efficiency of its damage control systems—damage control comprising prevention, detection and repair or replacement. Damage control is expensive in biological resources. Resources used for damage control and longevity cannot be used for reproduction, so long-lived species breed more slowly than short-lived ones. Slower reproduction provides for opportunities to improve the survival of progeny to their own sexual maturity, for example by timing reproduction to seasonal availability of food or providing parental care. As it is successful reproduction that leads to evolutionary success, natural selection will favour longevity in species that live in safe environments.[3]

Ageing of the members of populations will be reflected in risk of death computed as the age-specific mortality rate of the population. In the human species, senescence first becomes apparent about the age of 12 and is a continuous process thereafter. It is indeed a lifelong process, not something that starts mysteriously around the age of retirement; determinants of disease and disability in middle age can be identified in childhood and even fetal life.

Differences between younger and older people

A starting point for the scientific appraisal of human ageing is to compare young people with older people and the general view of ageing is derived, explicitly or implicitly, from such comparisons.[4] However, the result can be deceptive because differences between young and old people can arise through processes other than ageing (Table 26.1).

Differences not attributable to ageing

Some differences have come about, not because the old people have changed due to ageing, but because they have always been different from the young, with whom they are being compared.

- **Selective survival** is the result of people with advantageous genes or social environment, or healthy life-styles, surviving longer than the less fortunate people born at the same time. This effect can be important in extreme old age but is likely to have only a minor impact in middle or late middle life.

Table 26.1 Differences between young and old

Non-ageing

◆ Selective survival

◆ Cohort effects

◆ Differential challenge

True ageing

◆ Primary

  • intrinsic

  • extrinsic

◆ Secondary

  • individual adaptation

  • specific adaptation

◆ **Cohort effects** are the differences between generations of people born at different times and therefore exposed, especially in developing societies, to different influences and experiences, particularly early in life. Such cohort differences can be considerable. A study in the 1960s demonstrated that a major part of what appears in cross-sectional studies to be age-associated change in some types of psychological functioning was due to cultural, especially educational, differences between generations.[5] Although prominent in the sphere of psychological function, which reflects educational standards and practices during childhood, cohort effects will contribute to cross-sectional estimates of age-associated variation in physical variables such as height, serum lipids, and obesity, as well as to risk of diseases such as lung cancer. Cohort differences reflect differences between generations in their life-style and behaviour as well as in changes in the physical environment.

◆ **Differential challenge.** If ageing is to be defined in terms of reduced adaptability, it can only be assessed by offering equal challenges to people at different ages. Social policy often leads to our offering more severe challenges to older people than to younger and then attributing differences in outcome to the effects of ageing. Differential challenge is a feature of health services, in the UK as elsewhere, where older patients receive poorer quality care than is provided for younger people.[6] Ageism, in its various guises, is so deeply engrained in British society that discrimination against older people is universal, in the workplace, as in government and society at large.

Differences attributable to ageing (true ageing)

There has long been debate about distinguishing 'diseases' from 'normal ageing', but the distinction is meaningless in scientific terms.[7] True ageing comprises all the ways in which individuals change as time passes. Some of the responsible processes, for reasons that range from the medical to the political, may come to be called 'diseases'.

Primary ageing is loss of adaptability due to the effects of many different processes in the tissues and organs of the body. These ageing processes are the product of interactions between **extrinsic** (environmental and life-style) influences and **intrinsic** (genetic) factors. Some of these interactions may be specific: for example, it is likely that excess dietary salt raises blood pressure only in people with particular genes. Other interactions are more general: habits of physical exercise, for example, affect a wide range of body systems, presumably through genetically determined pathways. Diet is important in healthy ageing, notably through deficiencies and imbalance.

Dietary factors are also probably involved in ageing effects, due to the generation and insufficiently rapid destruction of free radicals (highly active oxygen molecules) generated in mitochondria that damage cell components including DNA.

Secondary ageing is a term usefully reserved to designate those adaptations made by individuals—or by a species through natural selection—that counter the effects of ageing. At the individual level, secondary ageing is most obvious in the realm of psychological and behavioural functioning. Mildly obsessional behaviour making an ordered environment substitute for memory is a common and successful adaptation. (If we always put our car keys on the hall table, we do not have to waste brain-power remembering where we have left them today.) Older workers may develop apparently idiosyncratic ways of carrying out familiar tasks that are efficient—for them—in conserving effort and circumventing specific problems, such as a stiff joint.

Social factors Social factors are important extrinsic determinants of ageing. One of the most significant correlates of healthy ageing is higher educational level.[8] This will partly reflect the health benefits of relative affluence and occupations that are less damaging physically. Education will also be relevant to the ability of the individual to know of medical advances and to understand their implications for prevention or therapy, and to profit from them. Education is one component in social class effects, much studied in the UK. Social class effects on health and disability are highly complex and there may be subtle psychosocial and work-related determinants of health in middle and later life. People in lower grade jobs have less sense of control over their patterns and pace of working, and this leads to chronic 'stress' arousal, associated with changes in endocrine and immune function, that may have pervasive effects on susceptibility to age-associated illness and disability, especially cardiovascular disease.[9]

Obviously, the effects of ageing processes on body functions depend in part on how good those functions were initially. Both men and women lose muscle tissue at the same rate with ageing but, because women start with less muscle (on average) than men, they are more likely (on average) to become immobile and dependent in later life.[10] A similar model applies to bone tissue, and to the high rates of fractures in older women, although women also experience a higher rate of bone loss with ageing.[11] Two determinants of how soon brain damage, produced by Alzheimer's disease, shows itself in the clinical syndrome of dementia, are the original intelligence and the education level of affected individuals.[12] The better the brain, it seems, the longer it can compensate for progressive damage.

Because we start from different baselines, carry different genes and live different lives, we age at different rates and in different ways. Although, on average, we deteriorate with age, some people in their eighties will be functioning better than would be regarded as normal for people in their thirties. It is therefore unscientific, as well as unjust, to make judgements about individuals' capabilities simply on the basis of their age—as unjust in fact as to make such judgements from their sex, skin colour or social class. In all the discussion of age-associated changes in health and function in this chapter, we describe what happens on average in the population; it must not be assumed that such changes affect every ageing individual.

Is the pattern of ageing changing?

Data from the USA indicate that, over the last two decades, people there have been living longer on average but that the prevalence of disability in later life has been falling.[8] This is presumably partly due to the adoption of healthier life-styles by significant sections of the population—notwithstanding a general increase in obesity—and partly due to better medical care, but there are probably other factors that have caused a decline in cardiovascular disease since the 1960s. It is not clear whether similar improvements in general health and function in middle and later life are occurring in the UK, although reductions in cigarette smoking among men and control of urban and industrial smoke pollution have reduced the prevalence of limiting pulmonary disease in the last three decades. Less reassuringly, British data suggest that social class differences in mortality and morbidity have been widening. The reasons for this are complex, and include changes over time in the composition of the various classes, but will also include failure of some members of the population to benefit as much as others from social and medical advances.[13]

There are encouraging signs that the epidemic of cardiovascular disease has peaked, although the incidence may still be rising in some population groups, notably immigrants from the Indian subcontinent.[14] If the improvements in the patterns of disability in older people seen in the USA could be made to happen here, there would be good prospects for people being fit enough to work longer for their pensions, while yet living to enjoy a sufficient and active period of retirement.

How old is an 'older worker'?

The World Health Organization has recommended that 'older people' should replace the potentially discriminatory term 'the elderly'. In the population at large the age at which one becomes 'older' has, quite properly, moved on with the growth in the expectation of life. Anxieties (largely ill-founded or tendentious) about the medical implications of ageing populations are usually expressed in terms of the numbers of people aged over 80. Certainly, in the developed world, the traditional male retirement age of 65 would now be regarded as a continuation of middle age rather than the onset of senility.

The retirement age of 65 for men was originally computed in nineteenth century Germany, on the assumption that pensions would be paid by a levy on the wages of men still working—a 'pay-as-you-go' system. Conceptually, the developed world is moving toward the assumption that future pensions will be based on an insurance model (private or social), in which individuals will in effect pay in advance for their own pensions. Logically this would lead to a system in which the average (not necessarily compulsory) retirement age would be adjusted to take account of the expectation of life in later years, so that a levy of 'x' per cent of one's earnings over an average of 'y' years would be seen as 'purchasing' an average of 'z' years of adequate income after retiring. Even more challenging than the actuarial intricacies of such a scheme would be equity issues raised by social class and occupation differences in life expectancy. Whatever happens, however, it is reasonable to expect that for the immediate future the 'older worker', of practical concern to occupational health services, will be aged 55–70, rather than over 75 years of age.

Age-associated changes in function

An attempt at a comprehensive catalogue of age-associated changes and illnesses easily fills a large textbook.[15] This chapter is necessarily restricted to major topics related to work capacity and to illustrative examples of how illnesses may present in a work-related context.

Physical activity

Muscle mass declines in both sexes from the third decade onwards. As already noted, because women start life with less muscle than men, they are more likely to suffer from limitation in muscle strength and power in later life.[10,16] This is part of the explanation for the paradox that although women on average live longer than men they are more likely to become physically disabled in old age.[17] In addition to muscular strength and power, endurance and joint flexibility also decline with age. The last can be partly compensated for by deliberately putting joints through a full range of movement before working.[18] The collective warm-up exercises required of workers in some Far Eastern factories have a physiological as well as ideological function.

Endurance, the ability to maintain high levels of physical activity over prolonged periods, is limited by muscular power and exercise tolerance, and also by pulmonary and cardiac function, all of which decline on average with age. Although breathlessness is usually the dominant symptom in strenuous activity, the limits on exercise capacity are usually muscular or cardiac rather than pulmonary, except in smokers or individuals with lung damage due to other causes.[19]

Older workers in physically strenuous jobs may be working closer to their physical limits than younger colleagues keeping to the same pace, and they may become more readily fatigued.[20] Older workers can cope with heavy muscular exertion,[21] so long as the work is interspersed with recovery periods sufficient in frequency and duration, but they find the demands of continuous fast paced lighter work more difficult to sustain.[10] Older workers may prefer to move away from externally paced or 'piecework' jobs into hourly paid jobs, if the choice is available. Part of the age-associated loss of muscular function observed in the population is due to lower levels of exercise in older age groups. Training can recover some of the loss by increasing muscle bulk and blood supply, as well as improving muscle metabolism.[22]

Hearing

Some age-associated loss of sensitivity to high frequencies is virtually universal in Western societies, and is probably largely due to chronic exposure to noise rather than intrinsic ageing processes.[23] Those who have worked in noisy industries for many years, with inadequate hearing protection, are almost certain to have significant hearing loss, by the time they reach their mid-fifties. High frequencies are important in the comprehension of speech but, before the process becomes severe enough to produce overt deafness, it can result in slower 'decoding' of speech. This in turn can produce functional cognitive impairment due to slowing of processing and the missing of some information.[24] (Detection and correction of 'minor' hearing loss, is a necessary first step in the assessment of someone suspected of early dementia.) In the workplace, this effect may be compounded by high ambient noise levels.[25]

Sufferers lose the ability accurately to distinguish particular consonants, notably 'b', 'd', 't', and 's' sounds. They may misidentify words or fail to make sense of what they are hearing. An additional problem is difficulty in reliably following one speaker when other voices are also audible, as in many social and work situations. The natural reaction when talking to someone perceived as deaf is to speak more loudly, but this may not help. The sufferer's cochlea may show a disproportionate response to increase in volume known as 'recruitment', and loud sounds can become both painful and distorted ('There is no need to shout, young man …'). In some working environments, loss of accurate comprehension of verbal instructions will have implications for safety and production costs, if process or other errors result. Some individuals can compensate for hearing loss by lip-reading, and colleagues can be helpful by making use of gesture and facial expression. In some working environments, more use of written material in the communication of crucial information can improve safety.

Up to a third of older people suffer from tinnitus, of which the commonest cause is sensorineural deafness due to previous noise exposure. Most people manage to ignore the problem but for others it can become distressing, at least intermittently. The clinician also needs to be alert to recognize depression when it presents as preoccupation with previously ignored tinnitus.[26]

Vision

There are age-associated changes in visual perception, due to both peripheral and central factors.[27] With increasing age, the lens becomes less elastic and the intrinsic muscles weaker, so that accommodation for near vision becomes limited. This effect can begin as young as the mid-forties in otherwise healthy workers and is sometimes a missed cause of what the older worker puts down to 'eyestrain.' The lens and vitreous of the eye become less transparent and acquire a yellowish tinge that can interfere with colour perception. Owing to the loss of transparency, and also because of changes in the retina, the older eye requires higher light intensities and greater contrast in print for accurate reading. This has important implications for the design of work environments for older employees. Cataracts become common, reducing acuity and also scattering incoming light, causing dazzle. This last factor is especially significant for night driving.

Also relevant to driving safety is a tendency for the functional visual field to contract, so that stimuli in the periphery of vision may not be noticed, even though formal static testing of the visual field shows no defect.[28] This is thought to be one factor in the increase with age in low-speed lateral car collisions at road intersections.[29] Some studies have found it possible to reverse this phenomenon by specific training, and it presumably represents some form of central inattention. Although less clear than in the case of hearing, minor degrees of visual impairment can manifest as slower or less accurate understanding of written material or misinterpretation of environmental cues that can present as apparent cognitive impairment.

Macular degeneration is a further affliction that an older worker may suffer. Treatment is at present unimpressive and access to advice on suitable visual aids less than perfect. Modifications to computer keyboards and visual display units, and scanning cameras to assist in reading are, however, available and may be of help in prolonging a sufferer's working life.

Touch and proprioception

Dexterity and fineness of touch may deteriorate over time, especially if chronic exposure to trauma leads to thickening of the skin and subcutaneous tissues of the hands. The risk of falls increases in both sexes after the age of 65. The risk is higher, at all ages, in women, who also show a bimodal risk with an earlier transitory peak around the age of 50.[30] Although the risk of falls is related to muscle strength and joint stiffness, as well as any neurological disease, there seems to be a general age-associated impairment of global proprioception.

Proprioception, as tested by standard clinical examination (joint position sense or Romberg test, for example), is unlikely to be manifestly impaired in the absence of specifically diagnosable conditions, such as vitamin B12 deficiency or cervical myelopathy. Global proprioception, in the sense of accurate awareness of the body's position and orientation in space, is the product of continuous integration of input from eyes, inner ear, and a range of peripheral proprioceptors, especially in cervical joints, the feet, and the Achilles tendons. As a consequence of degeneration in cervical joints and peripheral nerves, the information from these various sources may be attenuated or may not arrive simultaneously in the central nervous system. In later life, this probably underlies the common symptom of non-rotatory dizziness that is epidemiologically associated with a risk of falls.[31]

Mental function

Dementia is rare at ages under 70, except in people with a close family history of an early-onset form. There are, however, some differences in mental functioning between middle-aged people and young adults that may need to be considered in matching older workers to industrial tasks (by choosing the workers or designing the tasks) and in developing training programmes. As noted already, some of the differences observed between younger and older workers may be due to cohort effects rather than ageing and so will change with time. One of the first things we learn at school is how to learn, so cohort effects must be expected to be significant in designing training programmes for older workers.

The various processes and aptitudes that comprise human intelligence have been polarized between the 'crystalline' and the 'fluid'.[32] Crystalline intelligence solves problems by applying learned strategies or paradigms. Fluid intelligence solves problems by innovation and analysis from first principles. As we grow older, we tend to rely more on crystalline than on fluid processes.

As long as the paradigm chosen, often by recognition of analogies between present and past situations, is appropriate, crystalline intelligence is efficient. It may, however, fail, and indeed be a positive hindrance, in rising to a totally new challenge that requires original thinking. An older individual in a problem-solving situation may need to be made explicitly aware of the need for a new approach, not a ready-made solution from past experience.

Subjectively, the dominant problem in mental ageing is difficulty with memory. It is a clinically useful oversimplification to visualize human memory as comprising an immediate working memory, possibly subserved by active inter-neuronal transmission, linked to a long-term memory based on some permanent neuronal change such as modification of synapses. Some material from the first passes into the second, from whence if adequately filed and labelled, suitable cueing can bring it forth. Both types can show deterioration with age and difficulties with shorter-term memory are obvious enough. Minor loss of long-term memory can be difficult to assess because an examiner probing the long-term memory of someone older than himself may not know what should be there and so identify what the subject has forgotten. In age-associated memory impairment and in the early stages of Alzheimer's disease, a dominant feature is an apparent problem in the link between shorter-term and longer-term memory, so that material is not written into longer-term store or cannot be recalled from there. This difficulty is commonly, albeit somewhat misleadingly, labelled as a defect in short-term memory—even though the subject's ability to remember telephone numbers long enough to dial them ('digit span') may still be normal.

Increasing attention paid to Alzheimer's disease in the media has led to middle-aged people with subjective difficulties with memory becoming worried or even depressed, by a fear of incipient dementia. This is a particular concern for people with a family history of dementia, even though the risk for relatives of someone with late-onset dementia is very little higher than average. A middle-aged person manifesting or complaining of memory problems therefore needs skilled and empathetic care. Employers of older workers should encourage the appropriate use of memory supporting strategies—note-taking, notice boards, and electronic prompters, for example. This will help to prevent problems, both directly and also indirectly, so that individuals, fearful of memory loss, do not feel stigmatized by making use of supportive devices such as use of note-taking or pocket electronic organizers (suitably and regularly backed up to a computer in case of battery failure).

Ageing is also associated with a slowing of mental processing and a reduction in channel capacity—essentially the capacity to process several different sequences of data simultaneously. This is analogous to the difference between 'broadband' and single telephone line connections in home computer telephone linkages. Decisions may take longer and mistakes may be made in complex situations. These processes contribute to the rise in accident rates among older car drivers, for example. Compounding the channel capacity problem with ageing is a failure to identify and suppress irrelevant factors when analysing a situation or performing a complex task.[33,34]

Specific age-associated problems

Cardiovascular function

Age-associated changes are prominent in the structure and function of the cardiovascular system. Cardiovascular diseases increase in incidence and fatality with age and are leading causes of death and of premature retirement.

The heart With ageing, heart muscle becomes stiffer, so that diastolic filling may be impaired.[35] Perhaps partly in response to this change, the older heart functions as if, to some extent, under beta blockade. In response to exercise, it increases cardiac output less by increasing heart rate and more by increasing stroke volume, in comparison with a younger heart. Cardiac reserve reduces correspondingly with age, even in the absence of demonstrable ischaemic disease.

Ischaemic heart disease is common in middle age and beyond, especially so in men. Risk factors include hypertension, smoking, high low-density lipoprotein cholesterol, diabetes, obesity, and lack of exercise, all of which interact. Risk of ischaemic heart disease can be reduced by modification of risk factors at any age and there is no justification for excluding older people from preventive programmes. For reasons that are not yet clear, when ischaemic heart disease is present, pain may be a less prominent symptom in older people than at younger ages. In later life limited cardiac output, due to ischaemic disease or other causes, may present as a sensation of muscular fatigue on exertion rather than as dyspnoea.

Blood pressure In Western populations systolic blood pressure, on average, rises with age although this is associated with an increase in variance because some individuals show no rise. Blood pressure is positively associated with increase in risk of cardiovascular disease, especially stroke. The age-associated rise is due to both increased stiffness of the arterial walls, affecting chiefly systolic pressure, and arteriolar tension influencing diastolic pressure. The old notion that only diastolic pressure is relevant as a risk factor for cardiovascular disease is now discredited and high systolic pressure needs treatment even if the diastolic is 'normal'.[36]

Epidemiological evidence suggests that the rise with age is largely due to extrinsic factors. A high intake of dietary salt contributes, at least in genetically susceptible individuals, and obesity is another remediable factor. Other things being equal, the lower a person's blood pressure the better. Hypertension, as an indication for treatment, is best defined as that level of blood pressure above which treatment will, on average, do more good than harm.[37] This will vary with the drugs available and the doses necessary. As a risk factor for vascular disease, hypertension interacts powerfully with other risk factors such as smoking, and the combination of hypertension and diabetes is also particularly dangerous. Treatment for hypertension therefore requires a comprehensive review of an individual's cardiovascular risk status and not just pills to reduce blood pressure. The benefits of treatment are at least as great for older people as for younger. For older people, drug treatment is essentially along conventional lines but beta blockers are sometimes less effective and less well tolerated than with younger patients.

Cerebrovascular disease Epidemiological data suggest that cerebrovascular disease has been diminishing in incidence for many decades in Western populations,[38,39] but some specific forms have only been identified comparatively recently. Stroke with temporary or permanent neurological deficit, as a presenting feature of cerebrovascular disease, is well-recognized by both medical and lay members of the public. Diagnostic errors more often involve failure to identify non-cerebrovascular causes of an apparent stroke. Hypoglycaemia in a treated diabetic is an example requiring urgent exclusion; cardiac arrhythmia or hypotension, possibly iatrogenic, are others. An unwitnessed epileptic attack followed by Todd's paresis can have serious consequences, especially in a work situation, if mistaken for a transient ischaemic attack (see below). A cerebral tumour presenting as a stroke syndrome will usually come to light in the course of subsequent assessment, as will emboli from atrial fibrillation or valvular disease of the heart.

Cerebrovascular disease is a cause of dementia either through the accumulation of small strokes, or by the less well understood 'small vessel disease' thought to underlie the periventricular white matter damage (leucoaraiosis) seen on magnetic resonance imaging scan of the brain. Transient ischaemic attacks (TIAs) are often recurrent and need investigation and, usually, preventive treatment. They are characterized by focal neurological defects lasting less than 24 hours. It is not wise to assume that some kind of syncopal or confusional episode, without focal neurological signs, is a TIA; other conditions, especially cardiovascular syncope, need to be excluded. The increasingly recognized syndrome of transient global amnesia is probably not due to cerebrovascular disease—in the normal sense of the term—in the majority of cases. This condition, unrelated to hysterical amnesia and unlikely to be mistaken for it, consists of a sudden and temporary loss of recent memory and the ability to take in new information, lasting, usually, less than 24 hours.[40] Long-established skills such as driving are retained even if the driver has suddenly lost all knowledge of where he or she is or is meant to be going. The problem presumably lies in the temporal lobes or limbic structures of the brain, but the mechanism is usually obscure and in many cases attacks do not recur.

Peripheral vascular disease Peripheral vascular disease shares risk factors with other forms of vascular disease but smoking and diabetes are especially important. The typical presentation is intermittent claudication—pain in the lower legs induced by walking and passing off within 10 minutes of rest. The chief differential diagnosis is neurogenic intermittent claudication due to spinal stenosis (see below). If the lower aorta is involved in severe atherosclerotic disease some variant of the Leriche syndrome may occur, including buttock claudication and erectile dysfunction.

Neoplasms Recognition of cancer as a cause of health problems presenting in the workplace is a matter of normal clinical vigilance. Virtually all cancers increase in incidence with age,[41] a fact well-known to older patients for whom fear of cancer may be an unspoken element in any medical consultation. Lung, large bowel, prostate in men, and breast in women are currently the commonest sites of cancers in the UK.

It is to be hoped that cancers due to toxic substances at work are now a thing of the past but new industrial processes are constantly being developed and an ageing workforce risks longer periods of exposure. The occupational physician therefore still needs to be ready to respond appropriately and with due discretion to unusual types or frequencies of neoplasms in his or her workforce. Discretion is necessary as numbers are likely to be small and the statistical distinction between a true 'cluster' and the simple play of chance is strictly a matter for experts. Unnecessary induction of alarm in employers or workforce can have serious consequences.

Skeletal changes **Osteoarthritis** is a common problem in later middle age and beyond. One factor is damage due to overuse, an important issue in occupational, and therefore legal medicine, but the relative importance varies with the joint. The knee, shoulder, and hands are particularly susceptible to occupational damage, whereas the hip is more protected. Indeed it is suspected that many cases of osteoarthritis of the hip are consequent on pre-existing minor congenital or developmental abnormalities.[42] Obesity adds to the risk of arthritis in weight-bearing joints.

Good evidence for evolution by natural selection is the poor performance of the human spine in meeting the challenge of bipedal gait, over a lifespan that has increased in the recent history of our species. Apart from pain arising from damaged joints, cervical disk prolapse can produce acute and extremely painful entrapment neuropathies. Chronic disability due to other brachial neuropathies is also common, but the most damaging consequence of cervical spondylosis is cervical myelopathy, affecting the long tracts of the spinal cord. Among subtler effects of cervical spondylosis, as already mentioned, is the loss of proprioceptive feedback from cervical joint receptors that contributes to control of body stability and movement.

The lumbar spine is notorious as a cause of disability in the general population and loss of productivity in industry. It is disappointing that newer systems of body imaging have added little to our understanding of the mechanisms of lower backache. Acute syndromes involving spinal nerves may merit neurosurgical opinion, but for the great majority of chronic or recurrent lumbar pain not radiating down the legs, treatment remains initial analgesia with as little rest as is necessary to control pain before active exercise is gradually resumed. Obviously, with the older male worker, the possibility of metastatic prostatic disease needs to be borne in mind but until more specific tests for metastasizing prostatic cancer become available investigation has to be undertaken with care. The controversy associated with measuring for Prostate Specific Antigen

(P3A) in asymptomatic men exemplifies a general problem in testing for a condition that might, in some circumstances, be better left undiagnosed.[43]

Lumbar spine stenosis, especially in association with a midline disk protrusion may produce a syndrome of neurogenic intermittent claudication that can closely mimic vascular disease of the legs. An infrequent but suggestive feature is the association of paraesthesiae with the pain. The pain is produced because the vasa nervorum of the cauda equina nerves cannot dilate in response to increased neural activity associated with walking. Decompressive surgery can be effective for this condition.[44]

Osteoarthritis of the spine is more common in its cervical and lumbar regions than in the less mobile thoracic division. However, in occupations that involve much twisting of the upper body, pain radiating from thoracic spondylosis can cause diagnostic problems. In particular the discomfort may radiate to the anterior central chest and mimic cardiac pain. Other diseases of thoracic vertebrae, including metastases and osteoporotic collapse can cause a similar diagnostic problem.

Osteoporosis is largely but not exclusively a problem for older women, rather than men. Both sexes lose bone tissue on average throughout adult life but women start with less and experience accelerated loss following the menopause. In terms of mortality, the most serious consequence is proximal femoral fracture but that is rare until the eighth or ninth decade of life. The older female worker is more likely to suffer a forearm fracture in a fall,[45] or to experience the effects of spinal osteoporosis. Thoracic and lumbar vertebrae are vulnerable, the most commonly affected vertebrae being those near the thoracolumbar junction. Spinal osteoporosis may follow a painless and insidious course of kyphosis and loss of height. At the other extreme, acutely painful vertebral collapse may occur in a fall or follow apparently minor activity such as pushing a vacuum cleaner. As already noted, the pain of a thoracic vertebral collapse may occasionally mimic an acute cardiac syndrome. Although most spinal fractures in middle-aged women will reflect osteoporosis, the clinician has always to consider the possibility of metastatic disease, especially from the breast.

Some epidemiological evidence suggests that osteoporosis may become more common in women as a cohort phenomenon, owing to recent trends towards poor dietary calcium intakes and inadequate exercise, reducing bone formation in the years of adolescence. Increased use of hormone replacement therapy (HRT) in the postmenopausal period may partly counter such a trend, but in view of the current confusion about risks and benefits,[46] the likely pattern of the future of HRT use in the British population is uncertain.

Genitourinary problems Older men and women may experience various urinary difficulties. Urgency, frequency, and incontinence—or the fear of incontinence—can interfere with work as well as with sleep and social life.[47] Affected individuals may be loath to discuss their symptoms, even with their general practitioners (GP), and urinary difficulties are typically worsened by anxiety. Older workers with such problems will appreciate frequent rest periods from externally paced work. Surveys have indicated that people with incontinence in the general population have often not received expert advice on managing their problem. Incontinence advisors are now appointed in many districts.

Depression Opinions differ over whether the ageing brain is more or less susceptible to depression. Late middle age is, however, a time of life when particularly depressing experiences are liable to happen. Bereavements, awareness of lost opportunities and fading sexual attractiveness, anxiety about future (or present) income and vicarious involvement in the misfortunes of children are all part of the common lot. Although behaviour may change with the maturing of more recent age cohorts, older people are less willing than younger adults to countenance the idea of being mentally ill and tend to somatize their feelings of depression. Persistent pain, tinnitus, or paraesthesiae may become the focus of depressive rumination.

Suicide as a consequence of depression increases in risk with age. Middle-aged and older men, living alone, are particularly vulnerable to successful suicide when severely depressed. The presence of chronic symptomatic illness and higher social class are also recognized risk factors, as is accessibility of means of self-harm, such as a well-intentioned but too large a prescription of tricyclic antidepressants.[48]

Iatrogenic factors Geriatricians, traditionally the inheritors of other doctors' mistakes, have long recognized the high frequency of iatrogenic disorders among older people. The taking of a careful drug history is important for older workers. Most problems arise from lack of fine-tuning in prescribing and through interactions between multiple medications. With regard to pharmacokinetic issues, drugs excreted by mainly renal mechanisms can cause problems, but in the absence of unusual renal impairment this is unlikely to create problems at working ages. More relevant are some pharmacodynamic problems, especially an age-associated increased sensitivity to the effects of sedatives, such as benzodiazepines. Benzodiazepine prescription has been linked to road traffic accidents[49] and to falls,[50] and must be suspected as a probable cause of industrial accidents and errors. The drugs are addictive, and withdrawal effects can be unpleasant and sufficient often to interfere with work. Their duration varies with the actual benzodiazepine responsible. The so-called 'Z-drugs' are shorter acting than currently licensed benzodiazepines. Although chemically distinct from benzodiazepines and marketed as an alternative, they act on the same receptors in the brain and must be expected to have a similar profile of adverse effects and potential for dependency.

It is difficult for clinicians to keep up to date with all the possible adverse effects and interactions of modern drugs. The *British National Formulary*, now accessible on line, is an indispensable resource.[51] Among older patients, adverse effects from medications prescribed to control high blood pressure are common, and include hypotension, impotence, and depression. Impairment of exercise capacity by beta-blockers may be significant for older workers in physically demanding occupations, especially in externally paced work.

The possible involvement of over-the-counter or complementary medicines in causing problems is increasingly recognized, especially in their producing adverse effects through interactions with prescribed medication. GPs are often unaware of what non-prescribed remedies their patients are taking, and ethnic traditions are important determinants of self-treatment. The common, and arguably arrogant assumption among Western doctors that folk and herbal remedies are totally ineffective and can therefore do no harm, as well as no good, can mislead.

Alcohol Alcohol presents a range of challenges to the occupational physician. Alcohol-related health and behaviour problems can affect both sexes and all age groups. At a physiological level, tolerance of alcohol diminishes with age, owing in part to reduction in the size and blood supply of the liver, and many heavy social drinkers adjust their intake accordingly. Lowered tolerance can also result in habitual intakes starting to cause sleep disturbance in middle age, and drinkers may recognize this effect and reduce their intake. Not all heavy drinkers are dependent, and it has been often noted how workers in heavy industry may give up drinking abruptly and without difficulty, when they retire and can no longer afford the habit.

There is a particular risk of alcoholism being overlooked in older female workers, partly as a result of cultural expectations, but also because the volume of alcohol consumed need not be as great as for a male colleague with a similar problem. In general, however, the problems associated with alcohol and the means of dealing with them are the same for workers of all ages and are dealt with in Chapter 24 of this volume.

Drug problems Iatrogenic problems have been discussed above. Misuse of illegal 'recreational' drugs is still rare among older workers, and does not seem to have increased with the maturing of the generation that was young in the 1960s. This may be partly because use of illegal drugs is largely associated with the social ambience of late adolescence, and partly because individuals with a serious drug habit leave the workforce, one way or another. But culturally determined patterns of drug use must be expected to vary. Anecdotal evidence suggests that the present-day occupational physician is more likely to encounter a problem with cocaine among the managers than with heroin among the workers.

Health maintenance and service issues

Nutrition, diet, and exercise

Conventional wisdom has it that, as we age, we need less food and more exercise, less sleep and more rest. Few of today's older workers received any personal instruction or advice about diet and nutrition during their early lives. Many of them, while serving in the armed services in their youth, took advantage of the opportunity to overindulge themselves with cheap alcohol and tobacco. Barriers to older adults responding to nutrition education can be categorized as attitudinal, motivational, environmental, and related to lower levels of literacy and income. However, research suggests that older workers are likely to have a greater understanding of nutrition than younger workers.[52]

Evidence from the USA suggests that the most successful education interventions are aimed at families, neighbourhoods, and communities. Interventions are most likely to be successful when legislative, media, and marketing efforts support them. Within the ageing population, those with greatest health needs include members of minority groups and recent immigrants. These groups are often overlooked when designing and implementing health promotion programs.[53,54]

After food rationing was relaxed in the UK, in the mid-1950s, food preparation and storage methods allowed diversification of diets and, during the 1960s and 1970s, government health education encouraged the UK population to reduce salt, sugar, and fat in their diets. Quality protein, salads, and fruit were then more expensive than foods containing high concentrations of saturated fats. 'Ready-to-eat meals', often containing large quantities of salt, sugar, and saturated fats, became popular with the spread of home microwave ovens. The widening food and life-style habits of the different socio-economic groups in the population resulted in the wealthier groups eating a healthier diet. The effects of this diversity are seen in today's poorer older workers, in their higher rates of heart, lung, and liver disease, diabetes and bowel disorders and in their reduced life expectancy. Only those with particular eating habits (e.g. vegetarians and vegans) have bucked the trend of a widening gap between the life expectancy of rich and poor.

In the past 25 years, salads and fruit have become available all the year round and frozen food is now available to the majority, if not quite all, of the population. However, the habits (and the atheroma) developed in the 1960s and 1970s have been hard to change, with those in the poorer socio-economic groups changing the least. Tobacco smoking has continued longer in these same (poorer) groups, reducing their average life expectancy still further. Large quantities of toxins, such as the breakdown products of tobacco and alcohol, weaken the body's defences and addiction to them worsens the user's chances of a long and healthy life.

There is evidence that workers over 50 have more positive health behaviours, stronger beliefs about the value of healthy behaviour, and better self-assessed health. In addition, they have been found to be more likely to hold attitudes associated with participation in worksite health promotion activities. Physical activity should be continued in the older worker, even though strength may be diminished. Regular exercise is the key, continuing at least three times a week to raise the heart rate according to age and taking due account of concurrent medical conditions. There is evidence that those with a Body Mass Index (BMI—weight in kilograms divided by the square of the height in metres) of 30+ die earlier and that all age groups benefit from regular exercise. The BMI should ideally be kept under 25, even though there is a natural tendency for body weight to move centrally, with age. Accumulation of omental fat inside the abdomen is especially prominent in men.

Daily fruit and vegetables, adequate supplies of protein and a good intake of water (said to be ideally 1.5 litres per day, although there is no empirical evidence to support this recommendation) are essential for good health. For the older worker, keeping the immune system healthy, active, and effective against viruses, bacteria, and early cancers, may well be a matter of life and death. Adding vitamins and minerals, essential for proper nutrition, should be considered and the advice of a qualified nutritionist or dietician should be sought.[55]

Health surveillance

Studies in Scotland, more than four decades ago, demonstrated that much disease and disability among older people was unknown to their GPs. There were several reasons for this finding. One was that general practice then as now was response based; if patients did not complain they were assumed to be well. A second was that older people did not appreciate that some afflictions of later life were not simply due to ageing but were the consequence of potentially remediable disease. Thirdly, some older people dreaded the undignified and unpleasant processes of medical investigation and treatment more than the experience of illness and the prospect of premature death.

One response to this problem was to institute various kinds of what was initially called screening but is now better called surveillance. Screening is now narrowly but more usefully defined in terms of testing apparently well people for specific diseases or risk states using specific tests of known parameters (sensitivity, specificity) to be followed by specific treatment of known efficacy. Such screening, whether for cancer or any other condition, has the possibility of doing more harm than good and should not be undertaken without very great care and expert consultation. The National Screening Committee, accessible through its website, has defined criteria for establishing programmes and for the quality assurance standards that need to be applied in them. While it may be appropriate for an occupational physician to encourage workers to make use of national screening programmes, 'do-it-yourself' screening in the workplace is not to be recommended except where part of specifically required health surveillance (for more information on this topic, please refer to Chapter 29).

Surveillance, in contrast, is essentially an extension of clinical practice; people who have not presented themselves to a doctor are reviewed for problems they may be experiencing, problems that may have a variety of causes calling for a variety of interventions.

The issue of surveillance may arise in occupational medicine, with the increase in numbers of older workers, many of whom will not wish to seek medical attention if they thereby risk both investigation and possible loss of employment. While it might seem logical to consider special surveillance for older workers, both to safeguard their health and also to prevent accidents or loss of production due to unrecognized impairments, there are ethical questions. Nature is not equitable, but mankind, at least democratic mankind, is required to be. While Nature distributes impediments unequally between ages as between sexes and ethnic groups, equity should require that the chance of such impediment being recognized—with whatever beneficial and harmful consequences—should be equal for all individuals. It would not be equitable therefore to require surveillance over members of a particular age group, or ethnic group that was not provided for and required of all other members of the workgroup.

However, if we are anxious to do our best for the workforce as a whole, it is sensible to recognize that some problems are more likely to arise in some groups that in others. White women are more likely than black men to have difficulty with heavy physical activity because, on average, they have less muscle. Immigrants from the Indian subcontinent are more prone than the English to diabetes. Problems arising from low intelligence are more likely in some social classes than in others. It is prudent to be vigilant for problems that an older worker is more likely than a younger colleague to encounter, but only by surveillance procedures applied equally to workers of all ages.

This general issue of equity also holds for organizationally determined and legally required occupational health surveillance. If specific groups of workers are subject to regular review to ensure that they meet minimum physical and health standards for their particular assigned tasks and are not adversely affected by their work or the materials or processes involved, then both sexes, and all age and ethnic groups, should be treated equally.

Links with primary care

In recent years, many employers have become increasingly reluctant to accept without question the Form Med 3, issued by GPs, as a reliable indication of fitness to work. At the same time, GPs are now increasingly reluctant to continue supplying Med 3s. Employers are now more often obtaining (and following) the advice of a specialist occupational physician, working in the private healthcare sector. In addition, commercial organizations are using the private sector increasingly for healthcare services, to cut waiting times for investigations and treatment (and thereby reduce the length of periods of sickness absence). This sector will continue to expand, for obvious commercial reasons, if delays in the National Health Service (NHS) provision of diagnostic and treatment services persist.

The GP is (quite properly) the patient's advocate and will often feel obliged to take what the patient says about the workplace at face value. However, the GP seldom has access to the workplace and, commonly, no direct knowledge of working practices, corporate culture and what changes are possible to accommodate a worker returning to work after illness or injury. Graded schedules of reduced hours, modified work, shift alterations, and opportunities for periods of training, are now commonly advised by the occupational physician, as well as physical modification to the workplace. So long as the worker is 'adding value' and the graded return is reasonably time limited, employers will usually co-operate with the occupational physician's advice. Often, a short phone call by the GP to the manager or occupational physician will establish the true position at work and save much time (and money) for all parties.

There is often an implicit understanding between GP and hospital consultant, and an acceptance as to who is managing a patient's treatment, at any one time. This may not be the case between the GP and the occupational physician. Good communication, with patient consent, whenever relevant information needs to be shared, is the key to a productive synergistic relationship, with the objective being the best overall outcome for the patient. Healthy alliances (as described in the government documents *Health of the Nation*,[56] and *Our Healthier Nation*,[57]) will be especially necessary for effective and efficient patient care, in older workers, who are more likely to be taking regular long-term medication for chronic conditions.

There will therefore be a greater need for occupational health services and for more GPs to provide part-time occupational health services, in the future. The quality of these services will need to be monitored, through revalidation, to ensure appropriate standards are maintained. There is a need for faster, more accurate communication and wider dissemination of relevant medical information and knowledge (faxes, e-mail, health information credit-card style patient information cards and continuing medical education). There will, however, continue to be ethical and legal issues arising from GPs passing health information about their patients to occupational physicians, without obtaining patients' specific consent.

Workability and employability

Degenerative disease and the chronic illnesses of middle age, even if manageable and treatable, often impair working capacity and lead to restricted activity and reduced productivity at work. In the past, medical restrictions have been placed upon the work of individuals, advised by occupational physicians, with the aim of preventing exacerbation of existing conditions and avoiding injury, but employers find these onerous. Many large employers have responded to this challenge with a notable degree of responsibility, by investing heavily in lifting and handling aids and ergonomically improved workstations over the past decade. However, in the future, the sheer numbers of older workers may prove overwhelming to smaller employers, who have meagre resources with which to effect change.

The concept of 'workability', rather than 'disability', as recently advocated in the Faculty of Occupational Medicine position paper on 'Age and Employment', is the way forward and will require a change of 'mind set' on the part of employers, away from the concept of 'medical restrictions'.[2]

Workability is defined as the ability of workers to perform their jobs taking into account specific work demands, individual health conditions, and mental health resources.[58] This concept should be distinguished from workers' ability, which is related to competence to do the job. The ability to work is a function of health and functional capacities (physical, mental, social), education and competence, values and attitudes, motivation, work demands, work community, and the management culture.

Employability is a term used to describe the actions needed to improve rates of employment. At an individual level these processes include the promotion of good health and associated functional capacity. These are pre-requisites for prolonging the ability to work effectively. Adequate training to ensure competence to do the job and work scheduling to avoid overwork and exhaustion are also important.

Job analysis, skill assessment, job coaching (and retraining), and job matching are all components of an effective management system. There are now several job content and employee capability assessment computer programs under trial in Europe, e.g. the IMBA scheme, developed by the German government.[59,60] These consist of constructing a worker capability profile, against standardized ability measurements and matching this with a data bank of available job requirement profiles. The outcome is a list of jobs that the worker should be able to carry out, with minimal risk of exacerbating any existing medical conditions. Such programmes have several benefits, including transparency, supporting flexibility of labour, retaining older workers in suitable jobs within their capability, and producing an audit trail of effectiveness, for future reference. Substantial initial investment in job profiling is required, as is frequent re-assessment of workers recovering from recent incapacity (e.g. illness or surgery), but early signs are that the investment will prove worthwhile.

Ageing and recovery from illness or injury

Age-associated loss of adaptability not only increases the risk of disease and injury, it increases the risk of secondary complications and lengthens the time needed for healing and recovery. This can be compensated for by the deployment of enhanced rehabilitation programmes to speed an older employee's return to work. While a period of rest may be necessary to help in the control of pain after an accident, for example, inactivity is detrimental to older people, as any loss of fitness may bring them closer to their functional limits, on their return to work. Active rehabilitation and physiotherapy will prove a sound investment in restoring older individuals to the workforce. In addition, it may be necessary to pay attention to psychological, as well as physical, needs. In particular, an older worker may suffer loss of confidence following an accident or illness. Active *and repeated* encouragement and reassurance may prevent unnecessary invalidism.

On the subject of convalescence, George Bernard Shaw (1856–1950), the Irish Dramatist and Critic, has one of his characters in 'Back to Methuselah', Pt II, say 'I enjoy convalescence. It is the part that makes illness worth while.' Today, of course, we often take some of our convalescence at work, rather than at home, as part of a graded return to work.

Although on average older people recover more slowly than young people from illness, injury, or surgery, there is wide variation in the rate of recovery, dependent upon various factors, e.g. previous health, availability of suitable treatment, motivation, status and enjoyment of work, support of colleagues and family, managers' attitudes and the opportunity for a graded (part-time) return to work, monitored by trained medical staff.[61] Any delay can be compensated for by the deployment of enhanced rehabilitation programmes, to speed an older employee's return to work.

The myth that workers should be 'pain-free', before returning to (suitably restricted) work, should be actively debunked. Functional assessments in the work environment are key to early and successful reintegration into work, following absence due to illness or injury. This is especially true for acute musculoskeletal conditions.

Early access to assessment and treatment services, preferably on-site or close by the place of work and managed by a specialist occupational physician, will expedite a successful return. Active rehabilitation and physiotherapy will prove a sound investment in restoring older individuals to the workforce. Few employers today can afford the luxury of waiting weeks or months for such treatment to commence under the NHS and even fewer employees can afford the loss of income (or job) that results from such lengthy delays.

Where an employee's musculoskeletal symptoms indicate that strain is occurring at work, but this has not yet caused overt illness or injury, early proactive intervention using instruction by physiotherapists in individually tailored exercise programmes, reinforced by other medical and nursing staff, can reduce that risk of damage or deterioration.

It is the authors' experience that, if managers and supervisors are educated in the benefits (to them) of maintaining older workers' fitness, through the organization making available free physiotherapy assessment and treatment services on site and demonstrating their impact on manning levels (sickness absence reduction), supervisors will support such services, by proactive direct referral of workers. The benefit to supervisors is improved worker performance and overall attendance. Workers welcome early and easy access to assessment and treatment, enabling them to stay in work and avoid sickness absence (and the consequent loss of income). Both parties have improved control over their working lives, as a result, and the business reaps the benefit.

There is evidence that older workers may have longer absences from work due to illness, than younger workers, as common medical problems increase with age, but this is offset by a tendency to have fewer short-term spells of absence that are often more disruptive. On balance, older workers do not have more absence from the workplace than workers of other ages.[2] Indeed, there is evidence that older workers are careful to conserve sick leave as a 'cushion' for serious illness.[62] Older workers are also less prone to accidents. However, if absence due to illness has been prolonged, it is likely that colleagues, supervisors, working patterns, and the workplace itself will have changed, in the interim, thereby posing a greater challenge to the older worker, returning to what has effectively become a 'different' job, during their absence. Older workers are less confident and require more support when adapting to change.

In the authors' experience, an integrated approach comprising: (1) early completion of outpatient investigation and specialist assessment of the illness (ideally, within a planned maximum of 6 weeks); (2) a supportive treatment and work hardening plan (involving an individual physical or psychological training plan, to return the worker to their own work, or to suitable alternative work); and (3) a graded return to work on reduced hours, agreed with management, is the most cost-effective and efficient way of returning people safely to work. The by-product of this approach is a reduction in overall levels of long-term sickness absence. Ideally, this should be pursued with the co-operation of the GP and the occupational physician should keep the GP informed of progress throughout, as necessary. The objective should be to reach a decision point, regarding a return to work or (if appropriate) a medical ill health retirement, as soon as practicable.

The cost/benefit of proactive early completion of outpatient investigation and specialist assessment, taking into account all employment costs, can reach as high as 50:1, i.e. a saving of £50 for every £1 spent on early investigation and assessment, as opposed to waiting for NHS appointments, which can be delayed for many months, in some specialties. Followed over periods of 5–10 years, such policies can literally save large companies millions of pounds.

Retraining and redeployment

There is evidence that present generations of older workers are more reliable and make fewer mistakes than younger workers, once trained. In the initial phase of training it is prudent to help older workers to avoid making mistakes, as these may then have to be 'unlearned' before the correct track is established.

Time invested in training and re-training older workers is well spent, as lower staff turnover in the older age groups has financial benefits in reduced recruitment costs, and also in terms of better returns from training initiatives. The content and delivery of training of older workers needs to be structured differently from that of younger workers. This is definitely an area where one size does not fit all. Trainers need to understand and utilize the differing learning strengths and weaknesses of both groups and tailor their programmes accordingly.[63]

In this adaptive society, multiple career changes and continuous retraining will become the norm in a longer working life to age 70 and beyond. The 'cutting edge' new technologies of today will become 'routine' tomorrow and will be handed on to workers with specific skills. The latter will still require core skills, enabling them to adapt to new changes as they appear; otherwise their skill base will become obsolete, rendering them at a disadvantage. 'Ring-fenced' retraining funds will enable older workers to continue working, especially if they can no longer remain in their full-time job because of chronic illness or disability. These necessary costs will rise over the next 25 years.

Many 'retired' workers may seek part-time employment to supplement their pensions over a similar period. As is common in the southern USA, where a high proportion of the population is elderly, part-time and flexible work in the UK service industry sector now provides many jobs (but often low rates of pay). However, personal safety for older people in such employment, where direct contact with the public is an integral part of the work, is a growing concern. When handling cash is involved, the older worker may be physically more vulnerable to injury or threats than the younger worker; assaulting and robbing older people may be seen as relatively 'risk-free' by young assailants.

Older workers tend to be employed closer to their homes and presently tend not to travel as far to work as do younger workers. If these habits are to change, to satisfy demand for labour as the population ages, then improved public transport will be required, specifically designed to accommodate older workers with disabilities and special needs. As car travel to and from work becomes increasingly inefficient, costly and polluting, the need for better systems of public transport, which are both efficient and responsive to the needs of older workers, will increase steadily.

Ethical issues and 'retirement': duties to employers, responsibilities to employees

Expectations and norms will need to change for the manager, the worker, the GP, the occupational physician, the worker's family and dependents, and for all age groups in society.

Employment options for older workers may well become more varied, diffuse, and complicated, as the retirement age rises. Present patterns of the provision of primary medical care are likely to change, as more primary care is provided by alternative sources (NHS Direct etc.). An increased risk of confusion and the fragmentation of care may both have an adverse effect on the medical supervision of chronic conditions where, in an ageing population, the opposite would be desirable.

Ethical dilemmas will become more frequent and challenging for occupational physicians. The continuing desire of many larger employers for manpower reductions, to meet cost requirements ('downsizing', voluntary redundancy programmes, etc.), can result in both active and/or passive discrimination against the older worker.[64] Age discrimination is often based upon inaccurate and outdated assumptions and stereotypes about older workers or job applicants, which all work against the interests of both workers and their employers.[65,66]

The Faculty of Occupational Medicine position paper on Age and Employment (2004)[2] states:

> In addition, older workers often have accumulated experience or learned strategies that may be valuable in contributing to business success. The published literature does not support the popular misconception that work performance declines with age. Older workers are noted to perform generally more consistently and to deliver higher quality, matching the performance of younger colleagues. In practice, despite an age related decline in physical strength, stamina, memory and information processing, this rarely impairs work performance. Older workers may use knowledge, skills, experience, anticipation, motivation and other strategies to maintain their performance. Older workers also bring the benefits of often being more conscientious, loyal, reliable and hard working and having well developed inter-personal skills. On balance, older workers do not have more absence from the workplace than workers of other ages. Older workers are also less prone to accidents. Lower staff turnover in the older age groups has financial benefits in reduced recruitment costs, and also in terms of better returns from training initiatives.

In a recent survey by 'Maturity Works', it was reported that 80% of staff between the ages of 34 and 67 say they have been victims of age discrimination. Conversely, one major UK national retail store chain has made a virtue out of positive age discrimination, specifically recruiting older workers, for their greater experience in both using and advising customers about the products they sell. The UK is committed to implementing the EU Directive on Equal Treatment in Employment (Article 13) by December 2006. This will outlaw age discrimination in the workplace. A voluntary code is in place in the UK, from 2004, until then. However, whether employers will support this code remains to be seen.

Through lack of knowledge, some managers assume and promote the myth that all workers with cancers or those undergoing radiotherapy or chemotherapy will either die soon or will never return to productive work. This attitude is displayed more frequently by younger managers, with little or no personal experience of serious illness. Many older workers expect and want to stay in work, in spite of serious illness.[67–69] They appreciate that their work tasks may take more time to complete and that rehabilitation may be longer than average. They are often surprised and shocked when this is deemed unacceptable by their managers.[69]

The issue of ill health retirement is covered in detail in Chapter 27 of this volume. There are many differing definitions and criteria for 'ill health or medical' retirement, in different occupations and work environments. The criteria range from workers being no longer able to carry out the specified tasks for which they are employed for 'the foreseeable future', to their being 'permanently unfit for all work' (including part-time work). The terms of retirement schemes are usually laid down by a Pension Fund Trustees Committee, in larger organizations, or may be entirely at the discretion of operational managers in smaller enterprises. No two schemes are the same or are administered identically. Even in Local Government Authorities different employees are administered differently, in this respect, under different protocols and guidelines.

Under pressure from managers criteria for eligibility can become 'flexible', if organizational accommodations (reasonable adjustments) are believed by them to be too difficult. Older workers may then be judged to be failing in their jobs and can feel threatened if they are considered for dismissal on the grounds of capability.

The occupational physician must retain an independent and consistent position in such cases, always willing to consider and modify advice if and when relevant new evidence comes to hand, but resolute in the face of management pressure to remove an individual from the organization if he or she is simply perceived (in the manager's view) as being ill and unlikely to return to productive work.

All relevant information should be gathered from GPs, hospital consultants, and, if appropriate, independent specialists, to build up a complete picture of the patient's health and long-term prognosis. In practice, if a hospital consultant is adamant that the condition warrants a recommendation in favour of medical retirement, then unless the occupational physician is an expert in that discipline, the advice should be followed. However, until clear evidence of permanent (or, in some organizations/cases, 'prolonged') incapacity on medical grounds is available, the occupational physician should continue to seek out and to promote opportunities to rehabilitate the employee, whenever possible. In difficult circumstances it is often useful to discuss the case with a more experienced specialist occupational physician colleague.

If people expect to work longer, then the attitudes of society to career trajectories will need to change. The question of whether large employers, whose core business requires much heavy or repetitive externally paced work, should be required by government to make lighter work available, is as yet unanswered. Recent outsourcing by large organizations of non-core business, e.g. of caterers, janitors, and security staff, may in future be reversed, providing a possible method of keeping 'retired' workers in closer contact with the former employer. So can the placing of contracts with co-operatives of 'retired' workers aged over 50 years, providing a variety of services, ranging from engineering expertise to welfare services. These considerations are as valid for managers, at all levels, as they are for shop floor workers.

Pre-retirement courses, run by many large employers, are both popular and generally informative. They should always include a session on 'staying healthy in retirement, delivered by a competent and experienced occupational physician or occupational health nurse. Such courses provide a valuable opportunity to guide prospective retirees in life-style choices and to encourage them to remain active, to eat healthily, and avoid obvious (to the occupational physician) pitfalls.

Organizational issues

Management and social aspects

There is a perception among UK managers that older workers are more expensive than younger workers, but this is partly a product of past and present employer/employee structures. This may change, particularly with the growth in popularity among employers of the practice of offering fixed term contracts in which overhead costs are unaffected by the age of the employee.

Organizational 'downsizing', for which the driver may be cost reduction, can have a disproportionately adverse effect on a predominately older workforce. One study has demonstrated that when the proportion of employees who were older than 50 years was high, downsizing increased the individual risk of absence because of ill health by between three and 14 times, depending on diagnostic category.[64] This risk varies according to individual factors.

Trades Unions (TUs) can find themselves in a dilemma about older workers. There is an understandable ambivalence in the attitude of TUs to older workers, or to any development that may increase the availability of manpower, such as older workers remaining economically active into their later years. Governments, too, are happy to have a 'sink' of retirement in which to hide excessive unemployment. Society will need to address this issue and one option is for positive discrimination, in favour of the older worker. However, if it is perceived that older workers are receiving preferential treatment, within the group or company, at the expense of younger workers, TUs will feel a conflict of interest that may be difficult to resolve. The occupational physician may be asked for an opinion, as various interested parties seek to 'medicalize' what are essentially management issues, to their own group's advantage, and occupational physicians should be alert to this ploy.

Increasingly, retirement is anticipated as a time not to be wasted in rest and inactivity but used for new interests and the pursuit of new goals. Part-time working, job-sharing, 'five years' work in ten', and other innovative semi-retirement packages can all help the older worker to achieve what is for them an 'ideal' work pattern to suit their capability and personal circumstances as they move from full-time work into full-time retirement. However, in a mass production environment, this is often difficult to achieve where employers find job-sharing expensive (due to taxation, employment and training costs) and also time consuming, especially if illness or family responsibilities disrupt the agreed work pattern and employees require additional support.

Co-operatives of retired workers providing services to their former employer and annualized contracts, allowing seasonal flexibility for individuals, are two ways of retaining older workers in part-time work. These enable recently retired workers to retain the social contact and support network of the working environment without the pressure and commitment to full-time work.

Shift work

Many older workers find shift work more difficult as they age, especially night work and may seek medical approval for stopping night shifts.[70] Those aged over 40 starting shift work for the first time experience difficulty adapting to different sleep and eating times while those who have worked shifts for decades may suddenly notice fatigue at night and feel lethargic and less well. The performance of older workers may fall, relative to younger workers, on night shifts.[71] There is evidence that the time to exhaustion is reduced by a significant amount (20%) for older shift workers during the recovery period from night shift.[72] In addition, evidence exists that a fast forward rotating shift schedule is more suitable for older workers than a slower backward rotating system.[73]

Sleep disorders are more common in older workers.[74] In extreme cases the older worker may be at risk of losing his or her job if regular day shift work cannot be provided. However, a recent court judgment (see p 53) requires that a worker should be placed into a vacant higher grade job, if available, when no job at the same grade is available.

In addition, older workers, who travel regularly back and forth across several time zones by air either as aircrew or passengers, take longer to recover their circadian rhythm with increasing age. However, older individuals who have wider natural circadian rhythm swings and the apparent ability to 'reset' their body clocks more quickly appear to cope better than others with this work/life style. If performance is affected adversely, to an unacceptable degree, redeployment within the employing organization may prove difficult, e.g. for pilots. Employers should be sympathetic to making reasonable adjustments to accommodate such requests.

Temporary reorganization of shift patterns may be necessary for individual workers, e.g. after depressive illness or while still recovering on medication. This is especially necessary during the winter months at higher latitudes when 'Zeitgeber' (time-of-day) cues are reduced or absent and when the risk of relapse, after stopping medication at this time of year, may be increased. Diabetics and sufferers from seasonal affective disorder (SAD syndrome) will have their own additional difficulties with alterations in diurnal rhythm associated with shift changes. These can usually be overcome by good planning and a disciplined approach, both of which are more commonly observed in older workers. Bright desk lamps can be used by office workers with SAD syndrome to assist alertness and productivity.

Hours of work

The EU Working Time Directive (Council Directive 94/103/EC), adopted in 1993, requires written consent from workers required to work an average of more than 48 hours per week over a (normally 3-month) reference period. In addition, other requirements include a minimum daily rest period of 11 consecutive hours a day and that night working must not exceed 8 hours a night on average. The Working Time Directive is implemented in the UK by the Working Time Regulations 1998.[75]

A culture of long working hours is prevalent in the UK, more so than in other European countries. Additional hours of work (e.g. weekend overtime and additional shifts) are often welcomed by the younger worker for the earnings they bring. Older workers are often not so enthusiastic, especially those in poor health. The incentives for the self-employed to work longer hours and to take less time off for illness have always been more pressing than for employed workers. Access to occupational health services for the self-employed has been inferior to that for employed workers in the past. In order to reach and service the ageing self-employed population adequately these services may need to be expanded.

The Turner Report[76] urged the UK Government to consider incentives for both employers and workers to keep older workers in work for longer. Such incentives will need to be flexible, regarding part-time working, and accompanied by suitable alterations in taxation and employment legislation to ensure that they achieve the desired result. In addition, the older self-employed and teleworkers will need to be included in these arrangements.

'Upstream ergonomics': input into the design of processes

Mass production line job design requires early occupational health involvement and effective monitoring of process developments and changes. Feedback of information, learned on current job processes, into new and future product development and assembly (incorporating ergonomic improvements into new manufacturing/assembly processes) is in the interests of all workers, regardless of age.

Occupational physicians should make strong representation to be consulted regularly during the design phase of new components and products as this has been inconsistent in the past. In particular, the occupational physician **must** be involved at the earliest possible stage of repetitive assembly job design. Late design changes and alterations in the product should not be made without the occupational physician being consulted. Failure to involve the occupational physician, at the design stage, can lead to costly subsequent reworking of processes and/or legal claims from workers, affected by repetitive overuse injuries and other work-related musculoskeletal conditions. The older worker who develops such conditions is likely to take longer to recover than the younger worker, and is more likely to develop a chronic state, requiring permanent redeployment, always assuming that such alternative work is available.[20]

Ergonomic improvements should ideally be innovative, individual, and inexpensive. Adaptation of the majority of workplaces is needed to accommodate physically restricted older workers. Such improvements will also, coincidentally, allow increased flexibility and accommodate workers of all ages and most abilities. Ideally, job rotation needs to be 2–4 hourly, rather than daily or weekly, to accommodate all temporarily or permanently restricted and disabled workers. A worker who is recovering from an open laparotomy, a myocardial infarction, or a prolapsed intervertebral disc may be restricted with regard to manual handling for several weeks or months whatever their age. The introduction of robots or other mechanical equipment (preferably under the worker's control) and improved workplace and component design, and 'lazy seats' allowing the worker to move more easily around a production line while sitting, thereby avoiding standing and repeated bending, are examples of improvements that will preferentially protect older workers and improve their overall flexibility and status in the workforce.

While much functional back pain is now avoided by ergonomic workplace improvements, made over the past decade, ergonomic design aimed at preventing neck, shoulder, and upper limb pain and fatigue is only now in the ascendant. Additional training is needed for ergonomists to enable them to understand the abilities and limitations of older people in respect of capabilities and working 'envelopes', muscular strength, static loads, the risk of injury, and the effect of shift patterns and rest periods in relation to fatigue. Expert ergonomic input into process and risk assessments will ensure that both are relevant and appropriate for workers of all ages.

Older workers and younger managers

This is the first generation in which a majority of younger managers (and supervisors), in their 30s and early 40s, are commonly managing groups of people, of whom half or more are from their parents' generation. This increased prevalence of the generation gap at work has potential adverse consequences for communication and productivity. Commonly, the younger manager has no concept of what it feels like to hurt before you get out of bed in the morning and the effect that this has on performance and on a workers' enjoyment of work. If you find yourself nodding in agreement with this statement, you are probably an 'older worker' yourself!

Research has shown that managers rate older job applicants as less economically beneficial (to the organization) than younger applicants.[66] The older worker is sometimes seen by the younger manager as being slow, work-shy, uncooperative, and resistant to change. The younger manager, in turn, is sometimes seen as unpredictable, overbearing, inconsistent, and arrogant. Clumsy or inflexible handling of misunderstandings by the younger manager can lead to humiliation of the older worker, thus resulting in resentment, mistrust, and ultimately, de-motivation. Older workers may fear for their job security, especially if already coping with discomfort and disability associated with long-standing degenerative illness, either in themselves or in a spouse or partner.

This can lead to emotional crisis or depression and, commonly, to sickness absence. Aggressive or 'blame' cultures can exacerbate such situations. Individual productivity inevitably suffers. In an ageing population, such situations are likely to occur more frequently in the future. All parties can benefit from improved training in conflict resolution and in improved knowledge and understanding of the strengths, capabilities, and reasonable expectations of different age groups. Patience and great sensitivity on the part of the occupational physician is often required in such situations (assisted by human resources staff and expert counselling services, as necessary), to re-establish the older worker's self-esteem, if prolonged sickness absence is to be avoided.

Possible actions and solutions

The National Statistical Office estimates that the UK population will rise by about 5 million people over the next 25 years, with immigrants accounting for approximately two-thirds of this growth. Net migration into the UK, during this period, is projected to be about 135 000 a year. Labour market gaps and government spending on public services to support this increase will create a need for more nurses, teachers, doctors, and other skilled workers.

Importing young people indiscriminately from abroad may be thought, at first sight, to represent a solution. However, this can produce a net drain on resources if they do not have skills that enable them immediately to contribute to the manufacturing economy, engineering, construction, technology, 'invisible' overseas earnings, or to the essential services (e.g. transport, power genera-tion, health and financial services). In addition, once migrants are settled, they tend to adopt the fertility patterns, eating habits, and life-style of the host country; they have children and grow older. More new immigrants are then needed to support them in their retirement and the cycle is repeated.

For more than a decade, societal attitudes, consumer pressures and tastes, legislation and the desire of businesses to be the 'employer of choice' have all been driving business organizations towards becoming 'lean, mean, and young'. The importance of the resource of skill and experi-ence that older workers represent has been largely sidelined, by the movement of the primary source of information away from books and older people, into information technology sys-tems. This has been given added impetus by computerization, the (global) standardization of processes across businesses, and by the need to reduce manufacturing process variability, all driven by consumer pressures for higher quality and reliability of goods and services at reduced cost.

As the population ages further, social institutions now need to be re-based; expectations and norms will need to change. John Stuart Mill[77] recognized a tolerant society, which was funda-mentally individualist but in which individual members accepted obligations towards other people. In an increasingly competitive world, all age groups will need to provide for themselves and for one another, and for their own potential periods of low productivity and earnings (e.g. preg-nancy, sickness, retirement), throughout their lives. The expectation that the older (and retired) worker will be provided for by or be dependent upon other members of society can no longer be supported if, as expected, the cohort of younger workers becomes significantly smaller than that of their older worker colleagues over the next two decades.

Concepts of 'rights' and 'entitlements' will undergo necessary evolution, as Britain's earn-ing capacity in the world alters, relative to the developing economies, primarily in China, and the Far East. However, the global picture is complex; for example, China also has a large older segment of its population.[78] Economic competitiveness of the EU with the Asian and Far Eastern economies, many of which have significantly younger age profiles, will require the UK workforce to 'work smarter', as 'working harder' may not be practicable as the working population ages.

This change **can** be accommodated within a culture of inclusion for the older worker, at the same time as meeting and maintaining manufacturing and service industry requirements, but the change will not be swift or easy. Older workers with scarce skills will remain in demand and will be economically self-sufficient; those who cannot embrace the computer age or who suffer from chronic illness and/or live in areas of higher unemployment will fare less well. There is good evidence of a link between unemployment and ill health, with older economically inactive people between 50 and 65 years of age being less fit than their working counterparts.

In the future, people will have to work longer, but not necessarily harder, up to the age of 70 and, if they wish beyond, in order to provide for their old age. This concept is now promoted by the UK government and a retirement age of 70 is intended to be in place by 2030. In practice, the change will probably be driven forward by international market forces, to occur in the UK some 10–15 years earlier.

A recent survey of UK employers showed that 86% believe that care issues (for older relatives) will be a key concern in the future. As a result, the career expectations, earnings, savings, and work trajectories of older workers will all need to alter, as will training, legislation, age discrimi-nation, taxation, the provision for pensions, and arrangements for the care of older workers' eld-erly relatives living into their nineties. (See Boxes 26.1 and 26.2, after G. Glover, pers. comm. Society of Occupational Medicine Annual Scientific Meeting, 2003.)

Box 26.1 What businesses require of Government as the population ages

Businesses need the Government to:

- develop a strategic position on the demographic issue
- develop health services aimed specifically at supporting older workers remaining in work
- consider funding/subsidizing individuals who cannot cope with full-time (first tier) employment as they become older
- provide tax incentives and other means of support for employing organizations to safeguard training budgets, especially for older workers
- ensure that pension arrangements support worker mobility
- be aware of the pressures on organizations for 'ill health retirement' as the retirement age rises
- provide flexible labour policies enabling employers to release employees, often at short notice and for extended periods, for elder care (parents and relatives)

Box 26.2 What businesses need to do to accommodate an ageing workforce

Businesses need to:

- consider their most effective strategic plan and direction—as well as employment legislation
- examine and change individual and institutional attitudes towards older employees
- review all policies, procedures, practices, and then customise them to meet the needs of the older employee
- consider how best to support the rising number of staff caring for elderly parents and relatives
- regard flexibility as key for employees seeking changes, to maintain an acceptable work-life balance
- review methods needed to sustain employee motivation over longer careers and to transform organisation cultures away from a 'youth culture'
- increase the emphasis on improving health, safety, and well-being, as part of a drive towards greater productivity and efficiency, especially for the older worker
- refine and embed strategies in their organisation to deal with foreseeable absence and periods of prolonged illness in older workers
- challenge organizational norms about what workers can do, as they age
- challenge established national norms about when employees leave (and return to) organisations
- harness new technologies, innovative work practices and job design to support and keep older workers at work
- promote an environment and culture of continuous personal improvement and lifelong learning
- establish a position as an employer of choice, not just for the young but for all age groups

Prospects and requirements for the future

In summary therefore, in the interests of the older worker, both business and government must jointly and severally acknowledge their responsibilities for joint action in the future.

References

1 Eurostat, 2005. http://www.eustatistics.gov.uk.

2 Faculty of Occupational Medicine. Position paper on Age and Employment. 2004. London, Faculty of Occupational Medicine.

3 Kirkwood TBL, Rose MR. Evolution of senescence: late survival sacrificed for reproduction. *Phil Trans R Soc Lond B* 1991; **332**: 15–24.

4 Grimley Evans J. How are the elderly different? In *Improving the health of older people: a world view* (eds Kane RL, Grimley Evans J, Macfadyen D), pp. 50–68. Oxford: Oxford University Press, 1990.

5 Schaie KW, Strother CR. A cross-sequential study of age changes in cognitive behavior. *Psychol Bull* 1968; **70**: 671–80.

6 Peake MD, Thompson S, Lowe D, Pearson G, on behalf of the Participating Centres. Ageism in the management of lung cancer. *Age Ageing* 2003; **32**: 171–7.

7 Grimley Evans J. Ageing and disease. In *Research and the ageing population* (eds Evered D, Whelan J), pp 38–57. Chichester UK: John Wiley and Sons Ltd, 1988.

8 Manton KG, Gu X. Changes in the prevalence of chronic disability in the United States black and nonblack population above age 65 from 1982 to 1999. *Proc Natl Acad Sci USA* 2001; **98**: 6354–9.

9 Steptoe A, Marmot M. The role of psychobiological pathways in socio-economic inequalities in cardiovascular disease risk. *Eur Heart J* 2002; **23**: 13–25.

10 Harridge SDR, Young A. Strength and power. In *Oxford textbook of geriatric medicine* (eds Grimley Evans J, Williams TF, Beattie BL, Michel J-P, Wilcock GK), pp. 963–8. Oxford: Oxford University Press, 2000.

11 Riggs BL, Melton LJ. Involutional osteoporosis. *N Engl J Med* 1986; **314**: 1676–86.

12 Ott A, Breteler MB, van Harskamp F, Claus JJ, van der Cammen TJM, Grobbee DE *et al*. Prevalence of Alzheimer's disease and vascular dementia: association with education. The Rotterdam study. *BMJ* 1995; **310**: 970–3.

13 Marmot MG, McDowall ME. Mortality decline and widening social inequalities. *Lancet* 1986; **328**: 274–6.

14 Bhopal R. Epidemic of cardiovascular disease in South Asians. *BMJ* 2002; **324**: 6–7.

15 *Oxford textbook of geriatric medicine*. Oxford: Oxford University Press, 2000.

16 Aittomaki A, Lahelma E, Roos E, Leino-Arjas P, Martikainen P. Gender differences in the association of age with physical workload and functioning. *Occup Environ Med* 2005; **62**: 95–100.

17 Newman AB, Brach JS. Gender gap in longevity and disability in older persons. *Epidemiol Rev* 2001; **23**: 343–50.

18 Raab DM, Agre JC, McAdam M, Smith EL. Light resistance and stretching exercise in elderly women: effect upon flexibility. *Arch Phys Med Rehabil* 1988; **69**: 268–72.

19 Johnson BD, Dempsey JA. Demand vs. capacity in the aging pulmonary system. *Exerc Sport Sci Rev* 1991; **19**: 171–210.

20 Salvendy G, Pilitsis J. Psychophysiological aspects of paced and unpaced performance as influenced by age. *Ergonomics* 1971; **14**: 703–11.

21 Snook SH. The effects of age and physique on continuous-work capacity. *Hum Factors* 1971; **13**: 467–9.

22 Orlander J, Aniansson A. Effects of physical training on skeletal muscle metabolism, morphology and function in 70–75 year old men. *Acta Physiol Scand* 1980; **109**: 149–54.

23 Goycoolea MV, Goycoolea HG, Rodriguez LG, Martinez GC, Vidal R. Effect of life in industrialized societies on hearing in natives of Easter Island. *Laryngoscope* 1986; **96**: 1391–6.

24 Pichora-Fuller MK. Cognitive aging and auditory information processing. *Int J Audiol* 2003; **42** (Suppl. 2): S26–32.

25 Pichora-Fuller MK, Schneider BA, Daneman M. How young and old adults listen to and remember speech in noise. *J Acoust Soc Am* 1995; **97**: 593–608.

26 Zoger S, Svedlund J, Holgers KM. The Hospital Anxiety and Depression Scale (HAD) as a screening instrument in tinnitus evaluation. *Int J Audiol* 2005; **43**: 458–64.

27 Weale RA. The eye and senescence. In *Oxford textbook of geriatric medicine* (eds Grimley Evans J, Williams TF, Beattie BL, Michel J-P, Wilcock GK), pp. 863–73. Oxford: Oxford University Press, 2000.

28 Ball K, Owsley C, Beard B. Clinical visual perimetry underestimates peripheral field problems in older adults. *Clin Vis Sci* 1990; **5**: 113–25.

29 Owsley C, Ball K, McGwin G, Sloane ME, Roenker DL, White MF *et al.* Visual processing impairment and risk of motor vehicle crash among older adults. *JAMA* 1998; **279**: 1083–8.

30 Winner SJ, Morgan CA, Grimley Evans J. Perimenopausal risk of falling and incidence of distal forearm fracture. *BMJ* 1989; **298**: 1486–8.

31 Grimley Evans J. Transient neurological dysfunction and risk of stroke in an elderly English population: the different significance of vertigo and non-rotatory dizziness. *Age Ageing* 1990; **19**: 43–9.

32 Cattell R. *Intelligence: its structure, growth, and action.* New York: Elsevier Science Publishing Company, 1987.

33 Salthouse TA. *A theory of cognitive ageing.* Berlin: Springer-Verlag, 1985.

34 Salthouse TA. Memory aging from 18 to 80. *Alzheimer Dis Assoc Disord* 2003; **17**: 162–7.

35 Lakatta EG. Cardiovascular aging without a clinical diagnosis. *Dialogues Cardiovasc Med* 2001; **6**: 67–91.

36 Black HR. The paradigm has shifted to systolic blood pressure. *J Hum Hypertens* 2004; **18** (Suppl. 2): S3–7.

37 Grimley Evans J, Rose G. The epidemiology of hypertension. *Br Med Bull* 1971; **27**: 37–42.

38 Grimley Evans J. The decline of stroke. In *Stroke: epidemiological, therapeutic and socioeconomic aspects* (ed. Rose FC), pp. 33–8. London: Royal Society of Medicine, 1986.

39 Rothwell PM, Coull AJ, Giles MF, Howard SC, Silver LE, Bull LM *et al.* Change in stroke incidence, mortality, case-fatality, severity, and risk factors in Oxfordshire, UK from 1981 to 2004 (Oxford Vascular Study). *Lancet* 2004; **363**: 1925–33.

40 Sander K, Sander D. New insights into transient global amnesia: recent imaging and clinical findings. *Lancet Neurol* 2005; **4**: 437–44.

41 Doll R. The age distribution of cancer: implications for models of carcinogenesis. *J R Stat Soc (A)* 1970; **134**: 133–55.

42 Felson DT. Epidemiology of hip and knee osteoarthritis. *Epidemiol Rev* 1988; **10**: 1–28.

43 Albertsen PC. Is screening for prostate cancer with prostate specific antigen an appropriate public health measure? *Acta Oncol* 2005; **44**: 255–64.

44 Zucherman JF, Hsu KY, Hartjen CA, Mehalic TF, Implicito DA, Martin MJ *et al.* A multicenter, prospective, randomized trial evaluating the X STOP interspinous process decompression system for the treatment of neurogenic intermittent claudication: two-year follow-up results. *Spine* 2005; **30**: 1351–8.

45 Miller SWM, Grimley Evans J. Fractures of the distal forearm in Newcastle: an epidemiological survey. *Age Ageing* 1985; **14**: 155–8.

46 Writing Group for the Women's Health Initiative Investigators. Risks and benefits of estrogen plus progestin in healthy postmenopausal women. Principal results from the Women's Health Initiative randomized controlled trial. *JAMA* 2002; **288**: 321–33.

47 Wu EQ, Birnbaum H, Marynchenko M, Mareva M, Williamson T, Mallett D. Employees with overactive bladder: work loss burden. *J Occup Environ Med* 2005; **47**: 439–46.

48 Morgan O, Griffiths C, Baker A, Majeed A. Fatal toxicity of antidepressants in England and Wales, 1993–2002. *Health Stat Q* 2004; **23**: 18–24.

49 Skegg DCG, Richards SM, Doll R. Minor tranquillizers and road accidents. *BMJ* 1979; **1**: 917–9.

50 Grimley Evans J. Drugs and falls in later life. *Lancet* 2003; **361**: 448.

51 British National Formulary, 2005. http://www.bnf.org/bnf/bnf/current. Ref Type: Electronic Citation.

52 Meck Higgins M, Barkley MC. Barriers to nutrition education for older adults, and nutrition and aging training opportunities for educators, healthcare providers, volunteers and caregivers. *J Nutr Elder* 2004; **23**: 99–121.

53 Bagwell MM, Bush HA. Improving health promotion for blue-collar workers. *J Nurs Care Qual* 2000; **14**: 65–71.

54 Infeld DL, Whitelaw N. Policy initiatives to promote healthy aging. *Clin Geriatr Med* 2002; **18**: 627–42.

55 Bozzetti F. Nutritional issues in the care of the elderly patient. *Crit Rev Oncol Hematol* 2003; **48**: 113–21.

56 Secretary of State for Health. *The health of the nation. A strategy for health in England.* Cm1986. London: HMSO, 1992.

57 Secretary of State for Health. *Our Healthier Nation. A Contract for Health.* CM 3852. London: The Stationery Office, 1998.

58 de Zwart BHC, Frings-Dresen MHW, van Duivenbooden JC. Test-retest reliability of the Work Ability Index questionnaire. *Occup Med* 2002; **52**: 177–81.

59 Greve J, Jochheim KA, Schian HM. Assessment methods for vocational integration of disabled persons–from ERTOMIS methods to the IMBA information system [in German]. *Rehabilitation (Stuttg)* 1997; **36**: 34–8.

60 Greve J. Indications for evaluation scales in quality assurance in rehabilitation [in German]. *Rehabilitation (Stuttg)* 1998; **37**: 41–51.

61 Bongers PM, de Winter CR, Kompier MAJ, Hildebrandt VH. Psychosocial factors at work and musculoskeletal disease. *Scand J Work Environ Health* 1993; **19**: 297–312.

62 Cant R, O'Loughlin K, Legge V. Sick leave—cushion or entitlement? A study of age cohorts' attitudes and practices in two Australian workplaces. *Work* 2001; **17**: 39–48.

63 Wetherick NE. Changing an established concept: a comparison of the ability of young, middle-aged and old subjects. *Gerontologia* 1965; **11**: 82–95.

64 Vahtera J, Kivimäki M, Pennti J. Effect of organisational downsizing on health of employees. *Lancet* 1997; **350**: 1124–8.

65 McMullin JA, Marshall VW. Ageism, age relations, and garment industry work in Montreal. *Gerontologist* 2001; **41**: 111–22.

66 Finkelstein LM, Burke MJ. Age stereotyping at work: the role of rater and contextual factors on evaluations of job applicants. *J Gen Psychol* 1998; **125**: 317–45.

67 Kinne S, Probart C, Gritz ER. Cancer-risk-related health behaviors and attitudes of older workers. Working Well Research Group. *J Cancer Educ* 1996; **11**: 89–95.

68 Verbeek J, Spelten E, Kammeijer M, Sprangers M. Return to work of cancer survivors: a prospective cohort study into the quality of rehabilitation by occupational physicians. *Occup Environ Med* 2003; **60**: 352–7.

69 Spelten ER, Sprangers MA, Verbeek JH. Factors reported to influence the return to work of cancer survivors: a literature review. *Psychooncology* 2002; **11**: 124–31.

70 Harma MI, Ilmarinen JE. Towards the 24-hour society-new approaches for aging shift workers? *Scand J Work Environ Health* 1999; **25**: 610–15.

71 de Zwart BC, Bras VM, van Dormolen M, Frings-Dresen MH, Meijman TF. After-effects of night work on physical performance capacity and sleep quality in relation to age. *Int Arch Occup Environ Health* 1993; **65**: 259–62.

72 Tepas DI, Duchon JC, Gersten AH. Shiftwork and the older worker. *Exp Aging Res* 1993; **19**: 295–320.

73 Hakola T, Harma M. Evaluation of a fast forward rotating shift schedule in the steel industry with a special focus on ageing and sleep. *J Hum Ergol (Tokyo)* 2001; **30**: 315–19.

74 Reid K, Dawson D. Comparing performance on a simulated 12 hour shift rotation in young and older subjects. *Occup Environ Med* 2001; **58**: 58–62.

75 Working Time Regulations 1998 (*Statutory Instrument 1998/1833*). 1998. Ref Type: Statute

76 The Pensions Commission. Pensions. challenges and choices The first and second reports of the Pensions Commission. http://www.pensionscommission.org.uk/publications/2004/annrep/index.asp and http://www.dwp.gov.uk/publications/dwp/2005/pensionscommreport/annrep-index.asp

77 Mill JS. *On liberty*. London: John W Parker and Son, West Strand, 1859.

78 Zhai Z. Urbanization and the aging of urban population in China: trend and countermeasures. *Chin J Popul Sci* 1997; **9**: 35–44.

General reading

Adisesh A, Parker G. ABC of work related disorders: working with an occupational health department. *BMJ* 1996; **313**: 999–1002.

Bromley DB. *The psychology of human ageing*, (2nd edn). Harmondsworth: Penguin.

Buchan J. The 'greying' of the United Kingdom nursing workforce: implications for employment policy and practice. *J Adv Nurs* 1999; **30**(4): 818–26.

Davies W (1996) ABC of work related disorders: assessing fitness for work. *BMJ* 1996; **313**: 934–8.

Healy ML. Management strategies for an aging work force. *AAOHN J* 2001.

Hearnshaw LS. *The psychological and occupational aspects of ageing*. Liverpool researches. Liverpool: Medical Research Council, 1953–70.

Heron A. Ageing and employment. In: *Modern trends in occupational health* (ed. Schilling RSF). London: Butterworth, 1960.

Jamieson GH. Inspection in the telecommunications industry: a field study of age and other performance variables. *Ergonomics* 1966; **9**: 297–303.

McGee JP, Wegman David H. *Health and safety needs of older workers: Committee on the Health and Safety Needs of Older Workers…*: Washington, DC.: National Academies Press, 2004.

Macheath JA. *Activity, health and fitness in old age*. London: Groom-Helm, 1984.

Wegman DH. Older workers. *Occup Med* 1999; **14**(3): 537–57. Review.

Welford AT. *Ageing and human skill*. Oxford: Oxford University Press, 1958.

Woollams C. *Everything you need to know to help you beat cancer*, (2nd edn). Gawcott, Buckingham: Health Issues Ltd., 2003 (allyouneedtoknowaboutcancer.com).

Chapter 27

Ill health retirement

C. J. M. Poole and P. Litchfield

Demographics

In the UK over recent decades the number of people of pensionable age has been rising as life expectancy has increased. The number of employed people has remained fairly constant so the ratio of employed to retired, known as the support ratio has fallen. The crude ratio in the UK is currently 3.4. By 2040 a ratio of 2.4 is estimated and if the number of unemployed is removed from the equation, then the ratio falls to 2.1 and 1.5 respectively.[1] An example of a low support ratio for a large national pension scheme with many more pensioners than active members is shown in Figure 27.1. In recent years there has been a trend towards taking early retirement, which exacerbates the ratio. For example in 1971 more than 80% of men in the age group 60–64 were in employment; however, by 1996 this figure had fallen to 50%.

During the 1980s the rate of early retirement due to ill health rapidly increased, doubling in Local Government[2] and forming 20–40% of all retirements in the public sector. Similar changes were seen in other European countries where rates of early retirement due to ill health have varied between 15% in France and 50% in Germany.[3] The reasons for these changes are unknown but are likely to include changes to working practices such as computer technology and increased systems of control over work. Currently, only a small proportion of people work after the age of 65, but this is likely to increase with forthcoming legislation on age discrimination and relaxation

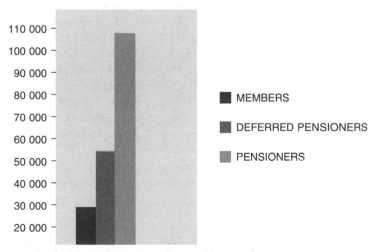

Fig. 27.1 Graph of a large UK pension scheme with a very low support ratio.

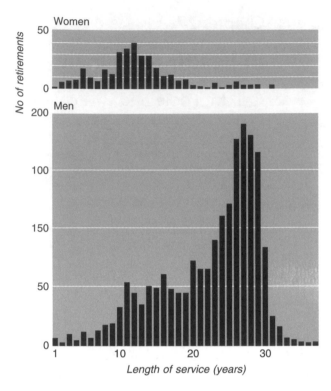

Fig. 27.2 Number of employees retiring on grounds of ill health by length of service and sex for 1994–5 in a large public sector organization. Enhancements in benefits are payable after 10 and 26.5 years of service.[4] Reproduced with permission from the BMJ Publishing Group.

of Inland Revenue rules on the receipt of pension benefits while continuing to work and the maximum number of pensionable years of service.

Wide variations in rates of early retirement have been reported between employers and even within different parts of the same organization.[4] While some variation is to be expected, such as a higher rate in jobs that require a high level of physical fitness, other variations are inexplicable on medical grounds alone. For example the concurrence of modes of ill health retirement with enhancements in benefits can only be satisfactorily explained by the influence of non-medical factors on decisions to retire (Figure 27.2). There is no plausible medical reason to explain why so much ill health (mainly in the form of minor psychiatric and musculoskeletal disorders) should occur at times that coincide with enhancements in pension benefits. It must be assumed that there are other reasons such as lack of motivation to remain at work, dissimulation, or illness deception.

In general rates of retirement due to ill health are higher in the public than private sector. The reason for this is likely to be multifactorial and may include a sharper focus by the latter on performance and attendance with a greater readiness to dismiss on incapability grounds, or to make jobs redundant. Despite anecdotal evidence that retirement is bad for physical health, the few longitudinal studies that have been undertaken of retirees and working controls have found no difference in the rate of decline in physical functioning between the two groups, but mental health has generally improved after retirement particularly among those with high socio-economic status.[5]

State pensions

The state scheme in the UK is two tier, consisting of a basic pension and an additional state pension known since April 2002 as the State Second Pension (previously SERPS); individuals may opt out of this additional scheme in favour of an occupational, stakeholder, or personal pension. It is funded directly from National Insurance contributions from both the employer and the employee. Currently the state pension is payable from age 65 for men and from age 60 for women but will increase gradually for women born after 1949 from 2010 until it has been equalized to age 65 in 2020. There is no facility for taking the state pension early (other than for widows or widowers), but the taking of a pension can be deferred until age 70, with a percentage increase for each week of deferment. The value of the basic pension has been declining since the link to earnings increases was replaced with inflation linkage some 20 years ago. Concerns about growing poverty in old age and the affordability of even the current level of benefits has resulted in a re-examination of the fundamental principles underpinning the current arrangements.[6]

Occupational and personal pensions

Occupational and personal pension schemes in the UK have traditionally been associated with larger and longer established employers. However, since October 2001 it has been mandatory for most employers of more than five people to offer a stakeholder pension if a suitable occupational or personal scheme is not in place (see the Welfare Reform and Pensions Act 1999); the take-up to date has been disappointing. It is estimated that 46% of employees belong to an occupational pension scheme with 25 million members (active, deferred, and retired) in private sector schemes and 9 million public sector scheme members.[7] They are generally funded by investment, though some large public sector schemes have no investment trust and are funded from taxation. They are run by representatives of the employer in the form of Trustees, with the help of administrators, investment managers, and external consultants such as auditors. Occupational and personal pension schemes tend to be more flexible than the state scheme, with the possibility of taking benefits early (e.g. sportsmen) or later up to age 75.

The rules for managing a scheme are contained in the Pensions Act 2004 and from April 2005 schemes have been overseen by the Pensions Regulator—formerly it was by the Occupational Pensions Regulatory Authority (OPRA). Trustees must be represented by current employees and by pensioners, at least one-third of whom must be elected from members of the scheme. Trustees have discretionary powers over eligibility to an early pension and in the case of ill health will base their decision on information obtained from selected medical practitioners. Schemes must have a formal internal dispute resolution procedure (IDRP) for complaints and appeals.

Pensions Advisory Service

Advice about pensions can be obtained in the UK from the Pensions Advisory Service (OPAS), an independent organization that is grant-aided by the Department of Social Security, and the Pensions Regulator. Complaints, disputes or appeals which cannot be resolved by an IDRP can be referred to OPAS who may in turn refer the case to the Pensions Ombudsman. He will determine whether Trustees or administrators have: (1) incorrectly interpreted the scheme regulations; (2) misdirected themselves in law; or (3) come to a perverse decision, i.e. one that no reasonable body would make. The Pensions Ombudsman receives 30–40 complaints per year about early retirement due to ill health, which represents about 7% of complaints referred to his office.[8]

Defined Benefit and Defined Contribution Schemes

The model for most occupational pension schemes through the twentieth century was that of Defined Benefits (DB). Individuals and employers pay a proportion of salary into a general fund from which pensions are then paid out. Characteristically each year of service with the organization would qualify the individual for a proportion (e.g. 1/80 or 1/60) of their final salary at retirement as a pension—such schemes are therefore sometimes referred to as Final Salary schemes. These arrangements favour individuals who accrue long service with a single organization and whose earnings peak at the end of their career. They also provide the individual scheme member with substantial certainty about the value of the pension they are likely to receive at retirement but employers carry the risk of pension funds being unable to meet their liabilities. Many schemes include a provision for compensating members who have to give up work early because of ill health and this is typically achieved by paying the pension immediately, rather than at the normal retirement age, without actuarial reduction of benefits and often with an enhancement to the pensionable years of service.

The main alternative model is the Defined Contribution (DC) scheme. Here individuals and employers pay a proportion of salary into a fund of which each member has a share dependent upon their contribution. Upon retirement the individual is free to use the sum accumulated to purchase an annuity that will provide an income—such schemes are therefore sometimes described as Money Purchase schemes. These arrangements are more favourable to individuals whose earnings do not vary substantially or whose peak income occurs some time before their retirement age. The value of the annuity is dependent upon market conditions at the time of purchase but employers have much greater certainty regarding their potential liability. There is no single predominant method for providing ill health cover within a DC arrangement. Approximately one-third of companies provide permanent health insurance, one-third offer an ill health pension from the pension plan, and one-third do not provide any benefit above the accumulated fund.[9]

In the first few years of the twenty-first century there has been a fundamental shift in the private sector away from DB to DC schemes. By 2004, 65% of UK companies were only offering DC schemes to new employees though most retained legacy DB schemes for existing employees.[10] The trend has been an accelerating one and DB schemes may well not be a feature of UK private sector employment in the next decade. Concern about the ongoing affordability of DB schemes has also led to a review in the public sector. The shift from DB to DC schemes has implications for ill health retirement, which is also a gateway to pension benefits. As shown above, only one-third of DC schemes offer ill health pensions from the pension plan and this has often been put in place to minimize the differences from DB schemes that they are replacing.

Criteria

Eligibility to an early or enhanced pension because of ill health is dependent on the member meeting various criteria as set out by the Trustees or administrators of the pension scheme. Criteria vary between schemes but most require the applicant to have permanent ill health or permanent incapacity due to ill health, illness, or injury. It is essential for doctors to understand the precise criteria for any scheme on which they are advising and the interpretation that is applied to the wording. Even the order in which words are placed can alter eligibility criteria (see Box 27.1) and reference should always be made to the scheme regulations or guidance notes.

Permanence is usually defined as until the scheme's normal retirement age, which can currently vary from, for example, 55 years for many emergency services workers to 65 years for most employees in local government. The Pensions Act 2004 introduces flexibility in allowing people to draw an occupational pension while continuing to work for the same employer and will normally make compulsory retirement ages unlawful from 2006 onwards. This should not affect the pensionable age currently defined by schemes but may well impact on ill-health retirement rates as older workers find it financially viable to 'step down' in their work rather than ceasing work altogether.

Box 27.1

Scheme A states that to qualify for ill health retirement an individual must be *incapable by virtue of permanent ill health* while Scheme B states that one must be *permanently incapable by virtue of ill health*. Someone experiencing an acute exacerbation of a chronic condition, such as diabetes or epilepsy, which renders them unfit for work now but which is expected to improve over time might arguably qualify for ill health retirement under the rules of Scheme A but not under those of Scheme B.

Most schemes require that the applicant has undergone a reasonable range of treatments before ill health is said to be permanent and a refusal to undergo reasonable treatment is likely to lead to the application failing. For legal reasons and for reasons of good practice, permanence should only be accepted when the applicant has been unable to work despite reasonable adaptations or aids in the workplace or to the job itself have been unsuccessful and redeployment to a comparable job has been unsuccessful for medical rather than non-medical reasons. Ill-health retirement (IHR) would not be justified under the Disability Discrimination Act unless all reasonable adaptations have been considered and IHR has been requested by the employee as opposed to being offered as an alternative to dismissal or redundancy by the employer.

A number of pension schemes in both the private and public sectors have a two tier system where eligibility to the lower tier characteristically includes the criterion of inability to do the job for which the member is employed and for the upper tier inability to do any gainful employment. A common arrangement is that, while a pension is paid immediately for both tiers, only upper tier benefits are enhanced and may be subject to review. The job may be defined in various ways, for example for NHS staff as their contracted duties for that employer (Trust rather than NHS); for teachers as teaching in any school (including part-time) and for police officers as the ordinary duties of a male or female member in any force and not just the one for which they are employed. In general, incapacity from all work is more clear-cut than incapacity from their own job but a much higher standard for the applicant to achieve. Determining incapacity from an individual's own job requires the advising doctor to have a good knowledge of that activity, working practices, and the adjustments that can reasonably be accommodated by that employer.

Terms such as ill health or infirmity of body or mind are rarely defined in regulations and doctors are advised to become familiar with the regulations or explanatory notes of the member's scheme before advising on eligibility. Illnesses that are not contained within the current International Classification of Diseases,[11] such as stress or burnout, should not be accepted as medical illnesses for the purpose of IHR. Care should also be taken to ensure that there is a direct causal link between any incapacity and ill health. Some applicants will declare incapability of carrying out tasks for which they are employed and incidental coexisting ill health may be convenient, for termination of employment on favourable terms funded by the pension scheme. An area of particular difficulty is that of secondary ill health. Individuals with performance, attendance or disciplinary problems may absent themselves from work citing 'stress' or some other self-limiting condition such as reactive depression and choose to pursue ill health retirement as the solution to their employment problems. Some schemes insist that the ill health qualifying for a pension must be primary (i.e. unrelated to any effects of a reasonable employment process) rather than secondary and require that issues related to employment be resolved before eligibility to a pension is considered.

Evidence

The optimum means of determining whether an individual is likely to meet the criteria for ill-health retirement will necessarily vary on a case by case basis. However, it will be usual for evidence to include an assessment of capability, matched to the requirements of the job, as well as objective medical evidence about the illness or injury that allows the formulation of a diagnosis and prognosis. In most cases sufficient objective medical evidence can be gleaned by examining the patient or from the patient's own medical practitioner but, where this is deficient, it may be necessary to commission an independent examination and/or investigations to provide the necessary quality of information. When requesting reports it should be made clear that it is medical fact and, where appropriate, opinion on prognosis which is being sought and not a view on employment issues or pension entitlement with which the doctor is unlikely to be familiar. In cases where the illness is terminal, prognosis should be ascertained as pension benefits may be commuted when life expectancy is less than 12 months.

Providing a professional opinion when a patient wishes to avoid work or to gain a financial benefit may in a few cases be problematic for the doctor. This is because the relationship between doctor and the patient is not a normal therapeutic one, but is for the purposes of providing specific advice to a third party and guidance on the ethical issues involved has been published by the Faculty of Occupational Medicine[12] (see also Chapter 5). In the process of examining the patient the doctor may identify inconsistencies in the history or examination, abnormal illness behaviour, entrenched beliefs or behaviours, undiagnosed psychological (rather than medical) ill health or illness deception. Such findings should be documented and taken into account when formulating a professional opinion so that the duties of the trustees can be discharged properly.

Conflicts of interest

Those charged with advising a pension scheme on ill health retirement must remember that their primary duty is to the trustees of the scheme and not to the individual scheme member or to the employer. Advice must be objective and evidence based and factors such as expediency or social circumstances should be disregarded. Doctors who are or may be involved in the treatment of the patient, or are the patient's general practitioner, should not advise the pension scheme about eligibility because of the inherent potential for a conflict of interests. Such a doctor may provide factual information about the patient's current or previous health but should not be asked whether eligibility criteria have been met and should avoid offering an unsolicited opinion on the patient's eligibility to an early pension. Pension scheme medical advisers or trustees may in our opinion reasonably disregard such opinions, as opposed to factual objective evidence.

In larger pension schemes it is usual to separate occupational health advice to the employer from that on pensions issues. Smaller schemes may have to rely on the employer's medical adviser as the only source of competent advice on health related to employment, so those undertaking such a role must be assiduous in acting impartially. For this reason it is good practice for two or more doctors to be involved in the process of early retirement due to ill health. Recommendations to the pension scheme should be given on the basis of a balance of probabilities rather than beyond reasonable doubt, i.e. what is likely, rather than what is possible or probable.

Competence

Advice on eligibility for ill-health retirement must only be given by doctors who have suitable and sufficient knowledge of the job and working environment of the scheme members. Many pension schemes require their medical advisers, rather than doctors solely providing information about the patient's health, to have a qualification in occupational medicine. The minimum quali-fication varies between schemes but should not be less than the Diploma in Occupational Medicine (DOccMed), supplemented by training in the application of the scheme criteria. It is recommended for such doctors to be overseen by an accredited specialist in occupational medi-cine (i.e. MFOM in the UK or equivalent qualification issued by a competent authority in an EEA State). An appeal against an initial decision should be considered by an accredited specialist in occupational medicine.

Appeals and complaints

All ill-health retirement assessment processes should have an appeal mechanism. The scheme member should be advised of the grounds on which the original decision was made and have the opportunity to provide additional medical evidence, usually within stipulated time limits. The appeal may be considered by a single doctor or a panel of doctors that should include an accred-ited specialist in occupational medicine with suitable and sufficient knowledge and experience to judge the issues. Some schemes require appellants to present for medical examination but most appeals are conducted on a 'papers only' basis, partly for logistical reasons but also because a fur-ther examination rarely provides new objective evidence. Appeal reports should demonstrate that all relevant evidence has been considered and should detail the rationale applied. It is essen-tial that appeal authorities articulate a clear decision on whether ill-health retirement criteria are met or not in plain language that can be readily understood by trustees and the appellant.

Assessment of eligibility for ill-health retirement may, like any other clinical activity, result in a complaint by the patient against the doctor. Such a complaint is most likely to occur if the appli-cation has been unsuccessful and may therefore be vindictive or malicious. It is essential not only to have a robust complaints procedure running alongside the appeals procedure but one which identifies this type of complaint. Requests by the patient to remove factually relevant material that is not supportive of their cases should be resisted, as should requests to assess a case without medical reports nominated by either side, or without sight of the medical report setting out a previous doctor's or panel's professional opinion.

Guidelines

No controlled trials have been undertaken on retirees and so the guidance that has been written is based on consensus opinions of senior occupational physicians arising from evidence and inferences about specific illnesses or diseases in relation to work.[2,13] Some large public sector pension schemes, such as the Civil Service, Home Office, and the Department of Education, have produced written guidance on the application of their criteria, which can be helpful. The occupa-tional physician should obtain all relevant information about the patient's illness to include diag-nosis, treatment (past and proposed), and prognosis, particularly in those cases that are unusual or complicated.

The *true* functional ability of the patient should be ascertained, as well as details of the patient's job or workplace. If the doctor is of the opinion that the true functional ability of the patient has not been ascertained, despite all reasonable efforts, or the degree of disability declared by the patient is more than would be normally expected for that illness or disease, it is recommended that the doctor bases his or her advice on what would normally be expected by way of function or prognosis in a patient with the same diagnosis but who is not seeking early retirement or financial benefit.

Reasonable adjustments or aids should have been tried to accommodate the patient's disability or illness, as well as opportunities for redeployment before a decision is made about medical

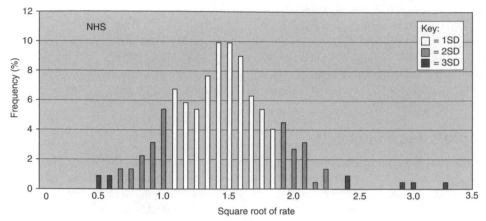

Fig. 27.3 Frequency distribution of square roots of rates with standard deviations (SD) of ill health retirements in NHS Trusts (2002–3).[13] (Reproduced with permission from the Society of Occupational Medicine.) The square root of retirement rates (number of retirals/1000 active members of a pension scheme, full and part-time/year) has a normal distribution, enabling occupational physicians to audit their practice.

retirement. Adjustments might include adaptive technology, involving the Access to Work team, 'permitted' or 'supported' employment. It should be remembered that medical retirement is a dismissal in law and failure to make reasonable adjustments may constitute grounds for a claim of unfair dismissal. Workplaces and the people who work in them are in a constant state of flux and refusal by an employee to return to a particular workplace should not merit medical retirement unless there is a demonstrable inability to do so caused by permanent incapacity due to ill health.

Advice should, whenever possible, be based on objective medical evidence and any non-medical factors that may be contributing to the patient's ill health (such as anger, embitterment, or disaffection with the employer or a lack of motivation to return to work) should generally be disregarded. Illnesses that are the most difficult to assess objectively are those that rely entirely on subjective complaints by the patient, such as chronic fatigue syndrome, fibromyalgia, post-traumatic stress disorder, and some mental health disorders. Specific advice on these illnesses is given elsewhere.[13]

Audit

There is much variability in the outcomes of judgements about early retirement due to ill health.[4,13] This is disconcerting for patients and the trustees or administrators of pension schemes. The medical standards to which the medical advisor(s) will be working should be made explicit to other doctors, the applicant, and other parties. Explanations of the meaning of the different components of the eligibility criteria and setting them in the context of examples may also be helpful. Audit should be undertaken of specific medical conditions against predetermined agreed standards for the management of these illnesses. Audit should also be routinely carried out of measurements such as rate of retirement for a particular pension scheme. Where possible, comparisons should also be made to national rates for the same pension scheme and similar types of employers. Individual practitioners or employers falling outside predetermined limits (such as two standard deviations from the mean) should warrant specific attention with a view to changing practice and re-auditing at a later date.

Medico-legal

Employees and managers often view ill health retirement as an alternative to resignation, redundancy or dismissal. In fact it is not an employment issue but rather the process of paying pension benefits once a decision to terminate an employee's service has been made. Even if the individual applies for the benefit, the employer must be satisfied that all decisions relating to employment have been made fairly and according to the organization's documented processes, otherwise a case for unfair dismissal may be justified.

The Disability Discrimination Act applies equally at the end of employment as it does at recruitment or during employment. If an employee has a physical or mental impairment that has substantial and a long-term adverse effect on his or her ability to carry out normal day to day activities, then the employer has an obligation to make reasonable adjustments for that employee rather than encouraging the employee to take ill health retirement. Examples of employers being found to have unlawfully discriminated against an employee by giving them an early retirement can be found in case law such as *Kerrigan* v. *Rover Group 1997* and *Meikle* v. *Nottinghamshire County Council 2004* (see Chapter 3).

Dismissing an employee with a work-related illness or injury without making reasonable adjustments or offering opportunities for redeployment may be grounds for unfair dismissal. In these circumstances doctors should be wary of advising an employee to apply for ill health retirement. On the other hand if an employee continues to expose himself to a hazard and the employer has taken all reasonable steps to limit the risks from that hazard, then the doctor should make sure that the patient understands the risks and confirms the advice to the patient in writing. It is important to recognize that ill health retirement benefits are not taken into account when assessing quantum for personal injury awards and any compensation will include loss of earnings arising from the early retirement.

Injury awards

These are benefits paid by pension schemes for injury, illness, or disease caused by the employee's work. They are confined entirely to the public sector and privatized public sector bodies. They are designed to compensate for loss of earning capacity, rather than loss of function, pain, or suffering for which Industrial Injury Benefit or a civil claim might be appropriate. Judgements about injury awards involve apportionment between illness or disability due to the injury and any pre-existing illness or disability, as well as calculations based on the applicant's pre-injury salary and current or projected earnings in the open job market. Access to the patient's medical records and experience in making these judgements is recommended.

Limited life expectancy

Most pension schemes allow commutation of benefits (replacement of monthly payments with an augmented lump sum) for members in employment, but not generally for deferred members, with a life expectancy of less than 12 months. This is a discretion that the trustees may apply if it is within the scope of their scheme but it is also governed by Inland Revenue rules. The tax rules clearly state that such commutation is intended for the benefit of the scheme member rather than their dependants or estate. Consequently, well-intentioned efforts to secure commutation for individuals who are clearly drawing their last breaths are potentially unlawful and, if repeated on a regular basis, could result in the withdrawal of the concession by the Inland Revenue for that scheme. Unfortunately, the patient or a relative has the task of requesting commutation that may create difficulties if the patient is unaware or particularly sensitive about their prognosis.

A doctor will be asked to confirm the prognosis in writing. Most schemes also offer some form of death benefit for the dependants of members still employed at the time of death. The taxation rules around commutation and death benefit are complex and occupational physicians should avoid acting as financial advisers even though they may be trying to act in their patients' best interests.

Conclusions

Doctors who give advice to pension scheme trustees or administrators should be aware of the eligibility criteria for that scheme and the meaning of the terms used in the Regulations or in explanatory notes published by the scheme. Most schemes now require that the doctors who act as their medical advisors have a minimum qualification in occupational medicine. The evaluation of the evidence in support of an application for ill-health retirement should be robust but fair and care should be taken to avoid conflicts of interest for doctors involved in the treatment of the patient or management of the case. The provision of a professional opinion about the merits of an application for financial benefits or for avoiding work may in certain circumstances be problematic for the doctor. The standards to which doctors who are making these judgements are working should be made explicit and audited if equitable decisions are to be made and confidence in the process maintained.

References

1 Office for National Statistics. *Labour Market Trends, 1997.*

2 Poole CJM *et al*. Ill health retirement—guidelines for occupational physicians. *Occup Med* 1996; **46**: 402–6.

3 *European Pensions Bulletin*, 4, 1999.

4 Poole CJM. Retirement on grounds of ill health: cross sectional survey in six organisations in United Kingdom. *BMJ* 1997; **314**: 929–32.

5 Mein G *et al*. Is retirement good or bad for mental and physical health functioning? Whitehall II longitudinal study of civil servants. *J Epidemiol Community Health* 2003; **57**: 46–9.

6 The Independent Pensions Commission. *Pensions: Challenges and choices, 2004.* www.pensionscommission.org.uk.

7 Occupational Pensions Regulatory Authority. Pension Schemes in the UK, 2004

8 Annual Report of the Pensions Ombudsman. London, 1999.

9 Watson Wyatt. Pension Plan Design Survey, 2004.

10 Towers Perrin. Defined Contribution Pension Arrangements, 2004.

11 ICD-10. *The International Statistical Classification of Diseases and Related Health Problems*, 10th revision. Geneva: WHO, 1992.

12 Faculty of Occupational Medicine. *Guidance on ethics for occupational physicians*, (5th edn). London, 1999.

13 Poole CJM *et al*. Ill health retirement: national rates and updated guidance for occupational physicians. *Occup Med* 2005; **55**: 345–8.

Chapter 28

Health and transport safety: fitness to drive

J. T. Carter, H. G. Major, A. R. Erlam, and S. B. Janvrin

Introduction

Fitness to work in all modes of transport, where this may put members of the public or other workers at risk, has long been an area of public concern. These are often termed 'safety critical' tasks, although the precise meaning of this term varies between different sectors. Because inadequate performance may put fellow workers, the public and expensive assets at risk, frameworks for statutory regulation have been developed. Each mode of transport has its own pattern of performance requirements and hence fitness standards but they have a number of features in common. This chapter reviews the common features, using fitness to drive as an example and also noting job requirements in the railway industry. Separate appendices cover fitness to work as a seafarer and in aviation.

This emphasis on risks to the safety of others posed by performance deficits has meant that decisions on fitness are frequently taken not for the benefit of the person examined but to safeguard those at risk as a consequence of their actions. Hence hard decisions often have to be taken. For this reason standards for medical aspects of fitness are usually formal and often published. They are usually applied by physicians who are acting on behalf of regulatory authorities and they have associated review or appeal mechanisms available to those who have been failed or restricted. Standards are necessarily based on the balance between public risk and potential loss of employment, with the former predominating.

The evidence base for current standards is of variable quality and depth and this is often a cause of contention.

In addition to long-term health problems that are handled by reference to these formal standards, workers in safety critical jobs may also have short-term decrements in performance from injury, minor illness, or medication. Management systems which recognize this and are supported by self awareness and advice from health professionals dealing with such conditions are an important part of risk reduction.

Safety critical tasks

The term 'safety critical task' can generally be taken to mean one where some forms of impairment in the person doing it can put other people at risk. It is a useful general concept but one open to slightly differing interpretations in different situations and so the rationale for its use should always be explored before assumptions are made. Driving provides a good example of a safety critical transport task. Information about the vehicle, other road users, and the road are perceived—mainly using vision. This is cognitively processed against a learned background of skills and intentions for the journey. Based on this the speed, direction, and signalling of the vehicle are determined by hand and foot controls. The results of these actions are, in turn, processed to determine subsequent control requirements. Lack of experience, inattention, behavioural traits such as risk taking and impairment, including that from a medical condition, may interfere with this loop. Interference will increase the risk of error and accident.

A similar perceptual, cognitive, and motor loop is relevant to rail drivers, air pilots, and seafarers when in charge of sailing a ship. However, the nature of the visual environment, the stimulation from the surroundings and the response to control actions all vary greatly. In addition there are differing safety support systems, both in human terms, as with a co-pilot in passenger aircraft, and engineered, such as protective signalling and automatic braking systems on the railways.

Health-related impairment is not an important contributor to road and other transport accidents, being identifiable in only about 1/250 of those events resulting in hospital admission. Other forms of impairment such as fatigue and alcohol are much more significant as is being an inexperienced driver, although this is hard to distinguish from the behavioural traits associated with youth! All forms of impairment and driver behaviour taken together are, however, much more important as causes of crashes than the condition of either the vehicle or the road.[1]

Box 28.1 Contributory factors for road crashes

Road conditions alone	2.5%
Road user alone	65%
Vehicle alone	2.5%
Road + user	24%
Road + vehicle	0.25%
User + vehicle	4.5%
Road + user + vehicle	1.25%

In some modes of transport, other workers undertaking safety critical tasks that are covered by fitness standards. These include air traffic controllers and rail signallers as well as those engaged in dangerous situations such as airside drivers at airports and lineside rail workers. In addition, most seafarers and some rail staff may have physically demanding emergency duties such as firefighting and passenger evacuation.

Impairing disabilities and medical conditions

Performance decrement may be a permanent feature, for instance the static disability of a fixed or amputated limb or a deficit in visual acuity or colour perception. It may also be episodic as in a seizure, cardiac event, or episode of hypoglycaemia. Many conditions also present with a mix of characteristics, for instance the fluctuating impairments of multiple sclerosis or the progression of a malignancy or of motor neurone disease. Recovery after an episode of illness, such as a stroke, can be variable and may sometimes take several months. A stroke will sometimes indicate an increased risk of sudden recurrence of the original conditions or of a related one, such as a myocardial infarction as both are effects of underlying arterial disease. Treatments frequently reduce risk, but some such as insulin, psychoactive medications, or warfarin can create new risks of their own. Any set of medical standards needs to accommodate this diversity in a rational way, which can be applied with demonstrable fairness.

The conceptual approaches to static and to episodic conditions are very different. In a static condition, given sufficient evidence linking the level of impairment to risk, it should be possible to make an assessment of the individual that includes any appliances used to reduce the impairment, such as corrective lenses, a prosthesis, or modified car controls. This can then be used to make a decision on the fitness of the individual. In practice the weak link is usually between the level of impairment and the excess risk of accident, which even for common conditions such as impaired visual acuity is poorly characterized.[2] An assessment of driving performance may be the most practically useful arbiter of safety and it has good face value for the participant, although its predictive value has not been formally evaluated.

When a condition is episodic it will not be possible to make an individual assessment of performance and the best that can be achieved is correct identification of a person's position in any stratification of risk which is available for the relevant condition. There is good information on recurrence rates for seizures and for cardiac events which can be used for stratification. This may be more difficult where there are important personal variables in disease management that are under individual control, as is the case with the risk of hypoglycaemia from insulin. One of the key features with an episodic condition is the time taken to become incapacitated and the level of awareness that this is happening. Thus, while a seizure may be instantly incapacitating with no warning, cardiac events usually only incapacitate once blood flow to the brain has been severely reduced and so there is frequently a warning period of perhaps half a minute. For drivers on roads this is, in most circumstances, sufficient to pull to one side of the road and stop. Where an incapacitating episode is not perceived, either through lack of awareness of the prodromal symptoms or because cognition is clouded by the early stages of the episode then cessation of driving may be less reliable. Both of these can sometimes arise with insulin.

In the longer term the period over which the incapacity arises can determine the scope for action by others. Incapacity in air pilots or watchkeepers on dual-manned ships' bridges should result in the command being taken over, while on the railways safeguards in the signalling system will come into play. A particular problem arises for seafarers in that illness, even when developing over several hours, cannot be referred for medical attention. Hence standards include restrictions on those at excess risk of a recurrence or complication, for instance from renal stones, strangulation of a hernia or dental abscess. While primarily aimed at reducing risk to the individual such restrictions also reduce risk to others as helicopter evacuation, diversion of a vessel and the operational consequences of having to nurse a seriously ill person on a modern ship with the minimum required crew can increase both risk and costs.

Work and leisure

In all modes of transport the space used is shared between those at work and those using the medium for leisure activities. The latter are, in general, required to meet less stringent fitness standards or, in some cases, none at all. The concept of employment and responsibilities for meeting standards is a complex one in transport. This is addressed in several ways. For road drivers there is no statutory distinction by employment category and vehicle size and use form the basis for differential standards. The categories are standardized across the EU[3] with more stringent fitness requirements for those vehicles, called Group 2, over 3.5 tonnes (recently reduced from 7.5 tonnes) or with more than eight passenger seats. The rationale for this is that there is good evidence of higher consequential damage from such vehicles. In addition the worst case accident when large numbers of passengers are carried will lead to more fatalities. These statutory standards are supplemented by a local licensing system for taxis, for which the more stringent Group 2 standards are recommended. In addition some employers have their own standards, in particular the emergency services where high speed driving may be anticipated.

For all other drivers the Group 1 standards apply. These do not, unlike those for Group 2, require periodic medical examinations but depend largely on self-declaration of medical conditions to the licensing authority. The basis for control in all cases is by the issue or revocation of the person's driving licence. This is only applicable to longer-term health conditions and it is up to the individual driver to avoid driving if they have a short-term impairment. This is something that many drivers find difficult to handle responsibly, especially when their livelihood depends on driving. It is one of the reasons why some employers have established corporate driving risk reduction programmes that include provision for declaration of short-term incapacity and temporary cessation of driving without penalty.[4]

Occupational driving

Many workers drive vehicles off the public roads as part of their job. These include farmers, dock workers, and forklift truck drivers in many sectors. There are also highly specialized vehicles used, for instance, in mines, quarries, airfield, and container ports. Where vehicles are operated occupationally, and the activities are not carried out on the public highway, there is often confusion as to the application of medical fitness standards. This would apply for instance to a wide range of lift trucks, cranes, construction site vehicles, etc.

The legal requirement of The Health and Safety at Work Act is that the employer has a safe system of work. Although there is no specific legal requirement for medical assessment, there is a clear implication that medical fitness may be a prerequisite of ensuring such a safe system. Health and safety law is applicable to all workplaces. The employer will normally require the advice and assistance of a competent person, in this case an occupational physician, for both the setting of medical fitness standards and their implementation

In setting standards, there is merit in using an existing set of fitness criteria for driving rather than setting new standards from scratch and a logical choice would be the Driver and Vehicle Licensing Agency (DVLA) Group 1&2 medical standards. It should be remembered, however, that these standards are developed for users of the public highway, and DVLA have no jurisdiction over driving on private property. If part or all of the driving activity takes place on the public highway, then of course, the DVLA standards apply.

In setting standards for occupational drivers who are not using the public highway, it is possible to use the DVLA Group 1&2 standards as benchmarks, and to deviate from them by the process of risk assessment applied to the specific work.[5] A risk assessment that uses DVLA standards for benchmarking is advised, as direct application of DVLA medical standards may not be suitable, resulting in challenges under such legislation as the Disability Discrimination Act.

Medical aspects of licensing

Each mode of transport has its own licensing arrangements. For aircrew and for seafarers the standards are linked to international agreements. A central authority is responsible for their oversight and there is a network of doctors approved by the authority who undertake medicals on all but the lowest risk groups (see Appendices 1 and 2). The arrangements for the railways are under review at present. For road drivers licensing is formally a responsibility of the Secretary of State for Transport. In practice in Britain it is delegated to the DVLA, where the medical aspects are the responsibility of the Drivers' Medical Group. There is a comparable agency in Northern Ireland. The legal basis for the standards and for their enforcement lies in the Road Traffic Act 1988.[6]

This specifies certain disabilities, known as 'relevant disabilities', which bar a person from driving, and 'prospective disabilities', which require regular medical licensing review. In both instances the fact of the disability places an obligation on the driver to notify the DVLA of the medical condition. The basis for medical standards in respect of these disabilities lies in the second EC driver licensing directive. While the standards are all derived from the same directive there are national variations in the ways in which they are applied and in which compliance is checked. Great Britain is unusual in having a single centre, with its own medical staff who make decisions based on clinical information obtained from drivers, their clinicians and sometimes from commissioned investigations and examinations. Records of about 33 million drivers are held, of whom just over 3 million have had contact with the medical group over the last decade. Over 400 000 new enquiries are received each year, with year on year growth well above 10%. About 80% of these are handled by administrative staff, while the more complex cases are assessed by one of the medical advisers. The advisers are also available to health professionals by telephone and written communication to discuss individual cases.[7]

The medical standards used are published in the *At a glance guide to medical standards*, which is revised every 6 months.[8] These standards are aligned with those in the EU driver licensing directive but are usually more detailed. There are six expert medical panels covering the commonest problem areas: vision, heart disease, diabetes, neurology, psychiatric illness, and the effects of drug and alcohol misuse. The members are appointed by the Secretary of State and they both advise on the medical standards and review any particularly difficult cases or ones where the standards are not working effectively.[9] Standard setting is also supported by review and research programmes undertaken within the Department[10] and by reports from elsewhere in the world literature.

A new applicant for a Group 1 licence has a legal obligation to declare that they do not suffer from an impairing illness. At the driving test vision is assessed based on reading a new style car number plate at a distance of 20 metres. The terms of the licence require drivers to inform the DVLA of any significant illness while they hold their licence. This remains their personal responsibility but the General Medical Council recommends a process for a doctor to go through if one of their patients does not notify when they have been advised to do so.[11] The Group 1 licence expires at the age of 70 (although the photo must be updated every 10 years) and then has to be renewed every 3 years with the submission of a new medical declaration.

Group 2 drivers (over 3.5 tonnes for a new licence and over 7.5 tonnes for those holding a current Group 1 licence issued prior to 1997) are required to supply a medical examination form (D4), which may be completed by any doctor, but usually comes from their general practitioner or occupational physician. This is needed on application, again at age 45, then every 5 years to 65 and annually thereafter. This does not absolve them from the requirement to self-declare in the interim.

Any declaration of a relevant illness on application, during the currency of a licence or found at the time of a Group 2 medical examination will be followed up by a medical enquiry. For Group 1 this normally involves the driver completing a factual questionnaire with similar questionnaire enquiry to the doctor(s) involved in their treatment. Specialist referral may be required, particularly for Group 2 licences. The information received is assessed by the staff of the DVLA Drivers Medical Group who will then reach a licensing decision. Options include whether to issue or continue a full licence, whether to issue one for a shorter period and review, to restrict a licence to the use of certain vehicles or use of vehicle adaptations or whether to refuse a licence application or revoke the existing licence. Appeals against any licensing decision are heard in the local Magistrates Court in England and Wales or the Sheriffs Court in Scotland. Such appeals are rare and only about 20 cases proceeded to full hearing in 2003–4.

Specific medical conditions

Details of the standards may be found in the *At a glance guide*. The evidence on which they are based is widely scattered in the literature but the evidence linking medical conditions to accidents has recently been reviewed in detail.[12] Other chapters of this book discuss most of the conditions of concern. The following are standards where there are important features specific to driving, and to a varying extent to other modes of transport.

Cardiac events and strokes

Arterial disease poses a risk of both progressive impairment and relatively sudden incapacity. Standards are based on current capabilities and especially on likelihood of recurrence. For Group 1 drivers little more than a period without driving after an event is required but for Group 2 the probability of recurrence is stratified based on the Bruce protocol exercise ECG test and allowing a return if this is satisfactorily completed. A cautious approach has been adopted to implanted defibrillators in any driver because they may discharge without warning. Their internal memories can be used to determine frequency of discharge and if this is very low may allow Group 1 driving. The need for an implanted defibrillator is at present a bar to Group 2 entitlement.

Seizures

There is good evidence about the probability of a repeat seizure at various times after the last one, both with and without medication. This has enabled standards to be set based on a quantitative risk of recurrence. The level used is a probability of <20% in the next year for Group 1 and <2% for Group 2. The difference reflects the time likely to be spent at the wheel and the consequential damage likely if an accident occurs. More generally, the scope for applying quantitative approaches to assessing the accident risk from medical conditions has been investigated but because of the inherent limitations of the data it will never be a precise tool.[13]

Diabetes

The major risk is from insulin-induced hypoglycaemia. Risk data on diabetes is complex. The medical causes of road accidents are not readily identifiable and, while there is no clear evidence that hypoglycaemia is a cause of overall excess risk, each year the DVLA receives some 300 police notifications of presumed impairment from this cause while driving. As noted the nature of impairment is multifaceted and there is some evidence that it changes over the lifetime of the person. This is an area of considerable concern as many otherwise fit people are affected and any threat of a restriction on driving may lead to less than optimal treatment of the disease because of the risks of 'hypos'.

Vision

Vision and the use of visual information is a complex process and the tests used are limited to the assessment of acuity and visual fields. There are few clear correlations between degree of impairment and accident risk. For on-road driving there is good evidence that colour vision is not a requirement. One of the most contentious areas is visual field loss, associated with glaucoma and certain retinopathies. Here decisions have to be taken on a wide variety of defects, each of which can be mapped in detail but for which the consequences in terms of current risk and progression are not predictable.

Sleep disorders

The majority of sleep-related road accidents are in those with sleep deficits that do not have a medical cause. However, two medical conditions: obstructive sleep apnoea and narcolepsy, are important. Sleep apnoea is particularly prevalent in the overweight middle-aged male and is reliably associated with an excess risk of road crashes. Treatment with continuous positive pressure ventilators during sleep is acceptable and has been shown to reduce the risk of accidents. The severity of narcolepsy may be reduced by medication and can sometimes be controlled sufficiently to permit Group 1 driving.[14]

Psychiatric illness, drugs, and alcohol

Severe psychoses are normally a bar but for less severe illness there may be other potentially debarring issues which relate to the side-effects of the medication used as much as to the risks from the disease. There are no good correlations between non-psychotic mental illness and fitness to drive. Substance abuse as a short-term impairment is normally handled by police sanctions. The assessment of longer-term dependency and misuse arises as a medical issue and there are provisions for certain classes of driving offences in 'high risk offenders' to require medical clearance before returning to driving.[15]

Fixed disabilities

People with fixed disabilities such as paralysis, cerebral palsy, spina bifida, and amputations can often drive safely once they have been trained to use a modified vehicle. Services for assessment and adaptation, as well as for assessment of other stable disabilities, are provided by a network of Mobility Centres.[16] Any clinician can arrange a referral.

The role of the occupational health professional

Clinicians, in furthering the wellbeing and return to work of their patient, often see a conflict between these considerations and giving sound advice on fitness to drive which may limit work and mobility. Those advising on return to work need to be aware of this and of the limited knowledge of fitness standards on the part of many clinicians, despite the ready access to information from the DVLA and elsewhere. OH advisers may need to have their own procedures in place to ensure that correct advice is given and that job adaptations are made if there is a temporary limitation to fitness to drive.

Medical factors, as currently controlled, appear to be only very small contributors to road accident risk. Any organization that has staff with driving duties needs to consider the introduction of policies on driving at work. While good health management is a part of such policies it is important to ensure that this does not just relate to the long-term conditions that may put the driving licence at risk. It also requires an approach to short-term issues of acute illness, injury, and the use of impairing medications.

Note on railway medical standards

This is not intended to be more than a general statement on the principal features. At the time of writing both structure and regulation of the industry are in a state of flux and transition, and for this reason the names of the responsible and regulatory bodies are not given.[17]

There is largely a non-statutory, self-regulatory approach within the industry to medical fitness standards, though this needs to be set in the broader context of a legislative requirement to ensure competence, of which medical fitness is one aspect. There is also a requirement that the arrangements for ensuring medical fitness be described in the statutory safety case made by operating companies for approval by the regulatory body.

Medical fitness standards are contained in 'Railway Group Standards'. These standards have been in place for a long time and originate from the time when all railways were operated by British Rail, a wholly publicly owned organization. The standards continue to be owned and operated by the industry, and are periodically updated.

The bulk of the infrastructure, including the track (excluding heritage railways, London Underground, and other privately owned track) is the responsibility of one body, Network Rail (formerly Railtrack). The operating companies (of which there are currently more than 25) are required to ensure that those using the track, specifically train drivers, signalling staff, and crossing keepers meet the fitness standards prescribed in the Railway Group Standards. Other Railway Group Standards set out detailed requirements for drug and alcohol testing, and additional standards to ensure the personal safety of those working on or near the track. The industry operates a system for approving doctors to undertake the medical examinations.

Notes and references

1   Taylor JF (ed.) *Medical Aspects of Fitness to Drive*, p. 7. London: Medical Commission on Accident Prevention, 1995.

2   Charman WN. Vision and driving—a literature review and commentary. *Ophthal Physiol* 1997; **17**: 371–91.

3   European Union Directive on driving licences 91/26/EC and amendments 97/26/EC.

4   Driving at work: managing work-related road safety. Department for Transport, Health and Safety Executive, 2004. www.hse.gov.uk/pubns/indg382.pdf

5   An example of how this can be applied is provided in the HSE publication *Safety in working with lift trucks*(HSG6). Appendix 2 deals with medical standards and explains the benchmarking process in relation to lift truck operators.

6   Road Traffic Act 1988 (Section 92). More detailed provisions are in the Motor Vehicles (Driving Licence) Regulations 1996.

7   Contact for use by medical professionals only. DVLA 01792 761119 or email via www.dvla.gov.uk. Driver and Vehicle Licensing Northern Ireland 028 703 41369.

8   At a glance guide to current medical standards of fitness to drive. Drivers Medical Unit DVLA, Swansea. Updated six monthly at www.dvla.gov.uk

9   Agendas, minutes and annual reports of the medical panels can be accessed on www.dvla.gov.uk

10 Research reports can be found at www.dft.gov.uk under science and research, road safety.

11 Confidentiality: protecting and providing information. London, General Medical Council 2004. para. 22–7.

12 Charlton J *et al. Influence of chronic illness on crash involvement of motor vehicle drivers*. Monash University Accident Research Centre Report 213. www.general.monash.edu.au/muarc

13 Spencer MB, Carter T, Nicholson AN. Limitations of risk analysis in the determination of medical factors in road vehicle accidents. *Clin Med* 2004; **4**: 50–3.

14 Carter T, Major H, Wetherall G, Nicholson A. Excessive daytime sleepiness and driving: Contribution of the Regulatory Authority to Road Safety. *Clin Med* (in press).

15 The Motor Vehicles (Driving Licences) Regulations 1999 S74.

16 Details of services and locations www.mobility-centres.org.uk .

17 The Association of Railway Occupational Physicians (ARIOPS), which is affiliated to The Society of Occupational Medicine www.som.org.uk can provide up to date information to members.

Chapter 29

Health screening

T-C. Aw and D. S. Q. Koh

Introduction

Health screening has been defined by the US Commission on Chronic Illness (1951) as 'the presumptive identification of unrecognized disease or defect by the application of tests, examinations or other procedures which can be applied rapidly.' The Commission describes screening tests as tests that 'sort our apparently well persons who probably have a disease from those who probably do not' and further cautions that 'A screening test is not intended to be diagnostic. Persons with positive or suspicious findings must be referred to their physicians for diagnosis and necessary treatment'.

There are several types of health screening, including:

◆ mass screening of the whole population;
◆ multiple or multiphasic screening, employing several tests on the same occasion;
◆ prescriptive screening for the early detection of specific diseases that would have better prognosis if detected and treated early.

Wilson and Jungner[1] suggested several principles on which screening should be based. These relate to the condition or disease to be screened, and the test to be used for screening (Table 29.1). The principles are applicable to screening for occupational diseases as well as non-occupational.

The US Preventive Services Task Force[2] evaluated several clinical conditions that can benefit from screening, and the screening tests that may be effective. The criteria used in the selection of conditions are similar to those proposed by Wilson and Jungner,[1] and include the burden of suffering caused by the condition, its suitability for early intervention to improve prognosis, and the characteristics of the screening procedures.

Sensitivity, specificity, and predictive value of screening tests

The sensitivity, specificity, and predictive value should be considered in the selection of screening tests.

Table 29.1 Characteristics of diseases and tests that are appropriate for screening

The disease	The screening test
◆ Clinically important	◆ Acceptable
—significant morbidity/mortality	◆ Safe
—prevalent	◆ Sensitive
◆ Has a recognizable latent or	◆ Specific
asymptomatic stage	◆ Easily done
◆ Amenable to treatment	◆ Relatively cheap

Table 29.2 Sensitivity, specificity, and positive predictive value

Test result	Disease or condition	
	Present (+)	Absent (−)
Positive (+)	a	b
Negative (−)	c	d

a = true positive, b = false positive, c = false negative, d = true negative

The **sensitivity** of a test is its ability to detect those with the condition being tested. A test with 100% sensitivity will produce a positive test result for everyone affected by the condition. In other words, it will not produce any false negative results.

The **specificity** of a test is its ability to detect those who do not have the condition for which testing is being done. A test with 100% specificity will produce a negative result for everyone not affected by the condition. In other words, it will not produce any false positive results.

No test is 100% sensitive and 100% specific. The likelihood of anyone with a positive test result actually having the disease, or the **positive predictive value** (PPV) of the test, depends on the prevalence of the disease in the population being tested. While sensitivity and specificity are constant characteristics of any screening test, the PPV of the test will vary with the population in which the test is being applied. If the disease prevalence is low in the population tested, there will be a greater likelihood of false positive results, so that a given positive test has only a low PPV.

The **negative predictive value** (NPV) of a test is the probability that a person is disease free in the presence of a negative screening test result. This value will also be affected by the disease prevalence in the population that is tested. For a rare disease, the NPV is expected to be high, as virtually all who are screened will be disease free. Besides the disease prevalence, the sensitivity and specificity of the test will also affect the predictive values (see below).

◆ **Sensitivity** $= a/(a + c) \times 100\%$

 is the probability of a positive test in people with the disease

◆ **Specificity** $= d/(b + d) \times 100\%$

 is the probability of a negative test in people without the disease.

◆ **PPV** $= a/(a + b) \times 100\%$

 is the probability of having the disease when the test is positive.

◆ **NPV** $= d/(c + d)$

 is the probability of not having the disease when the test is negative

The relationship between disease prevalence, sensitivity, specificity, and predictive value is shown in the worked example in Table 29.3.

PPV varies with disease prevalence, as well as the sensitivity and the specificity of the screening test.

In this example, we can see that:

◆ PPV increases with increasing disease prevalence
◆ PPV increases with increasing sensitivity of the screening test
◆ PPV decreases for a rare disease, but increases for a common disease with increasing specificity of the screening test

A similar example can be worked out for NPV.

Table 29.3 How disease prevalence, sensitivity and specificity of a screening test affect its positive predictive value. Consider screening tests for two diseases in a population of 1000 people

Let a = true positive, b = false positive and PPV = a/(a+b)

	True +ve *(a)*	False +ve *(b)*	PPV [*a/(a+b)*]
Rare disease (20 cases in 1000)			
Sensitivity low (20%)	4		
Specificity low (20%)		196	2.0%
Specificity 50%		490	0.8%
Specificity high (80%)		784	0.5%
Sensitivity and specificity 50%	10	490	2.0%
Sensitivity high (80%)	16		
Specificity low (20%)		196	7.5%
Specificity 50%		490	3.2%
Specificity high (80%)		784	2.0%
Specificity low (20%)		196	
Sensitivity low (20%)	4		2.0%
Sensitivity 50%	10		4.9%
Sensitivity high (80%)	16		7.5%
Specificity high (80%)		784	
Sensitivity low (20%)	4		0.5%
Sensitivity 50%	10		1.3%
Sensitivity high (80%)	16		2.0%
Common disease (400 cases in 1000)			
Sensitivity low (20%)	80		
Specificity low (20%)		480	14.3%
Specificity 50%		300	21.1%
Specificity high (80%)		120	40.0%
Sensitivity and specificity 50%	200	300	40.0%
Sensitivity high (80%)	320		
Specificity low (20%)		480	40.0%
Specificity 50%		300	51.6%
Specificity high (80%)		120	72.7%
Specificity low (20%)		480	
Sensitivity low (20%)	80		14.3%
Sensitivity 50%	200		29.4%
Sensitivity high (80%)	320		40.0%
Specificity high (80%)		120	
Sensitivity low (20%)	80		40.0%
Sensitivity 50%	200		62.5%
Sensitivity high (80%)	320		72.7%

Likelihood ratios

Likelihood ratios of tests indicate how many times more likely patients with the disease are to have that particular result, as compared with those without the disease. In other words, it is the ratio of the probabilities of specific test results among the diseased to those who are disease free.

Thus a test with a likelihood ratio above 1 indicates that it is associated with presence of the disease. Conversely, a test with a likelihood ratio below 1 is associated with absence of the disease. In general, a test with a likelihood ratio of 10 or more provides good evidence to rule in the disease, while a test with a likelihood ratio of less than 0.1 gives a good indication to rule out the disease.

Receiver operating characteristic (ROC) curves

There are often practical difficulties in the definition of a positive or negative screening result. Additionally, there are challenges to distinguish a true positive from a false positive among those with positive test results, and also to identify a true negative from a false negative among those who tested negatively.

If the screening test result is a variable measured on a continuous scale, the cut-off point for a positive result can be varied to produce a test with either a high sensitivity and low specificity, or a high specificity and low sensitivity. A pertinent question is 'How does one determine an appropriate cut-off point for the screening test?'

One method used to assist in the selection of an appropriate cut-off point for the screening test is to express these values of the screening test in a visual form as a receiver operating characteristic (ROC) curve. In a ROC curve, the vertical axis of such a plot is the sensitivity of the test, while the horizontal axis is (1– specificity). The individual points represent the sensitivity and specificity obtained using different cut-off values, and the optimal cut-off value for the screening test is the point that is furthest from the 45° diagonal.

An example:

> An occupational physician needs to determine an effective cut-off point for the blood level of chemical X as a test to screen and detect workers with clinically significant exposure and a high likelihood of developing toxic effects. He/she conducts a study in a group of workers who either have or do not exhibit clinically significant toxicity to chemical X. At the same time, the blood concentration of chemical X is measured in all the workers. From these data (Table 29.4), a ROC curve can be plotted (Figure 29.1). Based on the curve and the table:
>
> If a blood concentration of 41 is adopted as a cut-off point, the test would have a sensitivity of 64.7%, and a 15% false positive rate.
>
> If a blood concentration of 37.5 is adopted as a cut-off point, the sensitivity is increased to 76.5%, while the false positive rate remains at 15%.

However, this method to determine the most appropriate cut-off point is not applicable for a test with a dichotomous outcome. The method also assumes an equal weight (or value, or importance) for sensitivity and specificity. An equal weight given to sensitivity and specificity may not necessarily be desirable, depending on the nature and natural history of the disease being screened, and also the consequences of false positive and false negative results.

Disadvantages of health screening

Adverse effects of screening can arise with the indiscriminate use of screening tests. A false positive test result causes unnecessary anxiety and worry in the subject. Additionally, a false positive test often leads to further investigations, which incurs additional expense, and also may be potentially harmful—especially as a disease does not exist.

Table 29.4 Blood concentration of chemical X, presence of clinically significant toxicity, and sensitivity and false positive rate of a screening test at different cut-off points

Blood concentration of chemical X	Sensitivity	1 – Specificity (false positive)
21.5	941	550
24.0	882	500
27.5	882	300
32.5	765	200
37.5	765	150
41.0	647	150
43.5	588	150
46.5	412	100
49.0	412	050
52.5	294	050
55.5	235	050
57.0	176	050
59.0	059	050
61.0	000	000

On the other hand, false negative results may cause complacency and may even lead to the person ignoring future early warning symptoms. When this happens, early diagnosis and treatment therefore becomes less likely. A false negative result from screening may be viewed by the individual as an 'all-clear' until the next round of screening is conducted. This could provide false reassurance, as a negative result at one point in time does not guarantee an absence of occurrence of disease until the next screening occasion.

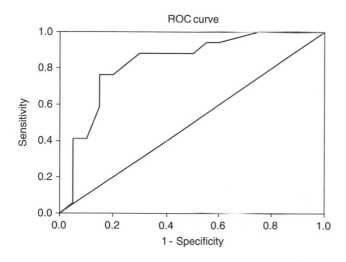

Fig. 29.1 ROC curve for blood concentration of X as a screening test

An example:

> The exercise electrocardiogram (stress ECG) is more sensitive (and also more expensive) than the resting ECG in screening for asymptomatic coronary artery disease. When used for screening coronary heart disease in an apparently healthy general population, the stress ECG has a PPV of less than 30%.[3]
>
> Thus, seven of 10 persons who are stress ECG positive are subjected to unnecessary and potentially harmful further investigations. In addition to causing anxiety in the person screened, a false positive stress ECG may also have negative consequences for occupational and insurance eligibility, and other opportunities.

There is a range of opinions on the use of the stress ECG for screening of asymptomatic persons for certain occupational groups.[2] For example, the American Academy of Family Physicians (AAFP)[4] recommends exercise electrocardiography for those whose jobs are linked to public safety (e.g. pilots, air traffic controllers) or occupations that require high cardiovascular performance (e.g. police officers, firefighters). The American College of Sports Medicine[5] recommends exercise ECG testing for men over age 40, women over age 50, and other asymptomatic persons with multiple cardiac risk factors, prior to beginning a vigorous exercise programme. The American College of Cardiology and the American Heart Association (ACC/AHA)[6] recognize that the exercise ECG is frequently used to screen asymptomatic persons in some high-risk groups but conclude that there is divergence of opinion with respect to its usefulness. The American College of Physicians (ACP)[7] does not recommend exercise testing with ECG as a routine screening procedure in asymptomatic adults.

Scope of the screening examination

Screening procedures could include symptom review, clinical assessment, medical examination, and special investigations. Apart from the detection of hypertension, the physical examination is unlikely to reveal significant abnormalities in an apparently healthy person. However, the consultation presents an opportunity to review life-style practices that impact on health, such as smoking habit, alcohol consumption, diet, and exercise behavior. The empathy that develops between the doctor/nurse and examinee would be advantageous when advice on life-style modification is given. Unfortunately, this aspect of the examination is often not fully capitalized upon. Also, health screening in the workplace for health promotion and prevention of common conditions, such as cardiovascular disease, should not be at the expense of controlling exposure to workplace hazards.

A wide range of ancillary tests and laboratory investigations are available to screen for health disorders such as vascular, neoplastic, and infectious diseases; metabolic, haematological, musculoskeletal, ophthalmological and otological disorders; mental disorders and substance abuse, and various prenatal conditions. Publications such as the Guides to Clinical Preventive Services[2] (second edition, 1996, and updated in sections to the third edition) prepared by the US Preventive Services Task Force, and the Canadian Task Force on Preventive Healthcare[8] are useful reference sources available on the internet. Website addresses:

- ◆ http://www.ncbi.nlm.nih.gov/books/bv.fcgi?rid=hstat3.part.19920
- ◆ http://www.ncbi.nlm.nih.gov/books/bv.fcgi?rid=hstat3
- ◆ http://www.ctfphc.org

These internet sites present updated information on the evidence-based clinical practice guidelines for screening.

Frequency of examination

The recommended frequency of examination varies with age and the natural history of the disease. Among adults, increasing age is associated with an increased likelihood of ill health. Frequency of examination may range from annually, or biennially, to once in 3–5 years, depending on the age group and the specific disease for which screening is done. In the case of occupational asthma, if sensitization to an inhaled agent in the workplace occurs, it is more likely in the early stages of employment and exposure. Hence the UK Health and Safety Executive (HSE) advice on lung function testing for workers exposed to asthmatogens puts emphasis on greater frequency of screening in the first few months of employment.

Ethical aspects and practical considerations

There is a major difference between clinical consultation and health screening. In the clinical consultation, the patient approaches the doctor for advice or treatment for a specific complaint or disease, and has to give consent to certain diagnostic procedures and therapy despite knowing that these may have some limitations or even possible adverse effects. In health screening, however, the doctor reviews an apparently healthy person for the possible presence of asymptomatic disease. In so doing, there must be a good understanding of the efficacy and safety of the screening tests, and patients should similarly be informed of the possible consequences of false positive and false negative results on screening.

It should also be noted that a test procedure that is ethically justifiable on diagnostic grounds may not be so when used for screening asymptomatic people. As Holland[9] points out, there is lack of evidence that some of the procedures are of benefit. On the other hand, there is positive evidence that they may lead to increased anxiety, illness behaviour, and also inappropriately utilize and deplete scarce healthcare resources.

For example, it could be argued that from a preventive medicine perspective, the energy and expense for health screening could perhaps be better diverted to promote measures to encourage proper diet, weight control, regular exercise, smoking cessation, moderation in alcohol consumption, and stress management, or control of exposure to workplace hazards for reduction of the likelihood of occupational diseases. Modifications in life-style behaviour require motivation and effort on the part of the individual, whereas health screening is essentially a passive process, where an individual is seemingly reassured that all is well after a negative examination. This perhaps is the reason why general health screening has a greater popular appeal.

However, the absence of abnormalities at the time of screening may well provide a false sense of security to the individual. The onset of illness could begin shortly after an apparently satisfactory screening, or the disease process may have already begun, but was not detectable at the time of screening by the methods used. This will create a major setback to the confidence of individuals participating in a screening programme, especially when disease appears in one or more participants within a short period of screening. Screening in itself does not prevent the occurrence of disease.

Screening in occupational health practice

In the occupational health setting, screening examinations are sometimes performed for specific purposes. The following are some examples.

Pre-placement examination

Pre-employment and pre-placement examinations are often required of persons embarking on a new job. The purpose of the examination is to determine whether there may be health reasons why an individual should not be placed in a particular job. The main reason for exclusion is that the safety of the individual or third parties may be compromised because of the health status of the prospective employee, e.g. a hepatitis B infectious carrier proposing to perform operations in a surgical specialty. In order to make a proper evaluation of fitness the examining doctor needs to be aware of the requirements of the job and the working environment, in addition to assessing the health status of the person. In some countries, there may be national regulations that stipulate pre-employment and periodic medical examination for specific occupational groups, or persons exposed to specific prescribed hazards at work, for example, lead exposed workers.

Another use of the pre-employment examination is to establish baseline health information for subsequent occupational health surveillance. It could also be used to assess health status for medical insurance purposes.

Many occupations do not require very high standards of physical fitness. The probability of discovering disease that might significantly impair job performance in apparently healthy job applicants, especially among young adults, is low. Thus, the rejection rate for fitness to work based on medical grounds is generally low. In a national audit of pre-employment assessments in the UK health service, it was determined that the rejection rate for applicants was less than 1%.[10]

In some instances, where medical conditions are detected that may have an effect on work, modification of the occupational functions, or special arrangements to accommodate the applicant's disability, might be required. In developed countries, there is often legislation such as the Disability Discrimination Act, to protect the employment rights of the disabled. Hence the components of any pre-employment assessment should be justified on the basis of necessity and risk, and based on sound evidence that the specific question asked or examination performed is warranted for the proposed job.

It would be appropriate to avoid subjecting every job applicant to the same general pre-employment screening. Instead, the screening examination should be tailored to the specific demands of the job. A self-administered health declaration or questionnaire that is processed by an occupational health adviser may be adequate for most clerical or administrative jobs. However, it has been advocated that more comprehensive screening be conducted for selected 'high flier' candidates, where substantial investment in training is required and grooming for positions of high office and responsibility is planned. This suggestion is not without controversy.

During pre-placement examinations, the opportunity to educate the potential employee on the health risks of the job, and the personal preventive measures that can be taken should not be missed. Counselling on changes to unhealthy life-style can also be offered.

Health screening prior to job transfers

Besides health screening for pre-employment job placements, health screening is often performed on employees prior to job transfers or job reassignment.

In cases of job reassignment involving posting to another country for a period of several years, the employee may be accompanied by his/her family, and therefore the examination may well be applied to accompanying family members. In addition to the health requirements of the job, the health services available in the country to which the employee is to be transferred need to be ascertained. This is especially important for medical conditions that may require treatment facilities unavailable in the host country. Possible medical complications that can arise which may require repatriation should also be considered. Another aspect to review is mental health. Adapting to life in a foreign country, where social support may be lacking, can be stressful. (See also Appendix 5.)

Health screening for return to work after prolonged or serious illness

Health screening can be conducted prior to return to work, especially after prolonged or serious illness. Knowledge of the natural history and prognosis of the illness is essential. It may be necessary to recommend an interim period of modified work, to allow time for the employee to readjust to the 'normal' work schedule and workload. For example, a person working in a hot environment who has been away from work for a prolonged period would require some time to become re-acclimatized to the work environment.

'Executive health screening'

The periodic medical examination is sometimes termed 'executive health screening' when applied to those in managerial posts. This is an example of multiphasic screening. It appears that the higher the manager is in the organizational hierarchy, the greater the frequency and extent of the examinations. It may be argued that the early detection of disease in highly paid executives has economic benefit to the company but there is nothing more than anecdotal evidence to support this. The screening processes may involve a wide range of biochemical profiles, exercise electrocardiograms, scans, and endoscopies. The utilization of some of these tests (especially those that may have been developed for assessment of diseased patients), for general screening of apparently healthy people with low prevalence of disease is inappropriate.

These annual medical examinations, often with the numerous screening tests, appear to be endorsed by primary care physicians.[11] This endorsement appears to be shared by patients as well, especially if the patients are not responsible for paying for these examinations and tests.[12] Why is there a discordance between the consensus statements recommending against routine annual physical examinations?[2,8] Some reasons could include the time gap for translation of evidence into practice, and also the change in practice in the intervening years between when the evidence was collected (30 years ago) and the present. Another could be the value placed by both doctors and patients on the development of the doctor–patient relationship, which occurs during such examinations.

As these examinations are usually offered on a voluntary basis, the tendency would be for the highly motivated and health conscious to participate in the examination. In contrast to these 'worried well', those who are less concerned with their personal health (and who may have a greater need for counselling and life-style interventions), often do not participate in the screening. Hence any illness that may be present in this latter group remains undetected. This paradoxical phenomenon has been called the 'inverse care law'.[13] Also executive medicals are seen as a benefit (if any) for selected groups within an organization. If there is any benefit in these screening procedures, then it should be made available for all.

Specific screening tests

In the UK, vision screening for staff doing work with visual display units is usually done using a Keystone machine. This is part of a process that also requires assessment of workstations where such work will be performed.

Audiometric screening is indicated under noise regulations in many countries, and also should be considered as a back-up process to detect temporary threshold shift, where noise exposure is intermittent and unpredictable, and/or where reduction of noise levels has not been completely successful or possible.

Screening for early hand–arm vibration syndrome (HAVS) is required under the Control of Vibration at Work Regulations 2005 for those exposed above an exposure action level of 2.5 m/s^2 A(8) (see p 681). This may include objective tests—e.g. simple two-point discrimination, aesthesiometry, and other tests aimed at detecting sensorineural effects from hand-transmitted vibration.

Spirometry, serial peak flow readings, and other tests of lung function are considered in workers exposed to the risk of obstructive or restrictive lung disease. Some of these tests are also used for diagnostic purposes, e.g. serial peak flow rates for occupational asthma, or for following up the efficacy of treatment or prevention (see Chapter 18).

Tests of liver or renal function are seldom indicated for routine screening in occupational health practice.

Periodic chest X-rays for workers exposed to fibrogenic dusts, e.g. asbestos and silica, and for divers and compressed air workers have been critically reviewed by the Health and Safety Laboratory.[14] The general consensus was that chest X-rays should be removed from occupational health statutory regulations, and only be performed following clinical indication. Subjecting workers to unnecessary radiation from repeated chest X-rays are not justified if the findings from these X-rays do not make any material difference to the management of the individual or where the X-rays are performed well within the latency period of the disease (e.g. for exposure to silica, if the intent is to detect early lung changes then chest X-rays in the first 10 years or so following initial exposure to silica is unlikely to be productive.) (See also Chapter 18.)

Genetic screening

Several methods have been developed that attempt to detect those at higher risk of disease following specific exposure. Examples are alpha-1-antitrypsin deficiency as an indicator of increased risk of emphysema in those exposed to cadmium, and human leucocyte antigen (HLA) gene markers, specifically HLA-DBP1, as a factor associated with the development of chronic beryllium disease.[15] There is no indication that these methods are sufficiently well-developed to warrant their use in occupational health practice.

The determination of atopic status for workers that may be exposed to asthmagens is of limited use for screening in occupational health, primarily because atopy in the general population is common and to use atopy as a criterion for exclusion would result in exclusion of a large majority of job applicants. It should only be considered where the actual risk of developing asthma or other allergic manifestations from occupational exposure is certain.

Screening for drugs and alcohol

In occupational health practice, this is best considered in the context of a clear organizational policy on the consequences of a positive result, on whether testing is voluntary or mandatory, and if it should apply to all levels of staff regardless of seniority. (See also Chapter 24.)

Biological monitoring and biological effect monitoring

Biological monitoring and biological effect monitoring are procedures used as part of screening in occupational health practice.[16] Biological monitoring screens for exposure, and biological effects monitoring attempts to detect early effects. As in other forms of screening, the principle is to detect adverse exposure or early alterations in biochemical parameters following workplace exposures, and to then take appropriate preventive measures to prevent the onset of overt health effects or clinical disease.

Biological monitoring in occupational health involves the analysis of biological samples (usually urine and/or blood, and occasionally breath or expired-air) for the presence of the chemical to which the individual worker is exposed, or for a metabolite. Examples of chemicals are metals such as lead and mercury, and organic solvents such as trichloroethylene (aliphatic) and xylene (aromatic). Metabolites of organic solvents that can be detected in urine samples are trichloroacetic acid for trichloroethylene and 1,1,1,-trichloroethane, and mandelic acid for styrene. Some metabolites are non-specific and can result from several different exposures, both occupational and non-occupational, e.g. hippuric acid in the urine can occur from benzoate in foods or from occupational exposure to toluene. Other metabolites are more specific, e.g. methyl-hippuric acid in urine for exposure to xylene.

Biological effect monitoring in occupational health attempts to detect changes in one or more biochemical parameters as an early effect from occupational exposure. Examples are the detection of an elevated free erythrocyte protoporphyrin level in blood for those exposed to inorganic lead, and depression of serum cholinesterase in workers exposed to organophosphates. Tests such as the detection of DNA adducts in biological samples for exposure to carcinogens are presently not sufficiently well-developed to be used for routine biological effect monitoring.

Health surveillance

The periodic clinical and physiological assessment of workers for exposure to workplace hazards,[17] or for monitoring general health status forms a large part of occupational medicine practice. For the prevention of work-related illness, emphasis should be on the former. Some of the components of health surveillance for specific purposes have been covered in the sections on health screening above.

Evaluation of screening programmes

A common error in evaluating the potential of a screening test is to adopt the sensitivity and specificity of a test when it is performed on people with the disease. As the screened population consists of asymptomatic persons who may or may not have the disease, the application of findings of the screening test in a diseased population to the general population may not be appropriate and could lead to erroneous conclusions.

Several other issues have to be considered when evaluating screening programmes. These include the potential for several biases to be present (Table 29.5).

Table 29.5 Possible biases in the evaluation of screening programmes

Selection bias	This bias may occur when those who participate in screening programmes are volunteers. Such volunteers are generally more health conscious than those who do not participate in screening programmes. As such, even without screening, these persons who volunteer for the screening test are more likely to have better health outcome from their disease as compared with the general population or those who do not participate in the screening
Lead time bias	The evaluation of the usefulness of screening examinations may sometimes be influenced by the apparent long survival of a patient (e.g. a patient with cancer) who is diagnosed early by screening. This long survival in fact may only be a manifestation of *lead-time bias*, where screening brings forward the time of diagnosis and thus lengthens the disease knowledge time without actually prolonging life
Length bias	There is a tendency for screening to detect the less serious or aggressive conditions. More rapidly advancing illnesses, by their nature, will only be present in the population for a relatively short time, and so miss being detected. As more slowly progressing illnesses than aggressive conditions are found on screening, this also gives the erroneous impression that detecting these conditions early has improved survival

Conclusions

Health screening is a useful tool in occupational health practice, but theoretical and practical considerations are essential before beginning such screening for any group of workers. Consideration of the legal requirements, and communication with the workforce, employer, and other occupational health and safety professionals is key to a successful health screening programme. Screening programmes should also be reviewed and audited periodically to ensure that the basis and procedures for such screening remain valid.

References

1 Wilson JMG, Jungner G. *Principles and practice of screening for disease.* Geneva: World Health Organisation, 1968.

2 US Preventive Services Task Force. *Guide to clinical preventive services,* (2nd edn). Washington DC: US Dept of Health and Human Services, 1968. http://www.ncbi.nlm.nih.gov/books/bv.fcgi?rid=hstat3.part.19920 (Accessed 1 Nov 2004)

3 Petch MC. Misleading exercise electrocardiograms. *Br Med J* 1987; **295**: 620–1.

4 American Academy of Family Physicians. *Age charts for periodic health examination.* Kansas City, MO: American Academy of Family Physicians, 1994.

5 American College of Sports Medicine. *Guidelines for exercise testing and prescription,* (4th edn). Philadelphia, PA: Lea & Febiger, 1991.

6 American College of Cardiology/American Heart Association. Guidelines for exercise testing. A report of the American College of Cardiology/American Heart Association Task Force on assessment of cardiovascular procedures (Subcommittee on Exercise Testing). *J Am Coll Cardiol* 1986; **8**: 725–38.

7 American College of Physicians. Efficacy of exercise thallium-201 scintigraphy in the diagnosis and prognosis of coronary artery disease. *Ann Intern Med* 1990; **113**: 703–4.

8 Canadian Task Force on the Periodic Health Examination. The periodic health examination: 1984 update. *Can Med Assoc J* 1984; **130**: 2–15.

9 Holland WW. Screening: reasons to be cautious. *BMJ* 1993; **306**: 1221–2.

10 Whitaker S, Aw TC. Audit of pre-employment assessments by occupational health departments in the National Health Service. *Occup Med* 1995; **45**(2): 75–80.

11 O'Malley PG, Greenland P. The annual physical: Are physicians and patients telling us something? *Arch Intern Med* 2005; **165**(12): 1333–4.

12 Oboler SK, Prochazka AV, Gonzalez R, Xu S, Anderson J. Public expectations and attitudes to annual physical examinations and testing. *Ann Intern Med* 2002; **136**: 652–9.

13 Hart JT. The Inverse Care Law. *Lancet* 1971; **i**: 405–12.

14 Health & Safety Laboratory. A critical review of the use of radiology in statutory medical examinations: Report from an HSE workshop held at the Lowry hotel 3rd-4th Dec 2001. Sheffield: HSL report HEF/02/02, 2002.

15 McCanlies EC, Ensey JS, Lefant Jr JS *et al.* The association between *HLA-DBP1*^{Glu69} and chronic beryllium disease and beryllium sensitization. *Am J Ind Med* 2004; **46**(2): 95–103.

16 Aw TC. Biological monitoring In: *Occupational hygiene* (eds Gardiner KG, Harrington JM), pp. 160–9. Oxford: Blackwell Publishing Ltd, 2005.

17 Koh DSQ, Aw TC (2003). Surveillance in occupational health. *Occup Environ Med* 2003; **60**(9):705–10.

Civil aviation

R. V. Johnston

Introduction

The civil aviation industry has a well-developed and tested system of medical standards that are regularly scrutinized and reviewed to preserve the safety of the travelling public. In the first instance this is addressed by the national authority responsible for air safety—in the UK the Civil Aviation Authority (CAA)—which is concerned to ensure that a licence holder can function effectively and is not likely to suffer sudden or subtle incapacitation during the period (6 months–1 year) for which their medical certificate is valid. An employer takes a more long-term view, seeking not only to satisfy the safety requirement, but also to recruit an employee who will remain fit throughout a full career. This is particularly important when the very high cost of training a professional pilot is considered. An individual with a progressive disability might be given a medical certificate subject to regular reviews and may gain a licence but would not be employed by a major airline. Guidance is often needed on this subject and would be given by the CAA.

Risk

Risk management is the main principle of aviation medical certification. It is not possible, nor is it policy, to seek a zero-risk environment. The best airlines operating the best aircraft now achieve a fatal accident rate close to or even better than the CAA safety target of 1 fatal accident in 10 million flights. Many factors contribute to accident causation; the flight crew may be considered to be one of the 'systems' on the aircraft, so the safety target for accidents from medical causes is now less than 1 in 100 million flights. This risk can be managed in larger aircraft by having two or more pilots, who have been exposed to incapacitation scenarios during routine simulator training, and by only certificating pilots with medical conditions that carry an incapacitation risk of 1% per year or less. This has become known as the '1% rule' and by using this approach the safety target can be met. With the advent of more sophisticated aircraft and improved training, it may be that this figure needs review. There is ongoing research to address this issue.

Risk mismatch

One issue of regular concern for occupational physicians practising aviation medicine is that patients' own doctors often advise applicants that the complications of a particular condition do not affect their fitness to hold a medical certificate. This misconception may arise from a lack of understanding of the aviation environment and a wish to reassure an individual on what is perceived as a low risk in terms of everyday life and work. This mismatch becomes manifest when a individual, with a very small risk of developing some medical complication, discovers that they fall outside the aviation risk criteria and is, therefore, denied a medical certificate. Dealing with such a situation demands experience, skill, and a degree of tact. An individual's career may be interrupted, albeit temporarily, for a reason that is self-evident to the aviation physician but is difficult for the patient to understand. A similar problem may arise when individuals present for examination to renew their medical certificates and an abnormality is found that has not caused any symptoms, e.g. ECG changes. Individuals in this situation often do not understand that such an abnormality may give rise to a risk of incapacitation in the future. Again, an occupational physician experienced in aviation medicine will be familiar with this scenario and will explain and discuss the situation with understanding and care.

Pilots

The medical standards for pilots (and for flight engineers and air traffic control officers) are internationally agreed and are contained in Annex 1 to the Convention on International Civil Aviation. A few, such as the visual requirements, are specific but many are couched in general terms such as 'cases of metabolic, nutritional or endocrine disorders likely to interfere with the safe exercise of the applicant's licence privileges shall be assessed as unfit'. There is also a waiver clause known as 'accredited medical conclusion', which allows a national authority to issue a medical certificate, even if the standards are not met, if it believes it is safe to do so. The International Civil Aviation Organization (ICAO), a United Nations organization, issues a manual of guidance material on the interpretation of the standards.

Possible exposure to a harsh environment, notably hypoxia, and sudden changes of pressure and temperature, requires very good cardiovascular function and freedom from conditions likely to be aggravated by sudden changes in pressure and volume such as middle ear and sinus disorders, lung bullae, and bowel herniation.

The special senses, especially vision, are clearly important. Uncorrected distant visual acuity must in some countries be 6/60 (20/200) or better. Correction to 6/9 (20/30) or better is required, and there are near and intermediate requirements. A correction of refractive error by the use of spectacles or contact lenses is allowed within certain limits. Normal colour vision is not always necessary provided the candidate can reliably distinguish signal red, white, and green.

Pilots with disabilities resulting from orthopaedic or neurological conditions are given a practical test in each aircraft type they wish to fly, which may require approved modifications.

The life-style of a professional pilot is necessarily irregular and this excludes applicants with some gastrointestinal and metabolic disorders. Type 1 diabetes is disqualifying due to the unacceptable risk of hypoglycaemia. Type 2 diabetes controlled by oral therapy does not preclude flying in trained professional pilots subject to regular follow-up and may be acceptable for initial fitness for private pilots.

Because the continual exercise of judgement and self-discipline is so vital to the pilot's task, significant mental and personality disorders are unacceptable. A history of psychosis is permanently disqualifying. Neurotic illness is assessed on the probability of recurrence, as is alcohol and drug abuse. HIV infection may first manifest itself with neuropsychiatric symptoms and is considered disqualifying in many countries.

A pilot's licence is temporarily suspended on presumption of pregnancy but flying in a two-pilot aircraft is usually possible in the middle trimester. Many airlines, however, ground pilots on declaration of pregnancy to minimize any potential exposure of the foetus to radiation.

The basic question in aviation medicine is: Will the disease or its treatment interfere with the safe execution of the flying task? Commonly used therapeutic agents are therefore often unacceptable because of their side-effects. Performance testing in a flight simulator may be carried out, if necessary, to assess this. In many cases the disorder requiring the therapy will be disqualifying, at least temporarily. For example the majority of antihypertensive agents are acceptable subject to satisfactory blood pressure control in the absence of side effects. Antidepressant therapy of any kind is not acceptable at present but this situation is currently under review, with protocols being developed to allow highly selected cases to be considered fit, subject again to close follow-up. Benzodiazepine hypnotics with a short half-life such as temazepam may be acceptable for short-term use depending on the indication. An aviation medicine specialist should assess such cases individually.

Conditions likely to cause incapacitation, either sudden or subtle, are usually disqualifying. Passenger aircraft smaller than 5700 kg (air-taxi size) sometimes only carry one pilot, whose incapacitation would inevitably result in an accident. Larger aircraft must carry two pilots. As mentioned earlier, incapacitation training in a simulator is now a routine practice and research has indicated that an accident may result on fewer than one in a hundred occasions of sudden pilot incapacitation.

Experience indicates that the risk of accidents increases directly as the total number of medical disabilities rises. It also falls dramatically with increasing age and experience up to age 60, when most professional pilots retire. Thus inappropriate removal of middle-aged pilots on medical grounds and their replacement by younger, less experienced pilots potentially may have an adverse effect on air safety.

The medical standards for pilots engaged in flying instruction and non-passenger-carrying activities, such as banner towing, were more relaxed than the standards described above but this is no longer the case with the introduction of harmonized European standards since July 1999.

In the UK, the Aeromedical Centre of the CAA carries out the initial medical examinations on professional pilots, flight engineers, and air traffic control officers. Airline transport pilots and commercial pilots below the age of 40 are examined annually and 6-monthly above the age of 40, the renewal examinations being undertaken by medical examiners who have had postgraduate training in aviation medicine and who are authorized by the CAA.

Flight engineers

Flight engineers play an important part in monitoring the actions of the pilots as well as controlling the systems on the aircraft. The required medical standards for these crew members are therefore essentially similar to those of pilots, but because they do not physically handle the flying controls at critical stages of flight, their sudden incapacitation does not present the same threat to safety as it would for pilots. They may, therefore, continue to fly with conditions that present a somewhat greater risk of incapacitation.

Air traffic control officers

The rise in air traffic movements means that air traffic control officers have responsibilities for maintaining safety that are similar to that of pilots. Medical fitness standards are therefore comparable. Many controllers work in teams and in these circumstances a risk of incapacitation identical to that for pilots of larger aircraft may be acceptable.

Cabin crew

Stewards and stewardesses do not hold licences and formal medical standards are not laid down. The Joint Aviation Regulations (see below) merely require airlines to ensure by 'medical examination or assessment' that cabin crew are fit to carry out their assigned duties. Good cardiorespiratory function and freedom from conditions aggravated by pressure changes and the effects of irregular working and world-wide travel are important. Visual acuity of at least 6/9 with or without correction is required.

For several years there has been a process of harmonization that covers all aspects of civil aviation in Europe. Licensing and medical certification are covered by this process and, since 1 July 1999, the European states known as the Joint Aviation Authorities (JAA), currently 38, have been required to establish identical licensing and medical standards [known as Joint Aviation Requirements—Flight Crew Licensing Part 3 (Medical)]. This will allow the states to accept each others' licences without further test or expense. A new code has assured primacy and States will not be allowed to vary the standard unilaterally. However, this does not limit national authorities' discretion under the waiver clause. An age limit of 65 has been established for two pilot and multi-crew operations. The standards for Air Traffic Controllers are currently being harmonized under the direction of Eurocontrol.

A European Community proposal has been adopted, leading to the establishment of a single European Aviation Safety Authority (EASA) with greater executive and enforcement powers than the current JAA. At present, under the JAA arrangements, each State will run the licensing and medical certification processes according to the harmonized requirements, the standards and policy being determined by committees made up of members of each States' authorities. With the establishment of EASA, there is likely to be a much stronger central policy unit with responsibility for setting, maintaining and enforcing the standards. The European States with major aviation industries will continue to have a major influence and involvement in this process.

Legislation

The Disability Discrimination Act does not apply to employment on board a ship, aircraft or hovercraft—(Section 68(3)). Civil aviation legislation, (The Civil Aviation Act 1982 and the Air Navigation Order 2000) specify the requirements for licensed jobs. The 'Joint Aviation Requirements—Flight Crew Licensing Part 3 (Medical)' is now effective in all JAA States.

Further reading

Bennett G. Pilot incapacitation and aircraft accidents. *Eur Heart J* 1988; **9** (Suppl. G): 21–4.

Bennett G. Medical-cause accidents in commercial aviation. In: First European workshop in aviation cardiology (ed. M. Joy). *Eur Heart J* 1992; **13** (Suppl. H): 13–15.

Chaplin JC. In perspective—the safety of aircraft pilots and their hearts. *Eur Heart J* 1988; **9** (Suppl. G): 17–20.

Evans ADB (in press). International Regulation of Medical Standards. In: *Ernstings aviation medicine* (eds Rainford DR and Gradwell DP), Chapter 36. London: Arnold.

International Civil Aviation Organisation. *Manual of civil aviation medicine*, (2nd edn). Montreal: International Civil Aviation Organisation, 1985.

International Civil Aviation Organisation. *Annex 1 to the Convention on international civil aviation*, (9th edn). Montreal: International Civil Aviation Organisation, 2001.

Tunstall Pedoe H. (1988). Acceptable cardiovascular risk in aircrew. In: Second United Kingdom workshop in aviation cardiology, (ed. M. Joy and G. Bennett). *Eur Heart J* 1988; **9** (Suppl. G): 9–11.

Appendix 2

Seafarer fitness

J. T. Carter

Seafaring is a job and a way of life. As a job it has both risks and performance requirements. As a way of life the consequences of being at sea in terms of diet, exercise, and social interactions, distance from healthcare facilities and, in some cases world-wide travel, are all important. The sector has complex international patterns of staffing, ownership of vessels, and employment contracts and these mean that any maritime country has limited freedom to set its own policies and standards.

Work demands on seafarers vary widely. Service may be world-wide, inshore, or on inland waterways. Vessel types include bulk carriers, container ships, cruise liners, ferries, commercial yachts, and canal boats. Responsibilities differ between officers and ratings, while the risks and performance requirements on the bridge, in the engine room and while catering or serving passengers have little in common. In an emergency physically and psychologically demanding tasks have to be undertaken, such as fire-fighting in restricted spaces, launching and manning lifeboats, or rescuing casualties from the sea.

Several major international organisations have a part to play in standard setting:

- The International Labour Organization (ILO), has a series of maritime labour conventions and recommendations that cover food, accommodation, medical standards, and care and welfare.[1]

- The International Maritime Organization, which is concerned with vessel safety and the contribution of human performance to this.[2]

- The World Health Organization is important in relation to infection control, port health agreements, emergency care of seafarers[3] and, jointly with ILO, guidance on medical fitness standards.[4]

- The European Union (EU) regulates working hours[5] and emergency medical supplies carried on EU vessels.[6]

- There is also a wide range of internationally integrated employer[7], trade union,[8,9] and professional bodies.[10]

Within each country a maritime authority implements these standards and may also be concerned with their enforcement. In UK the responsibility for this is with the Maritime and Coastguard Agency (MCA), an agency of the Department for Transport. Medical Standards for determining the fitness of seafarers are produced and regularly updated by the Agency.[11] These standards align with international requirements. Seafarers serving on UK flagged ships must have a medical certificate, issued within the last 2 years, showing that they meet these standards. Certificates of certain other countries are accepted as equivalent.[12]

The standards have been developed over more than a century in the light of experience, changes in medical practice and with a view to practicability and fairness in application. The rationale of the fitness criteria for each condition is specified and this is increasingly based on validated evidence of risk. There are two patterns of medical assessment against the standards, one for the majority of merchant seafarers who need to comply with international requirements[13] and another for the masters of small commercial craft such as yachts, work-boats, and passenger vessels in inland and estuarial waters.[14]

Merchant seafarer medicals are undertaken by doctors approved by the Agency. Approval is at the discretion of the MCA and is based on local need. There are about 240 approved doctors in UK and overseas. Most are available to any seafarer but a few are approved only in relation to a single company or for a range of company contracts.[15] Approved doctors are assisted by a procedural manual and have access to MCA administrative and medical staff for advice.[16] Standards of work are monitored and the majority of doctors now have relevant occupational medical or maritime experience.

Some 30 000 merchant seafarer medicals are done each year. Of these about 2000 lead to some form of restriction on service or to failure. Seafarers have the right to a review by a medical referee, of whom there are eight, and about 100 request a review each year.

Those who work on local commercial boats and yachts may alternatively go to any doctor registered in UK, but normally their general practitioner, who will complete a medical screening form (ML5). If there are no positive findings, an MCA marine office or the Royal Yacht Association will, subject to other tests of knowledge and competency, issue a Boatmaster's licence or commercial endorsement. If a possibly relevant medical condition is identified, an MCA appointed medical assessor will review the available medical information. They may fail the applicant or may issue a full or restricted ML5 certificate, which can then be used to support the licence application.

For some conditions fitness criteria are straightforward. Thus, in an environment where navigation lights are red, green, and white, anyone who cannot distinguish these colours cannot undertake lookout duties. Others may be very complex. Someone who has had a cardiac event may have continuing impairment to physical or cognitive performance—either of which could affect their ability to undertake routine or emergency duties. They have an increased risk of sudden incapacity—critical if they are navigating the ship or working alone. They may have a recurrence—a greater risk to them at sea as well as to others if evacuation is needed, and also posing operational problems if other crew members need to care for them or the ship has to be diverted. Fitness decisions will depend on the person's duties and where the ship is operating.

As seafarers live in close quarters and food is prepared on board, infection risks need to be identified, both in food handlers and in those who may spread infections such as tuberculosis. Formal standards are particularly contentious where they concern risk factors rather than disease; for instance those concerned with future cardiac risk such as hypertension and obesity—two of the commonest reasons for restriction. Related life-style interventions concerned with diet and smoking may be difficult for the individual to implement at sea unless there is commitment from owners and masters.

As a consequence of the variety of job requirements most standards depend on the job of the seafarer and on the part of the world in which the vessel sails.[17] Like any other statutory measure affecting employment and livelihood the fitness assessment system has to be demonstrably fair and credible, applied uniformly and such that there is an independent review procedure. The balance in standard setting is between public safety and employment opportunities for individuals.

Some maritime employers have additional fitness criteria but they may not go below the statutory minimum. Seafarers, to secure or maintain employment, sometimes fail to disclose health problems or may seek to avoid optimum treatment of conditions that require medications such as insulin or warfarin, which, because of their side-effects can be a bar to work at sea.

A wide range of health professionals can, from time to time, be involved in the care of seafarers and potential seafarers. In such situations there are a number of considerations:

1. Young people who want work at sea need to be aware that they have to meet certain medical standards. It is helpful to advise anyone who is unlikely to meet these standards that they may need to rethink their career options. Issues that commonly cause work limitation relate to vision—especially colour vision; asthma—usually better at sea but very dangerous in the event of a sudden exacerbation; congenital conditions—heart, limb function; seizures, and diabetes.

2. Immunizations and antimalarial prophylaxis may be needed. Seafarers should be advised of this and arrangements made for provision, usually by their employer, but they may seek advice or medications from others.[18]

3. Seafarers requiring elective surgery. Priority may need to be sought so that they can comply with medical standards and return to work.[19]

4. After a diagnosis of a significant illness such as heart disease, diabetes, or epilepsy the seafarer will need to obtain a new medical certificate but may have to wait until the condition is stabilized and may find that they are restricted or found unfit.

5. When continuing medication is needed. The acceptability of the person for sea service will need to be assessed and in some cases the medication itself will be the reason for restricting duties or finding the person unfit.

6. If cardiac risk factors are poorly controlled, especially weight and blood pressure, the patient will need to be reminded that failure to achieve control may lead to their career at sea being terminated even in the absence of a cardiac event.

Notes and references

1 International Labour Organization www.ilo.org

2 International Maritime Organization www.imo.org

3 WHO. *International medical guide for ships*, (2nd edn). Geneva: World Health Organization, 1988 (3rd edn in preparation).

4 WHO/ILO. *Guidelines for conducting pre-sea and periodic medical fitness examinations for seafarers* Geneva: WHO/ILO, 1997. www.ilo.org/public/english/standards/relm/gb/docs/gb271/stm-5a.htm

5 The Maritime Working Time Directive (1999/63/EC) www.europa.eu.int/eur-lex/en/index.html

6 Merchant Shipping Notice MSN 1768 (M+F). Ships' medical stores. Maritime and Coastguard Agency, 2003.*

7 International Shipping Federation www.marisec.org

8 International Transport Workers' Federation www.itf.org.uk

9 NUMAST—National Union of Marine Aviation and Shipping Officers www.numast.org

10 International Maritime Health Association www.imha.net

11 Merchant Shipping Notice MSN 1765 (M) Seafarer medical examination system and medical and eyesight standards. Maritime and Coastguard Agency 2002.*

12 MSN 1765(M) (Ref. 11 above) p8. List kept live on MCA's website.* www.mcga.gov.uk/seafarer information/health and safety/

13 Marine Guidance Note MGN 219(M). Seafarer medical examinations: guidelines for maritime employers and manning agencies. Maritime and Coastguard Agency, 2002.*

....

*Maritime and Coastguard Agency (MCA) publications are regularly updated and their reference numbers may change. Access to the current versions of those relevant to seafarer medicals can be obtained via: MCA's website: http://www.mcga.gov.uk/seafarer information/health and safety/

14 MGN 264(M)—Medical fitness requirements for those employed on boats certificated under MCA Codes of Practice ... Maritime and Coastguard Agency 2004.*

15 Merchant Shipping Notice MSN 1787 (M) AD list. Maritime and Coastguard Agency 2004.*

16 *Approved doctor's manual: seafarer medical examinations.* Maritime and Coastguard Agency. Controlled document periodic updates—current version on Agency website.*

17 Carter T. The evidence base for maritime medical standards. *Int Maritime Health* 2002; **53**: 1–4.

18 Marine Guidance Note MGN 257 (M). Prevention of Infectious disease at sea by immunisations and anti-malaria Medication (prophylaxis). Maritime and Coastguard Agency, 2003.*

19 Dreadnought Unit, Guy's and St Thomas' Hospital www.seabal.co.uk/dreadnought.htm (a service providing treatment for seafarers)

*Maritime and Coastguard Agency (MCA) publications are regularly updated and their reference numbers may change. Access to the current versions of those relevant to seafarer medicals can be obtained via: MCA's website: http://www.mcga.gov.uk/seafarer information/health and safety/

Appendix 3

Offshore workers

K. M. Doig

Introduction

Offshore oil and gas production is a global industry found in almost all the oceans of the world—shallow and deep water—arctic and tropical. In the UK, gas was first discovered in the southern North Sea in 1965 and brought ashore in 1967. In the northern North Sea the giant Forties Field was discovered in 1970 and the first oil from the Argyll Field came ashore in 1975.

Oil production generally has peaked, with the UK in 2004 producing 725 million barrels of oil and 95 billion m^3 of gas, with production expected to decline gradually. Both, however, will last well into the current century.

Further exploration continues encouraged by higher oil prices and new technology and mature developments are being given a new lease of life through enhanced recovery techniques such as steam injection, surfactant chemicals, and miscible gases and polymers to lower the viscosity of the oil.

At the peak of North Sea development activity in 1990, over 36 000[1] workers were employed in UK offshore fields. In 1994, with many more producing fields, about 27 000 workers were employed. By 2004, with a total of over 200 fields in production, about 20 000 people were employed offshore with more of the field processes being automated.

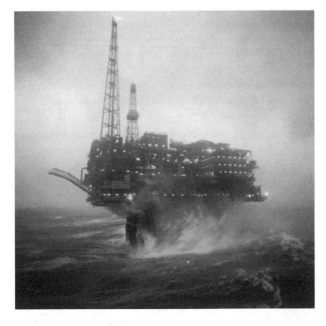

Fig. A3.1 Brent Charlie—Shell

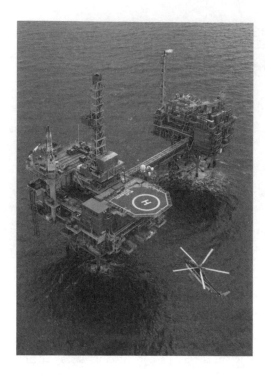

Fig. A3.2 Captain Field—Chevron

Offshore installations

There are currently over 260 fixed installations in the North Sea with a varying number of mobile drilling and accommodation rigs. They range in size from small exploration and drilling semisubmersibles to the massive fixed leg oil production and export installations. The latter represent a complex engineering feat fitting together all the processing plant required to receive the pressurized hot crude oil, process it, and then export it onshore under pressure through an undersea pipeline or to an adjacent holding vessel.

The production installations are usually fixed leg platforms, but occasionally floating moored facilities are used—more often in deeper water. As with fixed leg platforms they are connected to the seabed and hence the oilfields by large bore risers that carry the hot oil from deep subterranean reservoirs to the processing plant on the facility. The oil passes through separators cleaning it of water and sand that normally may be present, and it is then exported through a separate system, most often into a shared pipeline to the shore or, less commonly, into a storage vessel for uplifting by tanker. To enhance recovery rates there is often a high pressure compression system to pump treated seawater back into the field to replace the extracted oil and to maintain reservoir pressure. Production facilities normally depend on two to three large turbines for the production of electricity to supply the energy for all these processes and the needs of the service facilities, offices, and accommodation.

The offshore working environment

Located usually hundreds of miles offshore, these complex facilities pose a harsh working environment for the men and women of their workforce. Each offshore installation is a self-sufficient community where the workforce works, relaxes, and sleeps for the duration of their offshore tour—normally 2 or 3 weeks in duration.

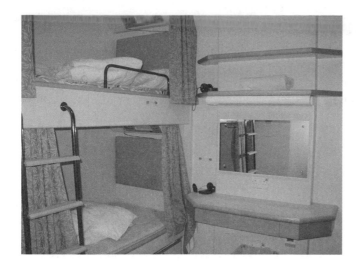

Fig. A3.3 Twin bunked accommodation Brae Field—Marathon

Logistic support is provided by helicopters and supply vessels transferring personnel and delivering food and equipment. Shift work is typical with workers allocated a 12-hour shift—most commonly daytime around 7 a.m.–7 p.m. with some reciprocal nightshifts of 7 p.m.–7 a.m. Living quarters offshore are compact but comfortable and usually shared with two, or less commonly, four bunks per cabin.

Food is of good quality and abundant at mealtimes—but no alcohol is allowed. There are recreational facilities normally including satellite television, a gym, and often a cinema. Isolation may be a factor for some of the workforce and many jobs are physically arduous. Manning levels and accommodation restraints are such that anyone becoming sick for any length of time will have to be returned onshore and replaced by another worker. An emergency medical evacuation can be expensive for the company and, if required in inclement weather conditions, can endanger the crew of the helicopter and any medical personnel involved.

Communication with the mainland can be fragile—telephone links are normally by radio and are subject to variations in quality related to weather conditions and downtime during maintenance. There are regular intervals where travel by helicopter may be impossible for 2–3 days, due to high winds in the winter or fog in the summer.

The regular visits by supply vessel can also be disrupted by the weather, interfering with the supply of engineering tools, service supplies, fresh food, and water from the mainland. It is essential that the close knit interdependent community of the offshore workforce can operate as a highly efficient and functional team.

Women as well as men work offshore but as yet remain a small minority in the UK sector of the North Sea.

Range of functions

The number of workers on a single installation is in the range of 150–250 core crew covering a wide range of duties to encompass all the functions associated with running, maintaining, and providing support services for a heavy engineering and oil production operation. Many of the tasks offshore still require a large degree of lifting and heavy manual handling and many valves are still manually operated. By the nature of the processes involved, equipment is very heavy and needs constant regular maintenance and repair, which often has to be done in a very confined working space. The compact nature of the oil installation dictates that the design is usually multilevel with access between levels normally by steep, open, external stairs. Because of the exposed environment and the need to contain potential fires and explosions there are ubiquitous fire and explosion proof safety doors that can be extremely heavy to open and close.

Among the specialized functions represented offshore are control room operators, chemists to test the oil and drill cuttings, health and safety professionals, caterers, drillers, geologists, electricians, instrument technicians, and an offshore medic.

Each installation comes under the authority and control of the offshore installation manager (OIM) who is deemed, for legislative purposes, to be the person in charge.

Health legislation

The Continental Shelf Act of 1964[2] extended petroleum exploration licensing arrangements offshore with provision for the safety, health, and welfare of persons employed on operations undertaken under the authority of any licence. The Health and Safety at Work Act,[3] Management of Health and Safety at Work,[4] Control of Substances Hazardous to Health (COSHH),[5] and Working Time Directives[6] have all been extended to cover the offshore workforce.

The provisions of the National Health Service do not extend offshore so private health providers supply the necessary medical resources to support the health requirements required by legislation, high industry standards, and the expectations of best practice.

Specific health legislation for the offshore workplace exists as the Offshore Installations and Pipeline Works (First Aid) Regulations 1989.[7] The regulations set out the requirements for the provision of healthcare facilities for everyone on an offshore installation. These define the minimal acceptable health requirements that should be in place offshore and use a wider definition of 'First Aid' to include the treatment of illness and injury and also define the title role and responsibilities of the dedicated on-site medical provider—the offshore medic.

The Offshore Installations (Prevention of Fire and Explosion, and Emergency Response) Regulations 1995 (PFEER)[8] set out requirements to secure an effective response including that of the medical team in the event of serious incidents on an offshore installation. In addition some functions of the team involving potential heavy physical loads have an industry defined specific

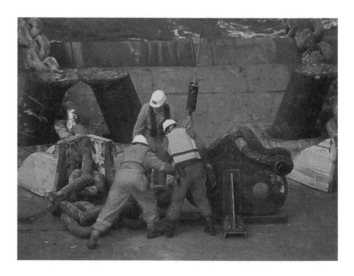

Fig. A3.4 Offshore workers Supply vessel—Maersk

medical fitness requirement described in the Emergency Response Team section of the industry medical fitness standards—UKOOA Guidelines for Medical Aspects of Fitness for Offshore Work.[9]

Offshore survival training

Because, as described, the normal transport to any offshore installation is by helicopter and, in a significant emergency, rescue is likely to involve evacuation by lifeboat into the sea, every employee offshore must hold a valid Certificate of Offshore Survival Training, approved by the Offshore Petroleum Industry Training Organization (OPITO) and valid for 4 years. The OPITO 'Standards of Competence for Emergency Response'[10] underpin the United Kingdom Offshore Operators Association (UKOOA) guidelines for 'The Management of Competence and Training in Emergency Response'[11] and define the competence requirements and safety training for the UK offshore Oil & Gas Industry.

The OPITO standards are competency-based and have been designed to ensure all personnel on board an offshore facility have the necessary skills and knowledge required to respond effectively in the event of an offshore emergency.

This physically demanding survival course initially takes 3 days, with some significant physical stressors such as embarking a life raft from the water, climbing rescue nets, and helicopter underwater escape simulation. Successful completion of this course alone requires a significant level of fitness and mobility. Refresher courses are required every 3 years.

Offshore health facilities—sickbay

Under the Offshore Pipelines legislation described above, all offshore installations are required to have a fully equipped sick-bay under the supervision of a health professional with an extended role. These dedicated facilities are required to be of a design suited to the needs of the installation and usually constitute an examination area, a small one or two bedded ward and a bath to treat hypothermia.

Sickbay medical equipment is usually very comprehensive with the basic recommended items defined in the industry first-aid and medical equipment guidelines[12] and normally includes an electrocardiograph, defibrillator, ventilators, autoclave, sphygmomanometers, and often even

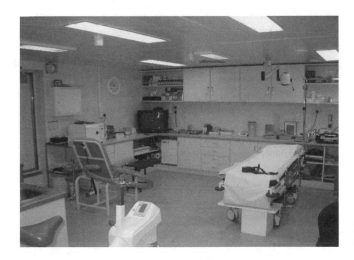

Fig. A3.5 Offshore sick bay Captain Field—Chevron

more sophisticated equipment such as pulse oximeters, which may be required for an appropriate emergency medical response and emergency evacuation. The medic will also have a wide range of drugs in stock—antibiotics, analgesics (including opiates) dyspeptic preparations, antihistamines, and a selection of emergency medication for use in cardiac arrest, poisoning by hydrogen sulphide, and thrombolytics for use following myocardial infarction. Again the basic recommended preparations are listed in these guidelines. The medic is not expected to have the level of training to be able to prescribe the complete range of stocked medication routinely, but when necessary their use can be authorized by a consulting onshore physician—'the topside doctor'—part of the 24-hour on-call service required for all installations with a medic. The patient's symptoms can be evaluated by the physician by teleconference and advice on treatment and clinical management can be given to the medic.

If necessary the topside physician will advise if he thinks medical evacuation should be considered, and he has the authority to mobilize a medical team to fly out to the installation according to the circumstances and severity of the medical condition.

The majority of these consultations are done by telephone—but management is being greatly improved by the use of more sophisticated communication tools. One example is the use of digital photographs sent as e-mail attachments, a facility that can be a great diagnostic aid to the advising physician, especially for external injuries and skin conditions. More sophisticated telemedicine equipment such as multiple parameter monitors encompassing blood pressure, oxygen saturation and ECG components have been developed, but the expense of the equipment, the restricted bandwidth of communication channels and the small number of patients with serious conditions has so far precluded their routine use.

The offshore medic

The offshore medics are usually trained nurses or sometimes armed services medical attendants who have all passed the specific HSE-approved medic training course as defined in the First Aid Regulations.[7] This 4-week intensive course extends the skills of the medic to a level that reflects the extra roles and skills they may need to act safely and effectively in the medical response to any sick or injured individual at the remote location. They must be able to initiate a wide range of medical interventions with no expectation of immediate medical back-up, relying only on the help of the first aid team and the advice of the on-call physician as already described.

The medic has a critical role on the offshore installation, being responsible for the treatment of any on-site illness or injury in the workforce and visitors. His or her duties include the provision of first-aid care to all personnel, the initiation and continued primary care of illness or injury, provision of a medical plan for emergency response, local medical surveillance of occupationally related conditions, general hygiene issues, and ongoing health promotion. There is normally only one medic per platform so that they are always on call for any medical conditions requiring advice or treatment. The medic may be given other functions if, as is often the case, the health-related duties do not occupy the full 12-hour shift, but these secondary duties must not conflict with the primary role of the medic to provide healthcare.

Principal duties of the medic include:

- primary care
- emergency medical care
- occupational health (health surveillance)
- environmental health audits
- emergency response plans

- emergency response team fitness evaluation
- ergonomic advice (display screen equipment programme)
- drug and alcohol policy support
- life-style evaluations
- statistics: recording and reporting of injury and illness
- health promotion

Clinical supervision by a suitably qualified medical practitioner, who is usually based onshore, must be available at all times to support the offshore medic. Suitably qualified implies, at minimum, a general practitioner with knowledge of the offshore environment and preferably with experience and qualifications in occupational medicine. This regular supervision of the medic includes the monitoring and ordering and supply of drugs and medical equipment, the application of medical policy and procedures, the provision of non-urgent medical advice and involvement in the continuing refresher training of the medic.

Offshore first-aiders

The offshore first aid team is determined by a needs assessment and will depend on the number of people normally on board the installation and the type of activity normally carried out. Workers at greater risk through the nature of their work and any special medical tasks, such as escort duties for sick or injured personnel, must also be considered. Some of the team may undergo further training as advanced first aiders and thereby become qualified for increased responsibility such as medical escort duties for medically evacuated personnel.

Medical screening and the UKOOA Medical Standards

First developed in June 1981, the regularly updated UKOOA Guidelines for Medical Aspects of Fitness for Offshore Work[9] recognize the special standards of physical and mental well-being required by this remote and specialized workplace. They also take account of the fact that some common medical conditions could, in these remote circumstances, pose a threat to the individual because of the inevitable delay in getting treatment in an emergency or be a potential safety hazard to other offshore workers.

Using the guidelines the examining physician will assess the physical and mental health of offshore employees in order to:

- anticipate and, where possible, prevent the avoidable occurrence of illness offshore which could place the individual, their colleagues or the emergency rescue services at undue risk, and
- ensure that so far as is reasonably practicable, designated offshore personnel are medically fit for their particular work at a remote and isolated location.

An individual's fitness for work offshore will be determined by:

- diagnosis, aetiology, and prognosis of any medical condition present
- efficacy or potential side-effects of current or proposed treatment
- risk of relapse or acute exacerbations requiring medical intervention
- risk of any adverse effects that could be precipitated by the offshore environment
- proposed frequency and duration of offshore visits

- restrictions in the availability of specialist medical support and supplies
- reasonable accommodations that could be made to the work or environment to mitigate risk.

The guidelines require that assessments of fitness to work offshore should only be carried out by, or under the supervision and direction of, examining physicians who are approved by UKOOA and have fulfilled minimum criteria related to clinical evaluation and can show that they have acquired through experience a knowledge and understanding of the offshore environment.

The UKOOA medical examination has an age-related periodicity at the time or writing—3-yearly to the age of 40, biannually to 50, and annually thereafter (but with proposals to move to a biannual examination across all ages during 2007). Audiometry is required as a baseline on entry to the industry, after 1 year to detect sensitive individuals and thereafter at every medical examination. In contrast to the modern practice of basing fitness for work on functionality, in the offshore environment the medical diagnosis, treatment and prognosis is, perhaps, more important.

Some of the conditions that may preclude someone from being given an offshore fitness certificate include:

- *Cardiovascular system*: congenital heart disease, valvular heart disease, ischaemic heart disease, myocardial infarction, cardiac arrhythmias, peripheral vascular disease, cerebrovascular disorders.
- *Gastrointestinal system*: peptic ulceration, inflammatory bowel disease, unrepaired hernia.
- *Nervous system*: any disorder causing significant defect of consciousness, cognitive function, power, balance, mobility, or co-ordination. Epilepsy with seizures, narcolepsy.
- *Musculoskeletal system*: any disorder impairing functional capacity including donning survival suit, mobilizing by helicopter and responding to emergency musters.
- *Respiratory system*: spontaneous pneumothorax, obstructive or restrictive pulmonary disease, active tuberculosis, moderate or severe asthma.
- *Genitourinary system*: renal calculi, renal failure, renal transplant, active sexually transmitted diseases.
- *Ear, nose and throat*: balance disorders, severe hearing loss.
- *Endocrine and metabolic*: insulin-dependent diabetes, adrenal disorders, morbid obesity.
- *Blood disorders*: significant anaemia, coagulation disorders, leukaemias, immunosuppressed.
- *Infectious diseases*: any active infectious disease.
- *Mental disorders*: acute depressive disorders, psychoses, personality disorders, drug or alcohol dependence.
- *Restricted medication:*
  - cytotoxics
  - immunosuppressants
  - oral steroids
  - antipsychotics
  - tricyclic antidepressants
  - benzodiazepines and other hypnotics
  - anticoagulants.

Emergency response team

Offshore installations are required to have arrangements in place to provide for an effective response in the event of an offshore emergency.[8] One element of the response is a specifically

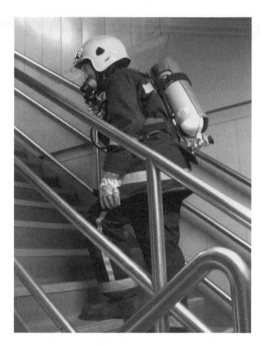

Fig. A3.6 Emergency Response Team member Alba Field—Chevron

trained emergency response team (ERT) that will have a variety of specialized roles including casualty rescue and fire fighting. These individuals have other full-time duties while on board and the ERT responsibilities are invariably part-time additional duties rather than a full-time responsibility. The Medical Guidelines stipulate specific task-related physical fitness guidelines for this group.

The exact duties of an ERT will depend upon the location and nature of the platform or vessel. A risk assessment must be carried out and decisions made upon the likely scenarios that may occur in an emergency. When this has been completed it is generally appropriate to designate a team as level 1 or 2 as described in the medical guidelines and reproduced below. The distinction is important as it will determine the level of fitness required for active participation in ERT duty.

All ERT members undergo the appropriate training, again at an OPITO approved facility. This in itself involves physical activity and a course requirement is that all participants be fit to a minimum of level 2.

Tasks may include:

- use of multiple cylinder breathing apparatus
- repeated or prolonged manual casualty lifting and carrying
- fire fighting including fire hose handling and boundary cooling
- search and rescue in smoke filled/hot environments
- manual casualty rescue from platform legs or vessel holds
- running out fire hoses
- moving foam barrels.

Level 1 ERT duty involves expected strenuous physical exertion lasting in excess of 30 minutes during a fire containment/casualty rescue scenario, which lasts for 1 or more hours. In these scenarios the total period of strenuous physical work will be in excess of 30 minutes.

Level 2 ERT duties may also involve strenuous physical exertion, but not exceeding 30 minutes total strenuous work within a total anticipated rescue scenario of 1 hour, at the end of which it is expected that the situation will be contained or the location will be abandoned.

Level 2 duties are essentially the same as those of level 1 with the distinction that the duration of the rescue activity is much shorter. It is this fact that permits a lower standard of physical fitness to be applied.

The health and fitness evaluation for participation in ERT duty

In addition to the standard offshore UKOOA Medical Fitness certificate the ERT members require additional medical and fitness assessment annually, including an ERT–Medical Assessment Questionnaire and any subsequent follow-up medical examination or screening process.

- a level 1 team member must demonstrate a minimum VO_2 max of 40 ml/kg per minute
- a level 2 team member must demonstrate a minimum VO_2 max of 35 ml/kg per minute.

Exercise capacity is measured by various submaximal tests. The Chester Step Test[13] or a bicycle ergonometer can be employed to estimate the available physical capability using an age-related predicted cardiovascular response. These tests can be employed as part of the UKOOA medical or, as is often the case, performed by the medic while the participants are offshore.

Medical fitness and disability

The Disability Discrimination Act[14] applies offshore and to offshore workers, but the demanding nature of the offshore environment means that it may be justified to exclude persons with significant disability that might reduce mobility in an emergency or impede the egress of others, including escape from a ditched helicopter. This is an important factor for consideration when assessing the fitness of any individual for an offshore position—even a sedentary job in administration will still be subject to these emergency requirements.

The final decision on anyone with a significant disability should always be made by an occupational physician who has a thorough knowledge of the offshore environment—possibly referring to the medical advisor of the operating oil company.

Occupational health

The offshore workforce is potentially exposed to a wide range of occupational exposures involved in heavy engineering, petrochemical processing, and drilling. These exposures can be compounded by the inherent lack of space on an offshore installation, which is often further diminished by the subsequent additional plant that has often been added during the life of a platform to extend or enhance recovery from the oil field.

As with any onshore engineering and chemical processing plant a wide range of potential hazards and toxic exposures need to be considered (Figure A3.7). These include:

- chemical hazards: toxic, corrosive, irritant, sensitizing, and potentially carcinogenic substances;
- physical hazards: noise, vibration, radiation, and thermal extremes;
- biological hazards: food poisoning, legionella;
- ergonomic hazards: manual handling, PC workstations;
- psychosocial hazards: work overload, shiftwork, tour patterns, work relationships, travel, isolation from home and family.

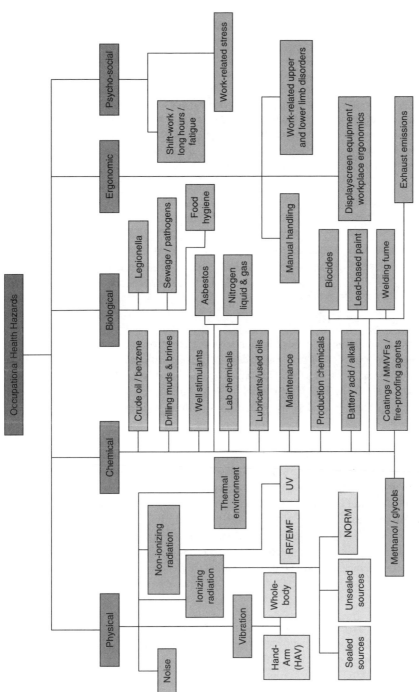

Fig. A3.7 Summary of occupational health hazards encountered on an offshore installation

Table A3.1 Example of a risk matrix used to rank safety and environmental issues on offshore installations

	Health/ safety risk	Threat to environment	Cost of threat to plant and equipment	1 Improbable/ remote	2 Occasional	3 Probable	4 Frequent
1	Slightly harmful/ minor	Negligible	<£10 000	L	L	M	M
2	Harmful/ serious	Minor	£10 000– £200 000	L	M	M	H
3	Very harmful/ major	Moderate	£200 000– £1 million	M	M	H	H
4	Extremely harmful/ fatality	Major	>£1 million	M	H	H	H

L: Acceptable but additional controls should be considered if cost effectve.

M: Should only proceed with management authorisation after additional controls are implemented.

H: Task must not proceed—must be redefined/further control measures put in place to reduce risk. The controls should be reassessed prior to the task commencing.

A robust strategy and policy is needed to identify, assess, control, and monitor these factors.

Potential hazards can then be risk-assessed using the same scale as that used to rank safety and environmental issues. (Table A3.1 provides an example of a typical risk matrix.)

In calculating exposure limits in the offshore environment allowance must be made for the 12-hour shift pattern. It is also an environment where multiple exposures—chemicals, noise, vibration, thermal extremes, manual handling—may be present together with potential interaction.

Health surveillance can be initiated where there is a known health effect and there is a reproducible and measurable decrement. This is a duty required by health and safety legislation[3–5] to be undertaken by the employer. As many of the offshore workforce are contractors, there is an implied duty on the operators to inform the contracting company of potential exposures and also to ensure there is access to any long-term health surveillance results such as audiometry so that the effectiveness of control measures can be evaluated.

Offshore installations are noisy places. Hearing should be monitored by annual audiometry to confirm that control measures are being successfully employed.

Catering

Food quality and safety is critical on an offshore installation. The installation has a single caterer for the whole workforce who must observe the highest food hygiene standards and comply with the Offshore Environmental Health Guidelines.[15] An episode of food poisoning offshore could be catastrophic for both the crew and production.

Mealtimes are a very important social occasion for the crew so the dining room, its layout and resulting social environment are an important part of maintaining psychosocial wellbeing on the platform.

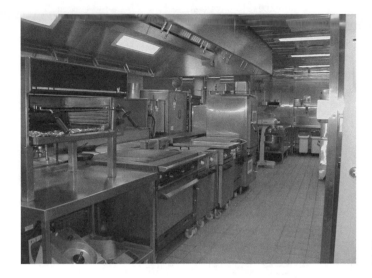

Fig. A3.8 Galley Brae Field—Marathon

Drilling

Drilling, whether exploratory or on established fields, is a high-risk activity with both physical and chemical hazards. Drill pipes are manhandled and fabricated into drill-stings many kilometres in length as they descend through the rock formations into the oil retaining sands. Although now highly mechanized, this part of the offshore operations continues to be one of the most hazardous with respect to manual handling and musculoskeletal injuries. Noise is also a constant hazard. Drilling mud circulates through the hole to remove the rock fragments but it also performs many functions—lubricating the drill string, cooling the bit, providing density and weight to counteract subterranean pressures and carrying materials downhole to stabilize the well wall. Some of the additives have in the past been particularly toxic through contact and inhalation although, in general, less toxic materials have now been developed and substituted.

Drilling is a round-the-clock operation involving heavy manual work, unpredictable hazards and constant exposure to potentially toxic materials.

Drugs and alcohol

By their very nature, processing flammable and explosive hydrocarbons under pressure, offshore oil and gas production facilities are very hazardous environments. Alcohol and drug use are therefore not tolerated on safety grounds alone. In addition, even while off duty, an emergency evacuation would require an immediate and very disciplined response from everyone on board. Many operating companies have strictly enforced drug and alcohol policies monitored by random testing and searches.

Infectious diseases

The close, intimate, and interdependent community of an offshore oil installation is the perfect environment for the potential spread of infectious diseases. The success of widespread vaccination programmes in Europe for the majority of common infectious diseases has in the past focussed any concern on food and water as the high risk vectors.

It is industry practice to report any cluster of more than three individuals with gastrointestinal illness to the company health advisor. Any suspected outbreak of food poisoning requires the

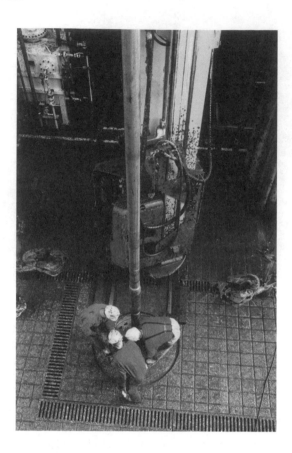

Fig. A3.9 Drill Floor—
Chevron

immediate isolation of infected individuals and possibly the testing of food samples offshore. The catering staff undergo regular catering medicals onshore as defined in the UKOOA Medical Guidelines and are required by the Environmental Health Guidelines to report any potential infectious illness and remove themselves from catering duties.

The recent impact of SARS, the increasing threat of avian influenza, and the potential use of biological agents by terrorists has led to the realization that offshore installations are potentially vulnerable. Many offshore operators now have an infectious disease protocol that defines the processes the company will implement to minimize the risk of the transfer of an infectious agent in a pandemic situation. This defines a screening process—such as aural temperature measurement for shift-change personnel travelling offshore—as well as identifying and isolating possibly infected individuals already working offshore. These protocols also recognize the function and potential exposure of the medic in conditions such as this, providing so far as is possible, a safe working environment primarily through scrupulous attention to hygiene, the use of good nursing practice, and also the use of appropriate specialized personal protective equipment.

Mental well-being

The isolation, demanding working environment, shift work, and separation from family and friends for up to 2 weeks at a time may all be stressors for mental well-being.

The spouse or partner who is expected to cope with the household and the family while the worker is away may also be under considerable stress, but the improved personal communications, using modern technology, have helped to mitigate this. However, many operating and contracting companies have stress awareness and management programmes for the benefit of offshore workers and their families.

Employee Assistance Programmes (EAPs) are now almost always provided by the major oil operators. The most common type in the UK provides confidential and free access to an information and counselling service that offers employees help with a broad range of problems from domestic and personal issues to more complicated financial and work-related concerns.

Where necessary the EAP provider will have access to company policies and processes and will provide advice and counsel on how work-related issues can be addressed effectively and in line with company procedures.

Additionally, these services will provide focused advice and support to business organizations managing the stressful consequences of redundancy or reorganization and traumatic incidents such as major accidents or workplace deaths.

Shift work

The 24-hour operation of an offshore installation requires that many workers are on shifts. Unmanaged circadian desynchrony can threaten safety.

Figure A3.10 shows the relationship between circadian rhythm and normal function in relation to a person working during the day. Note the fall in reaction time and alertness as melatonin levels increase at night.

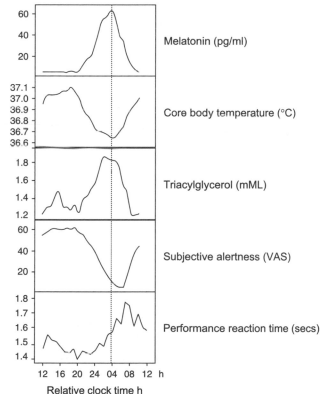

Fig. A3.10 Markers of health in a 24 hour society[16]

Following a shift change it takes several days for circadian–chronologic synchrony to occur and so workers on a new nightshift may not be at optimal performance for the first few nights. Some studies suggest that in some cases synchrony does not take place at all during the period of a nightshift, and this can lead to potential sleep disturbance, fatigue and performance decrement. Research continues into this subject, but there are some simple established strategies to help optimize the transition:

- only one shift change per offshore tour—preferably maintain all days or all nights
- use of the 7 a.m.–7 p.m./7 p.m.–7 a.m. shift pattern
- optimize sleeping conditions—full blackout, isolation from noise and disturbance
- employ normal time markers—'Zeitgebers'—arrange breakfast, lunch and dinner breaks at correct shift-related times.

Challenges for the future

The ageing workforce

When oil was first discovered in the North Sea there was no existing workforce in the UK to meet the industry's needs, so the resulting population of offshore workers that formed was comparatively young and relatively fit. Twenty-five years on, many of the same workforce are still working offshore with the average age now 47. This can raise significant issues in the physically demanding offshore environment.

Physical ability slowly decreases with age and will progress at a different rate in each individual. To some degree the initial loss of physical capability is masked by the acquisition of new skills but this more mature approach to problems will eventually be negated by declining physical ability. The older worker does not adapt so well to change, nor does he, or she, acquire new skills so readily, so failure to adapt to the evolution of the industry can lead to increased morbidity. The biological age of an individual rarely corresponds to chronological age so every person must be individually assessed.

Age related factors include:

- decreasing physical ability—decrease in muscle mass, decreased strength, wear and tear in joints, decreased aerobic capacity, decreased endurance, earlier fatigue, increased weight
- decrease in immunity and increase in pathology—older people have more illness
- slowing of healing mechanism so injuries take longer to recover
- psychological factors—older people may be less adaptive, slower, and less competitive than their younger colleagues.

Strategies that can be employed to maximize the worker-workplace fit:

1. Optimize health and physical fitness of the workforce—health education and life-style evaluation campaigns—access to fitness facilities.
2. Workplace design—minimize the physical requirements of all tasks as new processes are designed or old equipment replaced
3. Job content and design—classify and tier jobs within disciplines with agreed levels of physical job requirements to allow allocation of tasks to match measured ability
4. Functional capacity evaluation of the workforce to ensure individual capability matches task requirements.

Human factors: behavioural-based safety

Safety continues to be of greatest concern to the high profile offshore industry with constant efforts to minimize any work-related illness and injury. This is leading to greater focus on human factors and Behavioural Based Safety (BBS). Human factors looks at those aspects of health and safety where mistakes can be introduced by the human, through error or violation, in the safety critical process and in particular those factors which influence the critical decision making that is necessary to maintain a safe working environment. BBS sets out to change safety consciousness through the creation of a culture of modified health and safety sensitive behaviours. A greater understanding of these is likely to bring about a significant change in health and safety as it is realized how important it is to influence human behaviour to optimize performance.

In considering the interface of the individual, the job, and the organization five main factors are currently being considered: fatigue, communication, risk perception, risk-taking behaviour, and the health and safety culture of the organization.

Acknowledgement

Thank you to the following corporations for providing the photographs in this appendix: Shell Photographic Services, Royal Shell Dutch, Chevron UK, Marathon UK, and Maersk.

References

1 *United Kingdom Offshore Operators Association—Economic Reports 2004 and 2005*. London: UK Offshore Operators Association.

2 United Kingdom Continental Shelf Act 1964.

3 *Health and safety at Work Act 1974 (application outside Great Britain) Order 1995 SI 1995/263*. London: The Stationary Office, 1995.

4 *Management of Health and Safety at Work Regulations 1999 SI 1999/3242*. London: The Stationary Office, 1999.

5 *The Control of Substances Hazardous to Health Regulations 2002 SI 2002/2677*. London: The Stationary Office, 2002.

6 Working Time Directive 93/04/EC.

7 *Offshore Installations and Pipeline Works (First-Aid) Regulations 1989 SI 1989/1671*. London: The Stationery Office, 1989.

8 *The Offshore Installations (prevention of Fire and Explosion, and Emergency Response) Regulations 1995*. Approved Code of Practice and Guidance L65. London: HSE Books, 1995.

9 *Guidelines for medical aspects of fitness for offshore work*. Issue 5. London: UK Offshore Operators Association, 2003.

10 *Basic offshore safety induction and emergency training and further offshore emergency training*. Offshore Petroleum Industry Training Organisation, Aberdeen, 2003.

11 *The management of competence and training in emergency response for offshore installations*. London: UK Offshore Operators Association, 2004.

12 *Industry guidelines for first aid and medical equipment on offshore installations*. London: UK Offshore Operators Association, 2000.

13 Sykes K. Chester Step Test, Resource Pack (version 3). Cheshire UK: Chester College of Education, 1998.

14 *Disability Discrimination Act 1995*. London: HMSO, 1995.

15 *Environmental health guidelines for offshore installations*, Issue 3. London: UK Offshore Operators Association, 1996.

16 Rajaratnam SM, Arendt J. Health in a 24-h society. *Lancet* 2001; **358**(9286): 999–1005.

Appendix 4

The medical assessment of working divers

D. Bracher and N. K. I. McIver

Introduction

In the UK and, within the limits of the UK continental shelf, commercial diving must comply with the Diving at Work Regulations 1997[1] and for the purpose of the Regulations a person 'dives' if he enters water, or any other liquid; or a chamber that is part of a diving project, in which he is subject to a pressure greater than 100 millibars above atmospheric pressure; and in order to survive in such an environment he breathes in air or other gas at a pressure greater than atmospheric pressure.

The worksite for a commercial diving project can vary from a shallow stream, to a pool or aquarium, inland waters, inshore and offshore in deep open water.

The compressed air or gas for the diver may be in Self Contained Breathing Apparatus (SCUBA) or pumped from the surface by a hose.

Diving does not have to be the main work activity of the person. The activities undertaken by divers at work are very diverse and may include welding, maintenance work, and scientific study, acting and filming.

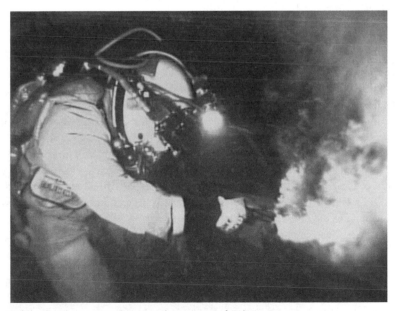

Fig. A4.1 Welding under water. Photograph courtesy of Subsea 7.

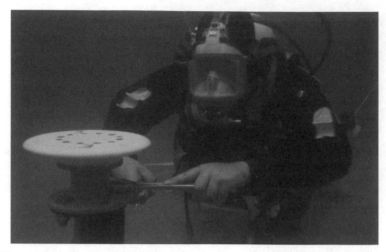

Fig. A4.2 Diver at work. Photograph courtesy of Stuart Jacques of the Diving and Marine Centre, the University of Plymouth.

The Health and Safety Executive has published five Approved Codes of Practice applicable to different sectors of the diving industry to accompany the Regulations. They are:

◆ commercial diving projects offshore

◆ commercial diving projects inland/inshore

◆ media diving projects

◆ recreational diving projects

◆ scientific and archaeological diving projects.

The journey through the water to the worksite may be by free descent or in a wet bell or cage, or in a closed bell supplied and pressurized with respirable gas. The bell is usually a particularly cramped piece of equipment.

In order to maximize the time at the worksite, by reducing the need for decompression from working at great depth, professional divers engaged in commercial diving projects may live in a pressure chamber and be 'stored' at a pressure equivalent to the depth at their worksite. The pressure chambers, called saturation chambers because the diver has reached the full saturation state for the pressure and breathing mixture being used, are relatively small and provide cramped living accommodation for several divers, often working on a shift basis. Several chambers on a ship are usually connected together by means of narrow tubular passages and pressure sealable hatchways to enable divers to move in a controlled way from one at living pressure to another to be stored for work at a different pressure. The linked chambers are called a saturation spread and all saturation chambers on ships must be linked to a hyperbaric lifeboat for evacuation under pressure in an emergency. Divers may live in these saturation chambers for several weeks at a time but only up to 28 days in UK waters.

Divers travel from their accommodation to the work site by a closed pressurized bell that locks on to the saturation chamber, usually on a dive ship, and are lowered to the worksite. The respirable gas mixture supplied to the divers in the saturation chamber and at the worksite is usually a mixture of helium and oxygen. This varies in proportion according to the pressure or depth.

Life support technicians outside the chamber care for divers in a saturation chamber. However, inside the saturation chamber it is a very isolated environment. If a diver is injured or becomes ill

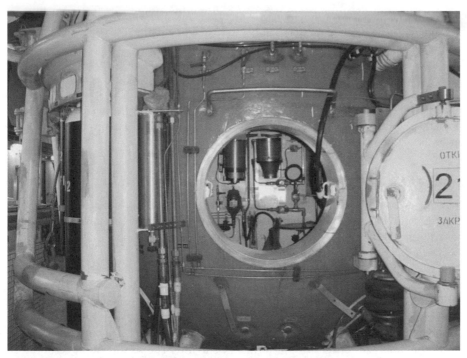

Fig. A4.3 View through open hatch of Closed Diving Bell (SDC) at surface on board DSV Akademik Tofig Ismayilov, off Baku, in Caspian Sea. Photograph courtesy of J Ray McDermott Diving Division.

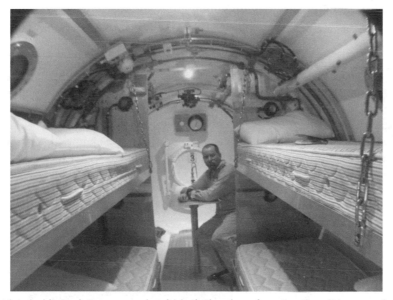

Fig. A4.4 View inside Deck Decompression (Living) Chamber of a saturation diving complex on board DSV Akademik Tofig Ismayilov. Photograph courtesy of J Ray McDermott Diving Division.

it can take several days of slow decompression in the chamber to remove the diver and send him for treatment. Doctors can enter the chamber to treat, but almost invariably are committed to remain in the chamber for the full time of the chamber decompression.

Treatment of acute medical or surgical conditions in a saturation chamber is difficult and management is conservative. Surface-orientated divers need to be physically and medically fit. Some types of diving require higher levels of fitness than others, but it is still essential that medical assessment, for fitness to dive, be performed prior to starting their career and at intervals through their working life in order to minimize the risk of a medical emergency occurring in the water or the saturation chamber.

Examination and certification mechanism

All working divers in the UK, including those who are self-employed, or receiving pay or 'favour or reward', perhaps as a recreational instructor, assistant or dive guide, are covered by the Diving at Work Regulations.

The Diving at Work Regulations apply when at least one diver is at work and therefore an unpaid 'volunteer', who is an essential member of a dive team that is also part of an 'undertaking' should also be examined by an HSE Approved Medical Examiner of Divers (AMED). An example would be a volunteer diver providing in-water standby cover for a paid instructor carrying out training if the project could not operate safely without that diver.

The Regulations stipulate that no person shall take part in any diving operation as a diver unless they have a valid certificate of medical fitness to dive. The validity of the certificate must not exceed 12 months and can be issued only after a medical examination in accordance with the HSE Guidelines, performed by an AMED.

The Regulations also impose a duty on people who have responsibility for, or control over, diving operations to ensure that diving is safe so far as reasonably practicable, and the divers have a responsibility to declare if they are unfit to dive on any diving operation.

Medical standards for divers at work vary from one country to another and standards for sports divers can also differ. In the UK the medical examination of divers should be carried out in accordance with the recommendations in the HSE document MA1 *The medical examination and assessment of divers*.[2]

AMEDs are located throughout the UK, the Channel Islands, and the Isle of Man. A list of AMEDs is available on the HSE website at www.hse.gov.uk/diving/information.htm. There is reciprocal recognition of the Norwegian medical examination and certification of divers, and it is envisaged that reciprocal arrangements will extend eventually throughout the member States of the European Union.

Before approval as an AMED by the HSE, a doctor must have knowledge of the different types of diving, diving work environments, and diving medicine. They must have attended a recognized course in the subject, show that they meet the continuing clinical requirements of the HSE and have access to the necessary equipment for special examinations including electrocardiography and audiometry. The AMED should be sufficiently knowledgeable to brief a novice diver on the occupational health hazards of diving before embarking upon training. The HSE audits the work and facilities of AMEDs every 1–5 years to ensure standards are being met. Currently, the HSE requires AMEDs to have 2 days refresher training every 5 years from the date of initial approval. This can also be fulfilled by 12 hours of individual academic work such as teaching or research or other appropriate activity related to diving medicine.

Medical considerations

Before the first diving medical examination the examining physician should obtain documentary evidence of the candidate's medical history from their general practitioner and a health questionnaire is in an annexe of MA1. At subsequent annual examinations the doctor must have a copy of the previous examination results. The diver should have a copy of these as the HSE medical examination form (MA2) is in duplicate; one copy is retained by the examining doctor and the other copy by the diver.

Diving requires superior levels of physical fitness, self-reliance, and aptitude with reserves to cope in an emergency. The effects of immersion, increased breathing resistance and exercise at depth produce physiological changes that require training for optimal performance. Once divers descend to their worksites the work they must perform may require strength, agility and judgement, observation and accuracy without distraction. These requirements are reflected in the demanding standards of fitness required for pre-employment selection to a career in diving. In general these standards are applicable to all divers. However, there may be divers who, although not meeting these standards fully, are fit for restricted diving, e.g. short shallow dives or within the confines of an aquarium or pool. Fitness to dive does not necessarily confer fitness for all the technical and manual tasks that can be performed by a diver. An AMED who is in doubt about a diver's fitness is recommended to obtain a further opinion from a second AMED or advice from a relevant specialist, preferably with knowledge of diving, or a diving medical specialist. Updated guidance is issued to AMEDs regularly.

Great importance is attached to the baseline medical examination. Individuals contemplating a career in diving, and their doctors, may obtain further information on medical fitness from the HSE website (www.hse.gov.uk/diving/information.htm).

The HSE does not specify any minimum age limit for diving at work, nor is any upper age limit specified providing that all the medical standards can be met.

The same general fitness criteria apply to both male and female divers apart from relating size and strength to the type of professional diving involved. Available evidence, however, supports the view that no pregnant woman should dive.

The decision on fitness to dive at work must take into account not only the safety of the diver but also the safety of others involved in the diving project. Divers going to the aid of a diver in trouble may be put at additional risk to their own safety.

Divers, who disagree with the AMED on their fitness to dive or any restriction on their diving activity may appeal to the HSE within 28 days of being informed of the AMEDs decision. The Head of the Employment Medical Advisory Service (EMAS) will consider the appeal.

Medical examination

There should be a standard enquiry into past and current health, occupational history, social history (including smoking and alcohol), and any details of past decompression illness (DCI).

Investigations that are required at the initial examination are: full blood count, urinalysis, audiometry, resting ECG, and spirometry. Sickle cell and thalassaemia assessment are required only when it is clinically indicated. Radiography is not required routinely and is based upon individual clinical assessment by the examining doctor.

At subsequent examination the following investigations should be included: urinalysis, spirometry, audiometry if there is a history of barotrauma or as part of a hearing conservation programme, and resting ECG 5-yearly if over the age of 40 years or more frequently if clinically indicated. Haematology and radiography of the chest and long bones are required only if clinically indicated.

Obesity

A commercial diver should not be obese. There is an association with an increased incidence of DCI with being overweight or obese. The height and weight of the diver, measured in underwear and bare feet, should be measured at every medical examination and the body mass index (BMI in kg/m^2) calculated. Where the BMI exceeds 30 further estimation of fat content should be made using skin impedance, or skin fold thickness of at least four anatomical sites.

Advice on diet and exercise should be given before the BMI reaches 30 in an attempt to avoid certification of unfitness. Where the BMI exceeds 30 then this may be a bar to diving, particularly if associated with lack of physical fitness.

If the physical fitness requirement of 13 Mets is reached and there is no other obesity related problem, such as diabetes and hypertension, then the AMED may wish to discuss the findings with the HSE Diving Medical Adviser. The examining doctor should be aware of other offshore work-related problems of obesity such as helicopter travel, which may be required to travel to the diving site. Emergency procedures require evacuation through the small windows of a helicopter and an obese individual becoming lodged will impede the escape of others.

Exercise testing

Exercise testing of commercial divers is routine. The safety and validity of exercise testing was considered by a HSE sponsored Workshop of AMEDS and Diving Medical Specialists in 2004.[3] It was decided that exercise testing should continue as it was better that an individual suffer a myocardial infarction in an environment with resuscitation facilities than during an actual dive or in a saturation chamber or other remote location. However, sensible precautions should be observed particularly in males over 45 years and 55 years for females, where there is an increased risk of myocardial infarction and ischaemic heart disease.

The authors recommend that these precautions should be extended to all age groups and medical assessment should be performed prior to exercise testing. This would include medical history, family history, coronary risk factors, clinical examination, and resting ECG if not already performed in the previous 5 years in those over 40 years, or in the initial examination for all ages. There is a short cardiac screening questionnaire in MA1. If there is any doubt then further advice should be sought from a cardiologist before proceeding to the exercise test.

Examining doctors have a legal duty to ensure the safety of divers undertaking exercise testing. It is advisable that resuscitation facilities are available but at a minimum that the examiner does not work alone, should have at least basic life support skills, and should be able to use a defibrillator. There should be a predefined procedure to follow in the event of collapse.

A diver must be able to meet the physical requirements of the task and those arising out of an emergency situation. An assessment of exercise capacity must be made at the preliminary examination and all subsequent examinations. Where possible an assessment of maximum oxygen uptake (either direct or indirect) should be made. A diver should be able to achieve an exercise level of 13 Mets or 45 ml/kg per min (lean body mass) oxygen consumption (equivalent to Stage 4 of the Bruce Protocol). These results should be considered in conjunction with general considerations such as blood pressure, obesity, and pulmonary function.

The HSE Exercise Workshop recommended the use of a validated step test including the appropriate protocol, which would be suitable for demonstrating HSE fitness requirements. Acceptable tests include the Army Physical Fitness Test, Master two-step test, and Chester step test. Ideally the same test should be performed at subsequent examinations for comparison.

Respiratory fitness

The integrity of the respiratory system is vital for diving.[4] The lung is responsible not only for gaseous exchange in aerobic activity including exercise response but also assists in buoyancy, and in decompression by acting as a filter for bubbles induced by standard decompression.

Any condition that might compromise gas exchange, or exercise response must be sought. Many accidents occur within the splash zone or 3 metres of the surface. Even more important is exclusion of any abnormality that may cause air trapping and could lead to barotrauma on ascent from depth.

Ideally the upper airways should be clear and the chest structure anatomically normal. Clinical assessment and pulmonary function testing should also be normal. There may be variations from normal and this is where the examining physician must, as in all systems, make an assessment based on sound knowledge, have discussion with peers or arrange appropriate onward referral.

The following may be contraindications to diving or require additional investigation:

- acute or chronic upper or lower respiratory disease or infection;
- abnormal chest or lung structure, or reduced exercise capability—examples would include mild chronic obstructive pulmonary disease (COPD), or inactive pulmonary sarcoidosis;
- pneumothorax.

Absolute contraindications

- These are conditions that may adversely affect lung function, and elastic recoil or lung compliance with risk of barotrauma[5] and would include:
- Significant COPD (with active obstructive or restrictive lung disease), active pulmonary sarcoidosis, active tuberculosis, cystic fibrosis, and pulmonary fibrosis.
- Bullous lung disease with attendant risk of barotrauma.
- Previous spontaneous pneumothorax unless treated by bilateral surgical pleurectomy and with normal lung function and thoracic imaging after surgery.
- Previous penetrating injury or chest surgery with pleural adhesions or scarring, unless healed and with normal lung function including flow volume loop and thoracic imaging.

Assessment of lung function

Routine spirometry is performed, but chest radiography, including low-dose computerized tomography, is only required if clinically indicated.

Conditions that require detailed pulmonary investigation should include FEV_1 and FVC as useful markers of progress rather than pass/fail criteria. The target should be an FEV_1 of >80% of predicted and >70% of predicted FEV_1/FVC ratio. An exercise test should not cause a drop of >15% of predicted FEV_1 postexercise.

Asthma

Safety of diving with asthma is controversial. There is no convincing evidence that asthma is a significant cause of pulmonary barotrauma but very careful initial assessment is necessary in a new candidate.

The British Thoracic Society (BTS) Guidelines advise against diving with active asthma requiring relief medication in the preceding 24 hours and where peak flow fall is greater than 10% from best values, or there is greater diurnal variation of peak flow than 20%. Also barred from diving are those with asthma induced by cold, exercise or emotion.[6] Diving may be permitted for asthmatics who are either at Step 1 or Step 2 of the BTS Asthma Guidelines, and who can comply with the foregoing. Asthmatics who dive should monitor their peak flow twice daily.

Ear, nose, and throat

Divers must be able to clear their ears in order to equalize the pressure across the tympanic membrane and to cope with the changing barometric pressures in the water or hyperbaric chamber. Complications of otitis media such as glue ear, deafness, perforation, and persistent discharge are contraindications to diving. Disease of the mastoid cavities is a contraindication. Nasal polyps and deviated septum should be treated.

A history of surgery of the ear is usually a contraindication and individual advice should be sought from a specialist. Stapedectomy is a contraindication to diving.

At each medical examination the external auditory meati should be examined and they should appear normal. Wax not completely obstructing the canal need not be removed. Exostoses are not a problem, providing they do not completely occlude the external auditory canal.

The tympanic membrane should be inspected; well-healed scars are acceptable. New entrants must demonstrate the ability to clear their ears. A similar requirement exists after infection or barotrauma.

The diver should be able to hear and understand normal conversation and communications systems. Vestibular function should be normal and Menière's disease is incompatible with diving.

Audiometry should be carried out at the preliminary examination and cover the frequencies 500–6000 Hz. Additional audiograms should be performed if there is a history of aural barotrauma or as part of a hearing conservation programme.

Vision

Effect of immersion on vision

There is an air/mask interface that maintains the one between air and the cornea when immersed. Without this a diver's vision would be unacceptably blurred.

There is progressive loss of ambient light with increasing depth. Only 20% of available surface light is perceived when at 10 metres of sea water (msw) and this is made worse by backscatter from suspended silt and particles. There is also progressive loss of colour; reds disappear at 10 msw and at 30 msw only blues and greens remain unless artificial light is used. Colour vision is not usually essential commercially apart from some specific job-related tasks. The full-face mask or helmet reduces the visual field very considerably.

Finally, the air/mask interface causes distortion such that objects appear about one-quarter nearer and magnified by about one-third.

A diver needs to be able to see well enough under water to orientate and function. The visual acuity should be 6/9 or 20/30 in both eyes. The diver should also be capable of reading dials, gauges, and text when out of the water and operating equipment or running the chamber.

Cornea

The cornea must be intact, and any acute corneal lesions must be allowed to heal. Refractive errors are correctable; soft, gas permeable, daily wear contact lenses may be used when diving albeit with some risk of infection. Hard lenses should be avoided. Prescription facemasks are also used. Myopic correction may now be accomplished in a number of ways using excimer laser keratotomy (e.g. photorefractive keratotomy, PRK). This heals rapidly and it does not compromise corneal strength; radial keratotomy (RK) is now thought possibly to put SCUBA divers at risk.[7]

Barotrauma or mask squeeze is unlikely to occur in professional divers wearing a full-face mask or helmet connected to the diver's breathing gas supply.

Cataract

The eye is fluid filled and can adjust to ambient pressure without its volume changing. Some surgical procedures involve insertion of gas into the eye and these will need careful assessment to avoid risk of barotrauma. Cataract surgery is common in the population and must be healed before further immersion. There are guidelines for appropriate periods for wound healing.[8]

Glaucoma

Glaucoma may cause problems, either as a result of medication or after surgery, when drainage blebs occasionally form superficially and may be prone to leakage and conjunctival infection. Progressive visual loss may occur.

Retina

Retinal repair by surgery may involve methods of volume reduction to improve adherence of the area of reattachment. This may be achieved by using plombs (either of foam or solid silicone) or by air or inert gas bubbles being inserted that are absorbed (e.g. a mix of air and Sulphur hexafluoride—SF6). Foam cells and air bubbles will follow Boyle's Law and diving is not permissible until any gas has disappeared. This may take from one to several weeks for gas bubbles. Foam plombs are not commonly used now but should be removed prior to commencing diving.

General risks

Any condition that leads to reduced vision or secondary infection may pose a hazard in diving.

Relative contraindications:

◆ Monocular vision.
◆ Any significant acute disorder causing pain, diplopia, or decreased visual acuity until resolved.
◆ Pathology reducing visual acuity to below ability to read a standard car number plate at 20.5 meters (using visual aid if appropriate).
◆ Postoperative gas in the eye.
◆ Hollow orbital implant.
◆ Recent eye surgery while within the recommended convalescent period.
◆ Glaucoma with significant visual loss or in the postoperative phase of a filter procedure.
◆ Residua from previous acute DCI.
◆ Risk of micro-embolism or vascular retinopathy.

Dental and alimentary

Dental care is important. Scuba divers need to be able to retain a mouthpiece. Dental caries and periodontal disease need to be treated. Unattached dentures should be removed during diving. Changes in pressure can cause pain in teeth that have been filled due to small pockets of air or gas being trapped within the tooth. This can lead to dental barotrauma.

Active peptic ulceration is not acceptable but the relapse rate after a course of triple therapy is sufficiently low to allow return to air diving.

Active inflammatory bowel diseases, symptomatic hiatus hernia, reflux oesophagitis, symptomatic haemorrhoids, fistula, anal fissures, cholelithiasis, abdominal wall hernia, chronic pancreatitis, and acute hepatitis are contraindications to diving. Asymptomatic cholelithiasis may not be a problem but the remote location of the dive site needs to be considered should symptoms occur. Saturation diving would be unsuitable. Chronic hepatic disease requires specialist assessment.

Stomas need to be individually assessed and free draining ones are compatible with diving. 'Continent' ones requiring a catheter to relieve pressure are not compatible with diving. However, they may not be suitable for saturation diving for social reasons, rather than medical ones, associated with living in confined spaces with several other divers.

Endocrine system

Most endocrine conditions are contraindications to professional diving. However, well controlled hypothyroidism is acceptable as is a history of hyperthyroidism, which has been successfully treated and is asymptomatic.

Conditions requiring cortisol replacement are contraindicated due to the risk of collapse associated with injury, stress, and infection.

Restricted sports diving may be allowed for certain diabetics in France.[9] In the UK diabetics may be allowed to dive subject to careful selection and rigorous control.[10]

Diabetes mellitus of any type and controlled by any means is usually a contraindication to commencing a career as a professional diver, but some restricted diving activities may be possible when the diabetes is controlled by diet alone. Generally, it should be a reason for failure of a new entrant because of the risk of ischaemic heart disease, peripheral vascular disease, hypertension, retinopathy, neuropathy, nephropathy, and other end organ damage causing unfitness at a later date. This could cause subsequent employment difficulties if diving is the principal activity of the job. However, in an existing diver with well-controlled diabetes it may be possible to give a certificate for certain diving activities. Diving under close supervision in a pool or aquarium may be acceptable. The examining doctor should discuss this with the HSE Diving Medical Adviser, or an appropriate Diving Medical Specialist.

Diabetes controlled by insulin or oral hypoglycaemic agents is generally a bar to diving because of the difficulty in maintaining good control under varying degrees of activity, which are often unpredictable during a dive. Hypoglycaemia in a professional diver with insulin-dependent diabetes and some oral hypoglycaemic agents, such as long-acting sulphonylureas, are a safety risk to the whole dive team as well as to themselves.

Cardiovascular system

A history, or finding on examination, of any type of heart disease including septal defects, cardiomyopathies, ischaemic heart disease, valvular disease, shunts, and dysrhythmias, except for sinus arrhythmia and infrequent ventricular extrasystoles, should lead to certification of unfitness for diving and the individual being referred for a cardiological opinion if they wish to pursue diving. The cardiologist should be one who has knowledge of diving medicine.

The preliminary assessment should include a resting ECG and this should be repeated 5-yearly after the age of 40 or more frequently if there are risk factors. However, if an exercise ECG has to be performed in individuals with specific risk factors for ischaemic heart disease then this should only be performed in an appropriately equipped and staffed centre. Referral to a cardiologist is the safest option for these individuals.

A history of successful conventional coronary bypass surgery is a contraindication to diving but some percutaneous procedures such as angioplasty, if successful, may be acceptable but require cardiological opinion and follow-up.

Conditions that permit intracardiac shunting from right to left, such as atrial septal defects are contraindications to diving. Patent foramen ovale (PFO) is common in the general population (27%) and most will not give rise to any problem; screening is not routinely conducted in either the preliminary or annual medical assessments. However, where there is a history of unexplained neurological, cardiorespiratory or cutaneous DCI,[11–13] particularly if there is also a history of migraine with aura, then contrast echocardiography should be performed by a cardiologist experienced in the procedure. There is a correlation between migraine with aura, and PFO and paradoxical gas embolism.[14] The PFO can now be effectively repaired through a percutaneous approach.[15]

Murmurs are not acceptable unless they are physiological. However, echocardiography or referral to a cardiologist may be required.

Peripheral vascular disease

Intermittent claudication or other evidence of ischaemia of the extremities is a bar to diving. Minor varicose veins may be acceptable but not if accompanied by varicose eczema, which is at risk of becoming infected and is also an indication of circulatory impairment. A history of deep vein thrombosis (DVT) may be a relative contraindication but current DVT is an absolute one.

Blood pressure

The resting, supine blood pressure at the preliminary examination should not exceed 140 mmHg systolic and 80 mmHg diastolic (fifth phase). However, the effect of age should be taken into account in older examinees. Mild hypertension not exceeding 160/100 is acceptable in subsequent assessments providing that there is no end organ damage and that it is not controlled by medication that is usually incompatible with diving (e.g. β-blockers).

The central nervous system

Assessment of the central nervous system (CNS) is extremely important initially and at subsequent intervals. A diver must have no functional disturbance of motor power and sensation, co-ordination, level of consciousness or cognition, special senses and balance, bowel, or bladder.

Any condition causing excessive daytime somnolence, unprovoked loss of consciousness or fainting is a contraindication to diving.

Neurological symptoms of acute DCI may present with loss or alteration of sensation, or with muscular weakness. Thus, any neurological condition with these symptoms may mimic DCI and if present in a diver may greatly complicate its management and should be a bar to diving.[16]

The assessment commences with a detailed neurological history. The following would also be contraindications to diving:

- Progressive neurological disease—Parkinson's disease, multiple sclerosis, cerebrovascular disease, muscular dystrophy, and motor neurone disease.
- Epilepsy or other seizure after the age of 5 years requiring treatment.
- Serious head injury with loss of consciousness or post-traumatic amnesia.

- Migraine with aura, which may be associated with a large PFO.[14]
- Severe motion sickness and claustrophobia.
- Any significant condition requiring continuous medication for its control such as attention deficit disorder.
- Chronic conditions such as myasthenia gravis, or chronic fatigue syndrome.

Examination of the CNS starts with observation of gait, speech and intellectual response. Detailed physical examination follows and the neurological findings must essentially be normal including:

- The cranial nerves, including visual fields.
- Sensation to light touch, pinprick, vibration sense, joint position sense, and two-point discrimination.
- Power, tone, and co-ordination of all limbs.
- Deep tendon reflexes, abdominal reflexes, and plantar response.

Where there is doubt an opinion must be sought from an appropriate specialist.

Specific problems that may be encountered

Epilepsy is a contraindication on grounds of safety if requiring medication for control. If there is a past history, but without seizure or need for treatment for at least 10 years, a candidate might be considered fit after individual specialist assessment and advice. A single seizure has a recurrence risk of between 23% and 80%.[17] Most second seizures occur within one year of the first. Enquiry must be made into predisposing factors (family history, EEG abnormality, or past history of febrile convulsion) and a specialist assessment is made. This is to exclude genetic or constitutional predisposition to seizures. Without recurrence after 10 years, diving may be reconsidered.

In **serious head injury** there is a significant risk of brain damage or post-traumatic epilepsy.[18] The diver should be excluded where:

- Period of unconsciousness or post-traumatic amnesia (PTA) is in excess of 30 minutes (PTA is the time from injury until time of sustained recall).
- There has been a depressed skull fracture, localizing neurological signs or intracranial haematoma.

After less severe head injury a 4-week suspension from diving and review by an AMED is required, before resumption.

Intracranial surgery is not an absolute contraindication to diving in the absence of epilepsy or persisting neurological deficit but would be subject to specialist assessment for a number of years.

Intracranial haemorrhage:

- subarachnoid haemorrhage would usually be a contraindication to diving.
- cerebrovascular accident would be a contraindication to diving because of concomitant cerebrovascular disease, risk of seizure and risk of recurrence, which is about 5% per year.

Hydrocephalus with ventriculo-peritoneal shunt would be a contraindication to all diving because of seizure risk, and possible areas of brain damage.

Psychiatric assessment

This includes psychological aspects and may be difficult at initial assessment unless there is a clear history.[19] The examination commences with general assessment of manner, attitude, and response. It should include some form of psychological aptitude testing and would continue at the dive school during initial training. There has been consideration of obtaining a neuropsychiatric baseline in view of reports of variations at a later date both with and without decompression 'events'. A mild subclinical finding of forgetfulness or loss of concentration has been identified in a study of commercial divers.[20] This was associated with significant impairment of health-related quality of life (HRQOL) and with periventricular hyperintensities on magnetic resonance imaging examination of the brain.

Evidence of psychological states that might affect the safety of the diver or others in the water must be sought. Diving itself will impose a specific stress depending upon the type of work, its location, and the operational risks involved. Divers should be free from psychiatric illness or impairment of cognitive function.

Absolute contraindications to diving even if successfully treated are:

+ schizophrenia
+ bipolar affective disorder
+ unipolar affective disorder
+ disorders rendered asymptomatic due to treatment, or
+ taking psychotropic medication.

More recently attention has been drawn to the relation between acute anxiety, panic attacks, and diving accidents.[21]

Alcohol or drug dependence would normally be a bar from diving unless there has been a period of abstinence of at least 1 year for alcohol and 3 years for drugs, off medication and without relapse. (UKOOA Guidelines).[22]

Disorders that may resolve and are subsequently compatible with diving unless they are of a recurring nature (e.g. within less than 2 years) include:

+ adjustment reaction
+ single episode of depression unless of severe nature
+ deliberate self-harm
+ isolated psychotic episodes, e.g. delusion
+ severe premenstrual syndrome, also known as premenstrual dysphoric disorder—but not diving during an active phase of the disorder.

Finally, a diver may be considered fit if suffering from simple phobia, other than agoraphobia or claustrophobia.

There should be referral for an opinion from a psychiatrist in any cases of doubt.

Genitourinary

Urinalysis should be performed routinely and any presence of blood, protein, or glucose investigated before diving is permitted. The presence of any urinary disease that causes abnormal renal function is usually a cause for rejection. Genitourinary infections including sexually transmitted diseases should be adequately treated before diving. The presence of a single kidney, which is functioning normally, is acceptable. Calculi should be investigated and some types of diving may be permitted if asymptomatic. However, the relative isolation of dive sites and dives that require decompression stops or saturation diving should be considered carefully as the calculi may become symptomatic.

Musculoskeletal

The diver's work requires strength, agility, and mobility both in the water and out. Generally, all joints should have the full range of movement but a more pragmatic approach can be adopted for experienced divers.

A history of recurrent back pain may be a reason for disqualification because of the need to perform heavy lifting when out of the water and because acute back pain can mimic DCI.[23]

The disabled diver

It is important to assess individuals in conjunction with their proposed work as divers. For example some substantially physically impaired divers with stable paralysis may be suitable to perform some types of diving. The assessment should include the individual's ability to look after themselves in the water and also the safety of other divers. Their mobility and physical fitness can be assessed by a timed swimming test in a pool. Full details of the restriction on the type of diving and other safety considerations should be recorded on the diving medical certificate (e.g. recreational diving only and must be accompanied by an unrestricted professional diver at all times). Approved Medical Examiners are advised to discuss fitness of disabled persons to dive with other AMEDs, diving medical specialists or the HSE Diving Medical Adviser before issuing a certificate of fitness to dive.

Haematological

Baseline haematological investigations, such as full blood count, are required routinely for professional divers at the initial examination but not subsequently unless clinically indicated. The sickle cell test and haemoglobin electrophoresis are not required routinely, but may be required depending on the medical and family histories. Sufferers of thalassaemia major and sickle-cell disease are not fit for diving. People with sickle-cell trait and thalassaemia minor are thought to be fit for diving if their haemoglobin level is satisfactory.[24]

Blood dyscrasias, even in remission, will usually be cause for rejection and polycythaemia will increase the risk of acute DCI.

Coagulation disorders are incompatible with diving.

Divers who have had splenectomy are at an increased risk of overwhelming infection from *Pseudomonas* and are not fit for saturation diving.

Malignancy

Cases of malignancy should be individually assessed for factors affecting in-water safety. If involved in saturation diving then suitability for an extended stay in an isolated environment needs to be assessed. Regular and frequent reviews of the diver's fitness are required.

Skin

Integrity of the skin is important for the diver. Immersion, use of diving suits and equipment, and raised temperature and humidity of saturation diving chambers can lead to skin damage and risk of secondary infection. Recent examples in professional divers include infections of divers' hands, ear canals, facial skin, and the most prevalent infection in saturation diving, *Pseudomonas aeruginosa*. Here the confined living space, hyperoxia and helium atmosphere also contribute to risk of bacterial skin contamination.[25] The daily hygiene and disinfection routine is essential in prevention of common skin infections spreading rapidly between members of a dive crew.

Relative contraindications

+ Active bacterial or viral skin infections
+ Active psoriasis and eczema.

The HSE has recently warned of microbiological hazards in relation to performing essential emergency procedures in a saturation diving environment.[26]

Communicable diseases

The medical examiner should be satisfied that the diver is not suffering from an infectious disease. Where there is doubt whether a person is infectious then further assessment and referral should be made to a medical microbiologist or specialist in infectious diseases.

There must be scrupulous attention to hygiene when diving and the usual precautions taken when dealing with any biological material, tissue damage or spillage of body fluids that may occur in the hyperbaric chamber. Blood and other body fluids should be treated as potentially infectious.[27]

Risk of cross-infection from blood-borne viruses must be considered and some authorities have advised that all commercial divers should be immunized against hepatitis B.

Diving during the acute phase of any type of hepatitis is contraindicated but diving after hepatitis A is permissible once the illness has ended. A diving candidate with a history of hepatitis B or hepatitis C may not be fit for some diving activities such as saturation diving, where divers live for up to 28 days in hyperbaric chambers. Good hygiene practices may not be followed and divers may share razors and toothbrushes. There is a risk of transmission of blood-borne viruses through mouth pieces that are contaminated by blood in saliva into abrasions of the mucous membrane of the mouth of another diver.[28] This may occur in scuba training for an emergency situation when one diver runs out of air and has to share the mouthpiece of a buddy, or when equipment is shared by a group of divers and may be inadequately cleaned. The risk in the first situation is probably small due to the cleansing action of the water.

There should be an established protocol such that oronasal diving equipment is locked out for disinfection in accordance with the procedure in the company operations manual and using preparations and methods recommended by the manufacturers of the diving equipment. The equipment should be dried after every disinfection.

Routine testing of all divers for blood-borne viral infections is not currently recommended, but it may be advisable to test a diver with a history of hepatitis B for e-antigen negativity and possibly viral load before resuming diving.

Both air and saturation diving are associated with an altered response to certain aspects of the immune system.[29] Whether this is relevant to blood-borne viral infection in the immuno-compromised individual is uncertain. Specialist advice would need to be sought for any diver presenting as HIV positive. A qualified diver who becomes HIV positive may continue for a time, subject to individual assessment and risk counselling. The development of AIDS-related complex symptoms would be a bar to diving because of the potential for neurocognitive impairment due to HIV/AIDS dementia, or because of the medication used to treat the condition. HIV-positive individuals would require frequent clinical cognitive assessment, which may be annually as currently required for HIV-positive pilots by the US Federal Aviation Administration (FAA).[30] Other measurements required by the FAA in the individual assessment include viral load performed at least quarterly and CD4 and full blood count and liver and renal function tests 6-monthly. For most divers this would be too onerous and expensive and there are practical considerations. For a HIV-positive saturation diver it would be impracticable to take regular anti-viral medication in the saturation chamber and for the medical problem to remain confidential.

Return to diving after acute decompression illness[31]

DCI is an occupational illness and once recovered the diver may be cleared as fit for work providing there has been response to treatment without residual symptoms or signs.

The so-called 'minor symptoms' include limb pain, skin rash or lymphatic swelling, non-specific headache, fatigue, anorexia, and nausea. After such a minor episode of DCI diving may be resumed 24 hours after an uncomplicated recovery. If there has been recurrence or relapse (with further therapy followed by recovery) a 7-day suspension from diving is required.

The major symptoms of DCI include neurological or pulmonary manifestations and must be assessed by an AMED. After an episode of 'serious' DCI a 7-day suspension is required if there has been sensory change in limbs only. If there have been other neurological, audiovestibular, or pulmonary manifestations a 28-day suspension is required and return only after clearance by an AMED with an opinion from a diving medical specialist, or after consultation with the hyperbaric doctor who treated the diver.

After pulmonary barotrauma with pneumothorax, mediastinal or subcutaneous emphysema, a layoff of at least 28 days is needed, with return only after clearance by an AMED in consultation with a diving medical specialist and only then, if complete recovery has occurred.

All other cases involving residua and re-treatment would usually be unfit and must be seen by an AMED and usually a diving medical specialist or the treating hyperbaric doctor before return to diving can be considered.

Long-term health effects

There has been much consideration of long-term effects but so far the only proven and potentially disabling condition is dysbaric osteonecrosis. This can, in most cases, be prevented through safe diving practice in the now standard procedures for regulated professional diving. It should be remembered that there is a statistical association between those that have suffered DCI and subsequent dysbaric osteonecrosis.[32]

Hyperbaric chamber workers

The Diving at Work Regulations 1997 covers the use of hyperbaric chambers within diving projects, and people who may be routinely subjected to hyperbaric conditions need to have the same level of medical fitness. In practice these chamber workers tend to be professional divers.

Hyperbaric chambers in hospitals are not covered by the Diving at Work Regulations but the British Hyperbaric Association (BHA) recommends that medical attendants working in such chambers undergo medical examinations and that the standards are similar to those for professional divers.[33]

Work in compressed air

The HSE has published *A guide to the Work in Compressed Air Regulations 1996* and this contains advice on medical fitness to work in compressed air in the construction industry (tunnelling) and the statutory requirement for medical surveillance. Generally the same level of medical fitness is required as in professional divers.

In Britain a doctor appointed by the HSE must provide statutory medical surveillance and should have the same level of training as a HSE Approved Examiner of Divers. Doctors providing a recompression treatment service on the construction site must be trained, or have suitable experience in hyperbaric medicine.

Conclusions

The statutory diving medical examination is designed to exclude factors that might affect the diver's safety in the water. To this is added the need to avoid danger to others who may become involved in a possible rescue. Finally, the long-term health effects should be monitored by comparing the results of each year's examination.

Divers have an obligation to declare any factor, of which they are aware, that might affect their own personal safety and the employer has the responsibility for ensuring that a diving operation is carried out in as safe a manner as is reasonably practicable.

The ability to forecast fitness to dive accurately by traditional fitness examination has been questioned in New Zealand. As Professor Des Gorman of Auckland, a leader in occupational health of divers in New Zealand, put it '... notwithstanding the biological nonsense of humans being "fit to dive"'. He conducted a survey of the outcome of the medical assessment of professional divers. The findings were that the outcome is more accurately determined by the free text actually written by the medical assessor and by the respiratory assessment performed. The questionnaire itself was more helpful in making a list of diagnoses rather than as a forecast of future fitness for diving.[34] Reform of the process was proposed, with restriction of this assessment to medical practitioners specifically trained in diving medicine to internationally accepted standards. The aim is to determine the level of health-related risk for a diving candidate who wishes to become a professional diver. This should be based more on a list of functional competencies than on a list of excluding diseases or diagnoses.

Information is being gathered to provide evidence-based advice on matters of fitness to dive in the future. The British Thoracic Society is dealing with pulmonary disease and the sport diving community with mild asthma and diabetes. The UK Sport Diving Medical Committee (UKSDMC) has also questioned the value of the traditional 'diving medical'. For the last 4 years there has been a more directly targeted self- assessment questionnaire. From this divers who require formal assessment are identified. This assessment and any subsequent investigation, examination or referral is performed by an appointed Medical Referee, who is a doctor trained in diving medicine and is also a practising sport diver.[35]

The HSE continues to require safe diving practice, the training of approved doctors (AMEDs) and the continuing medical assessment of commercial divers.

References

1 The Diving at Work Regulations (1997). *Statutory Instrument 1997* no. 2776.

2 *MAI The medical examination of divers.* London: The Health & Safety Executive, 2005. Available on line at www.hse.gov.uk/diving/ma1.pdf

3 Smith JS, Evans G. *HSE Workshop on exercise testing for divers, April 2004.* Health & Safety Laboratory Report, Broad Lane, Sheffield, 2004.

4 Mebane GY, McIver NKI. Fitness to dive. In: *The physiology and medicine of diving,* (4th edn) (eds Bennett PB, Elliott DH), pp. 60–3. London: WB Saunders, 1993.

5 Calder IM. Autopsy and experimental observations on factors leading to barotrauma in man. *Undersea Biomed Res* 1985; **12**(2): 165–82.

6 British Thoracic Society guidelines on respiratory aspects of fitness for diving. *Thorax* 2003; **58**: 3–13.

7 Le May M. Ophthalmological aspects of fitness to dive. *South Pacific Underwater Med Soc J* 1996; **26**(4): 253–9.

8 Butler FK Jr. Diving and hyperbaric ophthalmology. *Surv Ophthalmol* 1995; **39**(5): 347–66.

9 Tabah A, Dufaitre L, Grandjean B *et al*. Diving with diabetes is now allowed in France with selection rules and blood glucose based immersion procedures. UHMS ASM Abstract. *Undersea Hyperbar Med* 2005; (32) 4; 257.

10 Edge CJ, Grieve N, Gibbons N, *et al*. Control of blood glucose in a group of diabetic scuba divers. *Undersea Hyperbar Med* 1997; **24**(3): 201–7.

11 Wilmshurst PT, Pearson MJ, Walsh KP *et al*. Relationship between right-to-left shunts and cutaneous decompression illness. *Clin Sci* 2001; **100**: 539–42.

12 Torti SR, Billinger M, Schwerzmann M *et al*. Risk of decompression illness among 230 divers in relation to the presence and size of patent foramen ovale. *Eur Heart J* 2004; **25**(12): 1014–20.

13 Koch AE, Kampen J, Tetzlaff K *et al*. Incidence of abnormal findings in the MRI of healthy divers: Role of patent foramen ovale. *Undersea Hyperbar Med* 2004; **31**(2): 261–8.

14 Anzola GP, Magoni M, Guindani M *et al*. Potential source of cerebral embolism in migraine with aura: a transcranial Doppler study. *Neurology* 1999; **52**(8): 1622–5.

15 Walsh KP, Wilmshurst PT, Morrison WL. Transcatheter closure of patent foramen ovale using the Amplatzer septal occluder to prevent recurrence of neurological decompression illness in divers. *Heart* 1999; **81**: 257–61.

16 Dick DJ. Neurological assessment. In: *Medical assessment of fitness to dive* (ed. Elliott DH), pp. 224–9. Ewell, Surrey, UK: Biomedical Seminars, 1995.

17 Hauser *et al*. Seizure recurrence after a 1st unprovoked seizure: an extended follow-up. *Neurology* 1990; **40**: 1163–70.

18 Anneggers JF, Hauser WA, Coan SP *et al*. A population-based study of seizures after traumatic brain injuries. *N Engl J Med* 1998; **338**: 20–4.

19 Lunn B. Mental fitness to dive. In: *Medical assessment of fitness to dive* (ed. Elliott DH), pp. 215–21. Ewell, Surrey, UK: Biomedical Seminars, 1995.

20 Macdiarmid JI, Ross JAS, Taylor CL, Watt SJ, Adie W, Osman LM, Godden D, Murray AD, Crawford JR, Lawson A. Co-ordinated investigation into the possible long term health effects of diving at work. Examination of the long term health impact of diving: The ELTHI diving study. Research Report 230. London: HSE Books, 2004. Available online at www.hse.gov.uk/research/rrhtm/rr230.htm

21 Edmonds C. Stress response panic and fatigue. In: *Diving and subaquatic medicine*, (4th edn) (eds Edmonds C, Lowry C, Pennefather J, and Walker R), pp 465–72. London: Arnold, 2002.

22 *Guidelines for medical aspects of fitness for offshore work*. Issue No 5 October 2003. London: UK Offshore Operators Association, 2003.

23 Carter JT, Birrell LN (eds) *Occupational health guidelines for the management of low back pain at work—principal recommendations*. London: Faculty of Occupational Medicine, 2000.

24 Parker J. Haematology. In: *The sports diving medical* (ed. Parker J), pp. 100–2. Melbourne: JL Publications, 2002.

25 Ahlen C, Mandal LH, Iverson OJ. Identification of infectious Pseudomonas aeruginosa strains in an occupational saturation diving environment. *Occup Environ Med* 1998; **55**(7): 480–4.

26 HSE Diving Newsletter to AMEDS No. 8, August 2004, pp. 6–9.

27 HSE. *Blood-borne viruses in the workplace; guidance for employers and employees*. London: HSE Books, 2005. Available on line at www.hse.gov.uk/pubns/indg342.pdf

28 Piazza M, Chirianni A, Picciotto L *et al*. Blood in saliva of HIV seropositive drug abusers: possible implication in AIDS transmission. *Boll Soc Ital Biol Sper* 1991; **67**(12): 1047–52.

29 Pollock NW, Harris MF. Effect of daily exposure to compressed air on immune response. *Undersea Hyperbar Med* 2002; **29**(2): 129–30.

30 US Federal Aviation Administration Protocol on HIV Seropositivity (1997). Available online from: www.faa.gov, and search on HIV.

31 Diving Medical Advisory Committee. Assessing fitness to return to diving after decompression illness *Guidance note DMAC 13 Rev 1*. 5 Lower Belgrave Street, London SW1W 0NR, UK, 1994. www.dmac-diving.org/guidance

32 Elliott DH. Raised barometric pressure. In: *Hunter's diseases of occupation*, (9th edn) (eds Baxter PJ, Adams PH, Aw T-C, *et al.*), pp. 343–60. London: Arnold, 2000.

33 Colvin AP. Pre-employment assessment of hyperbaric healthcare workers. *Br Hyperbaric Assoc Newsl* June 1996; 10–18.

34 Greig P, Gorman D, Drewry A, Gamble G. The predictive power of initial fitness to dive certification procedures for occupational divers in New Zealand. *South Pacific Underwater Med Soc J* 2004; **33**(4): 182–7.

35 Glenn S, White S, Douglas JD. Medical supervision of sport diving in Scotland: reassessing the need for routine medical examinations. *Br J Sports Med* 2000; **34**: 375–8.

Further reading

Bove AA (ed.). *Bove and Davis' Diving Medicine*, (4th edn). WB Saunders, 2005.

Brubakk AO, Neuman TS (eds) *Bennett and Elliott's physiology and medicine of diving*, (5th edn). Bodmin, Cornwall, UK: Saunders, Elsevier Science Ltd, 2003.

Cox RAF (ed.) A code of good working practice for the operation and staffing of hyperbaric chambers for therapeutic purposes: *A report of the Faculty of Occupational Medicine of the Royal College of Physicians*. London: Faculty of Occupational Medicine, 1994.

Edmonds C, Lowry C, Pennefather J, Walker R (eds). *Diving and subaquatic medicine*, (4th edn). Arnold, 2002.

Elliott DH (ed.) *Medical assessment of fitness to dive*. Ewell, Surrey, UK: Biomedical Seminars, 1995.

Wendling J, Elliott DH, Nome T (eds). *Fitness to dive standards. Guidelines for medical assessment of working divers*. European Diving Technology Committee, 2003. (Note: Regular updates are available from website www.edtc.org.)

General aspects of fitness for work overseas

R. A. F. Cox

The general aspects of the comments in this appendix apply to companies and their employees overseas, but it must be remembered that many people are working overseas, often in hostile areas, without any support from well-organized parent organizations. Such people may include the self-employed, academics, missionaries, students, and professional adventurers. An excellent and fascinating account of the hazards facing anthropologists is given by Howell (see Further reading). Any person planning to work overseas should make careful preparation for the preservation of their health and the provision of medical care in the event of illness, before departure.

A list of centres from which essential medical advice can be obtained and useful books that may be consulted during planning of an overseas assignment can be found at the end of this appendix.

Thirty-five per cent of US international travel is on business.[1] Companies who send employees overseas, however long or short the assignment may be, retain a responsibility for them while they are abroad, as some companies have recently discovered to their cost. It is therefore essential that they ensure, as far as possible, that potential expatriates are fit for their overseas duties and that proper arrangements are in place to take care of them, if they are ill or injured.

Disability *per se* should not be a bar to travelling or working overseas though some medical conditions may not be compatible with some overseas locations. Those disabled by multiple sclerosis, for example, are likely to be worse in hot climates, though the progress of the disease is not affected. Each case must clearly be considered individually but employers would be expected to make 'reasonable adjustments' to enable disabled employees to travel or transfer overseas, especially where this is an integral part of their job or an important step in their career. 'Reasonable adjustment' might include, for example, providing transport to and from airports, making special arrangements with airlines, and if necessary, buying seats with more leg room or closer to the aircraft toilets, even if this means upgrading. Similarly, obtaining accommodation for a disabled employee close to the place of work, even if this were more expensive, would be regarded as a 'reasonable adjustment'. On the other hand, putting disabled employees' health at risk by posting them to a place where they are unable to obtain essential medical care would be regarded as unreasonable. Like any employees, those with disabilities should be carefully assessed by an occupational physician before a decision is made to allow them to travel or to transfer overseas. They should not be rejected, simply because they have a disability, without being given the opportunity of a skilled assessment by an occupational physician.

There are a great number of factors to be considered when the company is planning an overseas operation, and the medical requirements tend to be relegated to the end of the list even though concerns for general health will be a major anxiety of any potential expatriates and their families.

The company must, therefore, not only find out about diseases and medical conditions which may be prevalent in the area of their operations but it must also review the local medical and hospital facilities and services and appoint a local doctor to act on its behalf. In many areas of the world this will require a visit by a doctor from the home country on behalf of the company.

Any company that embarks on overseas operations should appoint a doctor at its home base, if it does not already have its own occupational physician. This is necessary not only so that they can determine whether employees are fit to transfer overseas but to liaise with the local overseas doctors and to advise on the numerous health queries that will inevitably arise in the course of a foreign operation.

No matter how thorough the pre-departure medical screening and examinations may have been, some illness will still occur, requiring decisions regarding treatment, possible repatriation, and liaison with doctors and relatives in the home country. Even if illness does not occur, injury, especially from road traffic accidents, is a constant risk and the commonest reason for emergency repatriations. Policies and procedures for dealing with such contingencies must be in place before the operation begins. It may be fatal to wait until such an emergency arises. Such policies must include the mechanism by which the costs of local medical care are to be met. It is essential that all overseas assignees and regular travellers have adequate medical insurance cover, which is available from any of the major health insurers. In most countries medical care has to be purchased and, in many places payment, or a guarantee of payment, is required before admission to hospital can be arranged or treatment commenced.

There are a number of air ambulance services available, but two of the largest established ones, Swiss Air Rescue Organization and SOS Assistance are based in Switzerland (addresses of these and other organizations in Appendix 8).

Before departure, or the establishment of an overseas operation, arrangements should be made with one of these, or a similar organization, for the emergency evacuation of sick and injured personnel, if this is not already fully covered through the medical insurer's policy.

People's behaviour changes as soon as they are overseas. The different culture, climate, food, and social activities include psychological and physiological changes, which often result in health effects. Even the most demure people seem to relax their usual standards of conventional sexual behaviour when abroad, particularly if they are not accompanied by their usual sexual partners. Ten per cent of 400 respondents of a survey reported having sexual intercourse with a new partner while abroad.[2] In a Canadian survey of returning business travellers 54% admitted not carrying a first aid travel kit, 21% drank more alcohol than they normally did, and 6–14% neglected food, water, and antimalarial precautions.[3] Stress in expatriates is likely to increase as world security deteriorates, religious and social cultures grow more divergent and travel becomes ever more stressful. The consequences of stress may be worsened as the opportunities for substance abuse increase.[4]

Some people will seek overseas employment to escape from domestic or financial crises or because they have drinking problems or established psychiatric conditions. Such people are likely to be disastrous choices for overseas assignments and should be rigorously excluded. The enquiries of the pre-departure medical examiner should be particularly oriented towards revealing these factors.

Staying well is taken for granted in Western countries, because of their excellent public health and medical care systems, but staying well in many undeveloped and tropical countries requires strict self-discipline and personal vigilance. Standards of personal and domestic hygiene must be greater, and risks that may be quite acceptable in Europe or North America may lead to dire consequences in tropical Africa. People who may have difficulty in adjusting to this very different environment should be counselled before departure. A trivial and easily managed illness in the

UK can be a major problem for the patient, their family, and their employers when it occurs overseas. In no other circumstance is the hackneyed cliché 'prevention is better than cure' more true. The emergency evacuation of a sick employee is often a hazardous experience for the patient and always an expensive, worrying, and very time-consuming exercise for those responsible for the organization of the repatriation.

In a survey of British Foreign and Commonwealth Office staff in 1995, 3.08% of those overseas required medical evacuation; 51% of these were considered to have been unpredictable and 70% were evacuated because the local medical facilities were unsuitable. Staff were found to be more likely to need medical evacuation than dependants and some staff, particularly young 'high flyers' seemed to be vulnerable to non-physical problems.[5]

The essential medical examination should be arranged well in advance of departure and should be conducted by a doctor experienced in travel medicine who is instructed to perform the examination on behalf of the company, to which they should make their report. This should preferably be in confidence to the company's own medical adviser but, if not, it should be in the form of a non-confidential report to the personnel manager or other appropriate senior person. As long as the report is made by a person who has not had clinical care of the employee it will not fall within the Access to Medical Reports Act.

The examining doctor must be aware of the local conditions at the overseas place of residence, preferably through first-hand experience. It may be quite acceptable to transfer someone with quite significant health problems to a location where medical care of an equivalent standard to that of the home base is available, although the same health problem would be an absolute bar to transfer to some other places. A totally different standard of medical fitness must be expected in a geologist who may be moving to an office job in Chicago, if they were instead to lead a survey party in Niger.

The medical examination should be designed and performed to reveal actual or potential health problems that may occur during the course of the overseas assignment. In this respect the examination for transfer overseas differs from an employment examination that is designed to determine only a person's fitness for work. Because of the different environmental and physiological demands, many employees who are perfectly fit to work in the UK would not be fit to do the same work overseas. The examination must also be performed sufficiently ahead of departure that remediable conditions can be treated.

Any person who is suffering from a medical condition that requires regular medical supervision should not be permitted to transfer overseas unless the examining doctor is quite certain that such supervision, and of an acceptable standard, is available.

If companies with international operations keep their employees under regular health surveillance they can be very rapidly processed for overseas service and may not even need an examination. However, unless the doctor who has to decide on the potential expatriate's fitness for overseas work is very familiar with their current medical state or has access to notes of a recent examination, the employee must have a comprehensive medical review including a physical examination. Screening by questionnaire is not in the experience of this author adequate.

Even more important is the examination of family members, if the employee is to be accompanied, though there is an increasing tendency for employees to transfer overseas on 'bachelor status' with 2 weeks home leave every 3 months. Children normally adapt to living overseas very well but may have medical conditions that could be a liability, and in many underdeveloped countries the facilities for the medical care of children are even less adequate than those for adults, so that children who are ill must either be nursed at home or repatriated. Expatriate mothers must, therefore, be not only capable, confident, resourceful, and very adaptable but they must also be very fit. A thorough and detailed review and examination of spouses is just as important as for employees.

When the family have been deemed 'fit to travel', appropriate prophylactic immunizations must be administered and essential emergency medical equipment in the way of drugs, dressings, and other items provided. Medicines and other medical items, readily available and taken for granted in the UK, are often unavailable or of very inferior quality in developing countries and every expatriate and family should carry essential supplies from their home base. The exact list should be recommended by the company medical officer and will depend on the location and the anticipated requirements of the family. The course of immunizations should also be completed in good time so that any untoward reactions are over before departure.

Although this is not the place for detailed advice about recommended immunizations, which changes regularly anyway, and can be obtained from any of the centres listed in Appendix 8, some comments on some of the latest vaccines is not out of place based on the assumption that the routine UK immunization schedule has been completed.

Hepatitis A vaccine should be given to all long-term assignees (i.e. more than 6 months stay) and travellers to areas where the food and water hygiene may be less than ideal.

Hepatitis B vaccine should be given to all regular travellers and long-term assignees (i.e. more than 6 months) to all areas of the world except North America, Australia, New Zealand, and northern Europe; also to travellers who may put themselves at risk because of their behaviour, or who may need medical or dental treatment abroad.

The modern **rabies** vaccine is safe and effective and it should be given to all longer-term travellers to developing areas of the world. Administering this vaccine prophylactically obviates the need for giving a blood product (rabies immunoglobulin) in the event of a bite, which is particularly reassuring in the current AIDS climate. However, the traveller must be warned that further doses of vaccine are always advised post-exposure.

Although **group B meningitis**, for which there is no available vaccine, is the commonest strain in the UK, the other strains, A and C W135 and Y, for which there is an effective vaccine, are commoner in some areas of the world. Meningitis vaccine should be given to overseas assignees or regular travellers to East, West, and Central Africa, and pilgrims to Mecca.

Vaccinations against **Japanese encephalitis** should be considered for people embarking on rural travel in Asia from India to Japan, but individual advice should be sought from one of the centres already mentioned.

Yellow fever vaccination is mandatory for many countries within the endemic zones of tropical Africa or South America. A single injection lasts for 10 years and it is so often neglected until immediately before urgent travel that it is mentioned here to emphasize the importance of taking the vaccine in advance, if there is any likelihood of travelling to a yellow fever area. Even where the vaccine is not mandatory, it is advised for personal protection for travel within the zones. The only exceptions are short trips to capital cities at high altitude.

AIDS is covered elsewhere in this book, but it is spreading rapidly in both sexes in some areas of Africa, Asia, the Caribbean, and eastern Europe and the importance of not taking risks cannot be overemphasized for the regular traveller or overseas assignee. (As a side issue, some international operators, in areas of the world where the prevalence of HIV positivity is reported to be as high as 40% of the population, may have to consider whether it would be any advantage to screen local employees for HIV prior to employment. For more detail on pre-employment screening see Chapter 29, p 619.)

The medical processing of potential overseas expatriates is an essential prerequisite that should be completed well in advance of departure and must include every member of the family who is travelling. The cost of such a procedure is small compared with the cost of medical repatriation, which such screening could have prevented.

Many international business travellers report travel related health problems. For example, in a sample of 140 employees from western Canada's oil and gas industry 74% had jet lag, 45% had travellers' diarrhoea and gastrointestinal complaints, 14% had climate adaptation problems, and 2% had accidents and minor injuries.[3] Returning expatriates should have a detailed physical examination and a basic set of laboratory tests, tailored to their specific history and exposures.[6]

Summary

- Local medical facilities must be reviewed.
- Appoint a local doctor.
- Establish liaison between the local overseas doctor and the company's occupational physician.
- Arrange adequate medical insurance cover.
- Prepare contingency plans for medical evacuation/repatriation.
- Arrange thorough medical examinations, well in advance of departure, for all members of the family who are going.

Acknowledgement

My grateful thanks are due to Dr Gil Lea of Trailfinders who kindly reviewed the latest immunization advice.

References

1 Rosselot Gail, Travel health nursing: expanding horizons for occupational health nurses. *J Am Assoc Occup Health Nurses* 2004; **52**: 28–41.

2 Bloor M *et al.* Differences in sexual risk behaviour between young men and women travelling abroad from the UK. *Lancet* 1998; **352**: 1664–8.

3 Rogers H, Lynn, Reilly Sandra M. A survey of the health experiences of international business travellers. *J Am Assoc Occup Health Nurses* 2002; **50**(10): 449–59.

4 Lei L, Liang,Y X Krieger Gary R. Stress in expatriates. *Clin Occup Environ Med* 2004; **4**: 221–9.

5 Patel D, Easmon CJ, Dow C, Snashall DC, Seed PT. Medical repatriation of British diplomats resident overseas. *J Travel Med* 2000; **7**(2): 64–9.

6 Hochberg, Natasha, Ryan Edward T. Medical problems in the returning expatriate. *Clin Occup Environ Med* 2004; **4**: 205–19.

Further reading
Generally for travellers

Dawood R (ed.) *Travellers' health.* Oxford: Oxford University Press, 1992.

Health advice for travellers. London: Department of Health (updated regularly and obtainable from www.dh.gov.uk).

Werner D. *Where there is no doctor.* London: Macmillan, 1993.

Wilson-Howarth J, Ellis M. *Your child's health abroad.* Chalfont St Peter: Bradt UK, 1998.

Generally for health professionals

Guidelines for malaria prevention travellers from the United Kingdom. *Commun Dis Public Health* 2001; **4**: 84–101.

Health information for international travel. Centre for Disease Control and Prevention, Atlanta, Georgia. 2005–2006 (The 'Yellow Book'). (Obtainable from www.us.elsevierhealth.com). **(Beware of significant differences in recommended practice between the USA and Europe.)**

Howell N. *Surviving fieldwork, a report on health and safety in fieldwork.* Washington, DC: American Anthropological Association, 1990.

Immunisation against infectious diseases (The Green Book). Dept of Health 2006 (Obtainable from www.dh.gov.uk).

Walker E, Williams G, Raeside F. *The ABC of Healthy Travel.* London: BMJ Books, 2002.

Workers exposed to hand-transmitted vibration: health surveillance and fitness for work

K. T. Palmer

Introduction

Exposure to hand-transmitted vibration (HTV) is very common in industry. According to one national survey an estimated 1.2 million men and 40 000 women in Britain have weekly exposures that could justify health surveillance.[1,2] Many sources are implicated, including concrete breakers, needle scalers, chainsaws, hand-held grinders, metal polishers, power hammers and chisels, powered sanders, hammer drills, and even powered lawnmowers. The main industries with exposure involve construction and heavy engineering, but significant exposures and health risks can arise in many trades, such as construction workers, metal-working and maintenance fitters, welders, foresters, shipbuilders, foundry workers, and male labourers.[1–4]

Adverse health effects are similarly common. The term **hand–arm vibration syndrome** (HAVS) has been used to define collectively the disorders thought to be associated with exposure,[3] which include secondary Raynaud's phenomenon (vibration-induced white finger or VWF) and digital neuropathy. It has been estimated that there are more than 220 000 cases of VWF[5] and over 300 000 cases of sensorineural HAVS[6] in the UK, while over 100 000 medico-legal claims have been processed among ex-miners from British Coal.[7] Users of hand-held powered tools often report a number of other symptoms (hand–arm pain, weakness of grip, loss of manual dexterity), and may be at somewhat greater risk of several upper limb disorders (carpal tunnel syndrome, osteoarthritis of the wrist or elbow, tendinitis, Dupuytren's contracture). Importantly, they are also at risk of hearing impairment, as vibrating equipment tends to be very noisy.

Thus, many occupational physicians care for workforces in which questions arise about heath screening and the management of HAVS. This appendix is presented in two main sections: the first (background) section reviews the problem of HAVS, with emphasis on diagnosis and clinical grading, while the second focuses on health surveillance and decisions of fitness for work. Collectively these activities are aimed at secondary prevention. The important aspect of primary prevention is touched on only briefly at the end.

Clinical features and diagnosis
Vibration-induced white finger

VWF is characterized by episodic cold-induced finger blanching (often a marble white appearance). Classically the disease is sharply demarcated, distal in its initial development, and affects the areas most closely in contact with vibrating tool parts. The thumbs are usually spared.

During an attack the affected parts become numb and cold, and sometimes cyanotic with a bluish tinge; during the recovery phase a reactive hyperaemia may cause the digits to appear fiery red and to tingle. Although the classical appearance is distinctive, other patterns can sometimes be seen. For example, blanching is normally circumferential, affecting all of the width of a digit, but sometimes it affects only the digit's lateral or medial aspect; and the extent of blanching may vary from one attack to another.

The diagnosis of VWF rests on a history of characteristic colour changes in the digits provoked by cold in a worker with a history of substantial occupational exposure to vibration, and exclusion of causes other than vibration. The subjectivity of this process is well recognized, there being several problems:

- Attacks are rarely witnessed by a doctor or nurse—reliance is placed primarily on the clinical history.

- Workers may have trouble in describing their symptoms: the pattern of the disease can vary naturally; development and progression tend to be insidious over a number of years; initial symptoms are minor and non-memorable—they may even be considered 'normal' by those who work in cold inclement conditions, especially if co-workers manifest similar problems; there is a need to distinguish diffuse physiological pallor from vasospastic attacks of blanching, but the distinction requires a good historian as well as a good history.

- Some workers may have a vested interest in concealing or exaggerating their symptoms—e.g. fear of job restriction or job loss, hope of gaining financial compensation.

- Primary Raynaud's phenomenon (RP) is quite common anyway, affecting some 5–10% of men who have never been exposed to vibration. VWF and RP are not sufficiently distinctive to distinguish the two reliably by appearance. Thus, while onset pre-dating first exposure is evidence of RP, an onset post-dating first exposure is no guarantee that the disease is secondary—attribution is a matter of probabilities rather than a certainty. (Other secondary causes of RP, such as SLE, although usually considered in the assessment process, are uncommon in the population: the main differential diagnoses are primary RP and physiological pallor.)

- Simple tests of cold challenge (e.g. immersing the hands in cold water) provoke blanching inconsistently. This means that while they could be useful if blanching is witnessed they do not reliably *exclude* the diagnosis. Moreover, they are uncomfortable, and in those with a compromised peripheral circulation they may even be harmful.

Hence, a lot of effort has been put into developing better objective methods of assessment. Current evaluative procedures for vascular disease include: plethysmography, Doppler ultrasonography, direct capillaroscopy (to assess the velocity of red blood cells in microcirculation), skin temperature and skin re-warming rates after cold challenge, and measurements of finger systolic blood pressure during cooling. The subject is a technical one and beyond the scope of this appendix. Further information on options and their test properties can be found elsewhere.[8–10] Instead, some general comments on the place of objective testing in health surveillance are provided later in the appendix.

Sensorineural hand–arm vibration syndrome

Transient digital paraesthesiae are common following use of powered vibratory tools. However, in those with sufficient long-term exposure they develop at other times—initially in an intermittent pattern, and then in protracted and troublesome spells that can disturb sleep. Transient and then permanent numbness is another frequent history. Physical examination may reveal abnormalities of light touch, temperature, and pinprick sensation in advanced cases of neurological disease; but in mild cases the clinical approach lacks sensitivity and repeatability, and HSE guidelines do not recommend their use in practice.

Electrophysiological tests suggest that a diffuse polyneuropathy of the digits and peripheral nerve entrapment can both arise. Disturbances of sensitivity to vibration, temperature, and touch can be demonstrated, as well as electrophysiological abnormalities of peripheral nerve conduction. Objective assessment methods for sensorineural HAVS include: aesthesiometry (to measure two-point discrimination and depth perception); thermo-aesthesiometry and temperature probe tests, to detect thermal thresholds; vibrometry, which measures vibrotactile thresholds using a vibrating probe; and a number of standardized tests of manual dexterity (see references 8–10 for further details). Vibration-associated carpal tunnel syndrome can be assessed in the usual fashion, by measurements of motor and sensory nerve conduction latencies.

Sensorineural and neuromuscular effects frequently coexist with vascular disease, but they can arise independently and progress at different rates.

Clinical grading

The vascular and neurological components are graded separately according to two scales that were developed by a workshop in Stockholm and published in 1987 (Table A6.1).[11,12] These scales have international currency and have been used at various times by HSE[13,14] and the UK Faculty of Occupational Medicine[15] to frame recommendations on career counselling.

Table A6.1 (a) The Stockholm workshop scale for the classification of cold-induced Raynaud's phenomenon in the hand-arm vibration syndrome (Gemne *et al.* 1987[11]). Reprinted with permission from the *Scandinavian Journal of Work, Environment and Health*.

Stage*	Grade	Description
0		No attacks
1	Mild	Occasional attacks affecting only the tips of one or more fingers
2	Moderate	Occasional attacks affecting distal and middle (rarely also proximal) phalanges of one or more fingers.
3	Severe	Frequent attacks affecting all phalanges of most fingers
4	Very severe	As in Stage 3, with trophic skin changes in the finger tips

*The staging is made separately for each hand. In the evaluation of the subject, the grade of the disorder is indicated by the stages of both hands and the number of affected fingers on each hand—for example: '2L(2)/1R(1)', '-/3R(4)', etc.

(b) Proposed sensorineural stages of the hand–arm vibration syndrome (Brammer *et al.* 1987[12]). Reprinted with permission from the *Scandinavian Journal of Work, Environment and Health*.

Stage*	Symptoms
0SN	Exposed to vibration but no symptoms
1SN	Intermittent numbness, with or without tingling
2SN	Intermittent or persistent numbness, reduced sensory perception
3SN	Intermittent or persistent numbness, reduced tactile discrimination, and/or manipulative dexterity

*The sensorineural stage is established separately for each hand.

Severity and prognosis

Attacks of cold-induced blanching are a source of discomfort, and work and leisure-time interference, but do not appear to cause much loss of working time. Neurological disturbance and muscle fatigue are more important causes of permanent disability.

Until the 1960s VWF was thought irreversible, but studies since have shown that vascular symptoms can improve (albeit slowly over several years) on withdrawal from exposure. Workers with advanced disease are less likely to recover. By contrast, the neurological effects of HAVS do not improve with time. Disabling and permanent impairment of hand function is thus the main morbidity to prevent.

In affected workers, both categories of disease tend to progress if the degree of exposure continues unchecked. However, the rate of progression varies between individuals, and is not entirely predictable. It depends on many factors, including vibration magnitude, operator technique, and (probably) personal susceptibility.

There is no well-established and really satisfactory treatment, although conservative measures (e.g. wearing of woollen gloves and warm clothing, avoidance of wet or draughty conditions), may alleviate some symptoms. In lieu of effective therapy, screening, early detection, and early withdrawal from exposure remain the most important practical interventions that can be offered. However, the decision to withdraw someone from exposure is not as simple as it might first appear, as discussed in the section that follows.

Health surveillance and fitness for work

Following some brief remarks on exposure assessment and the statutory framework, this section reviews several practical questions relevant to the provision of health surveillance for HAVS:

1. Who requires it and what are its aims?

2. Who should conduct it and what should it comprise?

3. What advice should be given to workers with symptoms?

4. Who requires work restrictions and when should exposures cease?

5. What is the role of objective testing?

Recent guidance from the HSE is summarized.

Exposure assessment

Vibration magnitude is measured in terms of its acceleration, averaged by the root-mean square method. Mounted accelerometers are used to measure frequency-weighted values (a_{hw}) in three axes relative to the tool handle and these are summated to produce the 'vibration total value', as defined in ISO standard 5349-1, 2001. Injury is assumed to relate to the total energy entering the hand, with a specific relation between time and vibration magnitude. Akin to the approach for noise, the dose or 'daily vibration exposure' can then be re-expressed in terms of the equivalent acceleration that would impart the same energy over an 8-hour reference period:

$$A(8) = a_{hw} \sqrt{(t/T_0)} \qquad (ms^{-2})$$

where:

$A(8)$ = the daily vibration exposure (eight-hour energy-equivalent vibration total value or $a_{hw(eq(8))}$

a_{hw} = the frequency-weighted vibration total value

t = duration of exposure in a day to the vibration a_{hw}

$T_0 - 8$ hours (in the same units as t).

Partial doses from several tools can be summed to an equivalent daily dose. In practice such information comes from an inventory of sources, data on vibration magnitude from equipment handbooks or suppliers' information sheets, and an estimate of hand-tool contact times. Tools may be conveniently grouped as 'high', 'medium', or 'low' risk (see http://www.hse.gov.uk/pubns/indg175.pdf). HSE provides an exposure ready-reckoner, to estimate A(8) from exposure time and vibration magnitude (http://www.hse.gov.uk/vibration/readyreckoner.htm), and an exposure calculator to facilitate the summation of doses from several tools (http://www.hse.gov.uk/vibration/hav/hav.xls).

The legal requirement: who should be under surveillance?

The Control of Vibration at Work Regulations 2005 came into force in the UK in July 2005. In addition to a general onus on employers to assess the risks from HTV and to provide information and training, this legislation specifies two sets of exposure limits:

1. An *Exposure Action Value* (EAV) A(8) of 2.5 m/s^2. This is the daily amount above which employers must act to reduce exposure.

2. An *Exposure Limit Value* (ELV) A(8) of 5 m/s^2. This is the most an employee may be exposed to on any given day. (The Regulations allow a transitional period, in certain circumstances, for tools in use before July 2007.)

A programme of health surveillance is mandated for those who remain regularly exposed above the EAV of 2.5 m/s^2. The HSE suggests a strategy and some rule of thumb guidelines (Table A6.2) for identifying workers with such exposures.[16]

The main aims of health surveillance are: (1) to aid early detection and counselling/job modification, and (2) to provide a check of workplace control measures—that is, to assist secondary and primary prevention. In addition, employers may wish to cite such services in medico-legal proceedings as evidence of their commitment to health and safety, so the boundaries between assessment for work fitness and assessment of legal liability sometimes become blurred.

What should such surveillance comprise? Who should do it?

The main elements of a health surveillance programme for HAVS comprise: (1) a system of symptom reporting; (2) periodic health inquiry and examination; (3) the formal clinical assessment of suspected cases; (4) the redeployment of affected individuals; and (5) statutory record keeping.

Table A6.2 Guidance from the HSE on exposures liable to lie above action limits defined in the Control of Vibration at Work Regulations 2005 (16)

'High risk' (above the ELV)	'Medium risk' (above the EAV)
Employees who regularly operate: hammer action tools for > about 1 hour/day; or some rotary and other action tools for >2 hours/day	Employees who regularly operate: hammer action tools for > about 15 minutes/day; or some rotary and action tools for >about 1 hour/day.
Employees in this group are likely to be above the ELV. The limit value could be exceeded in a much shorter time in some cases, especially where the tools are not the most suitable for the job	*Employees in this group are likely to be exposed above the EAV*

ELV, Exposure Limit Value; EAV, Exposure Action Value.

In practice the process begins with education and the encouragement of workers to report relevant symptoms to a responsible authority (doctor, nurse, line manager). In addition, for those exposed above the EAV a screening questionnaire is completed at regular intervals, at say the preplacement stage and then annually (with a check over the first 6 months to identify early and unusual susceptibility). Direct inquires are made about cold-induced finger blanching, sensorineural symptoms, problems of grip and dexterity, and sometimes other health effects.

The HSE suggests a tiered approach, as this is sparing of limited medical resource.[14] For such basic screening it says that employers may 'keep the costs down by carrying out this function for themselves or through a responsible appointee, referring any positive responses to an occupational health provider',[16] although the appropriateness of managers seeking such confidential health information directly like this seems open to question. As an alternative, the HSE suggests that confidential responses could pass directly to an occupational health (OH) professional.[14]

It further advises that health surveillance arrangements are unlikely to be considered adequate in the absence of services from an OH provider, a company occupational physician or similar services; but that any OH provider should be suitably qualified, with specific training and experience.[14] The Faculty of Occupational Medicine has adopted a syllabus of approved training for doctors and nurses involved in HAVS surveillance leading to a new certificate of competency, recognized by HSE inspectors; instruction is provided by approved training centres (see http://www.facoccmed.ac.uk/havs/index.jsp).

Several model questionnaires have been proposed for the initial screening stage.[13–15] In practice, such screens may be sensitive but not very specific and there has been very little assessment of their validity.[8,17,18] Hence, further evaluation by a clinician is needed for those with symptoms—to confirm the nature, pattern, and history of complaints, to perform a clinical examination, and to consider differential diagnoses and the need for further tests and care. Medical examination may suggest, for example, clinical evidence of carpal tunnel syndrome or a peripheral neuropathy or a coincidental connective tissue disorder. Face to face assessment by a clinician may also help to gauge the severity of a disorder (e.g. muscle wasting, trophic skin changes, significant sensory loss, or motor impairment), and is an essential precursor to any meaningful discussion of career changes. Diagnosis rests ultimately with the doctor.[14]

Pre-employment exclusions

The HSE recommends that individuals suffering from Raynaud's phenomenon or carpal tunnel syndrome should not be freshly employed in work involving exposure to HTV.[14] No firm evidence exists that such workers fare worse and deteriorate faster, but in practice many healthcare professionals share this pragmatic viewpoint.

Advice to those with symptoms

The HSE and the UK Faculty of Occupational Medicine have published several recommendations on counselling for affected workers.[13–15] It should be noted that the situation is not black and white (and this is well reflected in the latest guidance). In some workers disability may seem slight and the rate of progression slow. A need arises then to weigh the potential benefit against its cost in terms of limiting workers' earnings prospects prematurely. Advice tends to be titrated to the severity of disease, as determined using the Stockholm vascular and neurological scales. For those with mild disease (e.g. Stage 1 HAVS), work with vibratory tools is not ruled out provided that regular health checks are in place and proper thought is given to primary control measures; but at the other extreme, for those with advanced disease (Stage 3 HAVS), exposure should normally cease altogether. Where an outright ban is not mandated such factors as the individual's wishes, the length of remaining service, the scope to further limit exposures within the same job, the scope for redeployment to an alternative job, and the employer's attitude to medico-legal risk all feature in the judgement; different advice could legitimately be offered to young employees as to older workers approaching retirement.

At present, most experts feel that the dividing line between an acceptable and an unacceptable outcome lies somewhere along the continuum between early and late Stage 2 disease, the main challenge being not to allow progression from the former to the latter.

Information to employers

Whatever the doctor's decision on fitness for work, employers need to receive a written record confirming that surveillance has occurred and detailing any medical advice on restrictions. OH professionals will wish to keep separately from this their confidential clinical notes of assessment. Anonymized grouped results of health surveillance should, where practicable, be shared with the employer as these may be used as one check on the adequacy of control measures.

The role of objective testing

Standardized testing is not required as part of routine health surveillance provision,[14] although some OH professionals wish to use it to aid their assessment—especially to gauge severity and progression, and to substitute objective measures in place of subjective impressions. At present there are limited resources for testing nationally and these are applied mostly to help adjudicate in medico-legal disputes. These are all too common in workers exposed to HTV, and the distrust that sometimes exists between patient and doctor and between worker and manager has provided an impetus for services of objective testing to grow.

The properties of standardized tests are reviewed elsewhere.[7–10] It is noted here simply that no test is ideal (there being a lack of a clear gold standard), although several are well standardized and have acceptable/useful test properties; and where tests *are* applied that the methodology needs to be controlled carefully.[10]

Other legal issues

Industrial Injuries Benefit

In the UK, VWF (A11) is prescribed for Industrial Injuries Benefit in employed earners, provided that it occurs the year round, is extensive, and arises in a listed occupation (see http://www.dwp.gov.uk/advisers/ifpa/techguides/2004/db1_apr.pdf). State benefit may be claimed irrespective of fault and without a requirement for the individual to quit their job. Vibration-associated carpal tunnel syndrome (A12) is also prescribed. The Industrial Injuries Advisory Council has recommended prescription of the sensorineural component of HAVS, but at the time of writing its advice has still to be implemented.

Reporting of Injuries, Diseases, and Dangerous Occurrences Regulations (RIDDOR)

Under separate legal provisions (the RIDDOR Regulations), employers have a statutory duty to notify cases of VWF and sensorineural HAVS to the appropriate enforcing authority (HSE or local authority), once they become aware of them.

Role of the occupational physician

Occupational physicians have a specific role here in information sharing and advice. They should make affected employees aware of the opportunity to claim industrial injuries benefit, and should remind employers about their statutory duty to report on each doctor-confirmed case under RIDDOR.

Primary prevention

Although this account deals primarily with secondary prevention and fitness for work, it would be remiss not to emphasize the importance of primary prevention and the several steps that can be taken to mitigate risks in exposed workforces. These may be broadly summarized as: avoidance (e.g. doing the job another way); substitution (of tool or material worked); interruption of the pathway (by isolation or vibration-damping); and safer systems of work. Some options include: (1) the routine replacement of worn out tool parts; (2) proper selection of tools for the task; (3) the redesign of tools to avoid the need to grip high vibration parts, or to reduce grip force; and (4) rest breaks to limit exposure times. Advice on these important issues has been published in several places[3,13,16–18] and is strongly recommended as further reading.

References

1 Palmer KT, Coggon DN, Bendall HE, Kellingray S, Pannett B, Griffin M, Haward B. Hand-transmitted vibration: Occupational exposures and their health effects in Great Britain. HSE Contract Research Report 232/1999. London: HMSO, 1999.

2 Palmer KT, Griffin MJ, Bendall H, Pannett B, Coggon D. Prevalence and pattern of occupational exposure to hand-transmitted vibration in Great Britain: findings from a national survey. *Occup Environ Med* 2000; **57**: 218–28.

3 Griffin MJ. *Handbook of human vibration*. London: Academic Press, 1990.

4 Palmer KT, Griffin MJ, Syddall H, Pannett B, Cooper C, Coggon D. Risk of hand-arm vibration syndrome according to occupation and sources of exposure to hand-transmitted vibration: a national survey. *Am J Ind Med* 2001; **39**: 389–96.

5 Palmer KT, Griffin MJ, Syddall H, Pannett B, Cooper C, Coggon D. Prevalence of Raynaud's phenomenon in Great Britain and its relation to hand-transmitted vibration: a national postal survey. *Occup Environ Med* 2000; **57**: 448–52.

6 Palmer KT, Griffin MJ, Bendall H, Pannett B, Cooper C, Coggon D. The prevalence of sensorineural symptoms attributable to hand-transmitted vibration in Great Britain: a national postal survey. *Am J Ind Med* 2000; **38**: 99–107.

7 McGeoch KL, Lawson IJ, Burke F, Proud G, Miles J. Use of senorineural tests in a large volume of medico-legal compensation claims for HAVS. *Occup Med* 2004; **54**: 528–34.

8 Mason H, Poole K. *Clinical testing and management of individuals exposed to hand-transmitted vibration: an evidence review*. London: Faculty of Occupational Medicine, 2004.

9 Tyler LE, Fox JE, Griffin MJ, Jayson MIV, Lawson IJ. The objective assessment of hand-arm vibration syndrome. In: *Hand-transmitted vibration: clinical effects and pathophysiology. Part 2: Background papers to the working party report* (eds Faculty of Occupational Medicine), pp. 29–53. London: Royal College of Physicians, 1993.

10 Lindsell CJ, Griffin MJ. *Standardised diagnostic methods for assessing components of the hand-arm vibration syndrome*. HSE Contract Research Report 197/98. London: HMSO, 1998.

11 Gemne G, Pyykkö I, Taylor W, Pelmear, PL. The Stockholm Workshop scale for the classification of cold-induced Raynaud's phenomenon in the hand-arm vibration syndrome (revision of the Taylor Pelmear scale). *Scand J Work Environ Health* 1987; **13**: 275–8.

12 Brammer AJ, Taylor W, Lundborg G. Sensorineural stages of the hand arm vibration syndrome. *Scand J Work Environ Health* 1987; **13**: 279–83.

13 Health and Safety Executive. *Hand-arm vibration*. HS(G)88. Sudbury: HSE Books, 1994.

14 Health and Safety Executive. *The tiered system of health surveillance. Brief guidance for employers and health professionals.* http://www.hse.gov.uk/vibration/tieredsystem.pdf, HSE (accessed January 2006).

15 Faculty of Occupational Medicine. *Hand-transmitted vibration: clinical effects and pathophysiology.* Part 1: Report of a working party report, London: Royal College of Physicians, 1993.

16 Health and Safety Executive. *Control the risks from hand-arm vibration. Advice for employers on the Control of Vibration at Work Regulations 2005.* INDG 175. Sudbury: HSE Books, 2005. http://www.hse.gov.uk/pubns/indg175.pdf (accessed January 2006).

17 Health and Safety Executive. *Vibration solutions—practical ways to reduce the risk of hand-arm vibration injury.* Sudbury: HSE Books, 1997.

18 Health and Safety Executive. *Hand arm vibration: control of vibration at work, Regulations 2005. Guidance on Regulations.* L140. Sudbury: HSE Books, 2005.

Returning to work after intensive care treatment

E.S.M. Ziegler and J.M. Dixon

The scope of intensive care has increased over the last decade and many patients are admitted for observation to prevent potential problems. They pass through intensive care units (ICU) because of the higher level of nursing care available. The vast majority are discharged to a general ward after 1–2 days and subsequently home without complication. This appendix will cover the common sequelae of an extended requirement for intensive care. Considering the importance, as well as the expense of intensive care treatment there is little detailed work on the clinical recovery or follow-up support from the long-term effects of this medical therapy. An extended stay in ICU is frequently associated with serious physical, psychological, and social problems for patients and their families.

Significant improvements in survival rates in ICU have occurred in the last two decades; however, the 5-year mortality rate for patients following intensive care is over three times that of the general population. This increased mortality largely occurs in the first 2 years after which survival rates are parallel.

The majority of morbidity and deaths in patients in intensive care is caused by sepsis leading to multiple organ failure. The source of this infection may be the primary pathology (such as community acquired pneumonia or bowel sepsis) but frequently the specific source of infection is unknown. The term systemic inflammatory response syndrome (SIRS) is often used to describe a clinical reaction that is indistinguishable from sepsis but occurs in the absence of infection (for example, acute pancreatitis). The significance of both sepsis and SIRS is that they are associated with disordered vascular endothelial activity, which normally regulates the microvascular blood flow to organs. Disruption of this microcirculation causes organ hypoxia and failure.

Demographics

Critical illness can occur at any age though of 460,000 admissions 41% were people of working age*. While the prevalence is similar in all age groups the impact in terms of mortality is greatest at the extremes of age because of the limited reserve these patients have to cope with the insult of multiple organ failure. There are approximately 23,000 cases of sepsis admitted to ICUs per year in the UK. There is a 44.7% hospital mortality rate associated with severe sepsis; there are an estimated 12,000 survivors per year in the UK.

Long term problems following ICU (Table A7.1)

The most common post-discharge physical problems reported by patients are severe muscle weakness, fatigue, immobility, and breathlessness. Psychological problems are common and

*Pers.comm. David Harrison, Research Director of Intensive Care National Audit and Research Centre.

Table A7.1 Long-term ICU sequelae

General	Tracheostomy and tracheal stenosis
Change in physical appearance	**Cardiovascular**
Muscle loss (myopathy and neuropathy)	New or worsened heart failure
Psychiatric/ psychological	Myocardial infarction
Nightmares	Septic cardiomyopathy
Delusions/hallucinations	Postural hypotension
Post-traumatic stress disorder	Autonomic neuropathy
Anxiety/depression	**Joint contractures**
Panic attacks	Neck, ankle, knees, fingers
Cognitive impairment	**Needle injuries**
Sleep disorder	Radial artery damage
Sexual dysfunction	Nerve injury
Respiratory	**Other**
Resolving acute respiratory distress syndrome	Alopecia
Restrictive pulmonary function (mild)	Chronic pain
Weak respiratory musculature	Itching

include depression, anxiety, and post-traumatic stress disorder (PTSD). These health problems affect daily activities including work, home, and social life. Although recent years have seen an expansion of interest in these issues, much of the data comes from single centre studies.

Physical

Muscle weakness and fatigue

All survivors of critical illness report muscle weakness and fatigue. At 2 months following ICU discharge almost half of all survivors either cannot manage stairs or have difficulty climbing more than a few steps and one-third still use a wheelchair outside the house.[1] Other more specific problems with muscle weakness affect activities of daily living such as poor grip strength and inability to turn taps and keys; weak quadriceps muscles make getting out of a chair or car difficult. The fear of falling and not being able to get back up again is common.

At 3 months post-discharge fatigue is high in both men (63%) and women (60%) and remains high at 1 year (32% of men and 38% of women).[2]

This weakness and fatigue is caused by a combination of severe muscle catabolism and muscle atrophy secondary to an acute axonal neuropathy. Muscle mass is lost very rapidly by septic patients at about 2% per day. Although some of this muscle breakdown will be to release usable metabolic substrate it is clear that substrate deficiency alone does not explain the severity of muscle breakdown. Assessing myopathy in patients recovering from sepsis is difficult. Serum creatinine kinase is usually normal. Muscle biopsy may show structural abnormalities but is invasive and, as there is at present no specific therapy, will not lead to a change in management. Rebuilding this muscle is slow and can take over a year.

Acute axonal neuropathy is less frequent but is easier to assess using nerve conduction studies. However, like the myopathy, there is no specific therapy. In less severe cases recovery can be anticipated in a few months following discharge from hospital. In more severe cases these effects can be devastating. One study of 19 patients with severe neuropathy following sepsis at 2 years post-discharge showed that 11 had recovered completely, two had died and six remained quadriplegic.[3] A mixed picture of neuropathy and myopathy is common.

If a patient continues to have weakness sufficient to hinder return to work referral for neurophysiology tests to assess the extent of the neuropathic element of the weakness may be useful, not least to help the patient understand the nature of the problem.

Muscle contractures may develop in patients who remain on intensive care for long periods. These particularly affect the ankles, fingers, and neck. Treating patients in the prone position to improve ventilation has led to some patients developing chronic neck and shoulder pain. Follow-up studies have found that joint immobility affects 5–10% of patients. Immobility of large joints is the third most common reason, after persistent weakness and fatigue, for failure to return to work.[4]

Respiratory sequelae

Sepsis is frequently complicated by the development of diffuse bilateral pulmonary infiltrates. The patient usually requires support with mechanical ventilation and high concentrations of oxygen. The severest form of this acute lung injury, acute respiratory distress syndrome (ARDS), may lead to fibrotic changes within the lung as the initial inflammatory injury resolves. However, recovery of respiratory function as assessed by routine pulmonary function tests is surprisingly good. At 1 year patients may have a mild restrictive pattern on lung function testing and a mild to moderate reduction in carbon monoxide diffusion capacity. Median lung volume and spirometric values are within 80% of normal by 6 months. Persistent sensation of breathlessness in these patients is likely to be due to muscle weakness rather than persisting lung disease. However, a very small proportion of patients have persisting lung injury and scarring, with some requiring domiciliary oxygen after discharge.

Tracheal stenosis is a potential but uncommon complication of tracheostomy. It occurs in approximately 2–5% of surviving patients. Referral to an ENT specialist may be required if persistent airways narrowing is suspected. Other local complications such as tethering of skin scar tissue to the underlying trachea, and skin tags at the tracheostomy site may require correction.

Psychological dysfunction

Psychological dysfunction following discharge from ICU is common and can include nightmares, delusions, hallucinations, PTSD, anxiety, depression, panic attacks, and cognitive impairment. Factors that contribute to development include sepsis, opiate and sedative use and withdrawal, lack of sleep and circadian disruption and constant noise.

The recall of events on ICU has a major effect on the subsequent development of psychological distress. Prolonged periods of amnesia as well as specific traumatic memories have a significant impact. Between 22 and 79% of patients recall frightening adverse experiences (nightmares 63.8%, anxiety 41%, pain 40%, and respiratory distress 37.5%).[5] PTSD is more common in those who report two or more adverse experiences and especially in those with delusional memories. In a study of ICU patients with acute respiratory distress syndrome the incidence of PTSD was 27.5% compared with 11.9% in patients following maxillofacial surgery and 1.3% in United Nations' soldiers with prolonged service in Cambodia. Younger patients appear to be particularly vulnerable, perhaps because they metabolize or clear sedative drugs more rapidly and so may remember distressing events during their critical illness. Discussion of such problems can enable patients to create a coherent history of their illness rather than chaotic intrusive memories.

Twenty-eight to 45% of patients have little or no memory of their ICU experience which can make it difficult for patients to understand the severity of their illness. This leads to unrealistic expectations of the speed of recovery, which may take years rather than weeks. This is a further cause of frustration, irritability, and depression.

Affective disorders are common in survivors of critical illness. At 1 year, about half of all survivors will have clinically significant anxiety and depression.[6]

At discharge most patients who have had sepsis will have some degree of cognitive impairment as a result of sepsis-related encephalopathy. The severity of this encephalopathy is often masked by prolonged sedation with benzodiazepines and opioids, which themselves may alter brain receptor populations. The exact cause of this encephalopathy is unclear although periods of hypotension, hypoxia, or diffuse intravascular coagulopathy affecting small intracerebral vessels are possible aetiologies. A year after hospital discharge three-quarters of survivors of the acute respiratory distress syndrome have impaired memory, attention, and concentration or decreased processing speed. A quarter still have mild cognitive impairment 6 years after discharge.[7] A follow-up study of critically ill medical patients found a third had neuropsychological impairment equivalent to mild dementia; the impairment was generally diffuse but occurred primarily in areas of psychomotor speed, visual and working memory, verbal fluency, and visuo-construction.[8] Deficits of this severity are likely to impair social and occupational functioning but the sample in that study was of older patients (mean age 53.2 years).

Physical appearance is changed by prolonged illness. Both scarring and alopecia are common and may contribute to the psychological distress. Alopecia is more common in women (47% vs 8% of men). It usually resolves by 6 months.

The relatives of ICU patients, having witnessed the severity and complexity of the illness, can themselves be traumatized and may sometimes hinder recovery by being over-protective.

Daily activities

The Intensive Care National Audit and Research Council (ICNARC) looked at the quality of survival of 3474 patients following intensive care; 2147 were of working age. Six months postadmission to intensive care, only about a third of patients do not have problems with daily activities. ICU patients report more problems than survivors from other major surgery (heart/lung transplant, prostatectomy, CABG). A high proportion of patients of working age indicated that their health was affecting daily activities.[9]

◆ ability to look after the home: 41.7%

◆ social life: 39.5%

◆ interests and hobbies: 42.7%

◆ holidays: 37.9%

◆ sex life: 32.2%

◆ home life: 21.4%

◆ driving: 25%.

Work

The INARC study also looked at work and found of those who were working full or part-time prior to ICU admission, at 6 months postadmission, 42.2% were not working and in 79% this was for health reasons. Of those who had returned to work, 23.2% indicated their health affected their work. Individual data from other work show a decrease in full-time workers and an increase in part-time workers and those not working. There are reports that men may take longer to return to work than women (65% by 1 year compared with 75% of women by 6 months).[2] This may reflect gender difference in work. Overall, over half of those who survive to leave hospital will return to work within 1 year. The majority of these will return to their original work.

Critical care follow-up clinics

Over the last few years critical care follow-up clinics have been established in a number of hospitals in the UK. These have provided valuable information about the ongoing problems experienced by patients in the months following critical illness. Approximately 25% of UK intensive care units now run some kind of physician or nurse led follow-up clinic for most patients whose stay exceeded 4 days. Although the Department of Health review *Comprehensive critical care*[10] highlighted the need for follow-up clinics they continue to be very poorly funded.

A typical assessment is made at 2–3 months following discharge using a structured interview looking at morbidity and quality of life. Tools commonly used are based on the Hospital Anxiety and Depression Scale (HAD) and Short-Form 36 (SF36).

Additional specific areas of assessment are employment, ICU recollections, and sleep patterns, incidence of nightmares, fatigue, concentration, hair loss and evidence of neuropathy. Local referral for physiotherapy, clinical psychology and medical speciality review are organized from the follow-up clinic. Subsequent follow-up at 6 and 12 months is determined by need.

The role of the occupational physician

Patients reporting an extended stay in intensive care should alert the occupational physician (OP) to the common sequelae already mentioned. Employees who have access to an OP should make contact with him/her at the earliest opportunity. Hospital discharge letters may make only fleeting reference to a patient's stay in ICU. An OP seeing the patient some months after discharge may have difficulty identifying those patients who have had prolonged consequences from sepsis. Any patient who has spent more than 48 hours on an intensive care unit may be at risk. The common sequelae to sepsis typically become more significant after longer, more severe episodes of sepsis.

ICUs now often provide patients with information about their care, or may even compile diaries of the illness to aid recall and recovery. However, in one study only 16% of patients could remember receiving any information about their ICU stay and with few ICU follow-up clinics, the OP may need to advise on recovery and refer for further support, such as physiotherapy or clinical psychology.

Conclusions

Over the last decade information has been gathered as patients are followed up after leaving the intensive care unit. This has enabled intensive care outcomes to be viewed in a more sophisticated way than the previous focus on survival alone. This information has led to an understanding that the responses to severe illness can have long-term sequelae which may affect an individual's ability to work. Contact with the OP at the earliest opportunity will help to expedite rehabilitation.

References

1 Jones C, Griffiths RD. Identifying post intensive care patients who may need physical rehabilitation. *Clin Intens Care* 2000; **11**: 35–38.

2 Eddleston J, White P, Guthrie E. Survival, morbidity and quality of life after discharge from intensive care. *Crit Care Med* 2000; **28**: 2293–9.

3 de Seze M, Petit H, Wiart L, Cardinaud JP, Gaujard E, Joseph PA, Mazaux JM, Barat M. Critical illness polyneuropathy. A 2-year follow-up study of 19 severe cases. *Eur Neurol* 2000; **43**: 61–9.

4 Herridge MS, Cheung AM, Tansey CM *et al.* One year outcomes in survivors of the acute respiratory distress syndrome. *N Engl J Med* 2003; **348**: 683–93.

5 Scheeling G, Stoll C, Haller M, Briegel J, Manert W, Hummel T, Leihart A, Heyduck M, Polasek M, Meier M, Preubu, Bullinger M, Schuffel W, Peter K. Health-related quality of life and post traumatic stress disorder in survivors of the acute respiratory syndrome. *Crit Care Med* 1998; **26**: 651–9.

6 Scragg P, Jones A, Fauvel N. Psychological problems following ICU treatment. *Anaesthesia* 2001; **56**: 9–14.

7 Rothenhausler H-B, Ehrentraut S, Stoll C, Schelling G. The relationship between cognitive performance and employment and health status in long term survivors of the acute respiratory distress syndrome: results of an exploratory study. *Gen Hosp Psychiatry* 2001; **23**: 90–6.

8 Jackson JC, Hart RP, Gordon SM *et al.* Six month neuropsychological outcome of medical intensive care unit patients. *Crit Care Med* 2003; **31**: 1226–34.

9 Rowan KM. Outcome comparisons of intensive care units in Great Britain and Ireland using APACHE II method (DPhil Thesis). Oxford. University of Oxford, 1992

10 Comprehensive Critical Care. *A review of adult critical care services.* London: Department of Health, 2000.

Useful addresses

Chapters 1–5

EMAS (Employment Medical Advisory Service)
Offices located in each of HSE regions.
Details of local office in telephone directory.

Health and Safety Executive
Information Centre
Broad Lane
Sheffield S3 7H Q
Tel.: 08701 545 500
Tel.: 0845 345 0055 (Infoline)
Tel.: 01787 881165 (publications)

Health and Safety Executive
Rose Court
2 Southwark Bridge
London SE1 9HS

National Council for Voluntary Organisations (NCVO)
Regent's Wharf
8 All Saints Street
London N1 9RL
Tel.: 020 7713 6161
Voluntary sector helpdesk: 0800 2 798 798
Fax: 020 7713 6300

RADAR (The Royal Association for Disability and Rehabilitation)
12 City Forum
250 City Road
London EC1V 8AF
Tel.: 020 7250 3222
Fax: 020 7250 0212
Minicom: 0207 2504119
E-mail: radar@radar.org.uk

SKILL: National Bureau for Students with Disabilities
Chapter House
18–20 Crucifix Lane
London SE1 3JW
Info: 0800 328 5050 (voice)
Info: 0800 068 2422 (text)
Office voice/text: 020 7450 0620
Fax: 020 7450 0650
E-mail: skill@skill.org.uk

Employment Opportunities for People with Disabilities
53 New Broad Street
London EC2M 1SL
Tel.: 020 7448 5420
Fax: 020 7374 4913
Minicom: 020 7374 6684
E-mail: info@eopps.org

Disability Information Trust
Mary Marlborough centre
Nuffield Orthopaedic Centre
Headington
Oxford OX3 7LD
Tel.: 01865 227 592
Fax: 01865 227 596
E-mail: abilityonline@estateweb.net

Employers' Forum on Disability
Nutmeg House
60 Gainsford Street
London SE1 2NY
Tel.: 020 7403 3020
Fax: 020 7403 0404
Minicom: 020 7403 0040
E-mail: website.enquiries@
employers-forum.co.uk

Disabled Living Foundation
380–384 Harrow Road
London W9 2HU
Tel.: 020 7289 6111

Cancerbackup
Helpline: 0808 800 1234

Finchale Training College
Durham DH1 5RX
Tel.: 0191 386 2634
Fax: 0191 386 4962

**Queen Elizabeth's Training College
(training disabled adults 18–64 for work)**
Leatherhead Court
Woodlands Road
Leatherhead
Surrey KT22 0BN
Tel.: 01372 841100
Fax: 01372 844072
Web: www.qefd.org.uk

**St Loye's College (training disabled people
for employment)**
Topsham Road
Exeter EX2 6EP
Tel.: 01392 255428
Fax: 01392 420889

Rehab UK
Windermere House
Kendal Avenue
London W3 0XA

Faculty of Occupational Medicine
6 St Andrews Place
Regent's Park
London NW1 4LB
Tel.: 020 7317 5890
Fax: 020 7317 5899
Web: www.facoccmed.ac.uk

**British Occupational Health Research
Foundation**
6 St Andrews Place
Regent's Park
London NW1 4LB
Tel.: 020 7317 5898
Web: www.bohrf.org.uk

Chapter 6

**Parkinson's Disease Society of the United
Kingdom**
215 Vauxhall Bridge Road
London SW1V 1EJ
Tel : 020 7931 8080
Fax: 020 7233 9908/020 7963 9360
E-mail: enquiries@parkinsons.org.uk

Motor Neurone Disease Association
PO Box 246
Northampton NN1 2PR
Tel.: 01604 250505
Fax: 01604 638289/624726
Helpline: 08457 626262
E-mail: enquiries@mndassociation.org

Multiple Sclerosis Society
England and Wales
MS Society
MS National Centre
372 Edgware Road
London NW2 6ND
Tel.: 020 8438 0700

Scotland
National Office
Ratho Park
88 Glasgow Road
Ratho Station
Newbridge EH28 8PP
Tel.: 0131 335 4050
Fax: 0131 335 4051

Northern Ireland
The Resource Centre
34 Annadale Avenue
Belfast BT7 3JJ
Tel.: 02890 802 802

The ME Association
4 Top Angel
Buckingham Industrial Park
Buckingham
Buckinghamshire MK18 1TH
Tel.: 0870 444 8233
Fax: 01280 821602

The Stroke Association
Stroke Information Service
The Stroke Association
240 City Road
London EC1V 2PR
Tel.: 0845 3033 100
E-mail info@stroke.org.uk

British Guillain–Barrè Syndrome Support Group
Lincolnshire County Council Offices
Eastgate
Sleaford
Lincolnshire NG34 7EB
Tel.: 01529 304615
E-mail: webmaster@gbs.org.uk

Chapter 7

Mind
15–19 Broadway
London E15 4BQ
Tel.: 020 8519 2122
Fax: 020 8522 1725
E-mail: contact@mind.org.uk

The Samaritans
The Upper Mill
Kingston Road
Ewell
Surrey KT17 2AF
Tel.: 020 8394 8300
Tel. (24-hour confidential helpline): 08457 909090
Fax: 020 8394 8301
E-mail: admin@samaritans.org
Web: www.samaritans.org.uk

The British Stammering Association
15 Old Ford Road
London E2 9PJ
Tel.: 020 8983 1003
Fax: 020 8983 3591
E-mail: mail@stammering.org

Chapter 8

British Epilepsy Association
Epilepsy Action
New Anstey House
Gate Way Drive
Yeadon
Leeds LS19 7XY
Tel.: 0113 210 8800
Fax: 0113 391 0300
E-mail: epilepsy@epilepsy.org.uk

St Piers
St Piers Lane
Lingfield
Surrey RH7 6PW
Tel.: 01342 832 243
Web: www.ncype.org.uk

Park Road Hospital for Children
Churchill Hospital
Old Road
Headington
Oxford OX3 7LQ
Tel.:01865 741717

Bootham Park Hospital
Bootham Park
York YO30 7BY
Tel.: 01904 725274

Chapter 9

Royal National Institute of the Blind
105 Judd Street
London WC1H 9NE
Tel.: 020 7388 1266
Fax: 020 7388 2034
E-mail: helpline@rnib.org.uk

Royal National College for the Blind (RNC)
College Road
Hereford HR1 1EB
Tel.: 01432 265725
Fax: 01432 376628
E-mail: info@rncb.ac.uk

Queen Alexandra College
Court Oak Road
Harborne
Birmingham B17 9TG
Tel.: 0121 428 5050
Fax: 0121 428 5048
E-mail: enquiries@qac.ac.uk

Keeler Ltd
Clewer Hill Road
Windsor
Berkshire SL4 4AA
Tel.: 01753 857177
Fax: 01753 827145
E-mail: info@keeler.co.uk

International Glaucoma Association
Woodcote House
15 Highpoint Business Village
Henwood
Ashford
Kent TN24 8DH
Tel.: 0870 609 1870
Fax: 01233 64 81 79
E-mail: info@iga.org.uk

Chapter 10

**The Royal National Institute
for Deaf People**
19–23 Featherstone Street
London EC1Y 8SL
Tel.: 020 7296 8000
Fax: 020 7296 8199
Textphone: 020 7296 8001

RNID Court Grange College
Tel.: 01626 53401
Textphone: 01626 67677
Fax: 01626 60895

British Deaf Association
1–3 Worship Street
London EC2A 2AB
Tel.: 020 7588 3520
Fax: 020 7588 3527
E-mail: helpline@bda.org.uk
Minicom: 020 7588 3529

Medical Devices Agency (MDA)
Hannibal House
Elephant & Castle
London SE1 6TQ
Tel.: 020 7972 8000
E-mail: mail@medical-devices.gov.uk
Web: www.medical-devices.gov.uk

Chapters 11 and 12

National Ankylosing Spondylitis Society
PO Box 179
Mayfield
East Sussex TN20 6ZL
Tel.: 01435 873527
Fax: 01435 873027
E-mail: nass@nass.co.uk

Arthritis Research Council
Copeman House
St Mary's Court
St Mary's Gate
Chesterfield
Derbyshire S41 7TD
Tel.: 01246 558033
Fax: 01246 558007
E-mail: info@arc.org.uk
Web: www.arc.org.uk

Arthritis Care
18–20 Stephenson Way
London NW1 2HD
Tel.: 020 7380 6500
Fax: 020 7380 6505

National Back Pain Association
16 Elmtree Road
Teddington
Middlesex TW11 8ST
Tel.: 020 8977 5474
Fax: 020 8943 5318

**The Royal Society for the Prevention
of Accidents (RoSPA)**
RoSPA House
353 Bristol Road
Edgbaston
Birmingham B5 7ST
Tel.: 0121 238 2000
Fax: 0121 248 2001
E-mail: help@rospa.com

Chapter 14

British Colostomy Association
15 Station Road
Reading
Berkshire RG1 1LB
Tel.: 0118 939 1537
Web: www.bcass.org.uk

The Ileostomy and Internal Pouch Support Group
Web: www.the-ia.org.uk

The Coeliac Society
PO Box 220
High Wycombe
Buckinghamshire HP11 2MY
Tel.: 01494 437 278
Fax: 01494 474 349
Helpline: 0870 444 8804
E-mail: admin@coeliac.co.uk
Web: www.coeliac.co.uk

Digestive Disorders Foundation
3 St Andrews Place
Regent's Park
London NW1 4LB
Information: P O Box 251, Edgware,
Middlesex HA8 8HG
Web: www.digestivedisorders.org.uk

British Liver Trust
Central House
Central Avenue
Ransomes Europark
Ipswich IP3 9QG
Tel.: 01473 276 326
Fax: 01473 276 327
Information line: 01473 276 328

The National Association for Colitis & Crohn's Disease
4 Beaumont House
Sutton Road
St Albans
Hertfordshire AL1 5HH
Tel.: 01727 830 038
Fax: 01727 862 550
E-mail: nacc@nacc.org.uk
Web: www.nacc.org.uk

Chapter 15

British Diabetic Association
10 Queen Anne Street
London WIM 0BD
Tel.: 020 7323 3644
Fax: 020 7637 3644
Careline: 020 7636 6112 (for information about diabetes and diabetes care)

Chapter 16

Haemophilia Society
First Floor
Petersham House
57a Hatton Garden
London EC1N 8JG
Tel.: 020 7831 1020
Fax: 020 7405 4824
Freephone helpline: 0800 018 6068
(Monday to Friday 10 am–4 pm)
E-mail: info@haemophilia.org.uk

Sickle Cell Society
54 Station Road
London NW10 4UA
Tel.: 020 8961 7795
Fax: 020 8961 8346
E-mail: sicklecellsoc@btinternet.org
Web: www.sicklecellsociety.org

Leukaemia Research Fund
43 Great Ormond Street
London WIN 3JJ
Tel.: 020 7405 0101
Fax: 020 7405 3139

Chapter 17

British Heart Foundation
14 Fitzhardinge Street
London WIH 4DH
Tel.: 020 7935 0185
Web: www.bhf.org.uk

Heart Rhythm UK
(formerly The British Pacing and
Electrophysiology Group (BPEG))
9 Fitzroy Square
London W1T 5HW
Tel.: 020 7692 5413
E-mail: hruk@bcs.com

British Cardiovascular Society
9 Fitzroy Square
London W1T 5HW
Tel.: 020 7383 3887
Fax: 020 7388 0903
E-mail: enquiries@bcs.com

Chapter 18

Asthma UK
Summit House
70 Wilson Street
London EC2A 2DB
Tel.: 020 7786 4900
Fax: 020 7256 6075
E-mail: info@asthma.org.uk

Asthma UK Scotland
4 Queen Street
Edinburgh EH2 1JE
Tel.: 0131 226 2544
Fax: 0131 226 2401
E-mail: scotland@asthma.org.uk

Asthma UK Cymru
3rd floor
Eastgate House
34–43 Newport Road
Cardiff CF24 0AB
Tel.: 02920 435 400
Fax: 02920 487 731
E-mail: wales@asthma.org.uk

Asthma UK Northern Ireland
Peace House
224 Lisburn Road
Belfast BT9 6GE
Tel.: 02890 669736
Fax: 02890 669736
E-mail: ni@asthma.org.uk

Cystic Fibrosis Trust
11 London Road
Bromley
Kent BR1 1BY
Tel.: 020 8464 7211
Fax: 020 8313 0472
E-mail (for general enquiries):
enquiries@cftrust.org.uk
E-mail (for medical enquiries):
AskTheExpert@cftrust.org.uk

Action on Smoking and Health (ASH)
102 Clifton Street
London EC2A 4HW
Tel.: 020 7739 5902
Fax: 020 7613 0531
E-mail enquiries@ash.org.uk
Web: www.ash.org.uk
Quit: Tel.: 0800 00 22 00

Chapter 19

National Kidney Federation
6 Stanley Street
Worksop
Notts S81 7HX
Tel. (administration): 01909 487 795
Tel. (helpline): 01909 481 723
Fax: 0845 601 0209
Web: www.kidney.org.uk

**The British Kidney Patient
Association (BKPA)**
Bordon
Hants GU35 9JZ
Tel.: 01420 472 020/2
Fax: 01420 475 831
Web: www.britishkidney-pa.co.uk

The Continence Foundation
307 Hatton Square
16 Baldwins Gardens
London EC1N 7RJ
Tel. (administration): 020 7404 6875
Tel. (helpline 0930–1300 hours Mon–Fri):
0845 345 0165
E-mail: continence-help@dial.pipex.com
Web: www.continence-foundation.org.uk

Association for Continence Advice (ACA)
C/O Fitwise Management Limited
Drumcross Hall
Bathgate
West Lothian EH48 4JT
E-mail: info@aca.uk.com

Chapter 20

Wellbeing of Women
27 Sussex Place
Regent's Park
London NW1 4SP
Tel.: 020 7772 6400
Fax: 020 7724 7725
E-mail: wellbeingofwomen@rcog.org.uk

Breast Cancer Care
Kiln House
210 New King's Road
London SW6 4NZ
Tel. (administration): 020 7384 2984
Tel. (freephone helpline): 0808 800 6000
Tel. (textphone): 0808 800 6001
E-mail: info@breastcancercare.org.uk
Web: www.breastcancercare.org.uk

Women's Nationwide Cancer Control Campaign
Suna House
128–130 Curtain Road
London EC2A 3AR
Tel. (helpline): 020 7729 2229
Tel. (administration): 020 7729 4688
Web: www.wnccc.org.uk

Chapter 21

Cancerbackup
3 Bath Place
Rivington Street
London EC2A 3JR
Tel. (freephone 0900–2000 hours):
0800 800 1234
Tel. (0900–1730 hours): 020 7739 2280
Fax: 020 7696 9002
Web: www.cancerbackup.org.uk

Macmillan Cancer Relief
89 Albert Embankment
London SE1 7UQ
Tel. (freephone 0900–1800 hours Mon–Fri):
0808 808 2020
E-mail: cancerline@macmillan.org.uk
Web: www.macmillan.org.uk

Chapter 22

National Eczema Society
Hill House
Highgate Hill
London N19 5NA
Tel. (administration): 020 7281 3553
Tel. (helpline): 0870 241 3604
Fax: 020 7281 6395
E-mail: helpline@eczema.org
Web: www.eczema.org

The Psoriasis Association
Milton House
7 Milton Street
Northampton NN2 7JG
Tel. (0915–1645 Mon–Thurs, 0915–1615 Fri):
0845 676 0076
(Calls charged at local rate)
Fax: 01604 792 894
E-mail: mail@psoriasis.demon.co.uk
Web: www.psoriasis-association.org.uk

The Vitiligo Society
125 Kennington Road
London SE11 6SF
Tel. (freephone): 0800 018 2631
Web: www.vitiligosociety.org.uk

Acne Support Group
P O Box 9
Newquay
Cornwall TR9 6WG
Tel.: 0870 870 2263

Chapter 23

Terrence Higgins Trust
314–320 Gray's Inn Road
London WC1X 8DP
Tel.: 020 7812 1600
Fax: 020 7812 1601
E-mail: info@tht.org.uk
Web: www.tht.org.uk

National AIDS Map (NAM)
Lincoln House
1 Brixton Road
London SW9 6DE
Tel.: 020 7840 0050
Fax: 020 7735 5351
E-mail: info@nam.org.uk
Web: www.aidsmap.com

Chapter 24

Accept Services
724 Fulham Road
London SW6 5SE
Tel.: 020 7371 7477

Alcoholics Anonymous
PO Box 1
Stonebow House
Stonebow
York Y01 7NJ
Tel. (administration): 01904 644026
Tel. (national helpline, calls charged at local rate): 0845 769 7555
Web: www.alcoholics-anonymous.org.uk
Drink Aware: www.drinkaware.co.uk

Alcohol Concern
Tel.: 020 7928 7377
Web: www.alcoholconcern.org.uk
Drinkline: Tel.: 0800 917 8282
(24 hours)

Talk to Frank (national drugs awareness site)
Web: www.talktofrank.com

Chapter 25

British Airways Travel Clinics
213 Piccadilly
London W1J 9HQ
Tel.: 0845 600 2236
Web: www.britishairways.com/travel/healthclinintro

Chapter 26

Age Concern UK
Astral House
1268 London Road
London SW16 4ER
Tel. (administration): 020 8765 7200
Tel. (free helpline): 0800 00 99 66
Fax: 020 8765 7211
Web: www.ageconcern.org.uk

Department for Work and Pensions
Web: www.dwp.gov.uk

Chapter 28

Driver and Vehicle Licensing Agency (DVLA)
Drivers Medical Group
Swansea
SA99 1TU
Tel.: 0870 600 0301
Fax: 0845 850 0095
E-mail: eftd@dvla.gsi.gov.uk
Web: www.dvla.gov.uk

Appendix 1

Civil Aviation Authority
CAA House
45-59 Kingsway
London WC2B 6TE
Tel.: 020 7379 7311

Appendix 3

United Kingdom Offshore Operators Association (UKOOA)
UKOOA (London office)
2nd Floor
232–242 Vauxhall Bridge Road
London SW1V 1AU
Tel.: 020 7802 2400
Fax: 020 7802 2401
Web: www.ukooa.co.uk

UKOOA (Aberdeen office)
3rd Floor
The Exchange 2
62 Market Street
Aberdeen AB11 5PJ
Tel.: 01224 577 250
Fax: 01224 577 251
Web: www.ukooa.co.uk

Appendix 4

The Diving Medical Advisory Committee
5 Lower Belgrave Street
London SW1W 0NR
Tel.: 020 7824 5520
Fax: 020 7824 5521
E-mail: info@dmac-diving.org
Web: www.dmac-diving.org

Appendix 5

MASTA—Medical Advisory Service for Travellers Abroad
Web: www.masta.org
E-mail: enquiries@masta.org

The Hospital for Tropical Diseases
Mortimer Market Building
Capper Street
Tottenham Court Road
London WCIE 6AU
Tel.: 020 7387 4411 or 0845 155 5000
Fax: 020 7388 7645
Web: www.thehtd.org

Health Protection Agency (Travel Health)
Travel and Migrant Health Section
Health Protection Agency
Centre for Infections
61 Colindale Avenue
London NW9 5EQ
Tel.: 020 8200 6868
Fax: 020 8200 7868
E-mail: tmhs@hpa.org.uk
Web: www.phls.co.uk

HPA Malaria Reference library
London School of hygiene and Tropical Medicine
Keppel Street
London WCIE 7HT
Tel.: 020 7636 3924
Web: www.malaria-reference.co.uk

Swiss Air Rescue Organisation
Swiss Air-Rescue Rega
Rega Center
PO Box 1414
CH-8058
Zurich Airport
Tel. (emergency number): 00 41 333 333 333
Tel. (administration): 00 41 44 654 3311
Web: www.rega.ch

SOS Assistance
12 Chemin Riantbosson
1217 Meyrin 1
Geneva
Tel. (administration): 00 41 22 719 1100
Fax: 00 41 22 785 6426

Abbreviations

ABI	Association of British Insurers	BAC	blood alcohol concentration
ABR	auditory brainstem responses	BBS	Behavioural Based Safety
ACC	Accident Compensation Corporation (New Zealand); American College of Cardiology	BCG	Bacillus of Calmette and Guérin
		BCS	British Crime Survey
		BEA	British Epilepsy Association
ACE	angiotensin-converting enzyme	BHA	British Hyperbaric Association
ACL	anterior cruciate ligament	BM	bone marrow
ACOP	Approved Code of Practice	BMI	body mass index
ACP	American College of Physicians	BMT	bone marrow transplant
ADA	Americans with Disabilities Act	BNF	British National Formulary
ADL	activities of daily living	BP	blood pressure
AED	antiepileptic drug	BPH	benign prostatic hyperplasia
AHA	American Heart Association	BPT	bronchial provocation challenge test
AIDS	acquired immune deficiency syndrome	BSRM	British Society of Rehabilitation Medicine
ALAMA	Association of Local Authority Medical Advisers		
		BTS	British Thoracic Society
ALL	acute lymphoblastic leukaemia	CA	Court of Appeal
ALT	alanine transferase	CAA	Civil Aviation Authority
AMAS	activity matching ability system	CABG	coronary artery bypass grafting
AME	authorized medical examiner	CAPD	continuous ambulatory peritoneal dialysis
AMED	Approved Medical Examiner of Divers		
AML	acute myeloid leukaemia	CARDS	Collaborative Atorvastatin Diabetes Study
AMRA	Access to Medical Reports Act 1988		
ANHOPS	Association of National Health Occupational Physicians	CBI	Confederation of British Industry
		CBT	cognitive-behavioural therapy
APD	automated peritoneal dialysis	CCDC	Consultant in Communicable Disease Control
ARBs	angiotensin II receptor blockers		
ARDS	acute respiratory distress syndrome	CD	Crohn's Disease
ART	antiretroviral treatment	CD4 cells	T-helper lymphocytes (carry CD4 antigen)
AS	ankylosing spondylitis		
ASHRAE	the American Society of Heating, Refrigeration and Air Conditioning Engineers	CEDP	Committee for the employment of disabled people
		CEFEM	'Chance Encounter of Female Exceeding Male' strength
ATS-DLD	American Thoracic Society and the Division of Lung Disease	CEHR	Combined Equality and Human Rights Commission
AtW	Access to Work		
AVC	additional voluntary contribution	CFC	chlorofluorocarbons
AWT	all work test	CFS	chronic fatigue syndrome

CHD	coronary heart disease	DfEE	Department for Education and Employment
CI	confidence interval		
CIBSE	Chartered Institution of Building Services Engineers	DHA	docosohexaenoic acid
		DIP	distal interphalangeal joint
CISD	Critical Incident Stress Debriefing	DIT	Disability Information Trust
CJD	Creutzfeldt-Jakob disease	DLA	Disability Living Allowance
CKD	chronic kidney disease	DLF	Disabled Living Foundation
CLAW	The Control of Lead at Work Regulations	DMPA	depot medroxyprogesterone contraception
CLL	chronic lymphocytic leukaemia	DOccMED	Diploma in Occupational Medicine
CML	chronic myeloid leukaemia	DOTS	directly observed short-course treatment
CMP	Condition Management Programme		
CMV	cytomegalovirus	DPA	Data Protection Act 1998
CNS	central nervous system	DRG	dorsal root ganglion
COPD	chronic obstructive pulmonary disease	DRO	Disablement Resettlement Officer
COPIND	chronic organophosphate-induced neuropsychiatric disorder	DSA	Disablement Services Authority
		DSE	display screen equipment
CORAD	Committee on Restrictions against Disabled People	DSM IV	*Diagnostic and statistical manual of mental disorders* (American Psychological Association)
COSHH	Control of Substances Hazardous to Health	DSS	Department of Social Security
		DST	Disability Service Team
CPAP	continuous positive airways pressure	DVLA	Driving and Vehicle Licensing Agency
CPR	Civil Procedure Rules	DVT	deep venous thrombosis
CRE	Commission for Racial Equality	DWP	Department of Work and Pensions
CSAG	Clinical Standards Advisory Group	EAA	extrinsic allergic alveolitis
CSF	cerebrospinal fluid	EAGA	Expert Advisory Group on AIDS
CSII	continuous subcutaneous insulin infusion	EAP	Employee Assistance Programme
		EASA	European Aviation Safety Authority
CT	computed tomography	EAT	Employment Appeal Tribunal
CTEV	congenital talipes equinovarus (clubfoot)	EAV	Exposure Action Valve
		EBMT	European Group for Blood and Marrow Transplantation
CTS	carpal tunnel syndrome		
CVD	cardiovascular disease	ECG	exercise electrocardiogram
CVS	chorionic villus sampling	ECJ	European Court of Justice
DAS	Disability Advisory Service	ECSC	European Community for Coal and Steel
DB	Defined Benefits		
DBCP	1,2-dibromochloropropane	EDH	extradural haematoma
dB HL	decibels hearing level	EEG	electroencephalography
dB SPL	decibels sound pressure level	EFA	Epilepsy Foundation of America
DC	Defined Contribution	ELISA	enzyme-linked immunosorbent assay
DCU	Day Care Units	ELV	Exposure Limit Valve
DDA	Disability Discrimination Act 1995	EMAS	Employment Medical Advisory Service
DDAVP	desmopressin	EMG	electromyogram
DDH	developmental dysplasia of the hip	ENT	ear, nose, and throat
DEA	Disability Employment Adviser	EOC	Equal Opportunities Commission
DETR	Department of the Environment, Transport and the Regions	EPDS	Edinburgh Post Natal Depression Scale

ERC	Employment Rehabilitation Centres	HBeAG	hepatitis B e antigen
ERS	European Respiratory Society	HbIg	hepatitis B hyperimmune serum
ERT	emergency response team	HbS	haemoglobin S (sickle haemoglobin)
ESR	erythrocyte sedimentation rate	HBsAg	hepatitis B surface antigen
ESRD	end-stage renal disease	HbSC	sickle haemoglobin C disease
ETS	environmental tobacco smoke	HbSS	homozygous sickle cell anaemia (sickle haemoglobin allele)
EU	European Union		
EWC	expected week of confinement	Hbsßthal	sickle beta thalassaemia disease
EWDTS	European Workplace Drug Testing Society	HBV	DNA hepatitis B virus DNA
		HCV	hepatitis C virus
FCA	functional capacity assessment	HD	haemodialysis; Hodgkin's disease
FCE	functional capacity evaluation	HIV	human immunodeficiency virus
FEFC	Further Education Funding Council	HLA	human leucocyte antigen
FEVi	volume of gas expired in the first second	HNIG	human normal immunoglobulin
		HMFI	Her Majesty's Factory Inspectorate
FIX	factor IX of the blood clotting cascade	HMSO	Her Majesty's Stationery Office
		HPS	Heart Protection Study
FOM	Faculty of Occupational Medicine	HRT	hormone replacement therapy
FRC	functional residual capacity	HSAWA	Health and Safety at Work Act 1974
FVC	forced vital capacity	HSC	Health and Safety Commission
FVIII	clotting Factor VIII of the blood clotting cascade	HSE	Health and Safety Executive
		HTL	hearing threshold level
FXI	factor XI of the blood clotting cascade	HTLV1	human T-lymphotropic virus I
		HTLVII	human T-lymphotropic virus II
GBS	General Council of British Shipping	HTV	hand-transmitted vibration
G-CSF	granulocyte colony stimulating factor	IAP	intra-abdominal pressure
		IATA	International Air Transport Association
GCMS	gas chromatography–mass spectrometry	IB	Incapacity Benefit
		IBE	International Bureau for Epilepsy
GCS	Glasgow Coma Scale	IBS	irritable bowel syndrome
GFR	glomerular filtration rate	ICAO	International Civil Aviation Organization
GGT	gamma-glutamyl transferase		
GMC	General Medical Council	ICD	implantable cardioverter defibrillator
GOLD	Global Initiative for Chronic Obstructive Lung Disease	ICD-10	International classification of diseases (WHO)
GORD	gastro-oesophageal reflux disease		
GP	general practitioner	ICFDH	International classification of Functioning, Disability and Health
GvHD	graft versus host disease		
GvL	graft versus leukaemia	ICNARC	the Intensive Care National Audit and Research Council
HAART	highly active antiretroviral therapy		
HAD	Hospital Anxiety and Depression Scale	ICOH	International Commission on Occupational Health
		IDDM	insulin-dependent diabetes mellitus
HAVS	hand-arm vibration syndrome	IDH	intradural haematoma
HbAS	heterozygous sickle cell disease (one normal haemoglobin allele and one sickle haemoglobin allele)	IDRP	internal dispute resolution management
HBcAB	hepatitis B core antibody	IIDB	Industrial Injury Disablement Benefit

IIDTW	Independent Inquiry into Drug Testing at Work	MRC	Medical Research Council
ILO	International Labour Office; International Labour Organization	MRI	magnetic resonance imaging
		MRO	Medical Review Officer
IMiDs	immunomodulatory drugs	MRSA	methicillin-resistant *Staphylococcus aureus*
IMO	International Maritime Organization	MS	multiple sclerosis
INR	international normalized ratio	MTP	metatarsophalangeal joint
IOFB	intra-ocular foreign body	NA	nucleoside analogue reverse transcriptase inhibitor
IPSS	International Prostate Symptom Score		
IPV	inactivated polio vaccine	NASS	National Ankylosing Spondylitis Society
IT	information technology		
ITP	idiopathic thrombocytopenic purpura	NCYPE	National Centre for Young People with Epilepsy
IUATLD	International Union Against Tuberculosis and Lung Disease	NDDP	New Deal for Disabled People
		NGO	non-governmental organization
IUCD	intrauterine contraceptive device	NGPSE	National General Practice Study of Epilepsy
IUD	intrauterine death		
JAA	Joint Aviation Authorities	Nhanes III	Third National Health and Nutrition Survey
JCA	juvenile chronic arthritis		
JRA	juvenile rheumatoid arthritis	NHL	non-Hodgkin's lymphoma
JRRP	Job Retention and Rehabilitation pilots	NHS	National Health Service
KCO	carbon monoxide transfer coefficient	NI	National Insurance
KS	Kaposi's sarcoma	NICE	National Institute for Clinical Excellence
KSHV	Kaposi's sarcoma associated herpes virus		
		NIDDM	non-insulin dependent diabetes mellitus
LACS	lacunar syndromes		
LASIK	laser assisted *in situ* keratomilieusis	NIOSH	National Institute of Occupational Safety and Health (US)
LBP	low back pain		
LGV	large goods vehicle	NMC	Nursing and Midwifery Council
LLI	leg length inequality	NMR	nuclear magnetic resonance
LMWH	low molecular weight heparin	NNRTI	non-nucleoside reverse transcriptase inhibitor
LTD	long-term disability		
MAI	Mycobacterium avium intra cellulare	NPV	negative predictive value
MAOI	monoamine oxidase inhibitor	NRL	natural rubber latex
MCA	Maritime and Coastguard Agency	NRR	noise reduction ratio
MCH	mean corpuscular haemoglobin	NRTI	nucleoside analogue reverse transcriptase inhibitor
MCV	mean corpuscular volume		
MDS	myelodysplastic syndrome	NSAIDs	non-steroidal anti-inflammatory drugs
ME	myeloencephalitis	NSE	National Society for Epilepsy
MED3	medical statements	NSH	National Study of Hearing
METs	metabolic equivalents	NTD	neural tube defects
MHSW	Management of Health and Safety at Work Regulations 1992	nvCJD	new variant Creutzfeld–Jakob disease
MI	myocardial infarction	OA	osteoarthritis
MIT	multiple injection treatment	OH	occupational health
MND	motor neurone disease	OHA	oral hypoglycaemic agent
Mph	miles per hour	OHS	occupational health services
		OHSS	ovarian hyper stimulation syndrome

OPAS	Pensions Advisory Service	QMV	Qualified Majority Voting
OPCS	Office of Population Censuses and Surveys	RA	rheumatoid arthritis
		RADAR	The Royal Association for Disability and Rehabilitation
OPITO	Offshore Petroleum Industry Training Organization	RADS	reactive airways dysfunction syndrome
OR	odds ratio	RAST	Radio-Allergo-Sorbent test
ORIF	open reduction and internal fixation	RCGP	Royal College of General Practitioners
PACS	partial anterior circulation syndromes	RCOG	Royal College of Obstetricians and Gynaecologists
PACT	Placing, Assessment and Counselling Team	RECs	research ethics committees
PBSC	peripheral blood stem cell	RIDDOR	Reporting of Injuries, Diseases and Dangerous Occurrences Regulations 1995
PCP	pneumocystis carinii pneumonia		
PCR	polymerase chain reaction		
PCV	passenger carrying vehicle	RK	radial keratotomy
PD	peritoneal dialysis; Parkinson's disease; Psychological Debriefing	RNIB	Royal National Institute for the Blind
		RoC	receiver operating characteristic
PE	pulmonary embolism	RP	Raynaud's phenomenon
PEF	peak expiratory flow	RPE	respiratory protective equipment; retinal pigment epithelium
PEFR	peak expiratory flow rate		
PFEER	Prevention of fire and Explosion, Emergency Response	RRT	renal replacement therapy
		RSD	reflex sympathetic dystrophy
PFO	patent foramen ovale	RSI	repetitive strain injury
PFP	Positive Futures Partnership	RTI	reverse transcriptase inhibitor
PGL	persistent generalized lymphadenopathy	RTP	residential training provider
		RV	residual volume
PHI	permanent health insurance	SAMHSA	Substance Abuse and Mental Health Services Administration
PI	protease inhibitor		
PID	pelvic inflammatory disease; prolapsed lumbar invertebral disc	SARS	Severe Acute Respiratory Syndrome
		SCAT	standardized concussion assessment tool
PIP	proximal interphalangeal joint		
PMS	premenstrual syndrome	SCBA	self-contained breathing apparatus
PNH	paroxysmal nocturnal haemoglobinuria	SCD	sickle cell disease
		SCI	spinal cord injury
POBA	plain old balloon angioplasty	SCID	severe combined immune deficiency
POCS	posterior vertebrobasilar circulation syndromes	sCJD	sporadic Creutzfeldt-Jakob disease
		SCT	stem cell transplantation
PPE	personal protective equipment	SDA	Severe Disablement Allowance
PPI	proton pump inhibitors	SES	socio-economic status
PPV	positive predictive value	SIG	Sheltered Industrial Group
PRK	photorefractive keratectomy	SLE	systemic lupus erythematosus
PRV	polycythaemia rubra vera	S/N	signal-to-noise (ratio)
PSA	Prostate Specific Antigen	SOPHID	Survey of Prevalent HIV Infections Diagnosed
PTA	post-traumatic amnesia		
PTCA	percutaneous transluminal coronary angioplasty	SPB	spontaneous preterm birth
		SPL	sound pressure level
PTD	post-traumatic disorder	SSP	Statutory Sick Pay
PTSD	post-traumatic stress disorder	SSRI	serotonin selective re-uptake inhibitor

TACS	total anterior (carotid) circulation syndrome
TB	tuberculosis
TEC	Training and Enterprise Council
TED	thromboembolic deterrent
TENS	transcutaneous electrical nerve stimulation
TfW	Training for Work programme
THC	tetrahydrocannabinol
TIA	transient ischaemic attack
TLC	total lung capacity
TLCO	carbon monoxide transfer factor
TU	trades unions
TUC	Trades Union Congress
TVT™	tension-free vaginal tape
UC	ulcerative colitis
UKOOA	UK Offshore Operators Association
UKPDS	UK Prospective Diabetes Study
UV	ultraviolet
VA	visual activity
vCJD	variant Creutzfeld-Jakob disease
VCO_2	carbon dioxide production
VDE	visual display equipment
VDU	visual display unit
VR	vocational rehabilitation
VTE	venous thromboembolic disease
VZV	varicella zoster
VWF	Von Willebrand's factor; vibration-induced white finger
VO_2	oxygen consumption
VO_{2max}	maximum oxygen uptake
WAI	work ability index
WHO	World Health Organization
WRULD	work-related upper limb disorder
YOI	Young Offenders Institution
YMDD	tyrosine-methionine-aspartate-aspartate
ZDV	zidovudin

Index

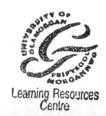